BLANCHARD & LOEB PUBLISHERS
Nurse's Choice for Better Care™

Nurse's Handbook of
Combination
Drugs

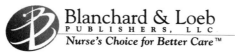

Blanchard & Loeb
PUBLISHERS, LLC
Nurse's Choice for Better Care™

San Francisco•Philadelphia•New York

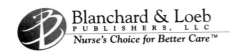

Blanchard & Loeb
P U B L I S H E R S ,   L L C
Nurse's Choice for Better Care™

Publishers: Ross Blanchard, Stanley E. Loeb
Clinical Director: Marlene Ciranowicz, RN, MSN, CDE
Book Editor: Catherine E. Harold
Copy Editor: Jenifer F. Walker, MA
Cover: Ray Keim

© 2007 Blanchard & Loeb Publishers, LLC

Printed in the United States of America

Blanchard & Loeb Publishers, LLC
454 Railroad Avenue
Shiremanstown, PA 17011

Contents

Reviewers and Clinical Consultants

Alison Calabrese, RPh.
Clinical Pharmacist
Lourdes Hospital
Binghamton, NY

Kimberly A. Couch, PharmD
Clinical Pharmacy Specialist,
  Infectious Diseases
Department of Pharmacy
Christiana Care Health System
Newark, DE

Thomas Forrest, RPh.
Clinical Pharmacist
Lourdes Hospital
Binghamton, NY

John P. Gatto, RPh.
Clinical Pharmacist
Eckerd Pharmacy
Owego, NY

Jeanne M. Hoff, RPh.
Clinical Pharmacist
Lourdes Hospital
Binghamton, NY

Mary Ann Klee, RPh.
Pharmacist
St. Joseph Hospital
Elmira, NY

Shannon M. Murray, PharmD, CGP
Clinical Pharmacy Specialist,
  Geriatrics
Christiana Care Health System
Newark, DE

Mirza E. Perez, PharmD, BCPS
Assistant Professor
Temple University, School of
  Pharmacy
Philadelphia, PA

HOW TO USE THIS BOOK

Blanchard & Loeb Publishers' *Nurse's Handbook of Combination Drugs* provides what today's nurses and nursing students need: accurate, concise, and reliable drug facts when administering combination products, with their more complicated and more numerous interactions, adverse reactions, and nursing considerations. This book emphasizes the vital information you need to know before, during, and after combination drug administration. And the information is presented in easy-to-understand language and organized alphabetically, so you can find what you need quickly.

What's Special

In addition to the drug information you expect to find in each entry (see "Drug Entries," below, for details), the *Nurse's Handbook of Combination Drugs* boasts these special features:

- **One concise, thorough drug entry for each formulation** puts the information you need right at your fingertips, whether the formulation contains two, three, or more drugs. No more having to look up the two or more drugs individually and then wonder if you have all the information you need for safe administration and care.

- **Practical trim size and good-size type** give you a book that's easy to carry, easy to read, and easy to handle. You can hold the book in one hand, see complete pages at a glance, and use your other hand to document or perform other activities.

- **No-nonsense writing style** that speaks everyday language and uses the terms and abbreviations you typically encounter in your practice and your studies—although a few abbreviations may not be used in certain facilities. (See Abbreviations, pages 727 to 730.) And to avoid sexist language, we alternate between male and female pronouns throughout the book.

- **Up-to-date drug information,** including the latest FDA-approved drugs, new and changed indications, new warnings, and newly reported adverse reactions.

- **Dosage adjustment,** highlighted in the text, alerts you to expected dosage changes for a patient with a specific condition or disorder, such as advanced age or renal impairment.

- **Warning,** highlighted in the text, calls attention to important facts that you need to know before, during, and after drug administration. For example, in the amplodipine and benazeprine entry, this feature informs you that the drugs may cause anaphylactoid reactions, including angioedema, especially after the first dose.

- **Useful appendices** give an overview of important drug facts and nursing considerations in antineoplastic combination drug therapy for selected common cancers and in combination oral contraceptives. You'll also find handy information you can use every day in your practice and studies, such as instructions for calculating drug dosages and checking which drugs are compatible in a syringe.

Drug Entries

Nurse's Handbook of Combination Drugs clearly and concisely presents all the vital facts on the combination drugs that you'll typically administer. To help you find the information you need quickly, entries are grouped first according to their general classification, listed alphabetically:

- Anti-infective Drugs
- Cardiovascular Drugs
- Central Nervous System Drugs
- Dermatologic Drugs
- Endocrine Drugs
- Eye and Ear Drugs
- Gastrointestinal Drugs
- Genitourinary Drugs
- Respiratory Drugs

Generic names

Each chapter lists its drugs alphabetically by generic name, making the first drug in the combination the one in the original FDA approval of the drug combination. For example, the combination drug glyburide and metformin hydrochloride is found in the chapter on Endocrine Drugs under the G listings, not the M listings. You can also find it in the index by looking up glyburide, metformin, or its trade name, Glucovance.

For consistency, details of the individual drug components within the entry present glyburide before metformin. In the dosage section of the entry, the combined dosage is given first but is followed in brackets, where appropriate, with the portion of the dosage for the first drug named in the combination generic name followed by the second drug.

Class, Category, and Schedule

Each entry lists the drug's chemical and therapeutic classes. With this information, you can compare drugs in the same chemical class but in different therapeutic classes—and vice versa.

The entry also lists the FDA's pregnancy risk category, which categorizes drugs based on their potential to cause birth defects. (For details, see *FDA pregnancy risk categories* on page viii.)

Where appropriate, the entry also includes the drug's controlled substance schedule. (For details, see *Controlled substance schedules* on page ix.)

Indications and Dosages

This section lists FDA-approved therapeutic indications. For each indication, you'll find the applicable drug form or route, age-group (adults, adolescents, or children), and dosage (which includes amount per dose, timing, and duration).

Mechanism of Action

Set off by a box, this section concisely describes how a drug achieves its therapeutic effects at the cellular, tissue, or organ level, as appropriate.

Incompatibilities

You'll be alerted to drugs or solutions that are incompatible with the topic drug when mixed in a syringe or solution, or infused through the same I.V. line.

Contraindications

An alphabetical list details the conditions and disorders that preclude administration of the topic drug.

Interactions

This section presents the drugs, foods, and activities (such as alcohol use and smoking) that can cause important, problematic, or life-threatening interactions with the topic drug. For each interacting drug, food, or activity, you'll learn the effects of the interaction. Listed interactions begin with the combination agent; then, the interactions unique to each drug follow, as needed.

Adverse Reactions

Organized by body system, this section highlights common, serious, and life-threatening adverse reactions in alphabetical order.

Nursing Considerations

Warnings, general precautions, and key information that you must know before, during, and after drug administration are detailed in

FDA PREGNANCY RISK CATEGORIES

Each drug may be placed in a pregnancy risk category based on the FDA's estimate of risk to the fetus. If the FDA hasn't provided a category, the *Nurse's Handbook of Combination Drugs* notes that the drug is "Not rated." The categories range from A to X, signifying least to greatest fetal risk.

A Controlled studies show no risk

Adequate, well-controlled studies with pregnant women have failed to demonstrate a risk to the fetus in any trimester of pregnancy.

B No evidence of risk in humans

Adequate, well-controlled studies with pregnant women haven't shown increased risk of fetal abnormalities despite adverse findings in animals, or—in the absence of adequate human studies—animal studies show no fetal risk. The chance of fetal harm is remoate, but remains possible.

C Risk can't be ruled out

Adequate, well-controlled human studies are lacking, and animal studies have demonstrated a risk to the fetus or are lacking as well. A chance of fetal harm exists if the drug is administered during pregnancy, but the potential benefits may outweigh the risk.

D Positive evidence of risk

Studies in humans, or investigational or post-marketing data, have demonstrated fetal risk. Nevertheless, the drug's potential benefits may outweigh its risks. For example, the drug may be acceptable for use in a life-threatening situation or serious disease for which safer drugs can't be used or are ineffective.

X Contraindicated in pregnancy

Studies in animals or humans, or investigational or post-marketing reports, have demonstrated positive evidence of fetal abnormalities or risks; these risks clearly outweigh any possible benefit to the patient.

this section. Examples include whether or not a pill can be crushed and how to properly reconstitute, dilute, store, handle, or dispose of a drug.

Patient teaching information is also included here. You'll find

CONTROLLED SUBSTANCE SCHEDULES

The Controlled Substances Act of 1970 mandated that certain prescription drugs be categorized in schedules based on their potential for abuse. The greater their abuse potential, the greater the restrictions on their prescription. The controlled substance schedules range from I to V, signifying highest to lowest abuse potential.

I High potential for abuse

No accepted medical use exists for Schedule I drugs, which include heroin and lysergic acid diethylamide (LSD).

II High potential for abuse

Use may lead to severe physical or psychological dependence. Prescriptions must be written in ink or typewritten and must be signed by the prescriber. Oral prescriptions must be confirmed in writing within 72 hours and may be given only in a genuine emergency. No renewals are permitted.

III Some potential for abuse

Use may lead to low-to-moderate physical dependence or high psychological dependence. Prescriptions may be oral or written. Up to five renewals are permitted within 6 months.

IV Low potential for abuse

Use may lead to limited physical or psychological dependence. Prescriptions may be oral or written. Up to five renewals are permitted within 6 months.

V Subject to state and local regulation

Abuse potential is low; a prescription may not be required.

important guidelines for patients, such as how and when to take each prescribed drug, how to spot and manage adverse reactions, which cautions to observe, when to call the prescriber, and more. To save you time, however, this section doesn't repeat basic patient-teaching points. (For a summary of those, see *Teaching your patient about combination drug therapy* on pages x and xi.)

TEACHING YOUR PATIENT ABOUT COMBINATION DRUG THERAPY

Your teaching about combination drug therapy will vary with your patient's needs and your practice setting. To help guide your teaching, each drug entry provides key information that you must teach your patient about those combined drugs. For all patients, however, you should also:

☑ Teach the generic and trade names for each drug component in the prescribed combination drug that he'll take after discharge—even if he took the combination before admission.

☑ Clearly explain why each combination drug was prescribed, how it works, and what it's supposed to do. To help your patient understand the drug's therapeutic effects, relate its action to her disorder or condition.

☑ Review the drug form, dosage, and route with the patient. Tell him whether the drug is a tablet, suppository, spray, aerosol, or other form, and explain how to administer it correctly. Also, tell him how often to take the drug and for what length of time. Emphasize that he should take the drug exactly as prescribed.

☑ Describe the drug's appearance, and explain that scored tablets can be broken in half for safe, accurate dosing. Warn the patient not to break unscored tablets because doing so may alter the drug dosage. If your patient has difficulty swallowing capsules, explain that she can open ones that contain sprinkles and take them with food or a drink but that she shouldn't do this with capsules that contain powder. Also, warn her not to crush or chew enteric-coated, extended-release, sustained-release, or similar drug forms.

☑ Teach the patient about common adverse reactions that may occur. Advise him to notify the prescriber at once if a dangerous adverse reaction, such as syncope, occurs.

☑ Warn her not to suddenly stop taking a drug if she's bothered by mild, unpleasant adverse reactions. Instead, encourage her to discuss the reactions with her prescriber, who may adjust the dosage or substitute a drug that causes fewer adverse reactions.

☑ Warn the patient that some adverse reactions, such as dizziness and drowsiness, can impair his ability to operate machinery, drive a car, or perform other activities that require alertness. Help him develop a dosing schedule that prevents adverse reactions from interfering with such activities.

☑ Inform the patient which adverse reactions resolve with time.

☑ Teach the patient how to store the drug properly. Let him know if the drug is sensitive to light or temperature and how to protect it from these elements.

☑ Instruct the patient to store the drug in its original container, if possible, with the drug's name and dosage clearly printed on the label.

☑ Inform the patient which devices to use—and which ones to avoid—for drug storage or administration. For example, instruct him to use a calibrated device when measuring a dose of liquid brompheniramine and pseudoephedrine.

☑ Teach the patient what to do if she misses a dose. Generally, she should take a once-daily drug as soon as she remembers—provided that she remembers within the first 24 hours. If 24 hours have elapsed, she should take the next scheduled dose, but not double the dose. If she has questions or concerns about missed doses, tell her to contact the prescriber.

☑ Provide information that's specific to the prescribed drug. For example, if a patient takes amiloride and hydrochlorothiazide to manage hypertension or heart failure, instruct him to weigh himself daily at the same time of day, using the same scale and wearing the same amount of clothing. Or if the patient takes niacin extended-release and lovastatin to treat primary hypersholesterolemia, urge him to have periodic eye examinations during therapy.

☑ Advise the patient to refill prescriptions promptly, unless she no longer needs the drug. Also instruct her to discard expired drugs because they may become ineffective or even dangerous over time.

☑ Warn the patient to keep all drugs out of the reach of children at all times.

FOREWORD

Patients have always found taking one drug simpler to manage than taking several. A patient taking several medications confronts issues of timing doses, daily planning and organization, personal understanding and memory—among others; and nurses and prescribers struggle with patient confusion and compliance in such situations. One simplifier in this complex situation comes from combination drug products.

With this problem in mind, drug manufacturers have devised, the FDA has approved, and more and more prescribers have endorsed increasing numbers of combination drug formulations. With the convenience of needing only one formulation to take two or more medications simultaneously, a patient's drug regimen simplifies. Also, patient safety may improve when the number of daily pills to be taken declines, resulting in fewer potential medication errors.

For the nurse, however, the convenience of combination drugs is linked with the added responsibility to provide safe, effective drug therapy and complete patient teaching about the medications. The combination product may be simpler to take, but its potential for adverse reactions and drug and food interactions is, if anything, more complex—not less—than dosages of individual drugs. A medication error or adverse reaction involving a combination drug product becomes compounded because it poses not just the threat of adverse effects with one drug but with two or more.

Your Responsibilities in Combination Drug Therapy

Your basic responsibilities in administering a combination drug product are similar to those in administering any drug, including:

- administering the right combination drug in the right dose by the right route at the right time to the right patient
- knowing the therapeutic use, dosage, interactions, adverse reactions, and warnings of each administered combination drug
- being aware of newly approved combination drugs that may be prescribed
- knowing about changes to existing combination drugs, such as new indications and dosages and recently discovered adverse reactions and interactions

- concentrating fully when preparing and administering combination drugs
- responding promptly and appropriately to serious or life-threatening adverse reactions, interactions, and other complications
- instructing each patient about the combination drug, how it's administered, which effects the drugs together may cause, and which reactions to watch for and report to you or to the prescriber.

Beyond these basic responsibilities, however, you also need additional nursing knowledge to meet the demands of today's combination drug therapy, such as knowing how the two or more drugs contained in the drug formulation will affect your care of the patient and the things he needs to know to self-administer the combination drug safely at home.

Meeting Your Needs

Nurses and students need a reliable, accurate, easy-to-use, quick-reference drug book on combination drug therapy. The book in your hands, Blanchard and Loeb's *Nurse's Handbook of Combination Drugs*, contains a wealth of reliable and easy-to-understand information on virtually all of the prescribed combination drug products you're likely to administer.

You can depend on the accuracy and reliability of the information contained in this Handbook because each entry has been written by nurses for nurses and reviewed by experts in nursing and pharmacology. What's more, every drug entry has been checked against the most respected drug references today, including the *American Hospital Formulary Service Drug Information*, *Drug Facts and Comparisons*, *Physician's Desk Reference*, and the *USP DI's Drug Information for the Health Care Professional*.

The *Nurse's Handbook of Combination Drugs* is practical and convenient, providing the information on the drugs included in each combination product in a single entry. It gives you the complete information you need and saves you from having to track down the information in any other handbook's two or more entries.

Organization

The *Handbook's* chapters are grouped by body system, giving you the advantage of finding all the combination drugs on cardiovascular disorders, for example, gathered together. Within each chapter, the entries are listed alphabetically by the generic name of the first drug in the combination—as defined by the manufacturer and approved by the FDA.

To speed you to each entry when you need it, the comprehensive index lists each generic drug, no matter whether it is the primary or a secondary drug in the combination, and no matter how many combinations it is part of. For example, neomycin sulfate appears in seven drug combinations in this book, and the index gets you to each one in a couple of seconds. Further, all trade names are indexed. So if you need to find Glucovance, you can do so whether or not you know it consists of glyburide and metformin. You can, of course, get to the Glucovance entry by looking up either glyburide or metformin in the index.

Two appendices cover combinations that do not receive entries in the main text: Antineoplastic Combination Drugs for Selected Cancers, and Combination Oral Contraceptives. Because drug regimens in cancer depend on the staging of the cancer, the absence or presence of metastasis, and the patient's physical status—among other important variables—coverage of this information is more efficiently presented in a table for your reference. Your relationship to patients taking oral combination contraceptives is probably advisory, and so the contraceptives table contains a good deal of patient teaching that is best concentrated in one place for your convenience.

Additional appendices include *Compatible Drugs in a Syringe*, *Drug Formulas and Calculations*, *Weights and Equivalents*, and *Abbreviations*.

Value in a Drug Reference

Whether you work in or are preparing to work in acute care, home care, long-term care, or another health care setting, you'll want your own copy of *Nurse's Handbook of Combination Drugs*. That's because this book will help you:

• reduce your risk of medication errors by giving you access to accurate, reliable drug information that's relevant to your practice
• stay current on the most up-to-date drug developments
• improve your drug administration skills and patient care during all stages of drug administration
• quickly detect and manage serious or life-threatening adverse reactions and complications—or prevent them from occurring
• save time because you won't have to sift through volumes of information or numerous web sites to find what you need, worry that the source you're using isn't timely, or juggle information from several sources on the component drugs in a combination
• increase your confidence about drug administration and enhance

your professional interactions with other health care team members
- ensure the delivery of safe, effective care
- improve the depth and quality of your patient teaching.

Your Rewards

You deserve the latest and most beneficial resources to support you in delivering the safest and most informed care that you can to your patients. And today, you face greater challenges than ever: more patients who are acutely ill, tighter budgets and staffing, and more complex drug therapy. The reference you hold now adds to your armamentarium and, as such, is a must for your professional nursing library. Blanchard & Loeb's *Nurse's Handbook of Combination Drugs* is a one-of-a-kind reference you'll want to have at your fingertips. It's a resource you'll use often and confidently because of its accurate, clearly written, and essential information—a vital nursing tool.

Kathleen A. Dracup, RN, FNP, DNSc, FAAN
Dean of Nursing
University of California, San Francisco

Anti-Infective Drugs

abacavir sulfate and lamivudine
Epzicom

Class and Category
Chemical: Synthetic nucleoside analogues (abacavir, lamivudine)
Therapeutic: Antiretroviral (abacavir, lamivudine)
Pregnancy category: C

Indications and Dosages
▶ *To treat HIV-1 infection*
TABLETS
Adults. 600 mg abacavir and 300 mg lamivudine (1 tablet) daily with other antiretrovirals.

Mechanism of Action
Abacavir, a carbocyclic synthetic nucleoside analogue, becomes converted inside cells to carbovir triphosphate, an active metabolite. Carbovir triphosphate stops the activity of HIV-1 reverse transcriptase required in viral DNA synthesis by competing with the natural substrate dGTP and by becoming a part of the viral DNA. This action ends formation of the DNA chain.

Lamivudine, a synthetic nucleoside analogue, becomes phosphorylated inside cells to lamivudine triphosphate, an active metabolite. The metabolite stops the activity of HIV-1 reverse transcriptase by becoming part of the viral DNA, thus ending formation of the DNA chain.

Contraindications
Hepatic impairment; hypersensitivity to abacavir, lamivudine, or any of their components

Interactions
DRUGS
abacavir component
methadone: Increased methadone clearance

lamivudine component
trimethoprim and sulfamethoxazole: Increased lamivudine exposure
zalcitabine: Possibly inhibited intracellular phosphorylation, making both drugs ineffective

Adverse Reactions

CNS: Abnormal dreams, anxiety, depression, dizziness, fatigue, fever, headache, insomnia, malaise, paresthesia, peripheral neuropathy, seizures, vertigo, weakness
CV: Elevated triglycerides
EENT: Pharyngitis, stomatitis
ENDO: Hyperglycemia
GI: Abdominal pain, diarrhea, elevated liver enzymes, gastritis, hepatic steatosis, hepatomegaly, nausea, pancreatitis, post-treatment exacerbation of hepatitis B, vomiting
HEME: Anemia, aplastic anemia, neutropenia, splenomegaly, thrombocytopenia
MS: Elevated CK, muscle weakness, rhabdomyolysis
RESP: Cough, dyspnea, wheezing
SKIN: Alopecia, erythema multiforme, rash, Stevens-Johnson syndrome, toxic epidermal necrolysis, urticaria
Other: Anaphylaxis, fat accumulation or redistribution, lactic acidosis, lymphadenopathy

Nursing Considerations

- Because dosages of individual drugs can't be adjusted, the combination drug shouldn't be given to a patient who has a creatinine clearance less than 50 ml/min/1.73 m^2, hepatic impairment, or dose-limiting adverse reactions. If any of these problems develop during therapy, notify prescriber and expect the patient to be switched to a different medication.
- **WARNING** Notify prescriber immediately at first sign or symptom of hypersensitivity to abacavir and lamivudine, such as abdominal pain, cough, diarrhea, dyspnea, fatigue, fever, nausea, pharyngitis, rash, or vomiting. Stop drug immediately if hypersensitivity is suspected, and notify prescriber. The drug should not be restarted after hypersensitivity reaction resolves because more severe symptoms will recur within hours and may be fatal. The prescriber should register the hypersensitivity reaction with the abacavir hypersensitivity reaction registry by calling 1-800-270-0425.
- Monitor patient's liver function routinely, as ordered, and assess patient for evidence of lactic acidosis and liver dysfunction that may result from abacavir and lamivudine therapy, especially in

women and patients with a history of prolonged nucleoside exposure. In patients with a history of hepatitis B, expect to monitor liver function for several months after therapy stops.

PATIENT TEACHING

- Advise patient that hypersensitivity reactions may occur with abacavir and lamivudine. Review the signs and symptoms listed on the warning card given with each prescription, and urge patient to stop the drug and seek immediate medical attention if hypersensitivity is even suspected. Warn patient never to take this or any abacavir-containing drug in the future if the drug is stopped because of hypersensitivity.
- Warn patient to take abacavir and lamivudine exactly as prescribed and not to interrupt therapy for any reason other than hypersensitivity because restarting the drug may cause a serious hypersensitivity reaction. Notify the prescriber immediately if interruption of therapy is unavoidable.
- Inform patients with a history of hepatitis B that it may worsen after abacavir and lamivudine therapy stops. Stress the need to monitor hepatic function for at least several months after therapy stops to detect an exacerbation that could warrant anti–hepatitis B therapy.
- Tell patient that abacavir and lamivudine may cause fat accumulation or redistribution. Advise patient to notify prescriber about central obesity, buffalo hump, limb or facial thinness, breast enlargement, or other signs of cushingoid appearance.
- Inform patient that taking drug therapy won't cure HIV infection and won't reduce the risk of transmitting HIV to others.

abacavir sulfate, lamivudine, and zidovudine
Trizivir

Class and Category
Chemical: Synthetic nucleoside analogues (abacavir, lamivudine, zidovudine)
Therapeutic: Antiretroviral (abacavir, lamivudine, zidovudine)
Pregnancy category: C

Indications and Dosages
▶ *To treat HIV-1 infection*
TABLETS
Adults and adolescents weighing 40 kg or more. 300 mg

abacavir, 150 mg lamivudine, and 300 mg of zidovudine
(1 tablet) b.i.d.

Mechanism of Action

Abacavir sulfate, lamivudine, and zidovudine are nucleoside analogues and are converted intracellularly to their respective active metabolites: abacavir to carbovir triphosphate, lamivudine to lamivudine triphosphate, and zidovudine to zidovudine triphosphate. These active metobolites inhibit the activity of HIV-1 reverse transcriptase by becoming incorporated into viral DNA. Carbovir triphosphate also inhibits the activity of HIV-1 reverse transcriptase by competing with the natural substrate, dGTP. These activities prevent the formation of a linkage essential for the viral DNA chain to elongate, thereby stopping viral DNA growth.

Contraindications

Hypersensitivity to abacavir, lamivudine, zidovudine, or their components

Interactions

DRUGS

abacavir component
methadone: Possibly increased methadone clearance
lamivudine component
trimethoprim and sulfamethoxazole: Possibly increased lamivudine exposure
zalcitabine: Possibly inhibited intracellular phosphorylation, making both drugs ineffective
zidovudine component
doxorubicin, ribavirin, stavudine: Increased risk of antagonistic relationship between zidovudine and doxorubicin, ribavirin, or stavudine
ganciclovir, interferon-alfa, and other bone marrow suppressive or cytotoxic agents: Possibly increased hematologic toxicity

Adverse Reactions

CNS: Depression, dizziness, fatigue, fever, headache, insomnia, malaise, neuropathy, paresthesia, peripheral neuropathy, seizures
CV: Cardiomyopathy, hypotension
EENT: Conjunctivitis, nasal congestion, oral mucous membrane pigmentation or ulceration, pharyngitis, stomatitis
ENDO: Gynecomastia, mild hyperglycemia
GI: Abdominal cramps or pain, anorexia, diarrhea, elevated liver

function tests, exacerbation of hepatitis B after treatment, hepatic failure or steatosis, nausea, pancreatitis, splenomegaly, vomiting
GU: Renal failure
HEME: Anemia, aplastic anemia, lymphopenia, neutropenia, pure red cell aplasia
MS: Arthralgia, muscle weakness, musculoskeletal pain, myalgia, myopathy, myositis, rhabdomyolysis
RESP: Acute respiratory distress syndrome, cough, dyspnea, respiratory failure, wheezing
SKIN: Alopecia, chills, erythema multiforme, rash, Stevens-Johnson syndrome, toxic epidermal necrolysis, urticaria
Other: Anaphylaxis, fat redistribution, hypersensitivity reactions, increased CK, lactic acidosis, lymphadenopathy

Nursing Considerations

- Use cautiously in patients with bone marrow suppression evidenced by a granulocyte count less than 1,000 cells/mm^3 or hemoglobin less than 9.5 g/dl because zidovudine can cause bone marrow suppression. Monitor patient's blood counts closely, as ordered.
- Be aware that because abacavir, lamivudine, and zidovudine are available only in a fixed-dose combination, patients who need a reduced dosage of lamivudine or zidovudine (such as those with a creatinine clearance less than 50 ml/min/1.73 m^2 and those who have impaired hepatic function of any degree) can't receive this drug combination. Likewise, patients who weigh less than 40 kg (88 lb) shouldn't receive this drug combination because dosage adjustments can't be made.
- **WARNING** Notify prescriber immediately at first sign or symptom of hypersensitivity, such as abdominal pain, cough, diarrhea, dyspnea, fatigue, fever, nausea, pharyngitis, rash, or vomiting. Expect to stop abacavir, lamivudine, and zidovudine. The drug should not be restarted after a hypersensitivity reaction resolves because more severe symptoms will recur within hours and may be fatal. The prescriber should register the hypersensitivity reaction with the abacavir hypersensitivity reaction registry by calling 1-800-270-0425.
- Monitor patient for fatigue or pallor because neutropenia and severe anemia have occurred with zidovudine use, especially in patients with advanced HIV disease. Notify prescriber if present.
- Monitor patient's hepatic function closely, including results of hepatic function studies, as ordered, because lactic acidosis and severe hepatomegaly have occurred with the use of nucleoside

analogues such as abacavir, lamivudine, and zidovudine. Patients at risk include women, obese patients, and patients who have had prolonged exposure to nucleosides. Notify prescriber and expect to stop the drug combination if patient develops any signs or symptoms that suggest lactic acidosis or hepatic dysfunction, such as a change in level of consciousness, fatigue, jaundice, nausea, or vomiting.

- Monitor patients receiving abacavir, lamivudine, and zidovudine closely for myopathy and myositis that may occur with prolonged use of zidovudine.
- Monitor patients who have both hepatitis B virus and HIV closely when the combination drug is discontinued because severe acute exacerbations of hepatitis B may occur up to several months after stopping the combination drug.

PATIENT TEACHING

- Caution patient to take abacavir, lamivudine, and zidovudine exactly as prescribed and not to stop and then restart therapy without consulting prescriber because severe hypersensitivity reactions can occur with re-introduction of the drug.
- Review signs and symptoms of hypersensitivity with patient, and instruct him to notify prescriber immediately if any occur, such as abdominal pain, cough, diarrhea, dyspnea, fatigue, fever, nausea, skin rash, sore throat, or vomiting.
- Alert patient that this drug combination may cause fat redistribution.
- Advise patient that abacavi, lamivudine, and zidovudine therapy doesn't HIV infection and doesn't reduce the risk of transmitting the virus to others.
- Instruct patient to avoid people with infections because this combination drug may increase his risk of infections.
- Remind patient to have his blood counts monitored, as prescribed, so that adverse effects of the combination drug can be detected early.

amoxicillin trihydrate and clavulanate potassium

Augmentin, Augmentin ES, Augmentin XR, Clavulin (CAN)

Class and Category

Chemical: Aminopenicillin, beta-lactamase inhibitor
Therapeutic: Antibiotic
Pregnancy category: B

Indications and Dosages

▶ *To treat otitis media, sinusitis, skin and soft-tissue infections, and UTI caused by susceptible strains of gram-positive and gram-negative organisms*

ORAL SUSPENSION, TABLETS

Adults and children weighing 40 kg (88 lb) or more. 500 mg q 12 hr or 250 mg q 8 hr.

Children age 12 wk and over weighing less than 40 kg. 25 mg/kg/day in divided doses q 12 hr or 20 mg/kg/day in divided doses q 8 hr.

Children under age 12 wk. 30 mg/kg/day q 12 hr.

▶ *To treat community-acquired pneumonia or acute bacterial sinusitis caused by beta-lactamase–producing pathogens and* Streptococcus pneumoniae *with reduced susceptibility to penicillin*

E.R. TABLETS

Adults. 4,000 mg in two divided doses daily at start of meals for 7 to 10 days for community-acquired pneumonia or 10 days for acute bacterial sinusitis.

▶ *To treat respiratory tract infections and severe otitis media and sinusitis caused by susceptible strains of gram-positive and gram-negative organisms*

CHEWABLE TABLETS, ORAL SUSPENSION, TABLETS

Adults and children weighing 40 kg or more. 875 mg q 12 hr or 500 mg q 8 hr.

Children age 12 wk and over weighing less than 40 kg. 45 mg/kg/day in divided doses q 12 hr or 40 mg/kg q 8 hr.

Children under age 12 wk. 30 mg/kg/day in divided doses q 12 hr.

DOSAGE ADJUSTMENT For a glomerular filtration rate (GFR) of 10 to 30 ml/min, dosage reduced to 250 or 500 mg q 12 hr, depending on the severity of the infection. For a GFR less than 10 ml/min, dosage reduced to 250 to 500 mg q 24 hr, depending on the severity of the infection. For hemodialysis patients, dosage reduced to 250 or 500 mg q 24 hr with another dose during and at the end of dialysis.

▶ *To treat acute otitis media caused by beta-lactamase–producing strains of* Haemophilus influenzae, Moraxella catarrhalis, *and* S. pneumoniae *(including penicillin-resistant strains)*

EXTRA-STRENGTH ORAL SUSPENSION

Children. 90 mg/kg/day in divided doses b.i.d. for 10 days.

Contraindications

History of amoxicillin and clavulanate–induced cholestatic jaundice or hepatic dysfunction; hypersensitivity to amoxicillin, clavulanate, penicillin, or their components; phenylketonuria (chewable tablets); severe renal impairment (E.R. tablets)

Mechanism of Action

Amoxicillin trihydrate kills bacteria by binding to and inactivating penicillin-binding proteins on the inner bacterial cell wall, weakening the cell wall and causing lysis.

Clavulanic acid inactivates bacterial beta-lactamase enzymes, thus protecting amoxicillin from degradation by these enzymes and making the drug effective against many bacteria normally resistant to amoxicillin.

Interactions

DRUGS

allopurinol: Increased risk of rash

aminoglycosides: Inactivation of both drugs

chloramphenicol, erythromycins, sulfonamides, tetracyclines: Reduced bactericidal effect of amoxicillin

heparin, oral anticoagulants: Possibly increased risk of bleeding with large doses of amoxicillin and clavulanate potassium

methotrexate: Risk of methotrexate toxicity

oral contraceptives with estrogen: Possibly reduced effectiveness of contraceptive

probenecid: Increased amoxicillin effects

Adverse Reactions

CNS: Agitation, anxiety, behavioral changes, confusion, dizziness, drowsiness, headache, insomnia, reversible hyperactivity

EENT: Black "hairy" tongue, glossitis, mucocutaneous candidiasis, stomatitis

GI: Diarrhea, enterocolitis, gastritis, hemorrhagic pseudomembranous colitis, indigestion, nausea, vomiting

GU: Hematuria, interstitial nephritis, vaginal candidiasis, vaginal mycosis

HEME: Agranulocytosis, anemia, eosinophilia, leukopenia, neutropenia, thrombocytopenia, thrombocytopenic purpura

SKIN: Erythema multiforme, exfoliative dermatitis, pruritus, rash, Stevens-Johnson syndrome, urticaria

Other: Allergic reaction, anaphylaxis, angioedema, serum sickness–like reaction (such as arthralgia, arthritis, fever, myalgia, rash, and urticaria)

Nursing Considerations

- Use amoxicillin and clavulanate cautiously in patients with hepatic impairment. Monitor hepatic and renal function and CBC, as ordered, in patients receiving prolonged therapy. Also use cautiously in patients who are breastfeeding or elderly.
- For children under age 12 weeks, expect to use 125-mg amoxicillin/5-ml clavulanate suspension because experience with 200-mg/5-ml suspension is limited.
- **WARNING** If allergic reaction occurs, stop drug immediately. Expect to give antihistamine and I.V. corticosteroid. If anaphylaxis occurs, expect to manage airway and give epinephrine, oxygen, and I.V. corticosteroid.
- Monitor patient closely for diarrhea, which may indicate pseudomembranous colitis. If diarrhea occurs, notify prescriber and expect to withhold drug. Expect to treat pseudomembranous colitis with fluids, electrolytes, protein, and an antibiotic effective against *Clostridium difficile.*
- Be aware that Augmentin 250-mg regular tablets should not be substituted for chewable or E.R. tablets because they contain different amounts of clavulanic acid.
- For a child weighing less than 40 kg (88 lb), expect to give 250-mg chewable tablets because the ratio of amoxicillin to clavulanic acid differs from that of Augmentin 250-mg regular tablets.

PATIENT TEACHING

- Tell patient to take amoxicillin and clavulanate with food to reduce GI upset.
- Instruct patient to refrigerate reconstituted suspension.
- Tell patient to chew or crush chewable tablets and not to swallow them whole.
- Teach patient to recognize and report adverse reactions and to seek emergency care if signs of anaphylaxis occur.
- Tell patient to notify prescriber if infection continues or worsens after 72 hours.
- Urge patient to tell prescriber about diarrhea that's severe or lasts longer than 3 days.

ampicillin sodium and sulbactam sodium
Unasyn

Class and Category
Chemical: Aminopenicillin, beta-lactamase inhibitor
Therapeutic: Antibiotic
Pregnancy category: B

Indications and Dosages
▶ *To treat skin and soft-tissue infections caused by beta-lactamase–producing strains of* Staphylococcus aureus, Escherichia coli, Klebsiella *species (including* K. pneumoniae*),* Proteus mirabilis, Bacteroides fragilis, Enterobacter species, *and* Acinetobacter calcoaceticus; *intra-abdominal infections caused by beta-lactamase–producing strains of* E. coli, Klebsiella *species (including* K. pneumoniae*),* Bacteroides *species (including* B. fragilis*), and* Enterobacter *species; gynecologic infections caused by beta-lactamase–producing strains of* E. coli *and* Bacteroides *species (including* B. fragilis*)*

I.V. INFUSION, I.M. INJECTION

Adults and children age 12 and over weighing 40 kg (88 lb) or more. 1.5 (1 g of ampicillin and 0.5 g of sulbactam) to 3 g (2 g of ampicillin and 1 g of sulbactam) q 6 hr, up to a maximum of 8 g of ampicillin and 4 g of sulbactam daily.

Children age 1 and over weighing less than 40 kg. 300 mg/kg (200 mg of ampicillin and 100 mg of sulbactam) daily in divided doses q 6 hr.

DOSAGE ADJUSTMENT Dosing frequency reduced to q 6 to 8 hr for patients with creatinine clearance of 30 ml/min/1.73 m^2 or more. Dosing frequency reduced to q 12 hr for patients with creatinine clearance of 15 to 29 ml/min/1.73 m^2. Frequency reduced to 1.5 to 3 g q 24 hr for patients with creatinine clearance of 5 to 14 ml/min/1.73 m^2.

Mechanism of Action
Ampicillin inhibits bacterial cell wall synthesis. The rigid, cross-linked cell wall is assembled in several steps. The drug exerts its effects on susceptible bacteria in the final stage of the cross-linking process by binding with and inactivating penicillin-binding proteins (enzymes responsible for linking the cell wall strands). This action causes bacterial cell lysis and death. When ampicillin is given alone, beta-lactamases may degrade it, making it ineffective. When it's combined with sulbactam, degradation can't occur. So sulbactam extends ampicillin's bactericidal effects to beta-lactamase–producing bacteria.

Incompatibilities

Don't mix ampicillin sodium and sulbactam sodium with any aminoglycoside in the same I.V. bag, bottle, or tubing; otherwise, both drugs will be inactivated. If patient must receive both drugs, give them in separate sites at least 1 hour apart.

Contraindications

Hypersensitivity to ampicillin sodium, sulbactam sodium, their components, or any penicillin

Interactions

DRUGS

allopurinol: Increased risk of rash, particularly in hyperuricemic patient

aminoglycosides: Possibly inactivated action of aminoglycoside and ampicillin sodium and sulbactam sodium when given together

heparin, oral anticoagulants: Increased risk of bleeding

oral contraceptives: Possibly breakthrough bleeding and reduced contraceptive effectiveness

probenecid: Possibly increased serum ampicillin level and ampicillin toxicity

tetracyclines: Possibly impaired action of ampicillin sodium and sulbactam sodium

Adverse Reactions

CNS: Chills, fatigue, fever, headache, malaise

CV: Chest pain, edema, thrombophlebitis

EENT: Black "hairy" tongue, epistaxis, glossitis, laryngeal stridor, mucocutaneous candidiasis, stomatitis, throat tightness

GI: Abdominal distention, diarrhea, enterocolitis, flatulence, gastritis, nausea, pseudomembranous colitis, vomiting

GU: Dysuria, urine retention, vaginal candidiasis

HEME: Agranulocytosis, anemia, eosinophilia, leukopenia, thrombocytopenia, thrombocytopenic purpura

SKIN: Erythema multiforme; erythematous, mildly pruritic maculopapular rash or other rash; exfoliative dermatitis; mucosal bleeding; pruritus; urticaria

Other: Anaphylaxis, facial edema, injection site pain

Nursing Considerations

- Avoid giving ampicillin sodium and sulbactam sodium to patients with mononucleosis because of the increased risk of rash.
- Administer I.V. dose by slow injection over 10 to 15 minutes or by infusion over 15 to 30 minutes in greater dilutions with 50 to 100 ml of a compatible diluent.

•Reconstitute drug for I.M. use with sterile water for injection or 0.5% or 2% lidocaine hydrochloride injection. For a 1.5-g vial, add 3.2 ml of diluent; for a 3-g vial, add 6.4 ml of diluent. Let solution stand until foaming dissipates. Inspect vial before withdrawing drug to ensure dissolution. After reconstituting solution, inject it within 1 hour.

•Administer by deep I.M. injection.

•Monitor patient closely for anaphylaxis, which may be life-threatening. Patients at greatest risk are those with a history of hypersensitivity to penicillin, multiple allergies, hypersensitivity to cephalosporins, or a history of asthma, hay fever, or urticaria.

•**WARNING** If drug triggers an anaphylactic reaction, stop giving drug, notify prescriber immediately, and provide appropriate therapy. Anaphylaxis requires immediate treatment with epinephrine as well as airway management and administration of oxygen and I.V. corticosteroids, as needed.

•Monitor patient closely for diarrhea, which may herald pseudomembranous colitis. If diarrhea occurs, notify prescriber. If pseudomembranous colitis is diagnosed, expect to stop treatment and, possibly, administer fluids, electrolytes, protein, and antibiotic effective against *Clostridium difficile.*

PATIENT TEACHING

•Warn patient that I.M. injection of drug is likely to cause discomfort.

•Instruct patient to report sudden or unusual symptoms, including diarrhea, immediately.

atovaquone and proguanil hydrochloride

Malarone

Class and Category

Chemical: Naphthalenedione (atovaquone), biguanide (proguanil)

Therapeutic: Antimalarial (atovaquone, proguanil)

Pregnancy category: C

Indications and Dosages

▶ *To treat acute, uncomplicated* Plasmodium falciparum *malaria when amodiaquine, chloroquine, halofantrine, or mefloquine resistance is suspected*

TABLETS, PEDIATRIC TABLETS

Adults and children weighing more than 40 kg (88 lb). 1 g atovaquone and 400 mg proguanil (4 tablets) daily for 3 consecutive days.

Children weighing 31 to 40 kg (68 to 88 lb). 750 mg atovaquone and 300 mg proguanil (3 tablets) daily for 3 consecutive days.

Children weighing 21 to 30 kg (46 to 66 lb). 500 mg atovaquone and 200 mg proguanil (2 tablets) daily for 3 consecutive days.

Children weighing 11 to 20 kg (24 to 44 lb). 250 mg atovaquone and 100 mg proguanil (4 tablets) daily for 3 consecutive days.

Children weighing 9 to 10 kg (20 to 22 lb). 187.5 mg atovaquone and 75 mg proguanil (3 pediatric tablets) daily for 3 consecutive days.

Children weighing 5 to 8 kg (11 to 18 lb). 125 mg atovaquone and 50 mg proguanil (2 pediatric tablets) daily for 3 consecutive days.

▶ *To prevent* P. falciparum *malaria when patient is traveling to areas where chloroquine-resistant* P. falciparum *malaria has been reported*
TABLETS, PEDIATRIC TABLETS

Adults and children weighing more than 40 kg. 250 mg atovaquone and 100 mg proguanil (1 tablet) daily starting 1 to 2 days before arrival in endemic area and continuing until 7 days after departure from endemic area.

Children weighing 31 to 40 kg. 187.5 mg atovaquone and 75 mg proguanil (3 pediatric tablets) daily starting 1 to 2 days before arrival in endemic area and continuing until 7 days after departure from endemic area.

Children weighing 21 to 30 kg. 125 mg atovaquone and 50 mg proguanil (2 pediatric tablets) daily starting 1 to 2 days before arrival in endemic area and continuing until 7 days after departure from endemic area.

Children weighing 11 to 20 kg. 62.5 mg atovaquone and 25 mg proguanil (1 tablet) daily starting 1 to 2 days before arrival in endemic area and continuing until 7 days after departure from endemic area.

Contraindications

Hypersensitivity to atovaquone, proguanil, or their components; severe renal impairment (creatinine clearance less than 30 ml/min/1.73 m^2.)

Mechanism of Action
Atovaquone selectively inhibits mitochrondial electron transport in the malarial parasite, which interferes with synthesis of pyrimidines needed for nucleic acid replication.

Proguanil mainly exerts its effects by inhibiting the enzyme dihydrofolate reductase, which disrupts deoxythymidylate synthesis in the malarial parasite. This action also interferes with synthesis of pyrimidines needed for nucleic acid replication, which prevents the malarial parasite from replicating.

Interactions
DRUGS

atovaquone component

metoclopramide, rifabutin, rifampin, tetracycline: Reduced plasma levels of atovaquone

Adverse Reactions
CNS: Anxiety, asthenia, depression, dizziness, fever, headache, insomnia, vivid dreams

EENT: Oral ulcers, visual disturbances

GI: Abdominal pain, anorexia, diarrhea, dyspepsia, gastritis, nausea, vomiting

MS: Back pain, myalgia

RESP: Cough, upper respiratory infection

SKIN: Erythema multiforme, photosensitivity, pruritus, rash, Stevens-Johnson syndrome, urticaria

Other: Flu syndrome

Nursing Considerations
• Use cautiously in elderly patients and in patients with hepatic or renal impairment.
• Determine if patient diagnosed with recrudescent malaria has been treated in the past with a combination of atovaquone and proguanil. If so, alert prescriber because atovaquone and proguanil may not be effective in this situation.

PATIENT TEACHING

• Instruct patient to take atovaquone and proguanil combination at the same time every day with food or a milky drink because the rate and extent of absorption is greater than when the drug is taken on an empty stomach.
• Inform patient that tablets may be crushed and mixed with condensed milk just before taking if he has trouble swallowing tablets.

• Tell patient to notify prescriber if vomiting occurs because an antiemetic may be needed. In addition, tell patient to repeat the dose if vomiting occurs within 1 hour of ingesting dose.

emtricitabine and tenofovir disoproxil fumarate

Truvada

Class and Category

Chemical: Synthetic nucleoside analog of cytidine (emtricitabine), acyclic nucleoside phosphonate analog of adenosine 5'-monophosphate (tenofovir)

Therapeutic: Antiretroviral (emtricitabine, tenofovir)

Pregnancy category: B

Indications and Dosages

▶ *To treat HIV-1 infection*

TABLETS

Adults. 200 mg emtricitabine and 300 mg tenofovir (1 tablet) daily with other antiretrovirals.

DOSAGE ADJUSTMENT For patients with a creatinine clearance between 30 and 49 ml/min/1.73 m^2, dosage interval increased to every 48 hours.

Mechanism of Action

Emtricitabine and tenofovir disoproxil are phosphorylated by cellular enzymes to form emtricitabine 5'-triphosphate and tenofovir diphosphatete respectively. These substances then compete with the natural substrate deoxycytidine 5'-triphosphate in the HIV-1 virus becoming a part of the DNA. This terminates the DNA chain resulting in viral death.

Contraindications

Hypersensitivity to emtricitabine, tenofovir or any of their components; severe renal impairment (creatinine clearance less than 30 ml/min/1.73 m^2) including patients receiving hemodialysis

Interactions

DRUGS

emtricitabine and tenofovir

nephrotoxic drugs such as acyclovir, adefovir dipivoxil, cidofovir, ganciclovir, valacyclovir, valganciclovir; renal competitors for active tubular se-

cretion: Increased serum levels of emtricitabine, tenofovir, and other drugs eliminated via the kidneys

emtricitabine component

lamivudine: Increased emtricitabine effect

tenofovir component

atazanavir, lopinavir and ritonavir: Increased serum tenofovir level, resulting in increased risk of adverse effects

didanosine: Increased serum didanosine level, resulting in increased risk of adverse effects

Adverse Reactions

CNS: Abnormal dreams, asthenia, depression, dizziness, fever, headache, insomnia, neuropathy, paresthesia, peripheral neuritis

CV: Chest pain, elevated triglycerides

EENT: Rhinitis

ENDO: Hyperglycemia, hypoglycemia

GI: Abdominal pain, anorexia, diarrhea, dyspepsia, elevated bilirubin or liver or pancreatic enzymes, flatulence, nausea, pancreatitis, vomiting

GU: Fanconi syndrome, renal insufficiency or failure

HEME: Decreased neurtophils

MS: Arthralgia, back pain, decreased bone density, elevated creatine kinase, myalgia,

RESP: Cough, dyspnea, pneumonia

SKIN: Diaphoresis, hyperpigmentation on palms or soles, pruritus, rash, urticaria

Other: Allergic reaction, hypophosphatemia, lactic acidosis, weight loss

Nursing Considerations

- Be aware that because dosage adjustments can't be made to emtricitabine and tenofovir combination, the drug shouldn't be given to a patient with a creatinine clearance less than 30 ml/min/1.73 m^2 or a patient undergoing hemodialysis. For patients with a creatinine clearance of 30 ml/min/1.73 m^2 or more, monitor creatinine and phosphorus level routinely throughout therapy.
- Test patient for the presence of hepatitis B virus, as ordered, before starting emtricitabine and tenofovir therapy. Expect to monitor the patient's liver function for several months after therapy stops because hepatitis B may worsen after emtricitabine and tenofovir are stopped.
- Monitor patient's liver function throughout therapy, as ordered, and assess patient for evidence of lactic acidosis and liver dys-

function that may occur as a result of emtricitabine and tenofovir therapy, especially in women, obese patients, and patients
with a history of prolonged nucleoside exposure.
• Be aware that bone monitoring should be done in a patient
with a history of pathologic bone fracture or who is at risk for
osteopenia. Expect to give supplemental calcium and vitamin D,
as ordered.

PATIENT TEACHING
• Inform patients with a history of hepatitis B that it may worsen
after emtricitabine and tenofovir therapy stops. Stress the need
to check hepatic function for at least several months after drug
therapy stops to detect an exacerbation that may warrant
anti–hepatitis B therapy.
• Tell patient that this combination drug may cause fat accumulation or redistribution. Advise him to notify prescriber about
central obesity, buffalo hump, limb or facial thinness, breast enlargement, or other signs of cushingoid appearance.
• Inform patient that emtricitabine and tenofovir therapy doesn't
cure HIV infection and doesn't reduce trhe risk of transmitting
HIV to others.

imipenem and cilastatin sodium

Primaxin (CAN), Primaxin ADD-Vantage, Primaxin IM,
Primaxin IV

Class and Category

Chemical: Thienamycin derivative (imipenem), heptenoic acid de-
rivative (cilastatin sodium)
Therapeutic: Antibiotic
Pregnancy category: C

Indications and Dosages

▶   *To treat severe or life-threatening bacterial infections (including
endocarditis, pneumonia, and septicemia as well as bone, joint, intra-
abdominal, skin, and soft-tissue infections) caused by gram-positive
anaerobic organisms, such as most staphylococci and streptococci and some
enterococci (including* Enterococcus faecalis*); most strains of
Enterobacteriaceae (including* Citrobacter *species,* Enterobacter *species,*
Escherichia coli, Klebsiella *species,* Morganella morganii, Proteus
mirabilis, Providencia stuartii, *and* Serratia marcescens*); and many
gram-negative aerobic and anaerobic species (including* Bacteroides
species, Campylobacter *species,* Clostridium *species,* Haemophilus
influenzae, Legionella *species,* Neisseria gonorrhoeae, *and*

Pseudomonas aeruginosa)
I.V. INFUSION (DOSAGES BASED ON IMIPENEM CONTENT)
Adults and adolescents. 500 mg q 6 hr to 1,000 mg q 6 to 8 hr. *Maximum:* 50 mg/kg or 4 g daily, whichever is lower.
Children age 3 months and over. 15 to 25 mg/kg q 6 hr. *Maximum:* 2,000 to 4,000 mg daily.
Infants ages 4 weeks to 3 months weighing 1,500 g (3 lb, 3 oz) or more. 25 mg/kg q 6 hr. *Maximum:* 2,000 to 4,000 mg daily.
Neonates ages 1 to 4 weeks weighing 1,500 g or more. 25 mg/kg q 8 hr. *Maximum:* 2,000 to 4,000 mg daily.
Neonates under age 1 week weighing 1,500 g or more. 25 mg/kg q 12 hr. *Maximum:* 2,000 to 4,000 mg daily.
▶ *To treat moderate infections caused by the organisms listed above*
I.V. INFUSION (DOSAGES BASED ON IMIPENEM CONTENT)
Adults and adolescents. 500 mg q 6 to 8 hr up to 1,000 mg q 8 hr. *Maximum:* 50 mg/kg or 4 g daily, whichever is lower.
Children age 3 months and over. 15 to 25 mg/kg q 6 hr. *Maximum:* 2,000 to 4,000 mg daily.
Infants ages 4 weeks to 3 months weighing 1,500 g or more. 25 mg/kg q 6 hr. *Maximum:* 2,000 to 4,000 mg daily.
Neonates ages 1 to 4 weeks weighing 1,500 g or more. 25 mg/kg q 8 hr. *Maximum:* 2,000 to 4,000 mg daily.
Neonates under age 1 week weighing 1,500 g or more. 25 mg/kg q 12 hr. *Maximum:* 2,000 to 4,000 mg daily.
I.M. INJECTION (DOSAGES BASED ON IMIPENEM CONTENT)
Adults and adolescents. 500 to 750 mg q 12 hr. *Maximum:* 1,500 mg daily.
Children. 10 to 15 mg/kg q 6 hr.
▶ *To treat mild infections caused by the organisms listed above*
I.V. INFUSION (DOSAGES BASED ON IMIPENEM CONTENT)
Adults and adolescents. 250 to 500 mg q 6 hr. *Maximum:* 50 mg/kg or 4 g daily, whichever is lower.
Children age 3 months and over. 15 to 25 mg/kg q 6 hr. *Maximum:* 2,000 mg (for fully susceptible organisms) to 4,000 mg (for moderately susceptible organisms) daily.
Infants ages 4 weeks to 3 months weighing 1,500 g or more. 25 mg/kg q 6 hr. *Maximum:* 2,000 to 4,000 mg daily.
Neonates ages 1 to 4 weeks weighing 1,500 g or more. 25 mg/kg q 8 hr. *Maximum:* 2,000 to 4,000 mg daily.
Neonates under age 1 week weighing 1,500 g or more. 25 mg/kg q 12 hr. *Maximum:* 2,000 to 4,000 mg daily.

I.M. INJECTION (DOSAGES BASED ON IMIPENEM CONTENT)
Adults and adolescents. 500 to 750 mg q 12 hr. *Maximum:* 1,500 mg daily.
Children. 10 to 15 mg/kg q 6 hr.
▶ *To treat uncomplicated UTI caused by the organisms listed above*
I.V. INFUSION (DOSAGES BASED ON IMIPENEM CONTENT)
Adults and adolescents. 250 mg q 6 hr. *Maximum:* 50 mg/kg or 4 g daily, whichever is lower.
▶ *To treat complicated UTI caused by the organisms listed above*
I.V. INFUSION (DOSAGES BASED ON IMIPENEM CONTENT)
Adults and adolescents. 500 mg q 6 hr. *Maximum:* 50 mg/kg or 4 g daily, whichever is lower.
DOSAGE ADJUSTMENT Dosage reduced based on creatinine clearance for patients with impaired renal function.

Mechanism of Action
During bacterial cell wall synthesis, imipenem selectively binds to penicillin-binding proteins responsible for cell wall formation. This action causes bacterial cells to rapidly lyse and die.

Cilastatin sodium inhibits imipenem's breakdown in the kidneys, thus maintaining a high imipenem level in the urinary tract.

Incompatibilities
Don't give imipenem and cilastatin through the same I.V. line as beta-lactam antibiotics or aminoglycosides.

Contraindications
Hypersensitivity to imipenem, its components, other beta-lactam antibiotics, or amide-type local anesthetics (I.M.); meningitis (I.V.); severe heart block or shock (I.M.)

Interactions
DRUGS
cyclosporine: Increased adverse CNS effects of both drugs
ganciclovir: Increased risk of seizures
probenecid: Slightly increased blood level and half-life of imipenem

Adverse Reactions
CNS: Confusion, dizziness, fever, seizures, somnolence, tremor, weakness
CV: Hypotension
EENT: Oral candidiasis
GI: Diarrhea, nausea, pseudomembranous colitis, vomiting

RESP: Wheezing
SKIN: Diaphoresis, pruritus, rash, urticaria
Other: Anaphylaxis, injection site thrombophlebitis

Nursing Considerations

- Obtain body fluid and tissue specimens for culture and sensitivity testing, as ordered, before giving first dose of imipenem and cilastatin. Expect to start therapy before results are available.
- For I.V. administration, add about 10 ml of diluent to each 250- or 500-mg vial and shake well. Transfer this reconstituted drug to at least 100 ml of prescribed I.V. solution. After the transfer, add another 10 ml of diluent to each vial, shake, and then transfer to infusion container. Shake infusion container until clear. To reconstitute piggyback bottles, add 100 ml of diluent to each 250- or 500-mg infusion bottle, and shake well.
- Administer reconstituted drug within 4 to 10 hours, depending on diluent used (24 to 48 hours if refrigerated). Color may range from clear to yellow; don't give solution that contains particles.
- Infuse 500-mg or smaller dose over 20 to 30 minutes and 750- to 1,000-mg dose over 40 to 60 minutes.
- Inject I.M. form into a large muscle mass.
- Expect increased risk of imipenem-induced seizures in patients with brain lesions, head trauma, or history of CNS disorders and in those receiving more than 2 g of drug daily.
- Assess patient for signs and symptoms of allergic reaction and bacterial or fungal superinfection.

PATIENT TEACHING

- Inform patient that imipenem and cilastatin must be given by infusion or injection.
- Instruct patient to report discomfort at I.V. insertion site.
- Advise patient to report itching, signs of superinfection (such as diarrhea and sore mouth), and hives.

lamivudine and zidovudine

Combivir

Class and Category

Chemical: Synthetic nucleoside analogues (lamivudine, zidovudine)
Therapeutic: Antiretroviral (lamivudine, zidovudine)
Pregnancy category: C

Indications and Dosages

▶ *To treat HIV infection with other antiretrovirals*
TABLETS
Adults. 150 mg lamivudine and 300 mg zidovudine (1 tablet)
b.i.d.

Mechanism of Action

Lamivudine and zidovudine as nucleoside analogues are converted intracellularly to their respective active metabolites: lamivudine to lamivudine triphosphate and zidovudine to zidovudine triphosphate. These active metobolites
inhibit the activity of HIV-1 reverse transcriptase by becoming incorporated
into viral DNA. Once incorporated, they prevent formation of a linkage essential for the viral DNA chain to elongate, thereby stopping viral DNA growth.

Contraindications

Hypersensitivity to lamivudine, zidovudine or any of their components

Interactions

DRUGS
lamivudine component
trimethoprim/sulfamethoxazole: Possibly increased lamivudine exposure
zalcitabine: Possibly inhibited intracellular phosphorylation of each
other, making both drugs ineffective
zidovudine component
doxorubicin, ribavirin, stavudine: Increased risk of antagonistic relationship between zidovudine and doxorubicin, ribavirin, or stavudine
*ganciclovir, interferon-alfa, and other bone marrow suppressive or cyto-
toxic agent:* Possibly increased hematologic toxicity

Adverse Reactions

CNS: Depression, dizziness, fatigue, fever, headache, insomnia,
malaise, neuropathy, paresthesia, peripheral neuropathy, seizures,
weakness
CV: Cardiomyopathy, hypotension, vasculitis
EENT: Conjunctivitis, nasal congestion, oral mucous membrane
pigmentation or ulcerations, pharyngitis, stomatitis
ENDO: Gynecomastia, mild hyperglycemia
GI: Abdominal cramps or pain, anorexia, diarrhea, dyspepsia, elevated liver function tests, exacerbation of hepatitis B after treat-

ment, hepatic failure or steatosis, nausea, pancreatitis, splenomegaly, vomiting

GU: Renal failure

HEME: Anemia, aplastic anemia, lymphopenia, neutropenia, pure red cell aplasia

MS: Arthralgia, muscle weakness, musculoskeletal pain, myalgia, myopathy, myositis, rhabdomyolysis

RESP: Acute respiratory distress syndrome, cough, dyspnea, respiratory failure, wheezing

SKIN: Alopecia, chills, erythema multiforme, rash, Stevens-Johnson syndrome, toxic epidermal necrolysis, urticaria

Other: Anaphylaxis, fat redistribution, hypersensitivity reactions, increased creatine phosphokinase, lactic acidosis, lymphadenopathy

Nursing Considerations

- Use cautiously in patients with bone marrow suppression evidenced by a granulocyte count less than 1,000 cells/mm^3 or hemoglobin less than 9.5 g/dl because zidovudine can cause bone marrow suppression. Monitor patient's blood counts closely, as ordered.
- Be aware that because lamivudine and zidovudine are available only in a fixed-dose combination, patients who need a reduced dosage of either one (such as those with a creatinine clearance less than 50 ml/min/1.73 m^2 and those who have impaired hepatic function of any degree) can't receive this drug combination. Likewise, patients who weigh less than 40 kg (88 lb) shouldn't receive this combination because dosage adjustments can't be made.
- Monitor patient for fatigue or pallor because neutropenia and severe anemia may occur with zidovudine use, especially in patients who have advanced HIV disease. Notify prescriber if present.
- Monitor patient's hepatic hepatic function studies, as ordered, because lactic acidosis and severe hepatomegaly have occurred with nucleoside analogues such as lamivudine and zidovudine. Those at risk include women, obese patients, and patients who have had prolonged exposure to nucleosides. Notify prescriber and expect to stop the drug combination if patient develops any signs or symptoms that suggest lactic acidosis or hepatic dysfunction, such as a change in level of consciousness, fatigue, jaundice, nausea, or vomiting.

- Monitor patients receiving this combination closely for myopathy and myositis, which may occur with prolonged use of zidovudine.
- Monitor patients infected with hepatitis B virus and HIV closely when lamivudine and zidovudine combination is stopped because severe exacerbations of hepatitis B may occur up to several months after therapy stops.

PATIENT TEACHING
- Caution patient to take lamivudine and zidovudine exactly as prescribed and not to stop and then restart therapy without consulting prescriber. Severe hypersensitivity reactions can occur when drug is restarted.
- Review signs and symptoms of hypersensitivity with patient and instruct him to notify prescriber immediately if any occur, such as abdominal pain, cough, diarrhea, dyspnea, fatigue, fever, nausea, skin rash, sore throat, or vomiting.
- Alert patient that this drug combination may cause fat redistribution.
- Advise patient that lamivudine and zidovudine therapy doesn't cure HIV infection and that he should continue taking precautions to reduce the risk of transmitting HIV to others.
- Instruct patient to avoid people with infections because the combination drug may increase his risk of infections.
- Remind patient to have his blood counts monitored as ordered so that adverse effects of combinaiton drug can be detected early.

lopinavir and ritonavir
Kaletra

Class and Category
Chemical: Protease inhibitors (lopinavir, ritonavir)
Therapeutic: Antiretrovial (lopinavir, ritonavir)
Pregnancy category: C

Indications and Dosages
▶ *To treat HIV infection with other antiretrovirals*
CAPSULES
Adults and children age 12 and over, or under age 12 and weighing 40 kg (88 lb) or more. 400 mg lopinavir and 100 mg ritonavir (three capsules) b.i.d with food.
DOSAGE ADJUSTMENT Increased in adults and children

over age 12 to 533 mg lopinavir and 133 mg ritonavir b.i.d. with food when given with amprenavir, efavirenz, nelfinavir, or nevirapine.

ORAL SOLUTION

Adults and children age 12 and over. 400 mg lopinavir and 100 mg ritonavir (5 ml) b.i.d with food.

DOSAGE ADJUSTMENT Increased in adults and children over age 12 to 533 mg lopinavir and 133 mg ritonavir b.id. with food when given with amprenavir, efavirenz, nelfinavir, or nevirapine.

Children under age 12 and weighing 40 kg or more. 400 mg lopinavir and 100 mg ritonavir (5 ml) b.i.d. with food

Children up to age 12 weighing 15 to 40 kg (33 to 88 lb). 10 mg/kg lopinavir and 2.5 mg/kg ritonavir b.i.d. with food.

Infants age 6 months to children up to age 12 weighing 7 to 15 kg (15 to 33 lb). 12 mg/kg lopinavir and 3 mg/kg ritonavir b.i.d. with food.

DOSAGE ADJUSTMENT Increased on individual basis in children age 12 or under who take amprenavir, efavirenz, or nevirapine.

TABLETS

Adults. 400 mg lopinavir and 100 mg ritonavir (2 tablets) b.i.d. with or without food

DOSAGE ADJUSTMENT Increased to 600 mg lopinavir and 150 mg ritonavir b.i.d. when given with efavirenz, nevirapine, fosamprenavir without ritonavir, or nelfinavir in treatment-experienced patients with decreased susceptibility to lopinavir

▶ *To treat HIV infection in patients who haven't received treatment previously and who won't be receiving amprenavir, efavirenz, nelfinavir, or nevirapine concurrently*

ORAL SOLUTION

Adults. 800 mg lopinavir and 200 mg ritonavir (10 ml) daily with food.

TABLETS

Adults. 800 mg lopinavir and 200 mg ritonavir (4 tablets) daily with or without food.

Contraindications

Co-administration with astemizole, cisapride, dihydroergotamine, ergonovine, ergotamine, methylergonovine, midazolam, pimozide, terfenadine, or triazolam; hypersensitivity to lopinavir, ritonavir, or any of their components

Mechanism of Action

Lopinavir inhibits the HIV protease by preventing cleavage of the Gag-Pol polyprotein. This causes production of immature, non-infectious viral particles, which abates replication of the HIV virus.

Ritonavir enhances lopinavir activity by inhibiting the CYP 3A–mediated metabolism of lopinavir, causing plasma lopinavir levels to increase.

Interactions

DRUGS

lopinavir and ritonavir

amiodarone, astemizole, bepridil, cisapride, flecainide, propafenone, pimozide, quinidine, terfenadine: Increased risk of life-threatening reactions, such as cardiac arrhythmias

amprenavir, atorvastatin, bupropion, carbamazepine, clarithromycin, clonazepam, clorazepate, cyclosporine, desipramine, dexamethasone, diazepam, dihydropyridine calcium channel blockers, diltiazem, disopyramide, dronabinol, estazolam, ethosuximide, flurazepam, fluticasone, HMG-CoA reductase inhibitors, indinavir, ketoconazole, immunosuppressants, itraconazole, lidocaine, methamphetamine, metoprolol, mexilitine, nefazodone, nelfinavir, nifedipine, perphenazine, prednisone, propoxyphene, quinidine, rapamycin, ,rifabutin, risperidone, saquinavir, selective serotonin reuptake inhibitors, sildenafil, sirolimus, tacrolimus, thioridazine, timolol, tramadol, tricyclics, verapamil, zolpidem: Increased levels and adverse effects of these drugs

atorvastatin, lovastatin, simvastatin and other HMG-CoA reductase inhibitors: Increased risk of myopathy, including rhabdomyolysis

atovaquone, ethinyl estradiol, methadone: Decreased plasma levels of these drugs

dihydroergotamine, ergonovine, ergotamine, methylergonivine: Increased risk of acute ergot toxicity

disulfiram, metronidazole: Possibly disulfiram-like reactions

itraconazole, ketoconazole: Increased plasma levels of these drugs

midazolam, triazolam: Increased risk of prolonged or increased sedation or respiratory depression

St. John's wort: Decreased effectiveness of lopinavir and ritonavir, with possible future resistance to these drugs or to drugs of the protease inhibitor class

warfarin: Altered concentrations of warfarin

lopinavir component

carbamazepine, dexamethasone, efavirenz, nevirapine, phenobarbital, phenytoin, rifamin: Decreased plasma lopinavir level

delavirdine: Increased lopinavir level
ritonavir component
atovaquone, divalproex, ethinyl estradiol, lamotrigine, methadone, pheny-toin, theophylline: Decreased levels and effectiveness of these drugs
fluticasone: Increased risk of adrenal suppression and Cushing's syndrome
meperidine: Increased analgesic activity and CNS stimulation
rifampin: Decreased ritonavir level
trazodone: Increased trazodone plasma level

Adverse Reactions
CNS: Asthenia, chills, depression, fever, headache, insomnia
CV: Increased cholesterol and triglyceride levels
EENT: Taste aversion
ENDO: Hyperglycemia
GI: Abdominal pain, anorexia, diarrhea, dyspepsia, dysphagia, flatulence, increased liver enzymes, nausea, pancreatitis, vomiting
HEME: Decreased platelet count, decreased neurtrophils
SKIN: rash
Other: Hypernatremia, hyponatremia, increased uric acid

Nursing Considerations
- Use cautiously in a patient with hepatic impairment because lopinavir and ritonavir are metabolized by the liver.
- Assess a patient with advanced HIV infection for hepatic dysfunction, and monitor liver enzymes, as ordered, for elevations, especially during the first several months of lopinavir and ritonavir therapy.
- Observe a hemophilic patient for bleeding tendencies. Although lopinavir and ritonavir haven't been known to increase bleeding risk, other drugs in their class (protease inhibitors) have.
- Determine patient's cholesterol and triglyceride levels, as ordered, before and periodically during therapy because cholesterol and triglyceride levels may rise markedly. Also, be aware that a patient with a markedly increased triglyceride level is at higher risk for pancreatitis while taking lopinavir and ritonavir.
- Monitor the patient's blood glucose level, as ordered, because hyperglycemia may develop in a patient with no history of diabetes mellitus and blood glucose level may increase in patients with diabetes mellitus.
- Be aware that diarrhea may be more common in patients that take the combination drug only once a day.

PATIENT TEACHING
- Emphasize the importance of the patient reporting all medications he takes, including OTC and herbal products, throughout lopinavir and ritonavir therapy because of the potential for drug interactions.
- Instruct patient to take lopinavir and ritonavir with food to decrease risk of stomach upset.
- Inform patient that lopinavir and ritonavir therapy doesn't cure HIV infection or reduce the risk of transmitting HIV to others.
- Instruct a diabetic patient to monitor his blood glucose level closely because lopinavir and ritonavir can cause blood glucose levels to rise above normal.
- Tell a patient who takes didanosine to take it 1 hour before or 2 hours after taking lopinavir and ritonavir.
- Instruct female patients of childbearing age who take estrogen-based hormonal contraceptives to use additional or alternative contraceptive measures while taking lopinavir and ritonavir.
- Inform patient that he may notice a redistribution or accumulation of body fat after starting lopinavir and ritonavir therapy, and urge him to notify the prescriber if this occurs.

penicillin G benzathine and penicillin G procaine

Bicillin C-R

Class and Category

Chemical: Penicillin (penicillin G benzathine, penicillin G procaine)
Therapeutic: Antibiotic (penicillin G benzathine, penicillin G procaine)
Pregnancy category: B

Indications and Dosages

▶ *To treat moderately severe streptococcal infections of the upper respiratory tract, scarlet fever, erysipelas, and skin and soft-tissue infections*

I.M. INJECTION

Adults and children weighing more than 27.5 kg (60 lb).
2.4 million units as a single injection. Alternatively, 1.2 million units given on day 1 and 1.2 million units given on day 3.
Children weighing 13.64 to 27.5 kg (30 to 60 lb). 900,000 to 1.2 million units as a single injection. Alternatively, 450,000 units given on day 1 and 450,000 units given on day 3.

Children weighing less than 13.64 kg (30 lb). 600,000 units as a single injection. Alternatively, 300,000 units given on day 1 and 300,000 units given on day 3.

▶ *To treat moderately severe pneumococcal infections (except pneumococcal meningitis)*

I.M. INJECTION

Adults. 1.2 million units q 2 or 3 days until body temperature is normal for 48 hours.

Children. 600,000 units q 2 or 3 days until body temperature is normal for 48 hours.

Mechanism of Action

Penicillin G benzathine and penicillin G procaine both inhibit the final stage of bacterial cell wall synthesis by competitively binding to penicillin-binding proteins inside the cell wall. Penicillin-binding proteins are responsible for various steps in bacterial cell wall synthesis. By binding to these proteins, penicillin leads to cell wall lysis.

Incompatibilities

Don't mix in the same syringe or container with aminoglycosides because aminoglycosides will become inactivated. Also, don't mix with drugs that may result in a pH below 5.5 or above 8.

Contraindications

Hypersensitivity to penicillin, procaine, or their components.

Interactions

DRUGS

penicillin G benzathine and penicillin G procaine

chloramphenicol, erythromycin, sulfonamides, tetracycline, thrombolytics: Possibly interference with penicillin's bactericidal effect

methotrexate: Decreased methotrexate clearance, increased risk of toxicity

probenecid: Increased blood penicillin level

Adverse Reactions

CNS: Anxiety, asthenia, chills, coma, confusion, dizziness, dysphasia, euphoria, fatigue, fever, hallucinations, headache, lethargy, myelitis, nervousness, neuropathy, neurovascular reaction, prostration, sciatic nerve irritation, seizures, somnolence, stroke, syncope, tremors

CV: Edema, labile blood pressure, palpitations, tachycardia, vasculitis, vasodilation, vasovagal reaction

EENT: Black "hairy" tongue, blindness, blurred vision, laryngeal edema, oral candidiasis, stomatitis, taste perversion

GI: Abdominal pain, blood in stool, diarrhea, elevated liver function test results (transient), indigestion, intestinal necrosis, nausea, pseudomembranous colitis, vomiting

GU: Elevated BUN and creatinine levels, hematuria, impotence, interstitial nephritis (acute), priapism, proteinuria, renal failure, vaginal candidiasis

HEME: Eosinophilia, hemolytic anemia, leukopenia, lymphadenopathy, thrombocytopenia

MS: Arthralgia, muscle twitching, rhabdomyolysis

RESP: Dyspnea, hypoxia, pulmonary hypertension or embolism

SKIN: Diaphoresis, exfoliative or maculopapular dermatitis, pruritis, rash, urticaria

Other: Anaphylaxis; electrolyte imbalances; elevated SGOT level; injection site necrosis, pain, or redness

Nursing Considerations

- Obtain body tissue and fluid samples for culture and sensitivity tests as ordered before giving first dose. Expect to start therapy before test results are known.
- Inject only deep into large muscle mass, such as the upper, outer quadrant of the buttock in an adult or the midlateral aspect of the thigh in small children.
- **WARNING** Don't inject intravenously because I.V. injection may be fatal and intra-arterial injection may cause extensive tissue and organ necrosis.
- Don't clear any air bubbles from the disposable syringe or needle because doing so may interfere with visualization of blood or discoloration during aspiration.
- Inject drug at a slow, steady rate; otherwise, the needle may become blocked because of the high concentration of suspended material in the solution. Stop injection at once if patient complains of sudden pain at the injection site or if a child shows signs of severe pain.
- Following injection, apply ice to the site for pain.
- Monitor patient closely for anaphylaxis, which may become life-threatening. Patients at greatest risk are those with a history of hypersensitivity to penicillin, cephalosporins, or multiple other allergies; those who have asthma or hay fever; and those who have developed urticaria in the past.
- **WARNING** If drug triggers an anaphylactic reaction, stop it immediately and notify prescriber. Provide appropriate ther-

apy. Anaphylaxis requires immediate treatment with epinephrine and airway management. It may also require administration of oxygen and I.V. corticosteroids.

• Be aware that giving the combination drug I.M. slows its absorbtion, which may make allergic reactions difficult to treat.

• Monitor patient closely for diarrhea, which may herald pseudomembranous colitis. If diarrhea occurs, notify prescriber. If the patient has pseudomembranous colitis, expect to stop the drug and possibly administer fluids, electrolytes, protein, and an antibiotic effective against *Clostridium difficile.*

PATIENT TEACHING

• Instruct patient to report previous allergies to penicillins and cephalosporins and to notify prescriber immediately about adverse reactions, such as a fever, rash and hives.

• Warn patient that injection will be uncomfortable; advise keeping ice on site for pain relief for length of time prescribed.

piperacillin sodium and tazobactam sodium

Tazocin (CAN), Zosyn

Class and Category

Chemical: Piperazine derivative of ampicillin, acylureidopenicillin (piperacillin); penicillinate sulfone (tazobactam)
Therapeutic: Antibiotic
Pregnancy category: B

Indications and Dosages

▶ *To treat moderate to severe gram-negative or anaerobic infections, such as appendicitis, community-acquired pneumonia, diabetic foot ulcers, intra-abdominal infections, pelvic inflammatory disease, peritonitis, postpartum endometritis, and uncomplicated or complicated skin or soft-tissue infections caused by susceptible organisms, such as* Bacteroides species *(including many strains of* Bacteroides fragilis*)*, Clostridium species, Enterobacter *species,* Enterococcus faecalis, Escherichia coli, Haemophilus influenzae, Klebsiella pneumoniae, Morganella morganii, Neisseria gonorrhoeae, Proteus mirabilis, Proteus vulgaris, Pseudomonas aeruginosa, *and* Serratia species

I.V. INFUSION

Adults and adolescents. 3.375 g q 6 hr. *Maximum:* 4.5 g q 6 to 8 hr.

▶ *To treat nosocomial pneumonia caused by susceptible organisms*
I.V. INFUSION
Adults and adolescents. 4.5 g q 6 hr in addition to aminoglycoside therapy for 7 to 14 days.
DOSAGE ADJUSTMENT Dosage possibly decreased to 2.25 g
q 6 hr for patients with creatinine clearance of 20 to 40 ml/
min/1.73 m^2 or to 2.25 g q 8 hr for those with creatinine clearance less than 20 ml/min/1.73 m^2.

Mechanism of Action

Piperacillin binds to specific penicillin-binding proteins and inhibits the third
and final stage of bacterial cell wall synthesis. It does this by interfering with
an autolysin inhibitor. Uninhibited autolytic enzymes destroy the cell wall and
result in cell lysis.

Tazobactam doesn't change piperacillin's action, but it protects piperacillin
against Richmond and Sykes types II, III, IV, and V beta-lactamases; staphylo-
coccal beta-lactamases; and extended-spectrum beta-lactamases.

Incompatibilities

Don't mix piperacillin and tazobactam in same container with
aminoglycosides because of chemical incompatibility (depending
on concentrations, diluents, pH, and temperature).

Contraindications

Hypersensitivity to beta-lactamase inhibitors, cephalosporins,
penicillins, piperacillin, tazobactam, or their components

Interactions

DRUGS

aminoglycosides: Additive or synergistic effects against some bacteria, possibly mutual inactivation
*anti-inflammatory drugs (including aspirin and NSAIDs), heparin, oral
anticoagulants, platelet aggregation inhibitors, sulfinpyrazone, thrombolytics:* Increased risk of bleeding
hepatotoxic drugs (including labetalol and rifampin): Increased risk of
hepatotoxicity
methotrexate: Increased blood methotrexate level and risk of toxicity
probenecid: Increased blood piperacillin level and risk of toxicity
vecuronium: Possibly prolonged neuromuscular blockade of vecuronium in perioperative period

Adverse Reactions

CNS: Chills, CVA, dizziness, fever, hallucinations, headache, lethargy, seizures

CV: Cardiac arrest, hypotension, palpitations, tachycardia, vasodilation, vasovagal reactions

EENT: Epistaxis, oral candidiasis, pharyngitis

GI: Diarrhea, elevated liver function test results, epigastric distress, intestinal necrosis, nausea, pseudomembranous colitis, vomiting

GU: Hematuria, impotence, nephritis, neurogenic bladder, priapism, proteinuria, renal failure, vaginal candidiasis

HEME: Eosinophilia, leukopenia, neutropenia, thrombocytopenia

MS: Arthralgia, prolonged muscle relaxation

RESP: Dyspnea, pulmonary embolism, pulmonary hypertension

SKIN: Erythema multiforme, exfoliative dermatitis, mottling, rash, Stevens-Johnson syndrome

Other: Anaphylaxis, facial edema, hypokalemia, hyponatremia

Nursing Considerations

- Obtain blood, sputum, or other samples for culture and sensitivity testing, as ordered, before giving piperacillin and tazobactam. Expect to begin therapy before results are available.
- Be aware that sunlight may darken powder for dilution but won't alter drug potency.
- Reconstitute with sterile water for injection, sodium chloride for injection, D_5W, or bacteriostatic water or normal saline solution that contains parabens or benzyl alcohol.
- For additional dilution (50 to 150 ml except as noted), use appropriate solution, such as sodium chloride for injection, sterile water for injection (no more than 50 ml), D_5W, or dextran 6% in normal saline solution.
- Shake solution vigorously after adding diluent to help drug dissolve, and inspect for particles and discoloration before administering.
- Administer over at least 30 minutes.
- Assess patient for bleeding or excessive bruising because drug can decrease platelet aggregation.
- Monitor serum potassium level to detect hypokalemia, which may result from urinary potassium loss.
- Assess patient for diarrhea during or shortly after drug therapy; it may signal pseudomembranous colitis.
- Administer aminoglycosides 1 hour before or after piperacillin and tazobactam, using a separate site, I.V. bag, and tubing.

PATIENT TEACHING
• Advise patient to consult prescriber before using OTC drugs during treatment with piperacillin and tazobactam because of the risk of interactions.
• Inform patient that increased bruising may occur if she takes anti-inflammatory drugs, such as aspirin and NSAIDs, during piperacillin and tazobactam therapy.
• Advise patient to notify prescriber about signs of superinfection, such as severe diarrhea or white patches on tongue or in mouth.

quinupristin and dalfopristin
Synercid

Class and Category
Chemical: Pristinamycin I and IIa derivative, streptogramin
Therapeutic: Antibiotic
Pregnancy category: B

Indications and Dosages
▶ *To treat serious or life-threatening infections, such as bacteremia caused by vancomycin-resistant* Enterococcus faecium
I.V. INFUSION
Adults and adolescents age 16 and over. 7.5 mg/kg q 8 hr.
▶ *To treat complicated skin and soft-tissue infections caused by methicillin-susceptible strains of* Staphylococcus aureus *or* Streptococcus pyogenes
I.V. INFUSION
Adults and adolescents age 16 and over. 7.5 mg/kg q 12 hr for at least 7 days.

Mechanism of Action
Quinupristin inhibits the late phase of protein synthesis by binding to the 50S ribosomal subunit.

Dalfopristin inhibits the early phase of protein synthesis by binding to the 70S or 50S ribosomal subunit.

Together, these drugs inhibit bacterial protein synthesis by irreversibly blocking ribosome function. Additionally, their combined activity inhibits transfer RNA (tRNA) synthetase activity, which decreases the amount of free tRNA in the cell. Without tRNA, bacterial cells can't incorporate amino acids into peptide chains, and the cells die.

Incompatibilities

Don't mix quinupristin and dalfopristin in saline solutions, including normal saline, half-normal (0.45%) saline, 3% sodium chloride, and 5% sodium chloride solutions, because drug is physically incompatible with these solutions.

Contraindications

Hypersensitivity to quinupristin or dalfopristin, other streptogramin antibiotics, or their components

Interactions

DRUGS

alfentanil, alprazolam, carbamazepine, delavirdine, diazepam, diltiazem, disopyramide, dofetilide, donepezil, erythromycin, ethinyl estradiol, felodipine, fexofenadine, indinavir, lidocaine, lovastatin, methylprednisolone, nevirapine, norethindrone, quinidine, ritonavir, saquinavir, simvastatin, tacrolimus, triazolam, trimetrexate, verapamil, vinblastine: Decreased elimination of these drugs, possibly resulting in toxicity
astemizole, cisapride, terfenadine: Decreased elimination of these drugs, possibly prolonged QT interval
cyclosporine, midazolam, nifedipine, terfenadine: Possibly increased blood levels of these drugs

Adverse Reactions

CNS: Anxiety, confusion, dizziness, fever, headache, hypertonia, insomnia, paresthesia
CV: Chest pain, palpitations, peripheral edema, thrombophlebitis, vasodilation
EENT: Oral candidiasis, stomatitis
GI: Abdominal pain, constipation, diarrhea, elevated liver function test results, indigestion, nausea, pancreatitis, pseudomembranous colitis, vomiting
GU: Hematuria, vaginitis
MS: Arthralgia, gout, muscle spasms, myalgia, myasthenia
RESP: Dyspnea, pleural effusion
SKIN: Diaphoresis, pruritus, rash, urticaria
Other: Injection site edema, inflammation, pain, or thrombophlebitis

Nursing Considerations

- Store unopened vials of quinupristin and dalfopristin in refrigerator.
- **WARNING** Reconstitute and further dilute with dextrose in water or sterile water for injection only. Don't use saline solutions because drug is physically incompatible with them.

- Dilute prescribed dose in 250 ml D_5W, and infuse over 1 hour through a peripheral I.V. line. If administered by central venous catheter, dilute prescribed dose in 100 ml of D_5W. Central venous administration may decrease incidence of infusion site reaction. Use an infusion pump or device to control rate of infusion.
- Further dilute reconstituted solution within 30 minutes. Vials are for single use only. Discard any unused portion.
- Don't flush I.V. catheter with saline or heparin flush solution because of possible incompatibility. Flush I.V. catheter only with D_5W before and after drug administration.
- Monitor patient for diarrhea, a possible indication of overgrowth of normal intestinal flora, such as *Clostridium difficile*. Be aware that pseudomembranous colitis may result from a toxin produced by *C. difficile.*
- If you suspect that patient has pseudomembranous colitis, notify prescriber and expect to stop drug immediately.
- If patient develops pseudomembranous colitis, be aware that drugs that inhibit peristalsis are contraindicated because of the risk of toxic megacolon.

PATIENT TEACHING
- Instruct patient to complete the full course of quinupristin and dalfopristin therapy, as prescribed.
- Advise patient to notify prescriber at once if he develops diarrhea or abdominal pains.
- Inform patient that if he requires long-term therapy, drug will be given in hospital or clinic or by a home health care nurse.

rifampin and isoniazid
Rifamate

Class and Category
Chemical: Semi-synthetic antibiotic derivative of rifamycin (rifampin), isonicotinic acid derivative (isoniazid)
Therapeutic: Antitubercular (rifampin, isoniazid)
Pregnancy category: C

Indications and Dosages
▶ *To treat pulmonary tuberculosis when initial therapy for tuberculosis has been ineffective*
CAPSULES
Adults. 600 mg rifampin and 300 mg isoniazid (2 capsules) daily.

Mechanism of Action
Rifampin inhibits bacterial and mycobacterial RNA synthesis by binding to DNA-dependent RNA polymerase, thereby blocking RNA transcription. Depending on the dose given, a bactericidal or bacteriostatic action results.

Isoniazid interferes with lipid and nucleic acid synthesis in actively growing tubercle bacilli cells. It also disrupts bacterial cell wall synthesis and may interfere with mycolic acid synthesis in mycobacterial cells, which halts the growth of tubercle bacilli.

Contraindications
Acute liver disease; concurrent use of nonnucleoside reverse transcriptase inhibitors or protease inhibitors (by patients with HIV); history of serious adverse reactions to isoniazid; hypersensitivity to rifampin, isoniazid, other rifamycins and their components

Interactions
DRUGS
rifampin and isoniazid
anesthetics (hydrocarbon inhalation, except isoflurane), hepatotoxic drugs: Increased risk of hepatotoxicity
ketoconazole: Possibly decreased blood ketoconazole level and resistance to antifungal treatment
rifampin component
aminophylline, oxtriphylline, theophylline: Increased metabolism and clearance of these theophylline preparations
beta blockers, chloramphenicol, clofibrate, corticosteroids, cyclosporine, dapsone, digitalis glycosides, disopyramide, hexocbarbital, itraconazole, mexiletine, oral anticoagulants, oral antidiabetic drugs, phenytoin, propafenone, quinidine, tocainide, verapamil (oral): Increased metabolism, resulting in lower blood levels of these drugs
bone marrow depressants: Increased leukopenic or thrombocytopenic effects
clofazimine: Decreased absorption of rifampin
diazepam: Increased elimination of diazepam, resulting in decreased effectiveness
estramustine, estrogens, oral contraceptives: Decreased estrogenic effects
methadone: Possibly impaired absorption of methadone, leading to withdrawal symptoms
probenecid: Increased blood level or prolonged duration of rifampin, increasing risk of toxicity

nonnucleoside reverse transcriptase inhibitors, protease inhibitors (indinavir, nelfinavir, ritonavir, saquinavir): Accelerated metabolism of these drugs by patients with HIV, resulting in subtherapeutic levels. Also delayed metabolism of rifampin, increasing the risk of toxicity

trimethoprim: Increased elimination and shortened elimination half-life of trimethoprim

isoniazid component

acetaminophen: Increased risk of hepatotoxicity and possibly nephrotoxicity

alfentanil: Decreased alfentanil clearance and increased duration of alfentanil effects

aluminum-containing antacids: Decreased isoniazid absorption

benzodiazepines: Decreased benzodiazepine clearance

carbamazepine: Increased blood carbamazepine level and toxicity; increased risk of isoniazid toxicity

corticosteroids: Decreased isoniazid effects

cycloserine: Increased risk of adverse CNS effects and CNS toxicity

disulfiram: Changes in behavior and coordination

enflurane: Increased risk of high-output renal failure

meperidine: Risk of hypotensive episodes or CNS depression

nephrotoxic drugs: Increased risk of nephrotoxicity

oral anticoagulants: Increased anticoagulant effects

phenytoin: Increased blood phenytoin level and risk of phenytoin toxicity

theophylline: Increased blood theophylline level

FOODS

isoniazid component

tyramine-containing foods, such as cheese and fish: Increased responses to tyramine contained in foods, possibly resulting in chills, diaphoresis, headache, light-headedness, and red, itchy, clammy skin

ACTIVITIES

rifampin and isoniazid

alcohol use: Increased risk of hepatotoxicity

Adverse Reactions

CNS: Chills, clumsiness, confusion, dizziness, drowsiness, encephalopathy, fatigue, fever, hallucinations, headache, neurotoxicity, paresthesia, peripheral neuritis, psychosis, seizures, weakness

CV: Vasculitis

EENT: Discolored saliva, tears, and sputum; mouth or tongue soreness; optic neuritis; periorbital edema

ENDO: Gynecomastia, hyperglycemia

GI: Abdominal cramps, anorexia, diarrhea, discolored feces, elevated liver function test results, epigastric discomfort, flatulence, hearburn, hepatitis, heptotoxicity, jaundice, nausea, pseudomembranous colitis, vomiting

GU: Discolored urine

HEME: Agranulocytosis, aplastic anemia, eosinophilia, hemolytic anemia, sideroblastic anemia, thrombocytopenia

MS: Arthralgia, joint stiffness, myalgia

SKIN: Discolored skin and sweat, pruritus, rash

Other: Angioedema, flulike symptoms, hypocalcemia, hypophosphatemia

Nursing Considerations

- Expect to also give pyridoxine (vitamin B_6) to patients who are malnourished or predisposed to developing neuropathy, such as diabetics.
- Monitor results of liver enzyme studies, which may be ordered monthly, because rifampin and isoniazid can cause hepatotoxicity. Monitor patient for evidence of hepatotoxicity, such as darkened urine, fever, jaundice, malaise, nausea, and vomiting.
- Be aware that about 50% of patients metabolize isoniazid slowly, which may lead to increased toxic effects of the combination drug. Monitor patient for such adverse reactions as peripheral neuritis; if they occur, notify prescriber and expect to decrease dosage.
- Be aware that patients with advanced HIV infection may experience more adverse reactions and in greater severity.

PATIENT TEACHING

- Instruct patient to take rifampin and isoniazid exactly as prescribed and not to stop taking it without consulting prescriber. Explain that interruptions can lead to increased adverse reactions. Remind patient that treatment may take months or years.
- Direct patient to take drug on an empty stomach 1 hour before or 2 hours after meals with a full glass of water. If GI distress occurs, instruct him to take drug with food or an antacid that doesn't contain aluminum.
- Advise patient to watch for and report signs of hepatic dysfunction, including darkened urine, decreased appetite, fatigue, and jaundice.
- Warn that drug may turn urine, feces, saliva, sputum, sweat, tears, and skin reddish orange to reddish brown.
- Caution patient against wearing soft contact lenses during therapy because drug may permanently stain them.

- Advise female patients who use an oral conceptive to use an additional form of birth control while taking rifampin and isoniazid.
- Caution patient not to drink alcohol while taking drug because alcohol increases the risk of hepatotoxicity.
- Provide patient with a list of tyramine-containing foods to avoid when taking rifampin and isoniazid, such as cheese, fish, salami, red wine, and yeast extracts. Inform him that consuming these foods during drug therapy may cause unpleasant adverse reactions, such as chills, pounding heartbeat, and sweating.
- Urge patient to keep appointments for periodic laboratory tests and physical examinations.
- Instruct patient to report fever, nausea, numbness and tingling in arms and legs, rash, vision changes, vomiting, and yellowing skin.

rifampin, isoniazid, and pyrazinamide
Rifater

Class and Category
Chemical: Semi-synthetic antibiotic derivative of rifamycin (rifampin), isonicotinic acid derivative (isoniazid), pyrazine analogue of nicotinamide (pyrazinamide)
Therapeutic: Antitubercular (rifampin, isoniazid, pyrazinamide)
Pregnancy category: C

Indications and Dosages
▶ *To treat pulmonary tuberculosis initially*
TABLETS
Adults weighing 55 kg (121 lb) or more. 720 mg rifampin, 300 mg isoniazid, and 1,800 mg pyrazinamide (6 tablets) daily.
Adults weighing 45 kg to 55 kg (99 to 121 lb). 600 mg rifampin, 250 mg isoniazid, and 1500 mg pyrazinamide (5 tablets) daily.
Adults weighing 44 kg (97 lb) or less. 480 mg rifampin, 200 mg isoniazid, and 1,200 mg pyrazinamide (4 tablets) daily.

Contraindications
Acute gout or liver disease; concurrent use of nonnucleoside reverse transcriptase inhibitors or protease inhibitors (by patients with HIV); history of serious adverse reactions to isoniazid; hy-

persensitivity to rifampin, isoniazid, pyrazinamide, other rifamycins and their components

Mechanism of Action

Rifampin inhibits bacterial and mycobacterial RNA synthesis by binding to DNA-dependent RNA polymerase, thereby blocking RNA transcription. Depending on the dose given, a bactericidal or bacteriostatic drug effect results.

Isoniazid interferes with lipid and nucleic acid synthesis in actively growing tubercule bacilli cells. It also disrupts bacterial cell wall synthesis and may interfere with mycolic acid synthesis in mycobacterial cells, which halts the growth of tubercle bacilli.

Pyrazinamide inhibits the growth of *Mycobacterium tuberculosis* organisms by decreasing the pH level. Depending on the blood pyrazinamide level, a bactericidal or bacteriostatic action results.

Interactions

DRUGS

rifampin and isoniazid

anesthetics (hydrocarbon inhalation, except isoflurane), hepatotoxic drugs: Increased risk of hepatotoxicity

ketoconazole: Possibly decreased blood ketoconazole level and resistance to antifungal treatment

rifampin and pyrazinamide

cyclosporine: Possibly decreased blood level and therapeutic effects of cyclosporine

rifampin component

aminophylline, oxtriphylline, theophylline: Increased metabolism and clearance of these theophylline preparations

beta blockers, chloramphenicol, clofibrate, corticosteroids, cyclosporine, dapsone, digitalis glycosides, disopyramide, hexocbarbital, itraconazole, mexiletine, oral anticoagulants, oral antidiabetic drugs, phenytoin, propafenone, quinidine, tocainide, verapamil (oral): Increased metabolism, resulting in lower blood levels of these drugs

bone marrow depressants: Increased leukopenic or thrombocytopenic effects

clofazimine: Reduced absorption of rifampin

diazepam: Enhanced elimination of diazepam and decreased effectiveness

estramustine, estrogens, oral contraceptives: Decreased estrogenic effects *methadone:* Possibly impaired methadone absorption, leading to withdrawal symptoms

probenecid: Increased blood level or prolonged duration of rifampin, increasing risk of toxicity

nonnucleoside reverse transcriptase inhibitors, protease inhibitors (indinavir, nelfinavir, ritonavir, saquinavir): Accelerated metabolism of these drugs in patients with HIV, resulting in subtherapeutic levels. Also delayed metabolism of rifampin, increasing the risk of toxicity

trimethoprim: Increased elimination and shortened elimination half-life of trimethoprim

isoniazid component

acetaminophen: Increased risk of hepatotoxicity and possibly nephrotoxicity

alfentanil: Decreased alfentanil clearance and increased duration of alfentanil's effects

aluminum-containing antacids: Decreased isoniazid absorption

benzodiazepines: Decreased benzodiazepine clearance

carbamazepine: Increased blood carbamazepine level and toxicity, and increased risk of isoniazid toxicity

corticosteroids: Decreased isoniazid effects

cycloserine: Increased risk of adverse CNS effects and CNS toxicity

disulfiram: Changes in behavior and coordination

enflurane: Increased risk of high-output renal failure

meperidine: Risk of hypotensive episodes or CNS depression

nephrotoxic drugs: Increased risk of nephrotoxicity

oral anticoagulants: Increased anticoagulant effects

phenytoin: Increased blood phenytoin level and risk of phenytoin toxicity

theophylline: Increased blood theophylline level

pyrazinamide component

allopurinol, colchicine, probenecid, sulfinpyrazone: Possibly increased blood uric acid level and decreased efficacy of antigout therapy

FOODS

isoniazid component

tyramine-containing foods, such as cheese and fish: Increased responses to tyramine contained in foods, possibly resulting in chills, diaphoresis, headache, light-headedness, and red, itchy, clammy skin

ACTIVITIES

rifampin and pyrazinamide

alcohol use: Increased risk of hepatotoxicity

Adverse Reactions

CNS: Chills, clumsiness, confusion, dizziness, drowsiness, enceph-alopathy, fatigue, fever, hallucinations, headache, neurotoxicity, paresthesia, peripheral neuritis, psychosis, seizures, weakness
CV: Vasculitis
EENT: Discolored saliva, tears, and sputum; mouth or tongue soreness; optic neuritis; periorbital edema
ENDO: Gynecomastia, hyperglycemia
GI: Abdominal cramps, anorexia, diarrhea, discolored feces, ele-vated liver function test results, epigastric discomfort, flatulence, hearburn, hepatitis, hepatotoxicity, jaundice, nausea, pseudomembranous colitis, vomiting
GU: Discolored urine, dysuria, interstitial nephritis
HEME: Agranulocytosis, aplastic anemia, eosinophilia, hemolytic anemia, porphyria, sideroblastic anemia, thrombocytopenia
MS: Arthralgia, gout, joint stiffness, myalgia
SKIN: Acne, discolored skin and sweat, photosensitivity, pruritus, rash, urticaria
Other: Angioedema, flulike symptoms, hypocalcemia, hypophos-phatemia

Nursing Considerations

- Review liver function test results before and every 2 to 4 weeks during rifampin, isoniazid, and pyrazinamide therapy because the drug can cause hepatotoxicity. Monitor patient for signs of hepatotoxicity, such as darkened urine, fever, jaundice, malaise, nausea and vomiting.
- Be aware that about 50% of patients metabolize isoniazid slowly, which may lead to increased toxic effects of the combi-nation drug. Monitor patient for such adverse reactions as pe-ripheral neuritis; if adverse reactions occur, notify prescriber and expect to decrease dosage.
- Be aware that patients with advanced HIV infection may expe-rience more adverse reactions and in greater severity.
- Expect to also give pyridoxine (vitamin B_6) to patients who are malnourished or predisposed to developing neuropathy, such as diabetics.
- Be aware that the pyrazinamide component of the drug can af-fect the accuracy of certain urine ketone strip test results.

PATIENT TEACHING

- Instruct patient to take rifampin, isoniazid, and pyrazinamide exactly as prescribed and not to stop without consulting pre-scriber. Explain that interruptions can lead to increased adverse

reactions. Remind patient that treatment may take months or years.
- Direct patient to take this combination drug on an empty stomach 1 hour before or 2 hours after meals with a full glass of water. If GI distress occurs, instruct him to take the drug with food or an antacid that doesn't contain aluminum.
- Advise patient to watch for and report signs of hepatic dysfunction, including darkened urine, decreased appetite, fatigue, and jaundice.
- Warn that drug may turn urine, feces, saliva, sputum, sweat, tears, and skin reddish orange to reddish brown.
- Caution patient against wearing soft contact lenses during therapy because drug may permanently stain them.
- Advise female patients who take an oral conceptive to use an additional form of birth control during therapy with rifampin, isoniazid, and pyrazinamide.
- Caution patient not to drink alcohol while taking drug because alcohol increases the risk of hepatotoxicity.
- Give patient a list of tyramine-containing foods to avoid while taking combination drug, such as cheese, fish, salami, red wine, and yeast extracts. Explain that consuming these foods during drug therapy may cause unpleasant adverse reactions, such as chills, a pounding heartbeat, and sweating.
- Instruct patient to keep appointments for periodic laboratory tests and physical examinations.
- Urge patient to report fever, nausea, numbness and tingling in arms and legs, rash, visual changes, vomiting, and yellow skin.
- Advise diabetic patient to use alternative methods of ketone determination while taking drug.
- Urge patient to minimize exposure to sun and to wear protective clothing, hat, sunglasses, and sunscreen when outdoors.

sulfadoxine and pyrimethamine
Fansidar

Class and Category
Chemical: Folic acid antagonist (sulfadoxine, pyrimethamine)
Therapeutic: Antimalarial (sulfadoxine, pyrimethamine)
Pregnancy category: C

Indications and Dosages
▶ *To treat acute, uncomplicated* Plasmodium falciparum *malaria*

when chloroquine resistance is suspected
TABLETS
Adults and adolescents age 18 and over. 1,000 mg sulfadox-ine and 50 mg pyrimethamine (2 tablets) as a single dose. Alter-natively, 1,500 mg sulfadoxine and 75 mg pyrimethamine (3 tablets) as a single dose.
Children over age 2 months weighing more than 45 kg (99 lb). 1,500 mg sulfadoxine and 75 mg pyrimethamine (3 tablets) as a single dose.
Children over age 2 months weighing 31 to 45 kg (68 to 99 lb). 1,000 mg sulfadoxine and 50 mg pyrimethamine (2 tablets) as a single dose.
Children over age 2 months weighing 21 to 30 kg (46 to 66 lb). 750 mg sulfadoxine and 37.5 mg pyrimethamine (1½ tablets) as a single dose.
Children over age 2 months weighing 11 to 20 kg (24 to 44 lb). 500 mg sulfadoxine and 25 mg pyrimethamine (1 tablet) as a single dose.
Children over age 2 months weighing 5 to 10 kg (11 to 22 lb). 250 mg sulfadoxine and 12.5 mg pyrimethamine (½ tablet) as a single dose.
▶ *To prevent* P. falciparum *malaria when patient is traveling to areas where chloroquine-resistant* P. falciparum *malaria is endemic and alternative drugs are not available or are contraindicated*
TABLETS
Adults and adolescents age 18 and over. 500 mg sulfadoxine and 25 mg pyrimethamine (1 tablet) 1 to 2 days prior to arrival in endemic area, followed by 500 mg sulfadoxine and 25 mg pyrimethamine (1 tablet) once weekly throughout stay and con-tinued for 4 to 6 weeks after departure from endemic area. Alter-natively, 1,000 mg sulfadoxine and 50 mg pyrimetha-mine (2 tablets) 1 to 2 days prior to arrival in endemic area, followed by 1,000 mg sulfadoxine and 50 mg pyrimethamine (2 tablets) q 2 wk throughout stay and continued for 4 to 6 weeks after de-parture from endemic area. Therapy should last no longer than 2 years.
Children over age 2 months weighing more than 45 kg. 750 mg sulfadoxine and 37.5 mg pyrimethamine (1½ tablets) as a single dose 1 to 2 days before arrival in endemic area, followed by 750 mg sulfadoxine and 37.5 mg pyrimethamine (1½ tablets) q wk throughout stay and continued for 4 to 6 weeks after leav-ing endemic area. Therapy should last no longer than 2 years.

Children over age 2 months weighing 31 to 45 kg. 500 mg sulfadoxine and 25 mg pyrimethamine (1 tablet) as a single dose 1 to 2 days before arrival in endemic area, followed by 500 mg sulfadoxine and 25 mg pyrimethamine (1 tablet) q wk throughout stay and continued for 4 to 6 weeks after departure from endemic area. Therapy should last no longer than 2 years.

Children over age 2 months weighing 21 to 30 kg. 375 mg sulfadoxine and 18.75 mg pyrimethamine (¾ tablet) as a single dose 1 to 2 days before arrival in endemic area, followed by 375 mg sulfadoxine and 18.75 mg (¾ tablet) pyrimethamine q wk throughout stay and continued for 4 to 6 weeks after departure from endemic area. Therapy should last no longer than 2 years.

Children over age 2 months weighing 11 to 20 kg. 250 mg sulfadoxine and 12.5 mg pyrimethamine (½ tablet) as a single dose 1 to 2 days before arrival in endemic area, followed by 250 mg sulfadoxine and 12.5 mg pyrimethamine (½ tablet) q wk throughout stay and continued for 4 to 6 weeks after departure from endemic area. Therapy should last no longer than 2 years.

Children over age 2 months weighing 5 to 10 kg. 125 mg sulfadoxine and 6.25 mg pyrimethamine (¼ tablet) as a single dose 1 to 2 days before arrival in endemic area, followed by 125 mg sulfadoxine and 6.25 mg pyrimethamine (¼ tablet) q wk throughout stay and continued for 4 to 6 weeks after departure from endemic area. Therapy should last no longer than 2 years.

Mechanism of Action
Sulfadoxine and pyrimethamine are both folic acid antagonists. Sulfadoxine inhibits the activity of dihydropteroate. Pyrimethamine inhibits the activity of dihydrofolate reductase, a folic acid enzyme. These actions take place during the asexual erythrocytic stages of malaria caused by *Plasmodium falciparum*, thus preventing the *P. falciparum* organism from replicating.

Contraindications
Breastfeeding; hypersensitivity to pyrimethamine, sulfadoxine, sulfonamides or their components; megaloblastic anemia caused by folate deficiency; pregnancy at term (prophylaxis use); prolonged use in patients with blood dyscrasias or renal or hepatic failure

Interactions
DRUGS
sulfadoxine and pyrimethamine

antifolic drugs such as sulfonamides, trimethoprim, trimethoprim-sulfamethoxazole: Increased risk of adverse reactions
chloroquine: Increased incidence and severity of adverse reactions
pyrimethamine component
antifolic drugs such as sulfonamides, trimethoprim, trimethoprim-sulfamethoxazole: Increased risk of bone marrow suppression
lorazepam: Increased risk of mild hepatotoxicity
p-aminobenzoic acid (PABA): Decreased effectiveness of pyrimethamine

Adverse Reactions

CNS: Apathy, ataxia, chills, depression, drug fever, fatigue, hallucinations, headache, insomnia, nervousness, peripheral neuritis, polyneuritis, seizures, vertigo
CV: Allergic myocarditis and pericarditis, periarteritis nodosa
EENT: Glossitis, periorbital edema, stomatitis, tinnitus
GI: Abdominal pain, bloating, diarrhea, hepatitis, hepatocellular necrosis, nausea, pancreatitis, transient liver enzyme elevation, vomiting
GU: Anuria, elevated BUN and serum creatinine levels, crystalluria, interstitial nephritis, oliguria, renal failure, toxic nephrosis
HEME: Agranulocytosis, aplastic anemia, eosinophilia, hemolytic anemia, hypoprothrombinemia, leukopenia, megaloblastic anemia, methemoglobinemia, purpura, thrombocytopenia
MS: Arthralgia, muscle weakness
RESP: Pulmonary infiltrates
SKIN: Alopecia, erythema multiforme, exfoliative dermatitis, generalized skin eruptions, photosensitivity, pruritus, Stevens-Johnson syndrome, toxic epidermal necrolysis, urticaria
Other: Anaphylaxis, lupus erythematosus phenomenon, Lyell's syndrome, serum sickness

Nursing Considerations

- Use cautiously in patients with impaired renal or hepatic function, possible folate deficiency, or severe allergy or bronchial asthma because of an increased risk of adverse effects.
- Monitor a patient who has glucose-6-phosphate dehydrogenase deficiency closely for pain, shortness of breath, and fatigue because hemolysis may occur when a sulfonamide drug such as sulfadoxine is administered.
- **WARNING** Stop sulfadoxine and pyrimethamine therapy and notify prescriber immediately if the patient shows any sign of a rash, if routine monitoring shows a significant reduction in any blood element, or if the patient develops an active bacte-

rial or fungal infection. Severe reactions such as Stevens-Johnson syndrome or toxic epidermal necrolysis may have occurred.

• Monitor patient's hematologic status, as ordered, and report any abnormalities. When sulfadoxine and pyrimethamine are used prophylactically for 2 months or longer, a mild but reversible leukopenia may occur. Although rare, severe reactions such as agranulocytosis, aplastic anemia, and other blood dyscasias may occur.

• If the patient has impaired renal function or if therapy is expected to last longer than 3 months, routinely monitor the patient's BUN and serum creatinine levels and obtain urine samples for microscopic examination.

PATIENT TEACHING

• Instruct patient to avoid excessive sun exposure.

• Stress the importance of stopping sulfadoxine and pyrimethamine therapy and notifying prescriber immediately at the first sign of a skin rash.

• Tell patient to drink at least 8 glasses of fluid daily to prevent crystalluria and stone formation.

• Instruct patient to notify prescriber immediately if he develops a sore throat, fever, achy joints, cough, shortness of breath, pallor, bruising, jaundice, or glossitis because the drug may need to be stopped and medical treatment given.

• Inform female patients of childbearing age to avoid pregnancy and not to breastfeed their infants during sulfadoxine and pyrimethamine therapy because sulfadoxine crosses the placenta and appears in breast milk, possibly causing kernicterus.

sulfamethoxazole and trimethoprim
(co-trimoxazole)

Apo-Sulfatrim (CAN), Bactrim, Bactrim-DS, Bactrim Pediatric, Cofatrim Forte, Cotrim, Cotrim DS, Cotrim Pediatric, Novo-Trimel (CAN), Nu-Cotrimox (CAN), Roubac (CAN), Septra, Septra DS, Septra Pediatric, Sulfatrim, Sulfatrim DS, Sulfatrim S/S, Sulfatrim Suspension

Class and Category

Chemical: Sulfonamide derivative (sulfamethoxazole), dihydrofolic acid analogue (trimethoprim)
Therapeutic: Antibiotic
Pregnancy category: C

Indications and Dosages

▶ *To treat acute otitis media, shigellosis, UTI, and other infections caused by gram-negative organisms (including* Enterobacter *species,* Escherichia coli, Haemophilus ducreyi, Haemophilus influenzae, *indole-positive* Proteus *species,* Klebsiella pneumoniae, Neisseria gonorrhoeae, Proteus mirabilis, Providencia *species,* Salmonella *species,* Serratia *species, and* Shigella *species) and gram-positive organisms (including group A beta-hemolytic streptococci,* Nocardia *species,* Staphylococcus aureus, *and* Streptococcus pneumoniae*)*

ORAL SUSPENSION, TABLETS

Adults. 800 mg of sulfamethoxazole and 160 mg of trimethoprim q 12 hr for 10 to 14 days (5 days for shigellosis).

Children age 2 months and over. 40 mg/kg of sulfamethoxazole and 8 mg/kg of trimethoprim daily in two divided doses q 12 hr for 10 days (5 days for shigellosis).

DOSAGE ADJUSTMENT If creatinine clearance is 15 to 30 ml/min/1.73 m^2, dosage reduced by one-half. If creatinine clearance is less than 15 ml/min/1.73 m^2, drug should be avoided.

I.V. INFUSION

Adults and children over age 2 months. 40 to 50 mg/kg of sulfamethoxazole and 8 to 10 mg/kg of trimethoprim daily in divided doses q 6, 8, or 12 hr for up to 5 days for shigellosis, 14 days for UTI.

▶ *To treat acute exacerbation of chronic bronchitis*

ORAL SUSPENSION, TABLETS

Adults. 800 mg of sulfamethoxazole and 160 mg of trimethoprim q 12 hr for 14 days.

▶ *To treat traveler's diarrhea*

ORAL SUSPENSION, TABLETS

Adults. 800 mg of sulfamethoxazole and 160 mg of trimethoprim q 12 hr for 5 days.

▶ *To prevent* Pneumocystis jiroveci (carinii) *pneumonia*

ORAL SUSPENSION, TABLETS

Adults. 800 mg of sulfamethoxazole and 160 mg of trimethoprim q 24 hr.

Children. 750 mg/m^2 of sulfamethoxazole and 150 mg/m^2 of trimethoprim daily in two divided doses on 3 consecutive days weekly. *Maximum:* 1,600 mg of sulfamethoxazole and 320 mg of trimethoprim daily.

▶ *To treat* P. jiroveci (carinii) *pneumonia*

ORAL SUSPENSION, TABLETS
Adults. 100 mg/kg of sulfamethoxazole and 15 to 20 mg/kg of trimethoprim daily in divided doses q 6 hr for 14 to 21 days.
I.V. INFUSION
Adults and children over age 2 months. 75 to 100 mg/kg of sulfamethoxazole and 15 to 20 mg/kg of trimethoprim daily in three or four divided doses q 6 to 8 hr for up to 14 days.

Mechanism of Action

Blocks two consecutive steps in the formation of essential nucleic acids and proteins in susceptible organisms. Sulfamethoxazole inhibits synthesis of dehydrofolic acid (a nucleic acid) by competing with para-aminobenzoic acid. Trimethoprim inhibits the action of the enzyme dihydrofolate reductase, thus blocking production of tetrahydrofolic acid.

Incompatibilities

Don't mix co-trimoxazole with other drugs or solutions.

Contraindications

Age under 2 months; hypersensitivity to sulfamethoxazole, sulfonamides, trimethoprim, or their components; megaloblastic anemia caused by folate deficiency

Interactions

DRUGS
ACE inhibitors: Possibly increased risk of hyperkalemia in elderly patients
cyclosporine: Decreased blood level and effectiveness of cyclosporine; increased risk of nephrotoxicity
digoxin: Possibly increased blood digoxin level and increased risk of digoxin toxicity
diuretics: Increased risk of thrombocytopenic purpura in elderly patients
indomethacin: Possibly increased blood co-trimoxazole level
methotrexate: Increased blood methotrexate level and risk of methotrexate toxicity
phenytoin: Possibly decreased hepatic clearance and prolonged half-life of phenytoin
pyrimethamine (dosage greater than 25 mg/wk): Increased risk of megaloblastic anemia
sulfonylureas: Possibly increased hypoglycemic effects of sulfonylureas

tricyclic antidepressants: Decreased effectiveness of tricyclic antidepressant

warfarin: Increased anticoagulant effects

Adverse Reactions

CNS: Anxiety, aseptic meningitis, ataxia, chills, depression, fatigue, hallucinations, headache, insomnia, seizures, vertigo

EENT: Glossitis, stomatitis

GI: Abdominal pain, anorexia, diarrhea, hepatitis, nausea, pancreatitis, pseudomembranous enterocolitis, vomiting

GU: Crystalluria, renal failure, toxic nephrosis

HEME: Agranulocytosis, eosinophilia, hemolytic anemia, leukopenia, methemoglobinemia, neutropenia, thrombocytopenia

RESP: Cough, dyspnea

SKIN: Dermatitis, erythema, photosensitivity, rash, Stevens-Johnson syndrome, toxic epidermal necrolysis, urticaria

Other: Anaphylaxis, hyperkalemia, injection site inflammation and pain

Nursing Considerations

- Use cautiously in patients with impaired hepatic or renal function, severe allergy or bronchial asthma, or possible folate deficiency (the elderly, long-term alcoholics, patients taking anticonvulsants, patients who are malnourished or have malabsorption).
- Expect to obtain culture and sensitivity test results before starting co-trimoxazole.
- For I.V. infusion, dilute each 5 ml of co-trimoxazole with 75 to 125 ml of D_5W before administration.
- When giving drug to neonates, don't mix with solutions that contain benzyl alcohol because this preservative has been linked to a fatal toxic syndrome involving circulatory, CNS, renal, and respiratory impairment and metabolic acidosis.
- Infuse slowly over 60 to 90 minutes.
- Watch for evidence of blood dyscrasia, including bleeding, ecchymosis, and joint pain, especially in elderly patients who are also taking a thiazide diuretic.
- Monitor elderly patients closely because they have an increased risk of bone marrow suppression, hyperkalemia, and severe skin reactions.

PATIENT TEACHING

- To minimize photosensitivity, advise patient to avoid direct sunlight and to use sunscreen.

• Instruct patient to notify prescriber immediately if rash, severe diarrhea, or other serious adverse reactions occur.

ticarcillin disodium and clavulanate potassium

Timentin

Class and Category

Chemical: Penicillin
Therapeutic: Antibiotic combination
Pregnancy category: B

Indications and Dosages

▶ *To treat moderate to severe infections, such as appendicitis, bacteremia, bone and joint infections (including osteomyelitis), diabetic foot ulcer, diverticulitis, gynecologic infections (including endometritis), infectious arthritis, intra-abdominal infection, lower respiratory tract infections (including pneumonia), peritonitis, septicemia, skin and soft-tissue infections (including cellulitis), and UTI caused by susceptible organisms; to manage febrile neutropenia*

I.V. INFUSION

Adults and children age 12 and over weighing 60 kg (132 lb) or more. 3.1 g (3 g of ticarcillin and 100 mg of clavulanic acid) infused over 30 min q 4 to 6 hr.

Adults and children age 12 and over weighing less than 60 kg. 200 to 300 mg/kg/day (based on ticarcillin content) in divided doses q 4 to 6 hr.

Children and infants over age 3 months. For mild to moderate infections, 200 mg/kg/day (based on ticarcillin content) in divided doses q 6 hr; for severe infections, 300 mg/kg/day (based on ticarcillin content) in divided doses q 4 to 6 hr.

▶ *To treat pulmonary infections caused by complications of cystic fibrosis, such as bronchiectasis or pneumonia*

I.V. INFUSION

Children. 350 to 450 mg/kg/day (based on ticarcillin content) in divided doses.

DOSAGE ADJUSTMENT For patients with renal impairment, loading dose of 3.1 g; then dosage adjusted based on creatinine clearance.

Incompatibilities

Don't give ticarcillin and clavulanate through the same I.V. line as amikacin, gentamicin, or tobramycin. Don't give within 1 hour of aminoglycosides.

Mechanism of Action

Ticarcillin inhibits bacterial cell wall synthesis by binding to specific penicillin-binding proteins located inside bacterial cell walls. In this way, the drug ultimately leads to cell wall lysis and death.

Clavulanic acid, which doesn't alter the action of ticarcillin, binds with bound and extracellular beta-lactamase, preventing beta-lactamase from inactivating ticarcillin.

Contraindications

Hypersensitivity to ticarcillin, clavulanic acid, or their components

Interactions

DRUGS

aminoglycosides: Additive or synergistic activity against some bacteria, possibly mutual inactivation
anticoagulants: Possibly interference with platelet aggregation
methotrexate: Prolonged blood methotrexate level, increased risk of methotrexate toxicity
probenecid: Prolonged blood ticarcillin level

Adverse Reactions

CV: Thrombophlebitis, vasculitis
GI: Elevated liver function test results, nausea, pseudomembranous colitis, vomiting
GU: Proteinuria
HEME: Anemia, eosinophilia, hemorrhage, leukopenia, neutropenia, prolonged bleeding time, thrombocytopenia
SKIN: Erythema nodosum, exfoliative dermatitis, pruritus, rash, toxic epidermal necrolysis, urticaria
Other: Anaphylaxis, hypernatremia, hypokalemia, infusion site pain

Nursing Considerations

- Keep in mind that 3.1 g of combination drug ticarcillin and clavulanate corresponds to 3 g of ticarcillin and 100 mg of clavulanic acid.
- Dilute reconstituted I.V. solution to 10 to 100 mg/ml with compatible I.V. solution. To minimize vein irritation, don't exceed 100 mg/ml. Concentrations of 50 mg/ml or greater are preferred. Infuse appropriate I.V. dose over 30 to 120 minutes.

- Know that ticarcillin and clavulanate may worsen symptoms in patients with a history of GI disease or colitis.
- For patients with renal impairment, implement seizure precautions according to facility policy because they're at increased risk for seizures.
- Assess patient for evidence of pseudomembranous colitis, such as abdominal cramps and severe watery diarrhea. Also watch for evidence of superinfection, such as oral candidiasis and rash in a breastfeeding infant.
- Monitor serum electrolyte levels for hypernatremia because of this drug's high sodium content. Monitor patient for hypokalemia from increased urinary potassium loss.
- **WARNING** Monitor patient's platelet count, PT, and APTT because drug may increase bleeding time and, in rare cases, may induce thrombocytopenia.
- Be aware that patient receiving high doses of ticarcillin may develop pseudoproteinuria.

PATIENT TEACHING

- Instruct patient taking ticarcillin and clavulanate to report past allergies to penicillins and to notify prescriber immediately about adverse reactions, including fever.
- Advise patient to decrease sodium intake to reduce the risk of electrolyte imbalance.

Cardiovascular Drugs

amiloride hydrochloride and hydrochlorothiazide
Moduretic

Class and Category
Chemical: Pyrazine-carbonyl-guanidine (amiloride), benzothiadi-azide (hydrochlorothiazide)
Therapeutic: Antihypertensive (amiloride, hydrochlorothiazide), potassium-sparing diuretic (amiloride), diuretic (hydrochlorothiazide)
Pregnancy category: B

Indications and Dosages
▶ *To manage hypertension or heart failure while preventing diuretic-induced hypokalemia*
TABLETS
Adults. 5 mg amiloride and 50 mg hydrochlorothiazide (1 tablet) daily; increased, as needed, to 10 mg amiloride and 100 mg hydrochlorothiazide (2 tablets) daily or 5 mg amiloride and 50 mg hydrochlorothiazide (1 tablet) b.i.d.

Mechanism of Action
Amiloride inhibits sodium reabsorption in the distal convoluted tubules and cortical collecting ducts of the kidneys. This results in sodium and water loss, which reduces blood pressure and enhances potassium retention.

Hydrochlorothiazide promotes the movement of sodium, chloride, and water from blood in the peritubular capillaries into the nephron's distal convoluted tubule. Initially, it may decrease extracellular fluid volume, plasma volume, and cardiac output, which helps explain blood pressure reduction. It also may reduce blood pressure by causing direct dilation of arteries. After several weeks, extracellular fluid volume, plasma volume, and cardiac output return to normal, and peripheral vascular resistance remains decreased.

Contraindications
Hypersensitivity to amiloride, hydrochlorothiazide, other sulfonamides or thiazides, or their components; impaired renal function; serum potassium level above 5.5 mEq/L; therapy with another potassium-sparing diuretic, such as spironolactone or
triamterene; or use of a potassium supplement

Interactions
DRUGS
amiloride and hydrochlorothiazide
antihypertensives: Increased antihypertensive effects
digoxin: Decreased effectiveness of digoxin
lithium: Reduced renal clearance of lithium and increased risk of
lithium toxicity
NSAIDs: Reduced diuretic effect of amiloride and hydrochlorothiazide
amiloride component
*ACE inhibitors, angiotensin II receptor antagonists, cyclosporine, potas-
sium products, spironolactone, tacrolimus:* Increased risk of hyperkalemia
hydrochlorothiazide component
amantadine: Possibly increased amantadine blood level and risk of
toxicity
amiodarone: Increased risk of arrhythmias from hypokalemia
amphotericin B, corticosteroids: Intensified electrolyte depletion, especially hypokalemia
barbiturates, opioids: May potentiate orthostatic hypotension
calcium: Possibly increased serum calcium level
cholestyramine, colestipol resins: Reduced GI absorption of hydrochlorothiazide
diazoxide: Increased antihypertensive and hyperglycemic effects of
hydrochlorothiazide
diflunisal: Possibly increased blood hydrochlorothiazide level
digoxin: Increased risk of digitalis toxicity from hypokalemia
dopamine: Possibly increased diuretic effects of both drugs
insulin, oral antidiabetics: Possibly increased blood glucose level
neuromuscular blockers: Possibly increased neuromuscular blockade
from hypokalemia
nondepolarizing skeletal muscle relaxants (such as tubocurarine): Possibly increased responsiveness to the muscle relaxant
pressor amines (such as norepinephrine): Possibly decreased response
to pressor amines
oral anticoagulants: Possibly decreased anticoagulant effects

sympathomimetics: Possibly decreased antihypertensive effect of hydrochlorothiazide
vitamin D: Increased risk of hypercalcemia
FOODS
amiloride component
high-potassium foods: Increased risk of hyperkalemia

Adverse Reactions

CNS: Confusion, depression, dizziness, drowsiness, encephalopathy, fatigue, headache, insomnia, nervousness, paresthesia, somnolence, tremor, vertigo, weakness
CV: Angina, arrhythmia, hypotension, palpitations, orthostatic hypotension, vasculitis
EENT: Blurred vision, dry mouth, increased intraocular pressure, nasal congestion, tinnitus, visual disturbances
ENDO: Hyperglycemia
GI: Abdominal pain, anorexia, constipation, diarrhea, GI bleeding, heartburn, indigestion, jaundice, nausea, vomiting
GU: Bladder spasms, decreased libido, dysuria, impotence, interstitial nephritis, nocturia, polyuria, renal failure
HEME: Agranulocytosis, aplastic anemia, hemolytic anemia, leukopenia, neutropenia, thrombocytopenia
MS: Arthralgia, leg pain, muscle spasms and weakness
RESP: Cough, dyspnea
SKIN: Alopecia, exfoliative dermatitis, photosensitivity, pruritus, purpura, rash, urticaria
Other: Anaphylaxis, dehydration, hypercalcemia, hyperchloremia, hyperkalemia, hyperuricemia, hypochloremia, hypokalemia, hyponatremia, hypovolemia, metabolic alkalosis, weight loss

Nursing Considerations

• Monitor blood pressure often to assess effectiveness of amiloride and hydrochlorothiazide therapy.
• Monitor fluid intake and output, daily weight, blood pressure, and serum levels of electrolytes, especially potassium, to detect volume depletion or electrolyte imbalance.
• **WARNING** Don't give amiloride and hydrochlorothiazide with other potassium-sparing diuretics.
• Watch for increased BUN and serum creatinine levels, especially in patients with impaired renal function, because drug may cause acute renal failure. If increases are significant or persistent, notify prescriber immediately.
• Monitor blood glucose level often in diabetic patients, and expect to increase antidiabetic dosage, as needed and ordered.

- If patient has a history of gouty arthritis, monitor patient for gout attacks during therapy.

PATIENT TEACHING
- Advise patient to take amiloride and hydrochlorothiazide with food in the morning or early evening to avoid the need to urinate during the night.
- Teach patient to monitor her blood pressure and to report consistently elevated measurements to prescriber.
- Direct patient to weigh herself at the same time each day wearing the same amount of clothing and to notify prescriber if she gains more than 2 lb (0.9 kg) per day or 5 lb (2.3 kg) per week.
- Instruct patient to avoid eating a diet high in potassium-rich foods, including citrus fruits, bananas, tomatoes, dates, and salt substitutes that contain potassium.
- To reduce the risk of dehydration and hypotension, advise patient to avoid exercise in hot weather and alcohol use. Also instruct her to notify prescriber if she has prolonged diarrhea, nausea, or vomiting.
- Advise patient to change positions slowly to minimize effects of orthostatic hypotension.
- Caution patient to avoid potentially hazardous activities until drug's CNS effects are known.
- Explain the importance of regular exercise, proper diet, and other lifestyle changes in controlling hypertension.
- Warn patient about possibility of reversible hair loss and for male patients the additional possibility of impotence.

amlodipine besylate and atorvastatin calcium
Caduet

Class and Category
Chemical: Dihydropyridine (amlodipine) and synthetically derived fermentation product (atorvastatin)
Therapeutic: Antianginal, antihypertensive (amlodipine); antihyperlipidemic, HMG-CoA reductase inhibitor (atorvastatin)
Pregnancy category: X

Indications and Dosages
▶ *To continue treatment of hyperlipidemia and either hypertension or angina previously treated individually; to continue treatment with one component and start treatment with a second component*

TABLETS

Adults. Highly individualized. Dosage may be equivalent to monotherapy with either drug, or both dosages may be higher than previously prescribed for additional effects, or dosage may be based on the component currently being prescribed plus the recommended starting dose for the added drug. (See monotherapy details below for usual adult dosages.)

Monotherapy with amlodipine

▶ *To control hypertension*

TABLETS

Adults. *Initial:* 5 mg daily, increased gradually over 10 to 14 days p.r.n. *Maximum:* 10 mg daily.

DOSAGE ADJUSTMENT Initial dosage of 2.5 mg daily for elderly patients or patients with impaired hepatic function. Increased gradually over 7 to 14 days based on response.

▶ *To treat chronic stable angina and Prinzmetal's (variant) angina*

TABLETS

Adults. 5 to 10 mg daily.

DOSAGE ADJUSTMENT 5 mg daily for elderly patients and patients with impaired hepatic function.

Monotherapy with atorvastatin

▶ *To control lipid levels as an adjunct to diet in primary (heterozygous familial and nonfamilial) hypercholesterolemia and mixed dyslipidemia*

TABLETS

Adults. *Initial:* 10 to 20 mg daily, increased according to lipid level. *Maintenance:* 10 to 80 mg daily.

DOSAGE ADJUSTMENT Initial dosage may be increased to 40 mg daily for patients who need significant reduction (more than 45%) of cholesterol levels.

▶ *To control lipid levels in homozygous familial hypercholesterolemia*

TABLETS

Adults. 10 to 80 mg daily.

▶ *To start treatment of hyperlipidemia and either hypertension or angina*

TABLETS

Adults. *Initial:* Dosage based on recommendations for monotherapies of amlodipine and atorvastatin. (See monotherapy details for usual adult dosages.) *Maximum:* 10 mg for amlodipine; 80 mg for atorvastatin.

Contraindications

Active liver disease; breastfeeding; hypersensitivity to atorvastatin, amlodipine, or their components; pregnancy; unexplained persistently elevated serum transaminase level

Mechanism of Action

Amlodipine binds to dihydropyridine and nondihydropyridine cell membrane receptor sites on myocardial and vascular smooth-muscle cells and inhibits the influx of extracellular calcium ions across slow calcium channels. This decrease in intracellular calcium level inhibits smooth-muscle cell contraction, relaxes coronary and vascular smooth muscles, and decreases peripheral vascular resistance and systolic and diastolic blood pressure. Decreased peripheral vascular resistance also reduces myocardial workload and oxygen demand, which may relieve angina. Also, by inhibiting coronary artery muscle cell contractions and restoring blood flow, amlodipine may relieve Prinzmetal's angina.

Atorvastatin reduces serum cholesterol and lipoprotein levels by inhibiting HMG-CoA reductase and cholesterol synthesis in the liver and by increasing the number of LDL receptors on liver cells, thus enhancing LDL uptake and breakdown.

Interactions

DRUGS

amlodipine component

beta blockers: Possibly excessive hypotension

fentanyl: Increased risk of severe hypotension and increased fluid volume requirements during surgery

atorvastatin component

antacids, colestipol: Possibly decreased blood atorvastatin level

cyclosporine, nicotinic acid: Increased risk of severe myopathy or rhabdomyolysis

digoxin: Possibly increased blood digoxin level, causing toxicity

erythromycin: Increased blood atorvastatin level

oral contraceptives (such as ethinyl estradiol and norethindrone): Increased hormone level

Adverse Reactions

CNS: Amnesia, anxiety, dizziness, emotional lability, facial paralysis, fatigue, fever, headache, hyperkinesia, lack of coordination, lethargy, light-headedness, malaise, paresthesia, peripheral neuropathy, somnolence, syncope, tremor, unusual dreams, weakness

CV: Arrhythmias, elevated serum CK level, hot flashes, hypotension, orthostatic hypotension, palpitations, peripheral edema, phlebitis, vasodilation

EENT: Amblyopia, altered refraction, cheilitis, dry eyes or mouth, epistaxis, eye hemorrhage, gingival hemorrhage, glaucoma, glossitis, hearing loss, pharyngitis, sinusitis, stomatitis, taste loss or perversion, tinnitus

ENDO: Hyperglycemia, hypoglycemia

GI: Abdominal cramps or pain, anorexia, bilary pain, colitis, constipation, diarrhea, duodenal or stomach ulcers, dysphagia, eructation, esophagitis, flatulence, gastroenteritis, hepatitis, increased appetite, indigestion, melena, nausea, pancreatitis, rectal hemorrhage, tenesmus, vomiting

GU: Abnormal ejaculation; cystitis; decreased libido; dysuria; epididymitis; hematuria; impotence; nephritis; nocturia; renal calculi; urinary frequency, incontinence, or urgency; urine retention; vaginal hemorrhage

HEME: Anemia, thrombocytopenia

MS: Arthralgia, back pain, bursitis, gout, leg cramps, myalgia, myasthenia gravis, myositis, neck rigidity, tendon contractures, tenosynovitis, torticollis

RESP: Dyspnea, pneumonia

SKIN: Acne, alopecia, contact dermatitis, diaphoresis, dry skin, ecchymosis, eczema, flushing, jaundice, petechiae, photosensitivity, pruritus, rash, seborrhea, ulceration, urticaria

Other: Allergic reaction, facial or generalized edema, flulike symptoms, infection, lymphadenopathy, weight gain or loss

Nursing Considerations

- Use amlodipine and atorvastatin cautiously in patients with heart block, heart failure, impaired renal function, or hepatic disorder.
- Monitor blood pressure when adjusting amlodipine, especially in patients with heart failure.
- If patient is receiving atorvastatin for the first time, obtain liver function tests before therapy starts, after 6 and 12 weeks, every 6 months thereafter, and whenever the dosage increases.
- Expect to measure blood levels 2 to 4 weeks after first atorvastatin dose and to adjust dosage, as directed. Repeat this process periodically until levels are within desired range.

PATIENT TEACHING

- Emphasize that drug is an adjunct to—not a substitute for—a low-cholesterol diet and any other prescribed dietary restrictions.
- Tell patient to immediately notify prescriber about dizziness, arm or leg swelling, trouble breathing, hives, or rash. Also advise patient to notify prescriber immediately if he develops unexplained muscle pain, tenderness, or weakness, especially if accompanied by fatigue or fever.

- Suggest taking drug with food to reduce GI upset that may be caused by the amlodipine component.
- Advise patient to routinely have his blood pressure checked and his blood monitored to verify the effectiveness of therapy with amlodipine and atorvastatin.

amlodipine besylate and benazepril hydrochloride
Lotrel

Class and Category
Chemical: Dihydropyridine (amlodipine), ethylester of benazeprilat (benazepril)
Therapeutic: Antihypertensive (amlodipine, benazepril)
Pregnancy category: C (first trimester), D (second and third trimesters)

Indications and Dosages
▶ *To treat hypertension in patients not adequately controlled with amlodipine or benazepril therapy alone*
CAPSULES
Adults. *Initial:* Depending on patient's previous dosage of amlodipine or benazepril, 2.5 mg amlodipine and 10 mg benazepril (1 capsule) to 10 mg amlodipine and 20 mg benazepril (1 capsule) daily. If dosage is started at lower end, may be gradually increased, as needed, based on response. *Maximum:* 10 mg amlodipine and 20 mg benazepril daily.
DOSAGE ADJUSTMENT Initial dosage of 2.5 mg amlodipine and 10 mg benazepril daily for elderly patients or patients with impaired hepatic function. Dosage increased gradually based on response.

Contraindications
History of hereditary or idiopathic angioedema; hypersensitivity to amlodipine, benazepril, other ACE inhibitors or their components; pregnancy

Interactions
DRUGS
amlodipine and benazepril
diuretics: Possibly excessive reduction of blood pressure when amlodipine and benazepril therapy starts.
lithium: Possibly increased serum lithium level and risk of toxicity

Mechanism of Action

Amlodipine binds to dihydropyridine and nondihydropyridine cell membrane receptor sites on myocardial and vascular smooth-muscle cells and inhibits the influx of extracellular calcium ions across slow calcium channels. This decreases the intracellular calcium level, inhibiting smooth-muscle cell contractions, relaxing coronary and vascular smooth muscles, decreasing peripheral vascular resistance, and reducing systolic and diastolic blood pressure.

Benazepril may reduce blood pressure by affecting the renin-angiotensin-aldosterone system. By inhibiting ACE, benazepril:

* prevents conversion of angiotensin I to angiotensin II, a potent vasoconstrictor that also stimulates adrenal cortex to secrete aldosterone.
* may inhibit renal and vascular production of angiotensin II.
* decreases serum angiotensin II level and increases serum renin activity. This decreases aldosterone secretion, slightly increasing serum potassium level and fluid loss.
* decreases vascular tone and blood pressure.
* inhibits aldosterone release, which reduces sodium and water reabsorption and increases their excretion, further reducing blood pressure.

---

potassium supplements, potassium-sparing diuretics: Possibly increased serum potassium level

amlodipine component

beta blockers: Possibly excessive hypotension

fentanyl: Increased risk of severe hypotension and increased fluid volume requirements during surgery

benazepril component

antacids: Possibly decreased benazepril bioavailability

capsaicin: Possibly induced or exacerbated ACE inhibitor cough

digoxin: Increased serum digoxin level

phenothiazines: Possibly increased intended and adverse benazepril effects

Adverse Reactions

CNS: Anxiety, asthenia, dizziness, fatigue, headache, insomnia, nervousness, somnolence, tremor

CV: Edema, orthostatic hypotension, palpitations

EENT: Dry mouth, pharyngitis

ENDO: Hot flashes

GI: Abdominal pain, constipation, diarrhea, dyspepsia, esophagitis, nausea

GU: Decreased libido, elevated plasma BUN and serum creatinine levels, impotence, polyuria

MS: Back pain, musculoskeletal pain or cramps
RESP: Cough
SKIN: Dermatitis, flushing, rash, skin nodule
Other: Anaphylaxis, angioedema, hypokalemia

Nursing Considerations

- Use amlodipine and benazepril cautiously in patients with heart block, heart failure, impaired renal function, or heptatic disorder because amlodipine can cause fluid retention.
- Before starting amlodipine and benazepril, evaluate blood pressure with patient lying down, sitting, and standing. Then monitor it throughout therapy to evaluate drug effectiveness.
- Check urine output and BUN and serum creatinine levels, as appropriate, before therapy begins. Be aware that the drug should not be used in patients with a serum creatinine level less than 30 ml/min/1.73 m^2.
- WARNING Be alert for anaphylactoid reactions, including angioedema, especially after the first dose of amlodipine and benazepril. If angioedema extends to larynx and patient has laryngeal stridor or signs of airway obstruction, prepare to give epinephrine subcutaneously immediately, as prescribed, and stop amlodipine and benazepril.
- Monitor WBC count periodically, especially in patients with collagen-vascular disease, to detect neutropenia and agranulocytosis. Although they aren't known to occur with benazepril, they have occurred with captropril, another ACE inhibitor.
- Check liver enzymes periodically and monitor patient for jaundice because hepatic failure, although rare, has occurred with other ACE inhibitors. If liver enzymes develop marked elevation or patient develops jaundice, notify prescriber and expect to stop amlodipine and benazepril.

PATIENT TEACHING

- Teach patient how to monitor blood pressure, if appropriate, and how to recognize signs of hypertension and hypotension.
- WARNING Strongly urge patient to contact prescriber before using any potassium supplements or OTC salt substitutes, which may contain potassium. These substances increase the risk of hyperkalemia.
- Inform patient that a persistent dry cough may develop and may not subside unless amlodipine and benazepril therapy is stopped. If cough becomes bothersome or interferes with sleep or activities, instruct patient to notify prescriber.
- WARNING Instruct patient to contact prescriber immediately

if she develops evidence of hypersensitivity, especially angioedema, (swelling of the face, eyes, lips, or tongue), difficulty breathing, hives, or rash.

- Urge patient to avoid sudden position changes and to rise slowly from a sitting or lying position to minimize orthostatic hypotension.
- Tell patient to notify prescriber if she is, could be, or is planning to become pregnant because amlodopine and benazepril may adversely affect fetal development; therapy should be stopped.

aspirin (buffered) and pravastatin sodium

Pravigard PAC

Class and Category

Chemical: Salicylate (aspirin), mevinic acid derivative (pravastatin)
Therapeutic: Antiplatelet (aspirin), antihyperlipidemic (pravastatin)
Pregnancy category: X

Indications and Dosages

▶ *To reduce the occurrence of cardiovascular events such as death, MI, and stroke in patients with cardiovascular or cerebrovascular disease*

TABLETS

Adults. *Initial:* 81 mg or 325 mg aspirin and 40 mg pravastatin daily. Pravastatin dosage may be increased q 4 wk, as needed. *Maintenance:* 81 mg or 325 mg aspirin and 40 to 80 mg pravastatin daily.

DOSAGE ADJUSTMENT For patients with significant renal or hepatic impairment, those taking immunosuppressants, and elderly patients, initial pravastatin dosage reduced to 10 mg daily. For elderly patients and those taking immunosuppressants, pravastatin maintenance dosage usually limited to 20 mg daily.

Contraindications

Active hepatic disease or unexplained, persistent elevated liver function test results; allergy to tartrazine dye; asthma; bleeding problems such as hemophilia; breastfeeding; hypersensitivity to aspirin, pravastatin, or their components; peptic ulcer disease; pregnancy

Interactions

DRUGS

aspirin and pravastatin

anticoagulants: Increased bleeding or prolonged PT
pravastatin component
cholestyramine, colestipol: Decreased pravastatin bioavailability
cyclosporine, erythromycin, gemfibrozil, immunosuppressants, niacin: Increased risk of rhabdomyolysis and acute renal failure
aspirin component
ACE inhibitors: Decreased antihypertensive effect
activated charcoal: Decreased aspirin absorption
antacids, urine alkalinizers: Decreased aspirin effectiveness
ascorbic acid, furosemide, para-aminosalicylic acid: Increased risk of aspirin toxicity
carbonic anhydrase inhibitors: Salicylism
corticosteroids: Increased excretion and decreased blood level of aspirin
heparin: Increased risk of bleeding
methotrexate: Increased blood level and decreased excretion of methotrexate, causing toxicity
nizatidine: Increased blood aspirin level
NSAIDs: Possibly decreased blood NSAID level and increased risk of adverse GI effects
oral antidiabetics, insulin: Increased risk of hypoglycemia
penicillins, sulfonamides: Increased blood levels of penicillins and sulfonamides probenecid, sulfinpyrazone:* Decreased effectiveness in treating gout
urine acidifiers (such as ammonium chloride and ascorbic acid): Decreased aspirin excretion
vancomycin: Increased risk of ototoxicity
ACTIVITIES
alcohol use: Increased risk of ulcers

Mechanism of Action

Aspirin inhibits platelet aggregation by interfering with production of thromboxane A2, a substance that stimulates platelet aggregation. It also blocks the activity of cyclooxygenase, the enzyme needed for prostaglandin synthesis. Prostaglandins, important mediators in the inflammatory response, cause local vasodilation with swelling and pain. By blocking cyclooxygenase and inhibiting prostaglandins, aspirin causes inflammatory symptoms to subside.

Pravastatin inhibits cholesterol synthesis in the liver by blocking the enzyme needed to convert hydroxymethylglutaryl (HMG)-CoA to mevalonate, an early precursor of cholesterol. When cholesterol synthesis is blocked, the liver increases breakdown of LDL cholesterol.

Adverse Reactions

CNS: Anxiety, confusion, depression, dizziness, fatigue, headache, nervousness, sleep disturbance
CV: Angina pectoris, chest pain
EENT: Blurred vision, diplopia, hearing loss, rhinitis, tinnitus
GI: Abdominal pain, constipation, diarrhea, flatulence, GI bleeding, heartburn, hepatotoxicity, indigestion, nausea, pancreatitis, stomach pain, vomiting
GU: Dysuria, nocturia, urinary frequency
HEME: Decreased blood iron level, leukopenia, prolonged bleeding time, shortened RBC lifespan, thrombocytopenia
MS: Arthralgia, musculoskeletal cramps or pain, myalgia, myopathy, rhabdomyolysis
RESP: Cough, dyspnea, upper respiratory tract infection
SKIN: Ecchymosis, rash, urticaria
Other: Angioedema, Reye's syndrome

Nursing Considerations

- Use aspirin and pravastatin cautiously in patients with renal or hepatic impairment and in elderly patients.
- Give aspirin and pravastatin 1 hour before or 4 hours after giving cholestyramine or colestipol.
- Monitor BUN and serum creatinine levels and liver function test results periodically for abnormal elevations.
- Monitor blood lipoprotein level, as indicated, to evaluate response to therapy.

PATIENT TEACHING

- Instruct patient to take aspirin with food or after meals because it may cause GI upset if taken on an empty stomach.
- Advise patient to consult prescriber before taking aspirin and pravastatin with any other prescription drug for blood disorder, diabetes, gout, or arthritis.
- Tell patient not to take aspirin that has a strong vinegar odor but to replace it with tablets that don't smell like vinegar.
- Instruct patient to notify prescriber immediately about muscle pain, tenderness, weakness, and other symptoms of myopathy.
- Urge female patient of childbearing age to use a reliable method of contraception during therapy and to notify prescriber at once if she becomes or suspects she might be pregnant.

atenolol and chlorthalidone

Tenoretic

Class and Category

Chemical: Cardioselective beta blocker (atenolol), phthalimidine derivative of benzenesulfonadmide (thiazide-like diuretic) (chlorthalidone)

Therapeutic: Antihypertensive (atenolol, chlorthalidone), diuretic (chlorthalidone)

Pregnancy category: D

Indications and Dosages

▶ *To treat hypertension*

TABLETS

Adults. 50 mg atenolol and 25 mg chlorthalidone (1 tablet) daily, increased, as needed, to 100 mg atenolol and 25 mg chlorthalidone (1 tablet) daily.

DOSAGE ADJUSTMENT For patients with creatinine clearance of 15 to 35 ml/min/1.73 m^2, atenolol dosage shouldn't exceed 50 mg daily. For patients with creatinine clearance below 15 ml/min/1.73 m^2, atenolol dosage shouldn't exceed 50 mg every other day.

Mechanism of Action

Atenolol inhibits stimulation of beta$_1$-receptor sites, which are located mainly in the heart, causing a decrease in cardiac excitability, cardiac output and myocardial oxygen demand. Atenolol also decreases release of renin from the kidneys, aiding in reducing blood pressure. At high doses, it inhibits stimulation of beta$_2$ receptors in the lungs, which may cause bronchoconstriction.

Chlorthalidone may promote sodium, chloride, and water excretion by inhibiting sodium reabsorption in the kidneys' distal tubules. Initially, chlorthalidone may decrease extracellular fluid volume, plasma volume, and cardiac output, which helps explain how it reduces blood pressure. It also may dilate arteries directly, which helps reduce peripheral vascular resistance and blood pressure. After several weeks, extracelllar fluid and plasma volume and cardiac output return to normal, but peripheral vascular resistance remains decreased.

Contraindications

Anuria; breastfeeding; cardiogenic shock; heart block greater than first degree; hypersensitivity to atenolol, chlorthalidone, other sulfonamide-derived drugs, or their components; overt cardiac failure: sinus bradycardia

Interactions
DRUGS
atenolol and chlorthalidone
antihypertensives, catecholamine-depleting drugs (such as reserpine): Increased antihypertensive effect leading to hypotension, marked bradycardia, or both
clonidine: Increased risk of rebound hypertension
atenolol component
calcium channel blockers (such as verapamil and diltiazem): Possibly symptomatic bradycardia and conduction abnormalities
chlorthalidone component
allopurinol: Increased risk of allopurinol hypersensitivity
amphotericin B, glucocorticoids: Intensified electrolyte depletion
anesthetics: Potentiated effects of anesthetics
anticholinergics: Increased chlorthalidone absorption
antidiabetics, methenamines, oral anticoagulants, sulfonylureas: Decreased effects of these drugs
antineoplastics: Prolonged antineoplastic-induced leukopenia
cholestyramine, colestipol: Decreased chlorthalidone absorption
diazoxide: Increased risk of hyperglycemia and hypotension
digitalis glycosides: Increased risk of digitalis-induced arrhythmias
lithium: Decreased renal lithium clearance and increased risk of lithium toxicity
loop diuretics: Increased synergistic effects, resulting in profound diuresis and serious electrolyte imbalances
methyldopa: Potential development of hemolytic anemia
neuromuscular blockers: Increased neuromuscular blockade
NSAIDs: Possibly reduced diuretic effect of chlorthalidone
vitamin D: Enhanced vitamin D action

Adverse Reactions
CNS: Depression, dizziness, dreaming, drowsiness, fatigue, hallucinations, headache, lethargy, light-headedness, paresthesia, psychosis, restlessness, tiredness, weakness, vertigo
CV: Bradycardia, orthostatic hypotension, Raynaud's phenomenon, sick sinus syndrome, vasculitis
EENT: Dry eyes or mouth, visual disturbance
ENDO: Hyperglycemia
GI: Abdominal cramping, anorexia, constipation, diarrhea, elevated bilirubin and liver enzymes, gastric irritation, jaundice, nausea, pancreatitis, vomiting
GU: Impotence

HEME: Agranulocytosis, aplastic anemia, leukopenia, thrombocytopenia
MS: Cold extremities, leg pain, muscle spasm
RESP: Dyspnea, wheezing
SKIN: Alopecia (reversible), cutaneous vasculitis, exacerbation of psoriasis, photosensitivity, psoriasis type rash, purpura, toxic epidermal necrolysis, urticaria
Other: Antinuclear antibody formation, hyperuricemia, hypochloremic alkalosis, hypokalemia, hyponatremia, lupus syndrome, Peyronie's disease

Nursing Considerations

- Use atenolol and chlorthalidone cautiously in patients with impaired hepatic function or progressive hepatic disease because minor changes in fluid and electrolyte balance may cause hepatic coma.
- Use atenolol and chlorthalidone cautiously in patients with heart failure controlled by cardiac glycosides, conduction abnormalities, or left ventricular dysfunction who take verapamil or diltiazem and in patients with arterial circulatory disorders, bronchospastic disease, or impaired renal function.
- Assess patient's blood pressure regularly to determine effectiveness of therapy.
- Monitor patient for evidence of heart failure. At first sign of heart failure, expect patient to receive a cardiac glycoside, a diuretic, or both and to be monitored closely. If failure continues, expect atenolol and chlorthalidone to be stopped.
- Assess BUN, serum electrolytes, uric acid, and blood glucose level before and periodically during therapy. Monitor patient for signs of fluid and electrolyte imbalance.
- Monitor diabetic patients closely because atenolol may mask tachycardia caused by hypoglycemia. Unlike other beta blockers, it doesn't mask other signs of hypoglycemia, cause hypoglycemia, or delay return of blood glucose to a normal level.
- Closely monitor patient with hyperthyroidism because atenolol may mask some signs of thyrotoxicosis. Avoid abrupt withdrawal of atenolol and chlorthalidone because it may prompt thyrotoxicosis or ischemic heart disease.
- Expect to stop atenolol and chlorthalidone several days before gradually withdrawing clonidine therapy, if prescribed. Then expect to restart atenolol and chlorthalidone several days after clonidine has been stopped because clonidine can cause rebound hypertension.

- Notify prescriber immediately if patient develops bradycardia, hypotension, or other serious adverse reactions.
- Stop atenolol and chlorthalidone, as ordered, before parathyroid function studies are performed because the chlorthalidone portion of the drug decreases calcium excretion.

PATIENT TEACHING

- Stress the importance of taking atenolol and chlorthalidone even when feeling well.
- Tell patient to take drug in the morning with food or milk to avoid gastric irritation.
- Caution patient not to stop taking atenolol and chlorthalidone abruptly because serious adverse effects may occur. Also tell him that while being weaned from the drug, he should perform minimal physical activity to prevent chest pain.
- Inform a diabetic patient that atenolol may alter his blood glucose level and mask a rapid heartbeat during a hypoglycemic reaction. Urge him to test his blood glucose level regularly.
- Instruct patient to rise slowly from a seated or lying position to minimize the effects of orthostatic hypotension.
- Teach patient to monitor his blood pressure and to report consistently elevated measurements to prescriber.
- Tell patient to protect his skin from the sun to avoid sunburn while taking atenolol and chlorthalidone.
- Urge patient to report sudden joint pain to prescriber immediately because drug can cause sudden gout attacks.
- Encourage patient to eat high-potassium foods, such as bananas, apricots, grapefruits, tomato juice, and orange juice.
- Advise patient to report symptoms of low potassium level (irregular heartbeat, muscle weakness, fatigue) or low sodium level (confusion, fatigue, irritability, muscle cramps).
- Advise female patient of childbearing age to notify prescriber if she is, could be, or plans to become pregnant or if she's breast-feeding because drug may cause serious adverse reactions in the fetus or newborn.

benazepril hydrochloride and hydrochlorothiazide

Lotensin HCT

Class and Category

Chemical: Ethylester of benazeprilat (benazepril), benothiadiazine (hydrochlorothiazide)

Therapeutic: Antihypertensive (benazepril, hydrochlorothiazide), diuretic (hydrochlorothiazide)
Pregnancy category: C (first trimester), D (second and third trimesters)

Indications and Dosages

▶ *To treat hypertension uncontrolled by benazepril or hydrochlorothiazide alone*

TABLETS

Adults. *Initial:* 10 or 20 mg benazepril and 12.5 mg (10-mg/ 12.5-mg tablet or 20-mg/12.5-mg tablet) hydrochlorothiazide daily, increased as needed based on response (hydrochlorothiazide increased only every 2 to 3 wk). *Maximum:* 20 mg benazepril and 50 mg hydrochlorothiazide daily

▶ *To treat hypertension for patients adequately controlled by hydrochlorothiazide but who develop significant potassium loss with monotherapy*

TABLETS

Adults. 5 mg benazepril and 6.25 mg hydrochlorothiazide (1 tablet) daily.

Mechanism of Action

Benazepril may reduce blood pressure by affecting the renin-angiotensin-aldosterone system. By inhibiting ACE, benazepril:

• prevents conversion of angiotensin I to angiotensin II, a potent vasoconstrictor that also stimulates adrenal cortex to secrete aldosterone.
• may inhibit renal and vascular production of angiotensin II.
• decreases serum angiotensin II level and increases serum renin activity. This decreases aldosterone secretion, slightly increasing serum potassium level and fluid loss.
• decreases vascular tone and blood pressure.
• inhibits aldosterone release, which reduces sodium and water reabsorption and increases their excretion, further reducing blood pressure.

Hydrochlorothiazide promotes movement of sodium, chloride, and water from blood in the peritubular capillaries into the nephron's distal convoluted tubule. Initially, it may decrease extracellular fluid volume, plasma volume, and cardiac output, which helps explain blood pressure reduction. It also may reduce blood pressure by dilating arteries. After several weeks, extracellular fluid volume, plasma volume, and cardiac output return to normal, and peripheral vascular resistance remains decreased.

Contraindications

Anuria; hypersensitivity to benazepril, other ACE inhibitors, hydrochlorothiazide, other sulfonamide-derived drugs or their components

Interactions

DRUGS

benazepril and hydrochlorothiazide
antihypertensives, diuretics: Increased antihypertensive effects
digoxin: Increased serum digoxin level and risk of toxicity
lithium: Increased serum lithium level and risk of toxicity

benazepril component
antacids: Possibly decreased bioavailability of benazepril
capsaicin: Possibly induced or worsened ACE inhibitor cough
indomethacin: Reduced hypotensive effects of benazepril
phenothiazines: Possibly increased therapeutic and adverse effects of benazepril
potassium-sparing diuretics (such as amiloride, spironolactone, triamterene), potassium supplements: Increased risk of hyperkalemia

hydrochlorothiazide component
amantadine: Possibly increased blood amantadine level and risk of toxicity
amiodarone: Increased risk of arrhythmias from hypokalemia
amphotericin B, corticosteroids: Intensified electrolyte depletion, especially hypokalemia
barbiturates, opioids: Possibly potentiated orthostatic hypotension
calcium: Possibly increased serum calcium level
cholestyramine, colestipol resins: Reduced GI absorption of hydrochlorothiazide
diazoxide: Increased antihypertensive and hyperglycemic effects of hydrochlorothiazide
diflunisal: Possibly increased blood hydrochlorothiazide level
dopamine: Possibly increased diuretic effects of both drugs
insulin, oral antidiabetics: Possibly increased blood glucose level
neuromuscular blockers: Possibly enhanced neuromuscular blockade from hypokalemia
nondepolarizing skeletal muscle relaxants (such as tubocurarine): Possibly increased responsiveness to the muscle relaxant
NSAIDs: Decreased diuretic effect of hydrochlorothiazide, increased risk of renal failure
pressor amines (such as norepinephrine): Possibly decreased response to pressor amines
oral anticoagulants: Possibly decreased anticoagulant effects
sympathomimetics: Possibly decreased antihypertensive effect of hydrochlorothiazide

vitamin D: Increased risk of hypercalcemia

Adverse Reactions

CNS: Anxiety, asthenia, dizziness, fatigue, fever, headache, hypertonia, insomnia, nervousness, parethesia, somnolence, syncope, vertigo, weakness

CV: Angina, chest pain, ECG changes, hypotension, orthostatic hypotension, palpitations, peripheral edema, vasculitis

EENT: Blurred vision, dry mouth, epistaxis, taste perversion, sinusitis, tinnitus, voice alteration

ENDO: Hyperglycemia

GI: Abdominal pain, anorexia, constipation, diarrhea, dyspepsia, elevated liver function test results, gastritis, jaundice, melena, nausea, pancreatitis, vomiting

GU: Decreased libido, elevated BUN and serum creatinine levels, impotence, interstitial nephritis, nephritic syndrome, nocturia, polyuria, proteinuria, renal insufficiency, urinary frequency, UTI

HEME: Agranulocytosis, aplastic anemia, decreased hemoglobin level, hemolytic anemia, leukopenia, neutropenia, thrombocytopenia

MS: Arthralgia, arthritis, muscle spasms and weakness, myalgia

RESP: ACE inhibitor cough, asthma, bronchitis, bronchospasm, dyspnea

SKIN: Alopeica, exfoliative dermatitis, diaphoresis, flushing, photosensitivity, purpura, rash, urticaria

Other: Anaphylaxis, angioedema, dehydration, flu syndrome, gout, hypercalemia, hyperuricemia, hypochloremia, hypokalemia, hyponatremia, metabolic alkalosis, weight loss

Nursing Considerations

- Use cautiously in patients with impaired renal function because benazepril and hydrochlorothiazide can alter renal function.
- Use cautiously in patients with impaired hepatic function because hydrochlorothiazide may alter fluid and electrolyte balance and precipitate hepatic coma.
- Use cautiously in patients with systemic lupus erythematosus because hydrochlorothiazide may activate or worsen it.
- Monitor blood pressure often to assess effectiveness of therapy.
- Watch for excessive hypotension, especially in patients with heart failure. If present, notify prescriber, place patient in supine position, and give normal saline intravenously if needed and ordered, until blood pressure is restored.
- **WARNING** Monitor patient closely for signs and symptoms of angioedema or allergic reactions such as rash, urticaria, or

difficulty breathing. If present, withhold drug, notify prescriber immediately, and expect to treat symptomatically. If airway obstruction threatens, promptly give 0.3 to 0.5 ml of epinephrine solution 1:1,000 subcutaneously, as prescribed.

• Provide adequate hydration, as appropriate, to help prevent hypovolemia.

• Monitor fluid intake and output, daily weight, and serum electrolyte levels (especially potassium) to detect volume depletion or electrolyte imbalance.

• Monitor patient for increased BUN and serum creatinine levels, especially in patients with impaired renal function, because drug may cause acute renal failure. If increases are significant or persistent, notify prescriber immediately.

• Monitor blood glucose level often in diabetic patients, and expect to increase antidiabetic dosage, as needed and ordered.

• Check WBC count periodically, especially in patients with collagen-vascular disease, to detect neutropenia and agranulocytosis. Although they aren't known to occur with benazepril, they have occurred with captropril, another ACE inhibitor.

• Assess liver enzymes periodically and monitor patient for jaundice because hepatic failure, although rare, has occurred with other ACE inhibitors. If liver enzymes develop marked elevation or patient develops jaundice, notify prescriber and expect to stop benazepril and hydrochlorothiazide.

PATIENT TEACHING

• Advise patient to take benazepril and hydrochlorothiazide in the morning or early evening to avoid the need to urinate during the night.

• Teach patient to monitor her blood pressure and pulse rate and to report consistently elevated measurements to prescriber.

• Direct patient to weigh herself at the same time each day wearing the same amount of clothing and to notify prescriber if she gains more than 2 lb (0.9 kg) per day or 5 lb (2.3 kg) per week.

• To reduce the risk of dehydration and hypotension, advise patient to avoid exercise in hot weather and to avoid alcohol. Also instruct her to notify prescriber if she has prolonged diarrhea, nausea, or vomiting.

• Caution patient to avoid potentially hazardous activities until drug's CNS effects are known.

• **WARNING** Strongly urge patient to contact prescriber before using any OTC salt substitutes, which may contain potassium or potassium supplements. These substances increase the risk of hyperkalemia.

- Advise female patient to notify prescriber immediately if she is or could be pregnant because benazepril and hydrochlorothiazide will need to be replaced with another antihypertensive that's safe during second and third trimesters of pregnancy.
- Warn patient with gout that drug may precipitate an acute gout attack.
- Inform patient that a persistent dry cough may develop and may not subside unless therapy is stopped. If cough becomes bothersome or interferes with her sleep or activities, instruct her to notify prescriber.
- **WARNING** Instruct patient to contact prescriber immediately if she has signs of hypersensitivity, especially angioedema, (swelling of the face, eyes, lips, or tongue), difficulty breathing, hives, or rash.
- Caution patient to avoid sudden position changes and to rise slowly from a seated or reclining position to minimize orthostatic hypotension.

bisoprolol fumarate and hydrochlorothiazide

Ziac

Class and Category

Chemical: Selective beta$_1$-adrenergic blocker (bisoprolol), benothiadiazide (hydrochlorothiazide)

Therapeutic: Antihypertensive (bisoprolol, hydrochlorothiazide), diuretic (hydrochlorothiazide)

Pregnancy category: C

Indications and Dosages

▶ *To treat hypertension uncontrolled by bisoprolol or hydrochlorothiazide alone; to treat hypertension in patients adequately controlled by hydrochlorothiazide alone but who develop significant potassium loss*

TABLETS

Adults. *Initial:* 2.5 mg bisoprolol and 6.25 mg hydrochlorothiazide (1 tablet) daily, increased as needed q 14 days based on response. *Maximum:* 20 mg bisoprolol and 12.5 mg hydrochlorothiazide daily.

Contraindications

Anuria; cardiogenic shock; heart failure unless caused by tachyarrhythmia; hypersensitivity to bisoprolol, hydrochlorothiazide, or their components; marked sinus bradycardia; overt heart failure unless compensated; second- or third-degree heart block

---

Mechanism of Action

Bisoprolol inhibits stimulation of beta$_1$-receptors mainly in the heart, which decreases cardiac excitability, cardiac output, and myocardial oxygen demand. Bisoprolol also decreases renin release from the kidneys, which helps reduce blood pressure.

Hydrochlorothiazide promotes movement of sodium, chloride, and water from blood in the peritubular capillaries into the nephron's distal convoluted tubule. Initially, it may decrease extracellular fluid volume, plasma volume, and cardiac output, which helps explain blood pressure reduction. It also may reduce blood pressure by dilating arteries. After several weeks, extracellular fluid volume, plasma volume, and cardiac output return to normal, and peripheral vascular resistance remains decreased.

Interactions
DRUGS
bisoprolol and hydrochlorothiazide
antihypertensives: Increased additive antihypertensive effect
clonidine: Rebound hypertension
bisoprolol component
aluminum salts, barbiturates, calcium salts, cholestyramine, colestipol, NSAIDs, penicillins, rifampin, salicylates, sulfinpyrazone: Possibly decreased therapeutic and adverse effects of bisoprolol
antiarrhythmics, calcium channel blockers (such as verapamil and diltiazem): Possibly symptomatic bradycardia and conduction abnormalities
calcium channel blockers: Possibly increased therapeutic and adverse effects of bisoprolol
catecholamine-depleting drugs (such as reserpine and guanethidine): Possibly enhanced reduction of sympathetic activity
ciprofloxacin, quinolones: Possibly increased bioavailability of bisoprolol
epinephrine: Possibly hypertension followed by bradycardia
ergot alkaloids: Possibly peripheral ischemia and gangrene
flecainide: Possibly increased therapeutic and adverse effects of either drug
lidocaine: Possibly increased risk of lidocaine toxicity
oral contraceptives: Possibly increased bioavailability and plasma level of bisoprolol

prazosin: Possibly increased orthostatic hypotension

quinidine: Possibly increased effects of bisoprolol

sulfonylureas: Possibly masked hypoglycemic symptoms

hydrochlorothiazide component

amantadine: Possibly increased blood amantadine level and risk of toxicity

amiodarone: Increased risk of arrhythmias from hypokalemia

amphotericin B, corticosteroids: Intensified electrolyte depletion, especially hypokalemia

barbiturates, opioids: May potentiate orthostatic hypotension

calcium: Possibly increased serum calcium level

cholestyramine, colestipol resins: Reduced GI absorption of hydrochlorothiazide

diazoxide: Increased antihypertensive and hyperglycemic effects of hydrochlorothiazide

diflunisal: Possibly increased blood hydrochlorothiazide level

digoxin: Increased risk of digitalis toxicity from hypokalemia

dopamine: Possibly increased diuretic effects of both drugs

insulin, oral antidiabetics: Possible increased blood glucose level

lithium: Decreased lithium clearance and increased risk of lithium toxicity

neuromuscular blockers: Possibly enhanced neuromuscular blockade from hypokalemia

nondepolarizing skeletal muscle relaxants (such as tubocurarine): Possibly increased responsiveness to the muscle relaxant

NSAIDs: Decreased diuretic effect of hydrochlorothiazide and increased risk of renal failure

pressor amines (such as norepinephrine): Possibly decreased response to pressor amines

oral anticoagulants: Possibly decreased anticoagulant effects

sympathomimetics: Possibly decreased antihypertensive effect of hydrochlorothiazide

vitamin D: Increased risk of hypercalcemia

Adverse Reactions

CNS: Anxiety, asthenia, confusion, depression, dizziness, emotional lability, fatigue, fever, hallucinations, headache, insomnia, malaise, nightmares, paresthesia, tremor, somnolence, vertigo, weakness

CV: Arrhythmia, bradycardia, chest pain, claudication, edema, heart block, heart failure, hypercholesterolemia, hyperlipidemia, hypotension, MI, orthostatic hypotension, palpitations, peripheral vascular insufficiency, renal and mesenteric artery thrombosis, vasculitis

EENT: Altered taste, blurred vision, dry mouth, eye pain or pressure, increased salivation, larynospasm, pharyngitis, rhinitis, sinusitis, tinnitus

ENDO: Hyperglycemia

GI: Abdominal cramps, constipation, diarrhea, dyspepsia, diarrhea, epigastric pain, gastritis, indigestion, jaundice, ischemic colitis, nausea, vomiting

GU: Cystitis, impotence, interstitial nephritis, loss of libido, nocturia, Peyronie's disease, polyuria, renal colic

HEME: Agranulocytosis, aplastic anemia, eosinophilia, hemolytic anemia, leukopenia, neutropenia, thrombocytopenia, thrombocytopenic purpura

MS: Arthralgia; muscle cramps, twitching, and weakness; myalgia; neck pain

RESP: Asthma, bronchitis, bronchospasm, cough, dyspnea, respiratory distress, upper respiratory infection

SKIN: Alopecia, diaphoresis, eczema, exfoliative dermatitis, flushing, photosensitivity, pruritus, purpura, rash, urticaria

Other: Anaphylaxis, angioedema, dehydration, gout, hypercalcemia, hyperkalemia, hyperuricemia, hypochloremia, hypokalemia, hyponatremia, hypovolemia, metabolic alkalosis, weight gain or loss

Nursing Considerations

- Use bisoprolol and hydrochlorothiazide cautiously in patients with heart failure, arterial circulatory disorders, bronchospastic disease, or impaired renal function.
- Use cautiously in patients with impaired hepatic function because hydrochlorothiazide may alter fluid and electrolyte balance, which may precipitate hepatic coma.
- Use cautiously in patients with systemic lupus erythematosus because hydrochlorothiazide may activate or worsen it.
- Monitor blood pressure often to assess effectiveness of bisoprolol and hydrochlorothiazide therapy.
- Provide adequate hydration, as appropriate, to help prevent hypovolemia.
- Monitor fluid intake and output, daily weight, blood pressure, and serum electrolyte levels (especially potassium) to detect volume depletion or electrolyte imbalance.
- Watch for increased BUN and serum creatinine levels, especially in patients with impaired renal function, because drug may

cause acute renal failure. If increases are significant or persistent, notify prescriber immediately.

- Monitor blood glucose level often in diabetic patients, and expect to increase antidiabetic dosage, as needed and ordered.
- Monitor patient for evidence of heart failure. At first sign of heart failure, expect patient to receive a cardiac glycoside, a diuretic, or both and to be monitored closely. If failure continues, expect bisoprolol and hydrochlorothiazide to be stopped.
- Monitor diabetic patient closely because bisoprolol may mask signs of hypoglycemia, cause hypoglycemia, or delay the return of blood glucose to a normal level.
- Monitor patient with hyperthyroidism closely because bisoprolol may mask some signs of thyrotoxicosis. Avoid abrupt withdrawal of bisoprolol and hydrochlorothiazide because it may precipitate thyrotoxicosis or ischemic heart disease.
- Expect to stop bisoprolol and hydrochlorothiazide several days before gradually withdrawing clonidine therapy, if prescribed. Then expect to restart bisoprolol and hydrochlorothiazide several days after clonidine has been stopped because clonidine can cause rebound hypertension.
- Notify prescriber immediately if patient develops bradycardia, hypotension, or other serious adverse reactions.

PATIENT TEACHING
- Advise patient to take bisoprolol and hydrochlorothiazide in the morning or early evening to avoid the need to urinate during the night.
- Warn patient to take bisoprolol and hydrochlorothiazide exactly as prescribed and not to abruptly stop therapy because serious adverse effects could occur, such as an MI or arrhythmia.
- Teach patient to monitor her blood pressure and to report consistently elevated measurements to prescriber.
- Direct patient to weigh herself at the same time each day wearing the same amount of clothing and to notify prescriber if she gains more than 2 lb (0.9 kg) per day or 5 lb (2.3 kg) per week.
- Instruct patient to eat a diet high in potassium-rich food, such as citrus fruits, bananas, tomatoes, and dates.
- To reduce the risk of dehydration and hypotension, advise patient to avoid exercise in hot weather and to avoid alcohol. Also instruct her to notify prescriber if she has prolonged diarrhea, nausea, or vomiting.
- Caution patient to avoid potentially hazardous activities until drug's CNS effects are known.

- Caution diabetic patient that the drug may mask some signs of hypoglycemia; tell her to test her blood glucose level regularly.

candesartan cilexetil and hydrochlorothiazide
Atacand HCT

Class and Category
Chemical: Angiotensin II receptor antagonist (candesartan), benothiadiazide (hydrochlorothiazide)
Therapeutic: Antihypertensive (candesartan, hydrochlorothiazide), diuretic (hydrochlorothiazide)
Pregnancy category: C (first trimester), D (second and third trimesters)

Indications and Dosages
▶ *To treat hypertension when candesartan or hydrochlorothiazide alone has failed to control blood pressure*
TABLETS
Adults whose blood pressure hasn't been controlled with 32 mg of candesartan. 32 mg candesartan and 12.5 mg hydrochlorothiazide (1 tablet) daily. Increased, as needed, to 32 mg candesartan and 25 mg hydrochlorothiazide (2 tablets) daily.
Adults whose blood pressure hasn't been controlled with 25 mg of hydrochlorothiazide or whose blood pressure has been controlled with 25 mg of hydrochlorothiazide but who develop hypokalemia as a result. 16 mg candesartan and 12.5 mg hydrochlorothiazide (1 tablet) daily.

Mechanism of Action
Candesartan selectively blocks binding of the potent vasoconstrictor angiotensin II to angiotensin 1 (a subtype of angiotensin II) receptor sites in many tissues, including vascular smooth muscle and adrenal glands. This inhibits vasoconstrictive and aldosterone-secreting effects of angiotensin II, which reduces blood pressure.

Hydrochlorothiazide promotes movement of sodium, chloride, and water from blood in the peritubular capillaries into the nephron's distal convoluted tubule. Initially, it may decrease extracellular fluid volume, plasma volume, and cardiac output, which helps explain blood pressure reduction. It also may reduce blood pressure by dilating arteries. After several weeks, extracellular fluid volume, plasma volume, and cardiac output return to normal, and peripheral vascular resistance remains decreased.

Contraindications

Anuria; hypersensitivity to candesartan, hydrochlorothiazide, other sulfonamide-derived drugs or their components

Interactions

DRUGS

candesartan and hydrochlorothiazide

antihypertensives, diuretics: Additive antihypertensive effects, possibly increasing risk of hypotension

lithium: Increased serum lithium level and risk of toxicity

candesartan component

cyclosporine, potassium-sparing diuretics, potassium supplements: Increased risk of hyperkalemia

hydrochlorothiazide component

amantadine: Possibly increased blood amantadine level and risk of toxicity

amiodarone: Increased risk of arrhythmias from hypokalemia

amphotericin B, corticosteroids: Intensified electrolyte depletion, especially hypokalemia

barbiturates, opioids: May potentiate orthostatic hypotension

calcium: Possibly increased serum calcium level

cholestyramine, colestipol resins: Reduced GI absorption of hydrochlorothiazide

diazoxide: Increased antihypertensive and hyperglycemic effects of hydrochlorothiazide

diflunisal: Possibly increased blood hydrochlorothiazide level

digoxin: Increased risk of digitalis toxicity from hypokalemia

dopamine: Possibly increased diuretic effects of both drugs

insulin, oral antidiabetics: Possibly increased blood glucose level

neuromuscular blockers: Possibly enhanced neuromuscular blockade from hypokalemia

nondepolarizing skeletal muscle relaxants, such as tubocurarine: Possibly increased responsiveness to the muscle relaxant

NSAIDs: Decreased diuretic effect of hydrochlorothiazide, increased risk of renal failure

pressor amines, such as norepinephrine: Possibly decreased response to pressor amines

oral anticoagulants: Possibly decreased anticoagulant effects

sympathomimetics: Possibly decreased antihypertensive effect of hydrochlorothiazide

vitamin D: Increased risk of hypercalcemia

FOODS

candesartan component

high-potassium diet, potassium-containing salt substitutes: Increased risk of hyperkalemia

Adverse Reactions

CNS: Anxiety, asthenia, dizziness, fatigue, headache, hypesthesia, insomnia, paresthesia, vertigo, weakness

CV: Abnormal ECG, angina, bradycardia, chest pain, depression, extrasystoles, hypotension, MI, orthostatic hypotension, palpitations, peripheral edema, tachycardia, vasculitis

EENT: Blurred vision, conjunctivitis, dry mouth, epistaxis, pharyngitis, rhinitis, sinusitis, tinnitus

ENDO: Hyperglycemia

GI: Abdominal pain or cramps, anorexia, constipation, diarrhea, dyspepsia, gastritis, gastroenteritis, hepatitis, increased liver enzymes, indigestion, jaundice, nausea, vomiting

GU: Acute renal failure, cystitis, decreased libido, hematuria, impotence, increased BUN and serum creatinine levels, interstitial nephritis, nocturia, polyuria, renal failure, UTI

HEME: Agranulocytosis, aplastic or hemolytic anemia, leukopenia, neutropenia

MS: Arthralgia, arthrosis, arthritis, back pain, muscle spasms or weakness, myalgia, leg cramps, sciatica

RESP: Bronchitis, cough, dyspnea, upper respiratory infection

SKIN: Alopecia, dermatitis, diaphoresis, eczema, exfoliative dermatitis, photosensitivity, pruritus, purpura, rash, urticaria

Other: Anaphylaxis, angioedema, dehydration, flulike symptoms, hypercalcemia, hyperuricemia, hypochloremia, hypokalemia, hyponatremia, hypovolemia, increased CK level, infection, metabolic alkalosis, viral infection, weight loss

Nursing Considerations

- Use cautiously in patients with impaired hepatic or renal function because candesartan and hydrochlorothiazide may cause acute renal failure or alter fluid and electrolyte balance, which may precipitate hepatic coma.
- Also use cautiously in patients with systemic lupus erythematosus because hydrochlorothiazide may activate or worsen it.
- If patient has known or suspected hypovolemia, expect to correct it with I.V. normal saline solution, as prescribed, before starting candesartan and hydrochlorothiazide.
- Provide hydration, as appropriate, during therapy to help prevent hypovolemia.
- Monitor blood pressure often to assess effectiveness of candesartan and hydrochlorothiazide therapy.

- If patient develops hypotension, expect to stop drug temporarily. Immediately place patient in supine position, and prepare to give I.V. normal saline solution, as prescribed. Expect to resume therapy after blood pressure stabilizes.
- Monitor fluid intake and output, daily weight, and serum electrolyte levels (especially potassium) to detect volume depletion or electrolyte imbalance.
- Check for increased BUN and serum creatinine levels, especially in patients with impaired renal function, because drug may cause acute renal failure. If increases are significant or persistent, notify prescriber immediately.
- Monitor blood glucose level often in diabetic patients, and expect to increase antidiabetic dosage, as needed and ordered.
- Check patient's CBC routinely, as ordered, for abnormalities. If they're significant or persistent, notify prescriber immediately.

PATIENT TEACHING

- Advise patient to take candesartan and hydrochlorothiazide in the morning or early evening to avoid nighttime urination.
- Teach patient to monitor her blood pressure and to report consistently elevated measurements to prescriber.
- Alert patient that full effects of therapy may take up to 4 weeks.
- Caution patient that light-headedness may occur, especially early in therapy, and should be reported to the prescriber.
- Direct patient to weigh herself at the same time each day wearing the same amount of clothing and to notify prescriber if she gains more than 2 lb (0.9 kg) per day or 5 lb (2.3 kg) per week.
- **WARNING** Strongly urge patient to contact prescriber before using potassium supplements or OTC salt substitutes, which may contain potassium. These substances increase the risk of hyperkalemia.
- To reduce the risk of dehydration and hypotension, advise patient to avoid exercise in hot weather and to avoid alcohol. Also tell her to notify prescriber if she has prolonged diarrhea, nausea, or vomiting.
- Caution patient to avoid potentially hazardous activities until drug's CNS effects are known.
- Explain the importance of regular exercise, proper diet, and other lifestyle changes in controlling hypertension.
- Advise female patient to notify prescriber immediately if she is or could be pregnant. Candesartan and hydrochlorothiazide will need to be replaced with another antihypertensive that's safe during the second and third trimesters.

captopril and hydrochlorothiazide
Capozide

Class and Category
Chemical: ACE inhibitor (captopril), benothiadiazide (hydrochloro-thiazide)

Therapeutic: Antihypertensive (captopril, hydrochlorothiazide), diuretic (hydrochlorothiazide)

Pregnancy category: C (first trimester), D (second and third trimesters)

Indications and Dosages
▶ *To treat hypertension uncontrolled with captopril or hydrochloro-thiazide alone*

TABLETS

Adults. *Initial:* 25 mg captopril and 15 mg hydrochlorothiazide (1 tablet) daily, increased as needed. *Maximum:* 150 mg captropril and 50 hydrochlorothiazide daily.

Mechanism of Action
Captopril may reduce blood pressure by affecting the renin-angiotensin-aldosterone system. By inhibiting ACE, captopril:
- prevents conversion of angiotensin I to angiotensin II, a potent vasocon-strictor that also stimulates adrenal cortex to secrete aldosterone.
- may inhibit renal and vascular production of angiotensin II.
- decreases serum angiotensin II level and increases serum renin activity. This decreases aldosterone secretion, slightly increasing serum potassium level and fluid loss.
- decreases vascular tone and blood pressure.
- inhibits aldosterone release, which reduces sodium and water reabsorption and increases their excretion, further reducing blood pressure.

Hydrochlorothiazide promotes movement of sodium, chloride, and water from blood in peritubular capillaries into the nephron's distal convoluted tubule. Initially, it may decrease extracellular fluid volume, plasma volume, and cardiac output, which helps explain blood pressure reduction. It also may reduce blood pressure by dilating arteries. After several weeks, extracellular fluid volume, plasma volume, and cardiac output return to normal, and peripheral vascular resistance remains decreased.

Contraindications
Anuria; hypersensitivity to captopril, hydrochlorothiazide, other ACE inhibitors or sulfonamide-derived drugs, or their components

Interactions

DRUGS

captopril and hydrochlorothiazide

antihypertensives, diuretics: Increased antihypertensive effects

digoxin: Increased blood digoxin level and risk of toxicity

lithium: Increased blood lithium level and toxicity

NSAIDs, sympathomimetics: Possibly reduced antihypertensive effects of captopril and hydrochlorothiazide and increased risk of renal toxicity

captopril component

allopurinol: Increased risk of hypersensitivity reactions, including Stevens-Johnson syndrome, skin eruptions, fever, and arthralgia; possibly increased risk of fatal neutropenia or agranulocytosis

antacids: Possibly impaired captopril absorption

bone marrow depressants (such as amphotericin B and methotrexate), procainamide, systemic corticosteroids: Possibly increased risk of fatal neutropenia or agranulocytosis

capsaicin: Possibly induced or worsened ACE inhibitor cough

cyclosporine, potassium-sparing diuretics, potassium supplements: Increased risk of hyperkalemia

probenecid: Increased blood level and decreased total clearance of captopril

hydrochlorothiazide component

amantadine: Possibly increased blood amantadine level and risk of toxicity

amiodarone: Increased risk of arrhythmias from hypokalemia

amphotericin B, corticosteroids: Intensified electrolyte depletion, especially hypokalemia

barbiturates, opioids: May potentiate orthostatic hypotension

calcium: Possibly increased serum calcium level

cholestyramine, colestipol resins: Reduced GI absorption of hydrochlorothiazide

diazoxide: Increased antihypertensive and hyperglycemic effects of hydrochlorothiazide

diflunisal: Possibly increased blood hydrochlorothiazide level

dopamine: Possibly increased diuretic effects of both drugs

insulin, oral antidiabetics: Possibly increased blood glucose level

neuromuscular blockers: Possibly enhanced neuromuscular blockade from hypokalemia

nondepolarizing skeletal muscle relaxants (such as tubocurarine): Possibly increased responsiveness to the muscle relaxant

pressor amines (such as norepinephrine): Possibly decreased response to pressor amines

oral anticoagulants: Possibly decreased anticoagulant effects
vitamin D: Increased risk of hypercalcemia
FOODS
captopril component
potassium-containing salt substitutes: Increased risk of hyperkalemia
ACTIVITIES
captopril component
alcohol use: Additive hypotensive effects

Adverse Reactions

CNS: Dizziness, fever, headache, insomnia, paresthesia, vertigo, weakness
CV: Chest pain, hypotension, orthostatic hypotension, palpitations, tachycardia, vasculitis
EENT: Blurred vision, dry mouth, loss of taste
ENDO: Hyperglycemia
GI: Abdominal cramps, anorexia, constipation, diarrhea, indigestion, jaundice, nausea, vomiting
GU: Decreased libido, dysuria, impotence, interstitial nephritis, nephritic syndrome, nocturia, oliguria, polyuria, proteinuria, renal failure, urinary frequency
HEME: Agranulocytosis, aplastic and hemolytic anemia, eosinophilia, leukopenia, neutropenia, thrombocytopenia
MS: Arthraliga, muscle spasms and weakness
RESP: Cough
SKIN: Alopecia, exfoliative dermatitis, photosensitivity, purpura, pruritus, rash, urticaria
Other: Anaphylaxis, angioedema, dehydration, hypercalcemia, hyperkalemia, hyperuricemia, hypochloremia, hypokalemia, hyponatremia, hypovolemia, metabolic alkalosis, positive ANA titer, weight loss

Nursing Considerations

• Use cautiously in patients with impaired hepatic function because hydrochlorothiazide may alter fluid and electrolyte balance, which may precipitate hepatic coma.
• Also use cautiously in patients with systemic lupus erythematosus because hydrochlorothiazide may activate or worsen the dieseae.
• Monitor blood pressure often to assess effectiveness of captropril and hydrochlorothiazide therapy. If hypotension occurs, keep patient supine until resolved.
• Provide adequate hydration, as appropriate, to help prevent hypovolemia.

- Monitor fluid intake and output, daily weight, and serum electrolyte levels (especially potassium) to detect volume depletion or electrolyte imbalance.
- Watch for increased BUN and serum creatinine levels, especially in patients with impaired renal function, because drug may cause renal dysfunction. If increases are significant or persistent or patient has renal symptoms such as oliguria, polyuria, or urinary frequency, notify prescriber immediately.
- Monitor blood glucose level often in diabetic patients, and expect to increase antidiabetic dosage, as needed and ordered.
- Monitor patient's WBC counts regularly, as ordered, especially in patients with collagen vascular disease or renal disease.
- **WARNING** Monitor patient closely for angioedema of the face, lips, tongue, glottis, larynx, or limbs. For angioedema of the face and lips, stop drug and give an antihistamine, as prescribed. If tongue, glottis, or larynx is involved, assess patient for airway obstruction, prepare to give epinephrine 1:1,000 (0.3 to 0.5 ml) subcutaneously, and maintain a patent airway.

PATIENT TEACHING

- Advise patient to take captropril and hydrochlorothiazide in the morning or early evening to avoid the need to urinate during the night. Also tell patient to take drug 1 hour before a meal.
- Teach patient to monitor her blood pressure and to report consistently elevated measurements to prescriber.
- Direct patient to weigh herself at the same time each day wearing the same amount of clothing and to notify prescriber if she gains more than 2 lb (0.9 kg) per day or 5 lb (2.3 kg) per week.
- To reduce the risk of dehydration and hypotension, advise patient to avoid exercise in hot weather and to avoid alcohol. Also instruct her to notify prescriber if she has prolonged diarrhea, nausea, or vomiting.
- Caution patient to avoid potentially hazardous activities until drug's CNS effects are known.
- Explain the importance of regular exercise, proper diet, and other lifestyle changes in controlling hypertension.
- Tell patient to avoid sunlight or to wear sunscreen in direct sunlight because photosensitivity may occur.
- Advise patient not to use salt substitutes that contain potassium and to consult prescriber before increasing dietary potassium intake to avoid increasing the risk of hyperkalemia.
- Stress importance of notifying prescriber about possible indicators of, such as a sore throat or fever occurs.
- Warn patient not to stop taking drug abruptly.

clonidine and chlorthalidone
Clorpres, Combipres

Class and Category
Chemical: Imidazoline derivative (clonidine), phthalimidine derivative of benzenesulfonamide (thiazide-like diuretic) (chlorthalidone)
Therapeutic: Antihypertensive, diuretic
Pregnancy category: C

Indications and Dosages
▶ *To treat hypertension uncontrolled with clonidine or chlorthalidone monotherapy*
TABLETS
Adults. *Initial:* 0.1 mg clonidine and 15 mg chlorthalidone (1 tablet) daily or b.i.d., increased as needed. *Maximum:* 0.6 mg clonidine and 30 mg chlorthalidone

---

Mechanism of Action
Clonidine stimulates alpha-adrenergic receptors in the brain stem to reduce sympathetic outflow from the CNS and a decrease in peripheral vascular resistance, heart rate, and systolic and diastolic blood pressure.

Chlorthalidone may promote sodium, chloride, and water excretion by inhibiting sodium reabsorption in the kidneys' distal tubules. Initially, chlorthalidone may decrease extracellular fluid volume, plasma volume, and cardiac output, which helps explain how it reduces blood pressure. It also may dilate arteries directly, which helps reduce peripheral vascular resistance and blood pressure. After several weeks, extracellular fluid and plasma volume and cardiac output return to normal, but peripheral vascular resistance remains decreased to lower blood pressure.

Contraindications
Anuria; hypersensitivity to clonidine, chlorthalidone, other sulfonamide-derived drugs, or their components

Interactions
DRUGS
clonidine and chlorthalidone
antihypertensives, diuretics: Increased antihypertensive effects
digoxin: Increased risk of digitalis toxicity from hypokalemia
clonidine component
barbituratres, other CNS depressants: Increased depressant effects of these drugs
beta blockers, calcium channel blockers: Additive effects, such as

bradycardia and AV block; increased risk of exacerbated hypertensive response when clonidine is withdrawn (beta blockers only)
levodopa: Decreased levodopa effectiveness
prazosin, tricyclic antidepressants: Decreased antihypertensive effect of clonidine

chlorthalidone component
allopurinol: Increased risk of allopurinol hypersensitivity
amphotericin B, corticosteroids: Intensified electrolyte depletion, especially hypokalemia
anesthetics: Potentiated effects of anesthetics
anticholinergics: Increased chlorthalidone absorption
antineoplastics: Prolonged antineoplastic-induced leukopenia
cholestyramine, colestipol resins: Reduced GI absorption of chlorthalidone
diazoxide: Increased antihypertensive and hyperglycemic effects of chlorthalidone
insulin, oral antidiabetics: Possibly increased blood glucose level
lithium: Decreased lithium clearance and increased risk of toxicity
loop diuretics: Increased synergistic effects, resulting in profound diuresis and serious electrolyte imbalances
methenamines: Decreased effects of methenamines
metyldopa: Potential development of hemolytic anemia
neuromuscular blockers: Possibly enhanced neuromuscular blockade
NSAIDs: Decreased diuretic effect of chlorthalidone
oral anticoagulants: Possibly decreased anticoagulant effects
sympathomimetics: Possibly decreased antihypertensive effect of clorthalidone
vitamin D: Enhanced vitamin D action
ACTIVITIES
clonidine component
alcohol use: Enhanced depressive effectives of clonidine

Adverse Reactions
CNS: Agitation, depression, dizziness, drowsiness, fatigue, headache, insomnia, light-headedness, malaise, nervousness, paresthesia, restlessness, sedation, vertigo, weakness
CV: Chest pain, orthostastic hypotension, vasculitis
EENT: Blurred or yellow vision, burning eyes, dry eyes and mouth
ENDO: Hyperglycemia
GI: Abdominal cramps or pain, anorexia, bloating, constipation, diarrhea, gastric irritation, mildly elevated liver function test results, nausea, pancreatitis, vomiting
GU: Decreased libido, impotence, nocturia

HEME: Agranulocytosis, aplastic anemia, hypoplastic anemia, leukopenia, thromboyctopenia
MS: Muscle spasms
SKIN: Cutaneous vasculitis, exfoliative dermatitis, jaundice, necrotizing vasculitis, photosensitivity, purpura, rash, urticaria
Other: Gout, hyperuricemia, hypochloremic alkalosis, hypokalemia, hyponatremia, weight gain, withdrawal symptoms

Nursing Considerations

- Use clonidine and chlorthalidone cautiously in patients with impaired hepatic function because minor changes in fluid and electrolyte balance may cause hepatic coma.
- Also use clonidine and chlorthalidone cautiously in elderly patients, who may be more sensitive to its hypotensive effect, and in patients with severe coronary insufficiency, recent MI, cerebrovascular disease, or chronic renal faiulre.
- Monitor blood pressure and heart rate often during clonidine and chlorthalidone therapy to assess effectiveness.
- Assess BUN, serum electrolyte, uric acid, and blood glucose levels before and periodically during therapy. Monitor patient for signs of fluid and electrolyte imbalance.
- **WARNING** Monitor renal function periodically to detect cumulative drug effects, which may cause azotemia in patients with impaired renal function.
- **WARNING** Be aware that stopping drug abruptly can elevate serum catecholamine level and cause such withdrawal symptoms as nervousness, agitation, headache, confusion, tremor, and rebound hypertension.
- If patient has had an allergic reaction to transdermal clonidine, be aware that he also may have an allergic reaction to oral clonidine. Monitor him closely.

PATIENT TEACHING

- Advise patient to take drug exactly as prescribed and not to stop taking it abruptly because withdrawal symptoms and severe hypertension may occur.
- Tell patient to take drug with food or milk and to take it earlier in the day to avoid the need to urinate during the night.
- Urge patient to eat high-potassium foods (such as bananas, apricots, grapefruits, tomato juice, and orange juice) and to report signs of a low potassium level (such as an irregular heartbeat, muscle weakness, and fatigue) or a low sodium level (such as confusion, irritability, and muscle cramps).

- Teach patient to monitor blood pressure and to report consistently elevated measurements to prescriber.
- Caution patient to avoid potentially hazardous activities until drug's CNS effects are known.
- Advise male patients about possibly decreased libido.
- Tell patient to report urine retention, vision changes, excessive drowsiness, rash, chest pain, and dizziness with position changes. Urge tell patient to rise slowly to avoid hypotensive effects.
- Instruct patient to protect his skin from the sun.
- Urge patient to immediately report sudden joint pain to prescriber because drug can cause sudden gout attacks.
- To reduce the risk of dehydration and hypotension, advise patient to avoid exercise in hot weather and to avoid alcohol. Also instruct her to notify prescriber if she has prolonged diarrhea, nausea, or vomiting.
- Advise diabetic patient to monitor blood glucose level closely because drug may cause hyperglycemia, which may warrant a change in treatment plan.

dipyridamole and aspirin
Aggrenox

Class and Category
Chemical: Salicylate (aspirin), pyrimidine (dipyridamole)
Therapeutic: Platelet aggregation inhibitor
Pregnancy category: NR (aspirin D, dipyridamole B)

Indications and Dosages
▶ *To prevent recurrence of thromboembolic stroke*
CAPSULES
Adults. *Initial:* 25 mg aspirin and 200 mg extended-release dipyridamole (1 capsule) b.i.d.

Mechanism of Action
Aspirin inhibits platelet aggregation by interfering with production of thromboxane A_2, a substance that stimulates platelet aggregation. Dipyridamole inhibits platelet uptake of adenosine, thus increasing the amount of adenosine in surrounding blood. The increased adenosine acts on platelet A_2 receptors, which stimulates the activity of intraplatelet adenylate cyclase. This action in turn increases the level of cyclic adenosine monophosphate in platelets, which decreases platelet activation and aggregation.

Contraindications

Allergy to NSAIDs or tartrazine dye; hypersensitivity to aspirin, dipyridamole, or their components

Interactions

DRUGS

aspirin component

ACE inhibitors, beta blockers: Decreased antihypertensive effect

acetazolamide: Increased blood acetazolamide level and risk of toxicity

activated charcoal: Decreased aspirin absorption

antacids, urine alkalinizers: Decreased aspirin effectiveness

carbonic anhydrase inhibitors: Salicylism

corticosteroids: Increased excretion and decreased blood level of aspirin

heparin: Increased risk of bleeding

methotrexate: Increased blood level and decreased excretion rate of methotrexate, causing toxicity

nizatidine: Increased blood aspirin level

NSAIDs: Possibly decreased blood NSAID level and increased risk of bleeding

oral anticoagulants: Increased risk of bleeding; prolonged bleeding time

phenytoin: Decreased blood phenytoin level

sulfonylureas: Possibly enhanced effect of sulfonylureas with large doses of aspirin

urine acidifiers (such as ammonium chloride and ascorbic acid): Decreased aspirin excretion

valproic acid: Increased blood valproic acid level

vancomycin: Increased risk of ototoxicity

dipyridamole component

adenosine: Increased blood adenosine level; potentiated effects of adenosine

cefamandole, cefoperazone, cefotetan, plicamyin, valproic acid: Possibly hypoprothrombinemia and increased risk of bleeding

cholinesterase inhibitors: Possibly counteracted effects of these drugs and aggravation of myasthenia gravis

heparin, NSAIDs, thrombolytics: Possibly increased risk of bleeding

ACTIVITIES

aspirin component

alcohol use: Increased risk of GI bleeding

Adverse Reactions

CNS: Amnesia, asthenia, headache, seizures, somnolence, syncope

EENT: Epistaxis
GI: Abdominal pain, anorexia, diarrhea, dyspepsia, esophageal irritation, GI bleeding, hemorrhoids, hepatic impairment, nausea, vomiting
HEME: Anemia
MS: Arthralgia, arthritis, back pain
SKIN: Purpura

Nursing Considerations

- Be aware that combination aspirin and dipyridamole isn't interchangeable with individual aspirin or dipyridamole tablets.
- **WARNING** Monitor patients with severe hepatic impairment for evidence of bleeding, such as easy bruising, tarry stools, and epistaxis. Monitor coagulation test results as appropriate, and notify prescriber immediately about significant changes. These patients already have an increased risk of bleeding, and platelet inhibition increases the risk further.
- Monitor liver function test results as appropriate if patient has hepatic impairment because dipyridamole may increase hepatic enzyme levels and cause hepatic failure.
- Monitor renal function test results, such as glomerular filtration rate (GFR), if patient has renal impairment. Because aspirin is excreted by the kidneys, it should be avoided in patients with a GFR below 10 ml/min. Otherwise, patient may develop aspirin toxicity.
- If patient consumes three or more alcoholic beverages daily or has hypoprothrombinemia, peptic ulcer disease, or vitamin K deficiency, monitor him closely for signs and symptoms of bleeding.
- If patient has coronary artery disease, assess for chest pain and hypotension because of dipyridamole's vasodilatory effect.

PATIENT TEACHING
- Advise patient to swallow capsule whole and not to break, chew, or crush it.
- Instruct patient to take drug with a full glass of water and to avoid lying down for 15 to 30 minutes afterward to prevent esophageal irritation.
- Warn patient to consult prescriber before taking any drug to treat pain, fever, or arthritis.
- Urge patient not to stop taking drug for any reason without first consulting prescriber.
- Advise patient to notify other health care providers that he takes aspirin and dipyridamole.

enalapril maleate and felodipine ER
Lexxel

Class and Category
Chemical: Dicarbocyl-containing ACE inhibitor (enalapril), dihy-dropyridine derivative (felodipine)
Therapeutic: Antihypertensive (enalapril, felodipine)
Pregnancy category: C (first trimester), D (second and third trimesters)

Indications and Dosages
▶ *To treat hypertension when enalapril or felodipine alone has failed to control blood pressure*
TABLETS
Adults. 5 mg enalapril and 5 mg felodipine (1 tablet) daily; increased as needed in 7 to 14 days to 10 mg enalapril and 10 mg felodipine (2 tablets) daily; increased again, as needed, in 7 to 14 days to 20 mg enalapril and 10 mg felodipine (4 tablets, each containing 5 mg enalipril and 2.5 mg felodipine) daily.

Mechanism of Action
Enalapril may reduce blood pressure by affecting the renin-angiotensin-aldosterone system. By inhibiting ACE, enalapril:
- prevents conversion of angiotensin I to angiotensin II, a potent vasocon-strictor that also stimulates adrenal cortex to secrete aldosterone.
- may inhibit renal and vascular production of angiotensin II.
- decreases serum angiotensin II level and increases serum renin activity. This decreases aldosterone secretion, slightly increasing serum potassium level and fluid loss.
- decreases vascular tone and blood pressure.
- inhibits aldosterone release, which reduces sodium and water reabsorption and increases their excretion, further reducing blood pressure.

Felodipine may slow movement of extracellular calcium into myocardial and vascular smooth-muscle cells by deforming calcium channels in cell membranes, inhibiting ion-controlled gating mechanisms, and interfering with calcium release from the sacroplasmic reticulum. The effect of these actions is a decrease in intracellular calcium ions, which inhibits contraction of smooth-muscle cells and dilates coronary and systemic arteries. As with other calcium channel blockers, felodipine increases oxygen to the myocardium and reduces peripheral resistance, blood pressure, and afterload.

Contraindications
Hereditary or idiopathic angioedema; history of angioedema from

previous ACE inhibitor; hypersensitivity to enalapril, felodipine, or their components

Interactions

DRUGS

enalapril and felodipine

antihypertensives, diuretics: Additive hypotensive effects

lithium: Increased blood lithium level and toxicity

NSAIDs, sympathomimetics: Possibly reduced antihypertensive effects of enalapril and felodipine

enalapril component

allopurinol, bone marrow depressants (such as amphotericin B and methotrexate), procainamide, systemic corticosteroids: Possibly increased risk of fatal neutropenia or agranulocytosis

cyclosporine, potassium-sparing diuretics, potassium supplements: Increased risk of hyperkalemia

felodopine component

anesthetics (hydrocarbon inhalation): Possibly hypotension

anticonvulsants: Decreased plasma felodipine level and effectiveness

beta blockers: Increased adverse effects of beta blockers

cimetidine, erythromycin, itraconazole, ketoconazole: Increased felodipine bioavailability

digoxin: Transient increase in blood digoxin level and risk of toxicity

estrogens: Possibly increased fluid retention and decreased therapeutic effect of felodopine

procainamide, quinidine: Increased risk of prolonged QT interval

tacrolimus: Possibly increased serum tacrolimus level

FOODS

enalapril component

potassium-containing salt substitutes: Increased risk of hyperkalemia

felodopine component

grapefruit juice: Doubled felodipine bioavailability

ACTIVITIES

enalapril component

alcohol use: Possibly additive hypotensive effect

Adverse Reactions

CNS: Asthenia, ataxia, confusion, depression, dizziness, dream disturbances, fatigue, headache, insomnia, nervousness, paresthesia, peripheral neuropathy, somnolence, stroke, syncope, vertigo, weakness

CV: Angina, arrhythmias, cardiac arrest, chest pain, edema, hypotension, MI, orthostatic hypotension, palpitations, Raynaud's phenomenon, tachycardia

EENT: Blurred vision, conjunctivitis, dry eyes and mouth, gingival hyperplasia, glossitis, hoarseness, lacrimation, loss of smell, pharyngitis, rhinorrhea, rhinitis, stomatitis, taste perversion, tinnitus

ENDO: Gynecomastia

GI: Abdominal cramps or pain, anorexia, constipation, diarrhea, hepatic failure, hepatitis, ileus, indigestion, melena, nausea, pancreatitis, vomiting

GU: Flank pain, impotence, oliguria, renal failure, UTI

HEME: Agranulocytosis

MS: Back pain, muscle spasms

RESP: Asthma; bronchitis; bronchospasm; cough; dyspnea; pneumonia; pulmonary edema, embolism, infarction, and infiltrates; upper respiratory tract infection

SKIN: Alopecia, diaphoresis, erythema multiforme, exfoliative dermatitis, flushing, pemphigus, photosensitivity, pruritus, rash, Stevens-Johnson syndrome, toxic epidermal necrolysis, urticaria

Other: Anaphylaxis, angioedema, herpes zoster, hyperkalemia

Nursing Considerations

- Use enalapril and felodipine cautiously in patients with heart failure, reduced ventricular function, or impaired hepatic or renal function.
- Monitor blood pressure during therapy and when dosage changes, especially in elderly patients, to assess effectiveness.
- Monitor laboratory test results to check hepatic and renal function, leukocyte count, and serum potassium level.
- Expect felodipine bioavailability to increase by up to twofold when taken with grapefruit juice.
- **WARNING** Be aware that felodipine may cause severe hypotension with syncope, which may lead to reflex tachycardia and angina in patients with coronary artery disease or a history of angina.
- **WARNING** Monitor patient closely for angioedema of the face, lips, tongue, glottis, larynx, or limbs. For angioedema of the face and lips, stop drug and give an antihistamine, as prescribed. If tongue, glottis, or larynx is involved, assess patient for airway obstruction, prepare to give epinephrine 1:1,000 (0.3 to 0.5 ml) subcutaneously, and maintain a patent airway.
- Monitor patient for signs of felodopine overdose, such as excessive peripheral vasodilation, marked hypotension, and possibly bradycardia. If you detect such signs, place patient in supine

position with legs elevated and give I.V. fluids, as prescribed. Expect to give I.V. atropine for bradycardia.

PATIENT TEACHING
• Instruct patient to swallow tablets whole and not to crush or chew them.
• Caution patient not to fluctuate her intake of grapefruit juice during therapy.
• Instruct patient to monitor her pulse rate and blood pressure and to report consistent changes to prescriber.
• Teach patient how to minimize gingival hyperplasia by following good dental hygiene practices.
• Advise patient to notify prescriber immediately if she has palpitations; pronounced dizziness; swelling of face, hands, or feet; or a persistent, dry cough.
• Advise female patient to notify prescriber immediately if she is or could be pregnant. Enalapril and felodipine will need to be replaced with another antihypertensive that's safe during second and third trimesters.
• Advise patient to change positions slowly and avoid potentially hazardous activities until the drug's effects are known.
• Tell patient to consult prescriber before using salt substitutes, potassium supplements, or other drugs (including OTC drugs) during therapy.
• Alert patient to notify prescriber about any signs of infection, such as a sore throat or fever.

enalapril maleate and hydrochlorothiazide

Vaseretic

Class and Category

Chemical: Dicarbocyl-containing ACE inhibitor (enalapril), benothiadiazide (hydrochlorothiazide)
Therapeutic: Antihypertensive (enalapril, hydrochlorothiazide), diuretic (hydrochlorothiazide)
Pregnancy category: C (first trimester), D (second and third trimesters)

Indications and Dosages

▶ *To treat hypertension not adequately controlled by enalapril or hydrochlorothiazide alone*

TABLETS
Adults. *Initial:* 5 mg enalapril and 12.5 mg hydrochlorothiazide

(1 tablet) daily. Alternatively, 10 mg enalapril and 25 mg hydrochlorothiazide (1 tablet) daily. Increased, as needed, q 2 to 3 wk. *Maximum:* 20 mg enalapril and 50 mg hydrochlorothiazide.

Mechanism of Action

Enalapril may reduce blood pressure by affecting the renin-angiotensin-aldosterone system. By inhibiting inhibiting ACE, enalapril:

* prevents conversion of angiotensin I to angiotensin II, a potent vasoconstrictor that also stimulates adrenal cortex to secrete aldosterone.
* may inhibit renal and vascular production of angiotensin II.
* decreases serum angiotensin II level and increases serum renin activity. This decreases aldosterone secretion, slightly increasing serum potassium level and fluid loss.
* decreases vascular tone and blood pressure.
* inhibits aldosterone release, which reduces sodium and water reabsorption and increases their excretion, further reducing blood pressure.

Hydrochlorothiazide promotes movement of sodium, chloride, and water from blood in the peritubular capillaries into the nephron's distal convoluted tubule. Initially, it may decrease extracellular fluid volume, plasma volume, and cardiac output, which helps explain blood pressure reduction. It also may reduce blood pressure by dilating arteries. After several weeks, extracellular fluid volume, plasma volume, and cardiac output return to normal, and peripheral vascular resistance remains decreased.

Contraindications

Anuria; hereditary or idiopathic angioedema; history of angioedema from previous ACE inhibitor; hypersensitivity to enalapril, hydrochlorothiazide, other sulfonamide-derived drugs or their components

Interactions

DRUGS

enalapril and hydrochlorothiazide
antihypertensives, diuretics: Additive hypotensive effects
lithium: Increased blood lithium level and toxicity
NSAIDs, sympathomimetics: Possibly reduced antihypertensive effects and increased risk of renal toxicity
enalapril component
allopurinol, bone marrow depressants (such as amphotericin B and methotrexate), procainamide, systemic corticosteroids: Possibly increased risk of fatal neutropenia or agranulocytosis

cyclosporine, potassium-sparing diuretics, potassium supplements: Increased risk of hyperkalemia

hydrochlorothiazide component

amantadine: Possibly increased blood level and risk of toxicity of amantadine

amiodarone: Increased risk of arrhythmias from hypokalemia

amphotericin B, corticosteroids: Intensified electrolyte depletion, especially hypokalemia

antihypertensives: Increased antihypertensive effects

barbiturates, opioids: May potentiate orthostatic hypotension

calcium: Possibly increased serum calcium level

cholestyramine, colestipol resins: Reduced GI absorption of hydrochlorothiazide

diazoxide: Increased antihypertensive and hyperglycemic effects of hydrochlorothiazide

diflunisal: Possibly increased blood hydrochlorothiazide level

digoxin: Increased risk of digitalis toxicity from hypokalemia

dopamine: Possibly increased diuretic effects of both drugs

insulin, oral antidiabetics: Possibly increased blood glucose level

neuromuscular blockers: Possibly enhanced neuromuscular blockade from hypokalemia

nondepolarizing skeletal muscle relaxants (such as tubocurarine): Possibly increased responsiveness to the muscle relaxant

pressor amines (such as norepinephrine): Possibly decreased response to pressor amines

oral anticoagulants: Possibly decreased anticoagulant effects

vitamin D: Increased risk of hypercalcemia

FOODS

enalapril component

potassium-containing salt substitutes: Increased risk of hyperkalemia

ACTIVITIES

enalapril component

alcohol use: Possibly additive hypotensive effect

Adverse Reactions

CNS: Asthenia, ataxia, confusion, depression, dizziness, dream disturbances, fatigue, headache, insomnia, nervousness, paresthesia, peripheral neuropathy, somnolence, stroke, syncope, vertigo, weakness

CV: Angina, arrhythmias, cardiac arrest, chest pain, hypotension, MI, orthostatic hypotension, palpitations, Raynaud's phenomenon, tachycardia, vasculitis

EENT: Blurred vision, conjunctivitis, dry eyes and mouth, glossitis, hoaseness, lacrimation, loss of smell, pharyngitis, rhinorrhea, stomatitis, taste perversion, tinnitus

ENDO: Gynecomastia, hyperglycemia

GI: Abdominal pain, anorexia, constipation, diarrhea, dyspepsia, flatulence, hepatic failure, hepatitis, ileus, indigestion, jaundice, melena, nausea, pancreatitis, vomiting

GU: Decreased libido, flank pain, impotence, interstitial nephritis, nocturia, polyuria, oliguria, renal failure, UTI

HEME: Agranulocytosis, aplastic anemia, hemolytic anemia, leukopenia, neutropenia, thrombocytopenia

MS: Arthralgia; muscle cramps, spasms, and weakness

RESP: Asthma; back pain; bronchitis; bronchospasm; cough; dyspnea; pneumonia; pulmonary edema, embolism, infarction and infiltrates; upper respiratory tract infection

SKIN: Alopecia, diaphoresis, erythema multiforme, exfoliative dermatitis, flushing, pemphigus, photosensitivity, pruritis, rash, Stevens-Johnson syndrome, toxic epidermal necrolysis, urticaria

Other: Anaphylaxis, angioedema, dehydration, gout, herpes zoster, hypercalcemia, hyperkalemia, hyperuricemia, hypochloremia, hypokalemia, hyponatremia, hypovolemia, metabolic alkalosis, weight loss

Nursing Considerations

- Use cautiously in patients with impaired renal or hepatic function because enalapril and hydrochlorothiazide may alter fluid and electrolyte balance and cause renal failure or hepatic coma.
- Also use cautiously in patients with systemic lupus erythematosus because hydrochlorothiazide may activate or worsen it.
- Monitor blood pressure frequently to assess effectiveness of enalapril and hydrochlorothiazide therapy.
- **WARNING** Be aware that drug may cause severe hypotension with syncope, leading to reflex tachycardia and angina in patients with coronary artery disease or a history of angina.
- **WARNING** Monitor patient closely for angioedema of the face, lips, tongue, glottis, larynx, or limbs. For angioedema of the face and lips, stop drug and give an antihistamine, as prescribed. If tongue, glottis, or larynx is involved, assess patient for airway obstruction, prepare to give epinephrine 1:1,000 (0.3 to 0.5 ml) subcutaneously, and maintain a patent airway.
- Provide hydration, as appropriate, to help prevent hypovolemia.
- Monitor fluid intake and output, daily weight, and serum electrolyte levels (especially potassium) to detect volume depletion or electrolyte imbalance.

- Watch for increased BUN and serum creatinine levels, especially in patients with impaired renal function, because drug may cause acute renal failure. If increases are significant or persistent, notify prescriber immediately.
- Monitor blood glucose level often in diabetic patients, and expect to increase antidiabetic dosage, as needed and ordered.
- Monitor WBC count periodically, especially in patients with collagen-vascular disease, to detect neutropenia and agranulocytosis. Although they aren't known to occur with enalapril, they have occurred with captropril, another ACE inhibitor.
- Assess liver enzymes periodically and monitor patient for jaundice because hepatic failure, although rare, has occurred with other ACE inhibitors. If liver enzymes develop marked elevation or patient develops jaundice, notify prescriber and expect to stop benazepril and hydrochlorothiazide.

PATIENT TEACHING

- Advise patient to take enalapril and hydrochlorothiazide in the morning or early evening to avoid the need to urinate during the night.
- Teach patient to monitor her blood pressure and to report consistently elevated measurements to prescriber.
- Direct patient to weigh herself at the same time each day wearing the same amount of clothing and to notify prescriber if she gains more than 2 lb (0.9 kg) per day or 5 lb (2.3 kg) per week.
- To reduce the risk of dehydration and hypotension, advise patient to avoid exercise in hot weather and to avoid alcohol. Also instruct her to notify prescriber if she has prolonged diarrhea, nausea, or vomiting.
- Caution patient to avoid potentially hazardous activities until drug's CNS effects are known.
- Explain the importance of regular exercise, proper diet, and other lifestyle changes in controlling hypertension.
- **WARNING** Strongly urge patient to contact prescriber before using potassium supplements or OTC salt substitutes, which may contain potassium. These products increase the risk of hyperkalemia.
- Advise female patient to notify prescriber immediately if she is or could be pregnant. Enalapril and hydrochlorothiazide will need to be replaced with another antihypertensive that's safe to use during second and third trimesters of pregnancy.
- Warn patient with gout that drug may precipitate an acute gout attack.

eprosartan mesylate and hydrochlorothiazide

Teveten

Class and Category

Chemical: Nonbiphenyl nontetrazole angiotensin II receptor antagonist (eprosartan), benothiadiazide (hydrochlorothiazide)

Therapeutic: Antihypertensive (eprosartan, hydrochlorothiazide), diuretic (hydrochlorothiazide)

Pregnancy category: C (first trimester), D (second and third trimesters)

Indications and Dosages

▶ *To treat hypertension uncontrolled by eprosartan or hydrochlorothiazide alone*

TABLETS

Adults. *Initial:* 600 mg eprosartan and 12.5 mg hydrochlorothiazide (1 tablet) daily; increased as needed to 600 mg eprosartan and 25 mg hydrochlorothiazide (1 tablet) daily.

Mechanism of Action

Eprosartan blocks the effects of angiotensin II (a potent vasoconstrictor that's part of the renin-angiotensin-aldosterone system) by blocking it from binding to angiotensin I receptors in vascular smooth muscles, adrenal glands, and other tissues. This action halts angiotensin II's negative feedback on renin secretion. Thus, circulating renin and angiotensin II levels rise and vascular resistance declines, reducing blood pressure.

Hydrochlorothiazide promotes movement of sodium, chloride, and water from blood in the peritubular capillaries into the nephron's distal convoluted tubule. Initially, the drug may decrease extracellular fluid volume, plasma volume, and cardiac output, which helps explain blood pressure reduction. It also may reduce blood pressure by dilating arteries. After several weeks, extracellular fluid volume, plasma volume, and cardiac output return to normal, and peripheral vascular resistance remains decreased.

Contraindications

Anuria; hypersensitivity to eprosartan, hydrochlorothiazide, other sulfonamide-derived drugs, or their components

Interactions

DRUGS

eprosartan and hydrochlorothiazide

diuretics, other antihypertensives: Increased antihypertensive effects
eprosartan component
cyclosporine, potassium-sparing diuretics, potassium supplements: Increased risk of hyperkalemia
hydrochlorothiazide component
amantadine: Possibly increased blood level and risk of toxicity of amantadine
amiodarone: Increased risk of arrhythmias from hypokalemia
amphotericin B, corticosteroids: Intensified electrolyte depletion, especially hypokalemia
antihypertensives: Increased antihypertensive effects
barbiturates, opioids: May potentiate orthostatic hypotension
calcium: Possibly increased serum calcium level
cholestyramine, colestipol resins: Reduced GI absorption of hydrochlorothiazide
diazoxide: Increased antihypertensive and hyperglycemic effects of hydrochlorothiazide
diflunisal: Possibly increased blood hydrochlorothiazide level
digoxin: Increased risk of digitalis toxicity from hypokalemia
dopamine: Possibly increased diuretic effects of both drugs
insulin, oral antidiabetics: Possibly increased blood glucose level
lithium: Decreased lithium clearance and increased risk of toxicity
neuromuscular blockers: Possibly enhanced neuromuscular blockade from hypokalemia
nondepolarizing skeletal muscle relaxants (such as tubocurarine): Possible increased responsiveness to the muscle relaxant
NSAIDs: Decreased diuretic effect of hydrochlorothiazide and increased risk of renal failure
pressor amines (such as norepinephrine): Possibly decreased response to pressor amines
oral anticoagulants: Possibly decreased anticoagulant effects
sympathomimetics: Possibly decreased antihypertensive effect of hydrochlorothiazide
vitamin D: Increased risk of hypercalcemia
FOODS
eprosartan component
high-potassium diet, potassium-containing salt substitutes: Increased risk of hyperkalemia

Adverse Reactions
CNS: Depression, dizziness, drowsiness, fatigue, headache, insomnia, paresthesia, vertigo, weakness
CV: Angina pectoris, atrial fibrillation, bradycardia, extrasystole,

hypertriglyceridemia, hypotension, orthostatic hypotension, palpitations, tachycardia, vasculitis

EENT: Blurred vision, dry mouth, pharyngitis, rhinitis

ENDO: Hyperglycemia

GI: Abdominal cramps or pain, anorexia, constipation, diarrhea, indigestion, jaundice, nausea, vomiting

GU: Decreased libido, impotence, interstitial nephritis, nocturia, polyuria, oliguria, renal failure, UTI

HEME: Agranulocytosis, aplastic and hemolytic anemia, leukopenia, neutropenia, thrombocytopenia

MS: Muscle spasms and weakness, myalgia, rhabdomyolysis

RESP: Cough, upper respirator tract infection

SKIN: Alopecia, exfoliative dermatitis, photosensitivity, purpura, rash, urticaria

Other: Anaphylaxis, angioedema, dehydration, hypercalcemia, hyperuricemia, hypochloremia, hypokalemia, hyponatremia, hypovolemia, metabolic alkalosis, weight loss

Nursing Considerations

- Use cautiously in patients with impaired hepatic function because hydrochlorothiazide may alter fluid and electrolyte balance and lead to hepatic coma.
- Also use cautiously in patients with systemic lupus erythematosus because hydrochlorothiazide may activate or worsen it.
- If patient has known or suspected hypovolemia, expect to correct it with I.V. normal saline solution, as prescribed, before starting eprosartan and hydrochlorothiazide.
- Monitor blood pressure often to assess effectiveness of eprosartan and hydrochlorothiazide therapy.
- If patient develops hypotension, expect to stop drug temporarily. Immediately place patient in supine position, and prepare to give I.V. normal saline solution, as prescribed. Expect to resume therapy after blood pressure stabilizes.
- Provide hydration, as appropriate, to help prevent hypovolemia.
- Monitor fluid intake and output, daily weight, and serum electrolyte levels (especially potassium) to detect volume depletion or electrolyte imbalance.
- **WARNING** Monitor patient closely for angioedema of the face, lips, tongue, glottis, larynx, or limbs. For angioedema of the face and lips, stop drug and give an antihistamine, as prescribed. If tongue, glottis, or larynx is involved, assess patient for airway obstruction, prepare to give epinephrine 1:1,000 (0.3 to 0.5 ml) subcutaneously, and maintain a patent airway.

- Watch for increased BUN and serum creatinine levels, especially in patients with impaired renal function, because drug may cause acute renal failure. If increases are significant or persistent, notify prescriber immediately.
- Monitor blood glucose level often in diabetic patients, and expect to increase antidiabetic dosage, as needed and ordered.

PATIENT TEACHING

- Advise patient to take eprosartan and hydrochlorothiazide in the morning or early evening to avoid the need to urinate during the night.
- Teach patient to monitor her blood pressure and to report consistently elevated measurements to prescriber.
- **WARNING** Strongly urge patient to contact prescriber before using potassium supplements or OTC salt substitutes, which may contain potassium. These products increase the risk of hyperkalemia.
- Direct patient to weigh herself at the same time each day wearing the same amount of clothing and to notify prescriber if she gains more than 2 lb (0.9 kg) per day or 5 lb (2.3 kg) per week.
- To reduce the risk of dehydration and hypotension, advise patient to avoid exercise in hot weather and to avoid alcohol. Also instruct her to notify prescriber if she has prolonged diarrhea, nausea, or vomiting.
- Caution patient to avoid potentially hazardous activities until drug's CNS effects are known.
- Explain the importance of regular exercise, proper diet, and other lifestyle changes in controlling hypertension.
- Advise female patient to notify prescriber immediately if she is or could be pregnant because eprosartan and hydrochlorothiazide will need to be replaced with another antihypertensive that's safe during the second and third trimesters of pregnancy.

ezetimibe and simvastatin
Vytorin

Class and Category
Chemical: Azetidinone (ezetimibe), synthetically derived fermentation product of *Aspergillus terreus* (simvastatin)
Therapeutic: Antihyperlipidemic
Pregnancy category: X

Indications and Dosages
▶ *To treat primary hypercholesterolemia*

TABLETS

Adults. *Initial:* 10 mg ezetimibe and 10 mg simvastatin daily for mild LDL cholesterol level reduction, 10 mg ezetimibe and 20 mg simvastatin daily for moderate LDL cholesterol level reduction, or 10 mg ezetimibe and 40 mg simvastatin daily for aggressive (more than 55%) LDL cholesterol level reduction. Dosage adjusted, as needed, after 2 or more weeks. *Maximum:* 10 mg ezetimibe and 80 mg simvastatin daily.

▶ *To treat homozygous familial hypercholesterolemia*

TABLETS

Adults. 10 mg ezetimibe and 40 mg simvastatin daily or 10 mg ezetimibe and 80 mg simvastatin daily h.s.

DOSAGE ADJUSTMENT For patients with severe renal insufficiency, ezetimibe and simvastatin are given only if patient has already taken simvastatin at a dose of 5 mg or higher. For patients taking cyclosporine, ezetimibe and simvastatin are given only if patient has already taken simvastatin at a dose of 5 mg or higher, and the dosage shouldn't exceed 10 mg ezetimibe and 10 mg simvastatin daily. For patients who take amiodarone or verapamil, dosage shouldn't exceed 10 mg ezetimibe and 20 mg simvastatin daily.

Mechanism of Action

Ezetimibe and simvastatin work together to decrease the serum cholesterol level. Normally, lipids in the intestinal lumen break down into cholesterol and other substances that create smaller droplets called micelles. Micelles enter intestinal epithelial cells (called enterocytes), where they combine with triglycerides, cholesterol, and other substances to form chylomicrons. Chylomicrons enter the lymphatic system and are carried to the bloodstream.

Ezetimibe blocks cholesterol absorption into enterocytes. This decreased movement of cholesterol through the intestinal wall decreases chylomicron and LDL cholesterol levels in the bloodstream.

Simvastatin interferes with the hepatic enzyme hydroxymethylglutaryl-coenzyme A reductase. This action reduces formation of mevalonic acid, a cholesterol precursor, thus interrupting cholesterol synthesis. When the cholesterol level declines in hepatic cells, LDLs are consumed, which in turn reduces the levels of circulating total cholesterol and serum triglycerides.

Contraindications

Active liver disease; breastfeeding; hypersensitivity to ezetimibe, simvastatin, or their components; pregnancy

Interactions
DRUGS
ezetimibe component
cholestyramine: Reduced ezetimibe effectiveness
cyclosporine, fenofibrate, gemfibrozil: Increased blood ezetimibe level
simvastatin component
amiodarone, clarithromycin, cyclosporine, danazol, erythromycin, gemfibrozil and other fibrates, itraconazole, ketoconazole, nefazodone, niacin at 1 g or more daily, protease inhibitors (amprenavir, indinavir, nelfinavir, ritonavir, saquinavir), telithromycin, verapamil: Increased risk of myopathy or rhabdomyolysis
azole antifungals, cyclosporine, gemfibrozil, immunosuppressants, macrolide antibiotics (including erythromycin), niacin, verapamil: Increased risk of acute renal failure
bile acid sequestrants, cholestyramine, colestipol: Decreased bioavailability of simvastatin
digoxin: Possibly slight elevation in blood digoxin level
diltiazem, verapamil: Possibly increased blood simvastatin level and increased risk of myopathy
oral anticoagulants: Increased risk of bleeding or prolonged PT
FOODS
simvastatin component
grapefruit juice (1 or more quarts/day): Possibly increased blood simvastatin level; increased risk of myopathy or rhabdomyolysis

Adverse Reactions
CNS: Asthenia, dizziness, fatigue, headache
CV: Chest pain
EENT: Pharyngitis, rhinitis, sinusitis, taste alteration
GI: Abdominal pain, cholelithiasis, cholecystitis, constipation, diarrhea, elevated liver function test results, flatulence, heartburn, hepatitis, nausea, pancreatitis, vomiting
HEME: Thrombocytopenia
MS: Arthralgia, back pain, myalgia, myopathy, rhabdomyolysis
RESP: Cough, upper respiratory tract infection
SKIN: Eczema, pruritus, rash
Other: Angioedema, viral infection

Nursing Considerations
- Use ezetimibe and simvastatin cautiously in elderly patients and those with hepatic or renal impairment.
- Monitor patient's liver function test results before and every 3 to 6 months during therapy, as ordered.

- Give ezetimibe and simvastatin 2 hours before or 4 hours after giving a bile acid sequestrant such as cholestyramine or colestipol).
- Monitor serum lipoprotein level, as ordered, to evaluate patient's response to therapy.

PATIENT TEACHING
- Advise patient to take ezetimibe and simvastatin in the evening.
- Encourage patient to follow a low-fat and low-cholesterol diet.
- Instruct patient who's taking a bile acid sequestrant (cholestyramine, colestipol) to take ezetimibe and simvastatin 2 hours before or 4 hours after taking the bile acid sequestrant.
- Urge patient to notify prescriber immediately if he develops symptoms of myopathy, such as muscle pain, tenderness, and weakness.
- Instruct female patient of childbearing age to use reliable contraception while taking drug. Instruct her to notify prescriber at once if she suspects pregnancy.
- Urge patient to avoid grapefruit juice to decrease risk of toxicity.

fosinopril sodium and hydrochlorothiazide
Monopril HCT

Class and Category
Chemical: Phosphinic acid derivative (fosinopril), benothiadiazide (hydrochlorothiazide)
Therapeutic: Antihypertensive (fosinopril, hydrochlorothiazide), diuretic (hydrochlorothiazide)
Pregnancy category: C (first trimester), D (second and third trimesters)

Indications and Dosages
▶ *To treat hypertension uncontrolled by fosinopril or hydrochlorothiazide alone*
TABLETS
Adults. *Initial:* 10 mg fosinopril and 12.5 mg hydrochlorothiazide (1 tablet) daily. Increased, as needed, to 20 mg fosinopril and 12.5 mg hydrochlorothiazide (1 tablet) daily.

Contraindications
Anuria; hypersensitivity to fosinopril, hydrochlorothiazide, other ACE inhibitors or sulfonamide-derived drugs, or their components

Mechanism of Action

Fosinopril may reduce blood pressure by affecting the renin-angiotensin-aldosterone system. By inhibiting ACE, fosinopril:

• prevents conversion of angiotensin I to angiotensin II, a potent vasoconstrictor that also stimulates adrenal cortex to secrete aldosterone.
• may inhibit renal and vascular production of angiotensin II.
• decreases serum angiotensin II level and increases serum renin activity. This decreases aldosterone secretion, slightly increasing serum potassium level and fluid loss.
• decreases vascular tone and blood pressure.
• inhibits aldosterone release, which reduces sodium and water reabsorption and increases their excretion, further reducing blood pressure.

Hydrochlorothiazide promotes movement of sodium, chloride, and water from blood in the peritubular capillaries into the nephron's distal convoluted tubule. Initially, it may decrease extracellular fluid volume, plasma volume, and cardiac output, which helps explain blood pressure reduction. It also may reduce blood pressure by dilating arteries. After several weeks, extracellular fluid volume, plasma volume, and cardiac output return to normal, and peripheral vascular resistance remains decreased.

Interactions

DRUGS

fosinopril and hydrochlorothiazide

antihypertensives, diuretics: Increased antihypertensive effects
digoxin: Increased serum digoxin level and risk of digitalis toxicity
lithium: Increased serum lithium levels and toxicity

fosinopril component

allopurinol, bone marrow depressants, procainaminde, systemic corticosteroids: Increased risk of potentially fatal neutropenia or agranulocytosis
antacids: Possibly decreased bioavailability of fosinopril from impaired absorption
cyclosporine, potassium-sparing diuretics (amiloride, spironolactone, triamterene), potassium supplements: Increased risk of hyperkalemia

hydrochlorothiazide component

amantadine: Possibly increased blood amantadine level and risk of toxicity
amiodarone: Increased risk of arrhythmias from hypokalemia
amphotericin B, corticosteroids: Intensified electrolyte depletion, especially hypokalemia
antihypertensives: Increased antihypertensive effects

barbiturates, opioids: May potentiate orthostatic hypotension
calcium: Possibly increased serum calcium level
cholestyramine, colestipol resins: Reduced GI absorption of hydrochlorothiazide
diazoxide: Increased antihypertensive and hyperglycemic effects of
hydrochlorothiazide
diflunisal: Possibly increased blood hydrochlorothiazide level
digoxin: Increased risk of digitalis toxicity from hypokalemia
dopamine: Possibly increased diuretic effects of both drugs
insulin, oral antidiabetics: Possibly increased blood glucose level
lithium: Decreased lithium clearance and increased risk of toxicity
neuromuscular blockers: Possibly enhanced neuromuscular blockade
from hypokalemia
nondepolarizing skeletal muscle relaxants (such as tubocurarine): Possibly increased responsiveness to the muscle relaxant
NSAIDs: Decreased diuretic effect of hydrochlorothiazide, increased risk of renal failure
pressor amines (such as norepinephrine): Possibly decreased response
to pressor amines
oral anticoagulants: Possibly decreased anticoagulant effects
sympathomimetics: Possibly decreased antihypertensive effect of hydrochlorothiazide
vitamin D: Increased risk of hypercalcemia
FOODS
fosinopril component
salt substitutes that contain potassium: Increased risk of hyperkalemia
ACTIVITIES
fosinopril component
alcohol use: Possibly additive hypotension

Adverse Reactions

CNS: Confusion, depression, dizziness, drowsiness, fatigue, fever,
headache, insomnia, mood swings, paresthesia, sleep disturbance,
syncope, tremor, vertigo, weakness
CV: Angina, arrhythmias (including AV conduction disorders,
bradycardia, and tachycardia), claudication, hypotension, MI, orthostatic hypotension, palpitations, vasculitis
EENT: Blurred vision, dry mouth, epistaxis, eye irritation,
hoarseness, rhinitis, sinus problems, taste perversion, tinnitus, vision changes
ENDO: Hyperglycemia
GI: Abdominal cramps, distention, or pain; anorexia; constipa-

tion; diarrhea; flatulence; hepatic failure; hepatitis; hepatomegaly; indigestion; jaundice; nausea; pancreatitis; vomiting
GU: Decreased libido, flank pain, impotence, interstitial nephritis, nocturia, polyuria, renal insufficiency or failure, urinary frequency
HEME: Agranulocytosis, aplastic and hemolytic anemia, leukopenia, neutropenia, thrombocytopenia
MS: Arthralgia, muscle spasms and weakness, myalgia
RESP: Asthma; bronchitis; bronchospasm; dry, persistent, tickling cough; dyspnea; tracheobronchitis; upper respiratory tract infection
SKIN: Alopecia, diaphoresis, exfoliative dermatitis, photosensitivity, pruritus, purpura, rash, urticaria
Other: Anaphylaxis, angioedema, dehydration, gout, hypercalcemia, hyperkalemia, hyperuricemia, hypochloremia, hypokalemia, hyponatremia, hypovolemia, metabolic alkalosis, weight gain or loss

Nursing Considerations

- Use cautiously in patients with impaired hepatic function because hydrochlorothiazide may alter fluid and electrolyte balance and cause hepatic coma.
- Also use cautiously in patients with systemic lupus erythematosus because hydrochlorothiazide may activate or worsen it.
- Monitor blood pressure often to assess effectiveness of fosinopril and hydrochlorothiazide therapy.
- Assess patient for hypotension for at least 2 hours after giving fosinopril and hydrochlorothiazide. If present, notify precriber and monitor patient until blood pressure stabilizes. Provide supportive measures, as indicated and ordered.
- If patient receives an antacid, separate administration times by at least 2 hours.
- **WARNING** Monitor patient closely for signs and symptoms of angioedema or allergic reactions such as rash, urticaria, or difficulty breathing. If present, withhold drug, notify prescriber immediately, and expect to treat symptomatically. If airway obstruction threatens, promptly give 0.3 to 0.5 ml of epinephrine solution 1:1,000 subcutaneously, as prescribed.
- Provide adequate hydration, as appropriate, to help prevent hypovolemia.
- Monitor fluid intake and output, daily weight, and serum electrolyte levels (especially potassium) to detect volume depletion or electrolyte imbalance.

- Watch for increased BUN and serum creatinine levels, especially in patients with impaired renal function, because drug may cause acute renal failure. If increases are significant or persistent, notify prescriber immediately.
- Monitor blood glucose level often in diabetic patients, and expect to increase antidiabetic dosage, as needed and ordered.
- Check WBC count periodically, especially in patients with collagen-vascular disease, to detect neutropenia and agranulocytosis. Although they aren't known to occur with fosinopril, they have occurred with captropril, another ACE inhibitor.
- Assess liver enzymes periodically, and monitor patient for jaundice because hepatic failure, although rare, has occurred with other ACE inhibitors. If liver enzymes develop marked elevation or patient develops jaundice, notify prescriber and expect to stop fosinopril and hydrochlorothiazide.

PATIENT TEACHING
- Advise patient to take fosinopril and hydrochlorothiazide in the morning or early evening to avoid the need to urinate during the night.
- Teach patient to monitor her blood pressure and pulse rate and to report consistently elevated measurements to prescriber.
- **WARNING** Instruct patient to contact prescriber immediately if she has evidence of hypersensitivity, especially angioedema (swelling of the face, eyes, lips or tongue), difficulty breathing, hives, or rash.
- Direct patient to weigh herself at the same time each day wearing the same amount of clothing and to notify prescriber if she gains more than 2 lb (0.9 kg) per day or 5 lb (2.3 kg) per week.
- To reduce the risk of dehydration and hypotension, advise patient to avoid exercise in hot weather and to avoid alcohol. Also tell her to notify prescriber if she has prolonged diarrhea, nausea, or vomiting.
- Caution patient to avoid potentially hazardous activities until drug's CNS effects are known.
- Explain the importance of regular exercise, proper diet, and other lifestyle changes in controlling hypertension.
- **WARNING** Strongly urge patient to contact prescriber before using potassium supplements or OTC salt substitutes, which may contain potassium. These products increase the risk of hyperkalemia.
- Advise female patient to notify prescriber immediately if she is or could be pregnant because fosinopril and hydrochloroth-

iazide will need to be replaced with another antihypertensive that's safe during the second and third trimesters of pregnancy.

- Warn patient with gout that drug may precipitate an acute gout attack.
- Inform patient that a persistent dry cough may develop and may not subside unless fosinopril and hydrochlorothiazide therapy is stopped. If cough becomes bothersome or interferes with her sleep or activities, instruct her to notify prescriber.
- Tell patient to avoid sudden position changes and to rise slowly from a seated or reclining position to minimize orthostatic hypotension.

hydralazine and hydrochlorothiazide
Apresazide, Hydra-Zide

Class and Category
Chemical: Phthalazine derivative (hydralazine), benzothiadiazide (hydrochlorothiazide)
Therapeutic: Antihyperthenisve (hydralazine, hydrochlorothiazide), diuretic (hydrochlorothiazide)
Pregnancy category: C

Indications and Dosages
▶ *To treat hypertension*
CAPSULES
Adults. 25 to 100 mg hydralazine and 25 to 50 mg hydrochlorothiazide (1 to 2 capsules depending on product) b.i.d.

Mechanism of Action
Hydralazine exerts a direct vasodilating effect on smooth muscle in arterioles, interferes with calcium movement in arteriole smooth muscle by altering cellular calcium metabolism, and dilates arteries to lower blood pressure.

Hydrochlorothiazide promotes movement of sodium, chloride, and water from blood in the peritubular capillaries into the nephron's distal convoluted tubule. Initially, it may decrease extracellular fluid volume, plasma volume, and cardiac output, which helps explain blood pressure reduction. It also may reduce blood pressure by dilating arteries. After several weeks, extracellular fluid volume, plasma volume, and cardiac output return to normal, and peripheral vascular resistance remains decreased.

Contraindications
Anuria; coronary artery or rheumatic heart disease; hypersensitiv-

ity to hydralazine, hydrochlorothiazide, other sulfonamide-derived drugs or their components; mitral valve disease

Interactions
DRUGS
hydralazine and hydrochlorothiazide
antihypertensives, diazoxide: Risk of severe hypotension
NSAIDs, sympathomimetics: Decreased antihypertensive effect
hydralazine component
beta blockers: Increased effects of both drugs
epinephrine: Possibly decreased vasopressor effect of epinephrine
hydrochlorothiazide component
amantadine: Possibly increased blood amantadine level and risk of toxicity
amiodarone: Increased risk of arrhythmias from hypokalemia
amphotericin B, corticosteroids: Intensified electrolyte depletion, especially hypokalemia
antihypertensives: Increased antihypertensive effects
barbiturates, opioids: May potentiate orthostatic hypotension
calcium: Possibly increased serum calcium level
cholestyramine, colestipol resins: Reduced GI absorption of hydrochlorothiazide
diazoxide: Increased hyperglycemic effects of hydrochlorothiazide
diflunisal: Possibly increased blood hydrochlorothiazide level
digoxin: Increased risk of digitalis toxicity from hypokalemia
dopamine: Possibly increased diuretic effects of both drugs
insulin, oral antidiabetics: Possibly increased blood glucose level
lithium: Decreased lithium clearance and increased risk of toxicity
MAO inhibitors: Risk of severe hypotension
neuromuscular blockers: Possibly enhanced neuromuscular blockade from hypokalemia
nondepolarizing skeletal muscle relaxants (such as tubocurarine): Possibly increased responsiveness to the muscle relaxant
NSAIDs: Increased risk of renal failure
pressor amines (such as norepinephrine): Possibly decreased response to pressor amines
oral anticoagulants: Possibly decreased anticoagulant effects
vitamin D: Increased risk of hypercalcemia
FOODS
hydralazine component
all foods: Possibly increased bioavailability of hydralazine
ACTIVITIES
hydralazine and hydrochlorothiazide

alcohol use: Potentiated hypotensive effect

Adverse Reactions

CNS: Chills, dizziness, fever, headache, insomnia, paresthesia, peripheral neuritis, vertigo, weakness

CV: Angina, edema, hypotension, orthostatic hypotension, palpitations, tachycardia, vasculitis

EENT: Blurred vision, dry mouth, lacrimation, nasal congestion

ENDO: Hyperglycemia

GI: Abdominal cramps, anorexia, constipation, diarrhea, indigestion, jaundice, nausea, vomiting

GU: Decreased libido, impotence, interstitial nephritis, nocturia, polyuria, proteinurea, renal failure

HEME: Agranulocytosis, aplastic and hemolytic anemia, leukopenia, neutropenia, thrombocytopenia

MS: Muscle spasms and weakness

RESP: Dyspnea

SKIN: Alopecia, blisters, exfoliative dermatitis, flushing, photosensitivity, pruritus, purpura, rash, urticaria

Other: Anaphylaxis, dehydration, gout, hypercalcemia, hyperuricemia, hypochloremia, hypokalemia, hyponatremia, hypovolemia, lupus-like symptoms, lymphadenopathy, metabolic alkalosis, weight loss

Nursing Considerations

- Use cautiously in patients with impaired hepatic function because hydrochlorothiazide component of drug may alter fluid and electrolyte balance, which may precipitate hepatic coma.
- Also use cautiously in patients with systemic lupus erythematosus because hydrochlorothiazide component of drug may activate or cause an exacerbation of the disorder and hydralazine component may cause lupus-like symptoms.
- Give drug with food to increase bioavailability.
- Monitor CBC, lupus erythematosus cell preparation, and ANA titer before and periodically during long-term treatment.
- **WARNING** Expect to stop drug immediately if patient develops lupus-like symptoms, such as arthralgia, fever, myalgia, pharyngitis, and splenomegaly.
- Check blood pressure often to assess effectiveness of hydralazine and hydrochlorothiazide therapy.
- Provide hydration, as appropriate, to help prevent hypovolemia.
- Monitor fluid intake and output, daily weight, and serum electrolyte levels (especially potassium) to detect volume depletion or electrolyte imbalance.

- Monitor for increased BUN and serum creatinine levels, especially in patients with impaired renal function, because drug may cause acute renal failure. If increases are significant or persistent, notify prescriber immediately.
- Monitor blood glucose level often in diabetic patients, and expect to increase antidiabetic dosage, as needed and ordered.
- Expect prescriber to withdraw drug gradually to avoid a rapid increase in blood pressure.
- Expect to treat peripheral neuritis with pyridoxine if it occurs.

PATIENT TEACHING

- Advise patient to take hydralazine and hydrochlorothiazide with food to increase absorption and in the morning or early evening to avoid the need to urinate during the night.
- Direct patient to weigh herself at the same time each day wearing the same amount of clothing and to notify prescriber if she gains more than 2 lb (0.9 kg) per day or 5 lb (2.3 kg) per week.
- Instruct patient to eat a diet high in potassium-rich foods, such as citrus fruits, bananas, tomatoes, and dates.
- To reduce the risk of dehydration and hypotension, advise patient to avoid exercise in hot weather and top avoid alcohol. Also instruct her to notify prescriber if she has prolonged diarrhea, nausea, or vomiting.
- Urge patient to change position slowly, especially in the morning. Caution her that hot showers may increase hypotension.
- Instruct patient to immediately notify prescriber about fever, muscle and joint aches, and sore throat.
- Urge patient to report numbness and tingling in her limbs, which may require treatment with another drug.
- Caution patient to avoid potentially hazardous activities until drug's CNS effects are known.
- Caution patient against stopping drug abruptly because doing so may cause severe rise in her blood pressure.
- Advise patient to avoid direct sunlight including ultraviolet light as much as possible and to wear protective clothing including a hat and use a sunscreen when exposure can not be avoided.

hydrochlorothiazide and triamterene
Dyazide, Maxzide

Class and Category
Chemical: benothiadiazide (hydrochlorothiazide), pterdine derivative (triamterene)

Therapeutic: Antihypertensive (hydrochlorothiazide, triamterene), diuretic (hydrochlorothiazide)
Pregnancy category: C

Indications and Dosages

▶ *To treat hypertension or edema in patients adequately controlled by hydrochlorothiazide alone but who develop significant potassium loss; to treat hypertension in patients uncontrolled with triamterene monotherapy*

CAPSULES

Adults. 25 mg hydrochlorothiazide and 37.5 mg triamterene (1 capsule) daily. Increased, as needed, to 50 mg hydrochlorothiazide and 75 mg triamterene (2 capsules) daily.

Mechanism of Action

Hydrochlorothiazide promotes movement of sodium, chloride, and water from blood in the peritubular capillaries into the nephron's distal convoluted tubule. Initially, it may decrease extracellular fluid volume, plasma volume, and cardiac output, which helps explain blood pressure reduction. It also may reduce blood pressure by dilating arteries. After several weeks, extracellular fluid volume, plasma volume, and cardiac output return to normal, and peripheral vascular resistance remains decreased.

Triamterene inhibits sodium reabsorption in distal convoluted tubules and cortical collecting ducts, causing sodium and water loss, which reduces blood pressure. It also enhances potassium retention.

Contraindications

Anuria; diabetic nephropathy or renal disease linked to renal insufficiency; hyperkalemia (potassium level of 5.5 mEq/L or more); hypersensitivity to hydrochlorothiazide, triamterene, other sulfonamide-derived drugs, or their components; severe hepatic dysfunction

Interactions

DRUGS

hydrochlorothiazide and triamterene

amantadine: Possibly increased blood level and risk of toxicity of amantadine

antihypertensives, diuretics: Increased antihypertensive effects

chlorpropamide: Increased risk of severe hyponatremia

exchange resins (such as sodium polystyrene sulfonate): Decreased serum potassium levels; increased fluid retention

insulin, oral antidiabetics: Possibly increased blood glucose level

lithium: Decreased lithium clearance and increased risk of toxicity

NSAIDs: Decreased diuretic effect of hydrochlorothiazide and triamterene, increased risk of renal failure

hydrochlorothiazide component

amiodarone: Increased risk of arrhythmias from hypokalemia

amphotericin B, corticosteroids: Intensified electrolyte depletion, especially hypokalemia

barbiturates, opioids: May potentiate orthostatic hypotension

calcium: Possibly increased serum calcium level

cholestyramine, colestipol resins: Reduced GI absorption of hydrochlorothiazide

diazoxide: Increased antihypertensive and hyperglycemic effects of hydrochlorothiazide

diflunisal: Possibly increased blood hydrochlorothiazide level

digoxin: Increased risk of digitalis toxicity from hypokalemia

dopamine: Possibly increased diuretic effects of both drugs

methenamine: Possibly decreased effectiveness of methenamine

neuromuscular blockers: Possibly enhanced neuromuscular blockade from hypokalemia

nondepolarizing skeletal muscle relaxants (such as tubocurarine): Possibly increased responsiveness to the muscle relaxant

pressor amines (such as norepinephrine): Possibly decreased response to pressor amines

oral anticoagulants: Possibly decreased anticoagulant effects

sympathomimetics: Possibly decreased antihypertensive effect of hydrochlorothiazide

vitamin D: Increased risk of hypercalcemia

triamterene component

ACE inhibitors, amiloride, angiotensin-II receptor antagonists, cyclosporine, heparin, potassium-containing drugs, potassium salts, potassium supplements, spironolactone: Increased risk of hyperkalemia

folic acid: Possibly antagonized action of folic acid

laxatives: Possibly reduced potassium-retaining effects of triamterene

Adverse Reactions

CNS: Dizziness, fatigue, headache, insomnia, paresthesia, vertigo, weakness

CV: Hypotension, orthostatic hypotension, vasculitis

EENT: Blurred vision, dry mouth

ENDO: Hyperglycemia, hypoglycemia

GI: Abdominal cramps, anorexia, constipation, diarrhea, indigestion, jaundice, nausea, vomiting

GU: Azotemia, decreased libido, impotence, elevated BUN and serum creatinine levels, interstitial nephritis, nocturia, polyuria, renal calculi, renal failure

HEME: Agranulocytosis, aplastic and hemolytic anemia, leukopenia, neutropenia, thrombocytopenia

MS: Muscle spasms and weakness

SKIN: Alopecia, exfoliative dermatitis, photosensitivity, purpura, rash, urticaria

Other: Anaphylaxis, dehydration, hypercalcemia, hyperkalemia, hyperuricemia, hypochloremia, hypokalemia, hyponatremia, hypovolemia, metabolic alkalosis, weight loss

Nursing Considerations

- Use cautiously in patients with impaired hepatic function because hydrochlorothiazide may alter fluid and electrolyte balance and lead to hepatic coma.
- Also use cautiously in patients with systemic lupus erythematosus because hydrochlorothiazide may activate or worsen it.
- Be aware that hydrochlorothiazide and triamterene shouldn't be given to patients with creatinine clearance below 10 ml/min/1.73 m^2 because they have an increased risk of drug-induced hyperkalemia.
- Check blood pressure often to assess effectiveness of hydrochlorothiazide and triamterene therapy.
- Provide hydration, as appropriate, to help prevent hypovolemia.
- Monitor fluid intake and output, daily weight, and serum electrolyte levels (especially potassium) to detect volume depletion or electrolyte imbalance.
- Monitor patient for evidence of hyperkalemia, such as irregular heartbeat (usualy the first sign), paresthesia, muscle weakness, fatigue, flaccid paralysis of the limbs, bradycardia, and shock. In suspected hyperkalemia, obtain an ECG tracing, as ordered. A widened QRS complex or an arrhythmia warrants prompt treatment. If hyperkalemia is confirmed, drug must be stopped.
- Watch for increased BUN and serum creatinine levels, especially in patients with impaired renal function, because drug may cause acute renal failure. If increases are significant or persistent, notify prescriber immediately.
- Monitor blood glucose level often in diabetic patients, and expect to increase antidiabetic dosage, as needed and ordered.
- Assess patient for evidence of metabolic or respiratory acidosis, which may occur suddenly in patients with cardiac disease or uncontrolled diabetes mellitus.

- Monitor patient's serum uric acid level, as ordered, because drug may reduce uric acid clearance and increase the risk of gout and hyperuricemia. It also may worsen hyponatremia.
- Monitor CBC with differential because hydrochlorothiazide may increase the risk of serious hematologic adverse effects and triamterene may increase the risk of megaloblastic anemia in a patient with folic acid deficiency.

PATIENT TEACHING
- Teach patient to monitor her blood pressure and pulse rate and to report consistent changes to prescriber.
- Advise patient to take hydrochlorothiazide and triamterene in the morning or early evening to avoid the need to urinate during the night.
- Instruct patient to take drug with milk or food to minimize stomach upset.
- Direct patient to weigh herself at the same time each day wearing the same amount of clothing and to notify prescriber if she gains more than 2 lb (0.9 kg) per day or 5 lb (2.3 kg) per week.
- To reduce the risk of dehydration and hypotension, advise patient to avoid exercise in hot weather and to avoid alcohol. Also instruct her to notify prescriber if she has prolonged diarrhea, nausea, or vomiting.
- Caution patient to avoid potentially hazardous activities until drug's CNS effects are known.
- Explain the importance of regular exercise, proper diet, and other lifestyle changes in controlling hypertension.
- Instruct patient to minimize exposure to sunlight.
- Explain to patient with a history of gout that drug may increase the risk of an attack.

irbesartan and hydrochlorothiazide
Avalide

Class and Category
Chemical: Nonpeptide angiotensin II antagonist (irbesartan), benothiadiazide (hydrochlorothiazide)
Therapeutic: Antihypertensive (irbesartan, hydrochlorothiazide), diuretic (hydrochlorothiazide)
Pregnancy category: C (first trimester), D (second and third trimesters)

Indications and Dosages

▶ *To treat hypertension uncontrolled by irbesartan or hydrochlorothiazide*
TABLETS
Adults. *Initial:* 150 mg irbesartan and 12.5 mg hydrochlorothiazide (1 tablet) daily. May be increased to 300 mg irbesartan and 12.5 mg hydrcholorothiazide (1 tablet) daily, as needed, in 2 to 4 wk. *Maximum:* 300 mg irbesartan and 25 mg hydrochlorothiazide daily.

Contraindications

Anuria; hypersensitivity to irbesartan, hydrochlorothiazide, other sulfonamide-derived drugs, or their components

---

Mechanism of Action

Irbesartan selectively blocks binding of the potent vasoconstrictor angiotension (AT) II to AT1 receptor sites in many tissues, including vascular smooth muscle and adrenal glands. This inhibits the vasoconstrictive and aldosterone-secreting effects of AT II, which reduces blood pressure.

Hydrochlorothiazide promotes movement of sodium, chloride, and water from blood in peritubular capillaries into the nephron's distal convoluted tubule. Initially, it may decrease extracellular fluid volume, plasma volume, and cardiac output, which helps explain blood pressure reduction. It also may reduce blood pressure by dilating arteries. After several weeks, extracellular fluid volume, plasma volume, and cardiac output return to normal, and peripheral vascular resistance remains decreased.

Interactions
DRUGS
irbesartan and hydrochlorothiazide
diuretics, other antihypertensives: Increased antihypertensive effects
hydrochlorothiazide component
amantadine: Possibly increased blood amantadine level and risk of toxicity
amiodarone: Increased risk of arrhythmias from hypokalemia
amphotericin B, corticosteroids: Intensified electrolyte depletion, especially hypokalemia
barbiturates, opioids: May potentiate orthostatic hypotension
calcium: Possibly increased serum calcium level
cholestyramine, colestipol resins: Reduced GI absorption of hydrochlorothiazide
diazoxide: Increased antihypertensive and hyperglycemic effects of hydrochlorothiazide
diflunisal: Possibly increased blood hydrochlorothiazide level

digoxin: Increased risk of digitalis toxicity from hypokalemia
dopamine: Possibly increased diuretic effects of both drugs
insulin, oral antidiabetics: Possibly increased blood glucose level
lithium: Decreased lithium clearance and increased risk of toxicity
neuromuscular blockers: Possibly enhanced neuromuscular blockade from hypokalemia
nondepolarizing skeletal muscle relaxants (such as tubocurarine): Possibly increased responsiveness to the muscle relaxant
NSAIDs: Decreased diuretic effect of hydrochlorothiazide, increased risk of renal failure
pressor amines (such as norepinephrine): Possible decreased response to pressor amines
oral anticoagulants: Possibly decreased anticoagulant effects
sympathomimetics: Possibly decreased antihypertensive effect of hydrochlorothiazide
vitamin D: Increased risk of hypercalcemia

Adverse Reactions

CNS: Anxiety, dizziness, fatigue, headache, insomnia, nervousness, paresthesia, vertigo, weakness
CV: Chest pain, hypotension, orthostatic hypotension, peripheral edema, tachycardia, vasculitis
EENT: Blurred vision, dry mouth, pharyngitis, rhinitis
ENDO: Hyperglycemia
GI: Abdominal cramps or pain, anorexia, constipation, diarrhea, heartburn, indigestion, jaundice, nausea, vomiting
GU: Decreased libido, impotence, interstitial nephritis, nocturia, polyuria, renal failure, UTI
HEME: Agranulocytosis, aplastic and hemolytic anemia, leukopenia, neutropenia, thrombocytopenia
MS: Muscle spasms and weakness, musculoskeletal pain
RESP: Upper respiratory tract infection
SKIN: Alopecia, exfoliative dermatitis, photosensitivity, purpura, rash, urticaria
Other: Anaphylaxis, angioedema, dehydration, hypercalcemia, hyperuricemia, hypochloremia, hypokalemia, hyponatremia, hypovolemia, metabolic alkalosis, weight loss

Nursing Considerations

• Use cautiously in patients with impaired hepatic function because hydrochlorothiazide may alter fluid and electrolyte balance and lead to hepatic coma.
• Also use cautiously in patients with systemic lupus erythematosus because hydrochlorothiazide may activate or worsen it.

- If patient has known or suspected hypovolemia, expect to correct it with I.V. normal saline solution, as prescribed, before starting irbesartan and hydrochlorothiazide. Provide hydration as needed during therapy to help prevent hypovolemia.
- Monitor blood pressure often to assess effectiveness of therapy with irbesartan and hydrochlorothiazide.
- If patient develops hypotension, expect to stop drug temporarily. Immediately place patient in supine position, and prepare to give I.V. normal saline solution, as prescribed. Expect to resume therapy after blood pressure stabilizes.
- **WARNING** Monitor patient closely for angioedema of the face, lips, tongue, glottis, larynx, or limbs. For angioedema of the face and lips, stop drug and give an antihistamine, as prescribed. If tongue, glottis, or larynx is involved, assess patient for airway obstruction, prepare to give epinephrine 1:1,000 (0.3 to 0.5 ml) subcutaneously, and maintain a patent airway.
- Monitor fluid intake and output, daily weight, and serum electrolyte levels (especially potassium) to detect volume depletion or electrolyte imbalance.
- Watch for increased BUN and serum creatinine levels, especially in patients with impaired renal function, because drug may cause acute renal failure. If increases are significant or persistent, notify prescriber immediately.
- Monitor blood glucose level often in diabetic patients, and expect to increase antidiabetic dosage, as needed and ordered.

PATIENT TEACHING
- Advise patient to take drug in the morning or early evening to avoid the need to urinate during the night.
- Teach patient to monitor her blood pressure and to report consistently elevated measurements to prescriber.
- Direct patient to weigh herself at the same time each day wearing the same amount of clothing and to notify prescriber if she gains more than 2 lb (0.9 kg) per day or 5 lb (2.3 kg) per week.
- To reduce the risk of dehydration and hypotension, advise patient to avoid exercise in hot weather and to avoid alcohol. Also instruct her to notify prescriber if she has prolonged diarrhea, nausea, or vomiting.
- Caution patient to avoid potentially hazardous activities until drug's CNS effects are known.
- Explain the importance of regular exercise, proper diet, and other lifestyle changes in controlling hypertension.
- Advise female patient to notify prescriber immediately if she is or could be pregnant; irbesartan and hydrochlorothiazide will

need to be replaced with another antihypertensive that's safe to use during second and third trimesters of pregnancy.

lisinopril and hydrochlorothiazide
Zestoretic

Class and Category
Chemical: Lysine ester of enaprilat (lisinopril), benothiadiazide (hydrochlorothiazide)
Therapeutic: Antihypertensive (lisinopril, hydrochlorothiazide), diuretic (hydrochlorothiazide)
Pregnancy category: C (first trimester), D (second and third trimesters)

Indications and Dosages
▶ *To treat hypertension uncontrolled by lisinopril or hydrochlorothiazide*
TABLETS
Adults. *Initial:* Depending on current lisinopril or hydrochlorothiazide therapy, 10 mg lisinopril and 12.5 mg hydrochlorothiazide (1 tablet) or 20 mg lisinopril and 12.5 mg hydrochlorothiazide (1 tablet) daily. May be increased, as needed q 2 to 3 wk. *Maximum:* 20 mg lisinopril and 25 mg hydrochlorothiazide daily.

Mechanism of Action
Lisinopril may reduce blood pressure by affecting the renin-angiotensin-aldosterone system. By inhibiting ACE, lisinopril:
- prevents conversion of angiotensin I to angiotensin II, a potent vasoconstrictor that also stimulates adrenal cortex to secrete aldosterone.
- may inhibit renal and vascular production of angiotensin II.
- decreases serum angiotensin II level and increases serum renin activity. This decreases aldosterone secretion, slightly increasing serum potassium level and fluid loss.
- decreases vascular tone and blood pressure.
- inhibits aldosterone release, which reduces sodium and water reabsorption and increases their excretion, further reducing blood pressure.

Hydrochlorothiazide promotes movement of sodium, chloride, and water from blood in peritubular capillaries into the nephron's distal convoluted tubule. Initially, it may decrease extracellular fluid volume, plasma volume, and cardiac output, which helps explain blood pressure reduction. It also may reduce blood pressure by dilating arteries. After several weeks, extracellular fluid volume, plasma volume, and cardiac output return to normal, and peripheral vascular resistance remains decreased.

Contraindications
Anuria; hereditary or idiopathic angioedema; history of angioedema from previous ACE inhibitor; hypersensitivity to lisinopril, hydrochlorothiazide, other ACE inhibitors, other sulfonamide-derived drugs, or their components

Interactions
DRUGS
lisinopril and hydrochlorothiazide
antihypertensives, diuretics: Increased antihypertensive effects
lithium: Increased blood lithium level and toxicity
NSAIDs, sympathomimetics: Possibly reduced antihypertensive effects of lisinopril and hydrochlorothiazide and increased risk of renal toxicity
lisinopril component
allopurinol, bone marrow depressants (such as amphotericin B and methotrexate), procainamide, systemic corticosteroids: Possibly increased risk of fatal neutropenia or agranulocytosis
cyclosporine, potassium-sparing diuretics, potassium supplements: Increased risk of hyperkalemia
hydrochlorothiazide component
amantadine: Possibly increased blood level and risk of toxicity of amantadine
amiodarone: Increased risk of arrhythmias from hypokalemia
amphotericin B, corticosteroids: Intensified electrolyte depletion, especially hypokalemia
antihypertensives: Increased antihypertensive effects
barbiturates, opioids: May potentiate orthostatic hypotension
calcium: Possibly increased serum calcium level
cholestyramine, colestipol resins: Reduced GI absorption of hydrochlorothiazide
diazoxide: Increased antihypertensive and hyperglycemic effects of hydrochlorothiazide
diflunisal: Possibly increased blood hydrochlorothiazide level
digoxin: Increased risk of digitalis toxicity from hypokalemia
dopamine: Possibly increased diuretic effects of both drugs
insulin, oral antidiabetics: Possibly increased blood glucose level
neuromuscular blockers: Possibly enhanced neuromuscular blockade from hypokalemia
nondepolarizing skeletal muscle relaxants (such as tubocurarine): Possibly increased responsiveness to muscle relaxant
pressor amines (such as norepinephrine): Possibly decreased response to pressor amines

oral anticoagulants: Possibly decreased anticoagulant effects
sympathomimetics: Possibly decreased antihypertensive effect of hydrochlorothiazide
vitamin D: Increased risk of hypercalcemia
FOODS
lisinopril component
potassium-containing salt substitutes: Increased risk of hyperkalemia
ACTIVITIES
lisinopril component
alcohol use: Possibly additive hypotensive effect

Adverse Reactions

CNS: Asthenia, ataxia, confusion, CVA, depression, dizziness, dream disturbances, fatigue, headache, insomnia, nervousness, paresthesia, peripheral neuropathy, somnolence, syncope, vertigo, weakness
CV: Angina, arrhythmias, cardiac arrest, chest pain, hypotension, MI, orthostatic hypotension, palpitations, Raynaud's phenomenon, tachycardia, vasculitis
EENT: Blurred vision, conjunctivitis, dry eyes and mouth, glossitis, hoarseness, lacrimation, loss of smell, pharyngitis, rhinorhea, stomatitis, taste perversion, tinnitus
ENDO: Hyperglycemia
GI: Abdominal pain, anorexia, constipation, diarrhea, dyspepsia, flatulence, hepatic failure, hepatitis, ileus, indigestion, jaundice, melena, nausea, pancreatitis, vomiting
GU: Decreased libido, flank pain, impotence, interstitial nephritis, nocturia, polyuria, oliguria, renal failure, UTI
HEME: Agranulocytosis, aplastic anemia, hemolytic anemia, leukopenia, neutropenia, thrombocytopenia
MS: Arthralgia; muscle cramps, spasms, and weakness
RESP: Asthma; back pain; bronchitis; bronchospasm; cough; dyspnea; pneumonia; pulmonary edema, embolism, infarction and infiltrates; upper respiratory tract infection
SKIN: Alopecia, diaphoresis, erythema multiforme, exfoliative dermatitis, flushing, pemphigus, photosensitivity, pruritis, rash, Stevens-Johnson syndrome, toxic epidermal necrolysis, urticaria
Other: Anaphylaxis, angioedema, dehydration, gout, herpes zoster, hypercalcemia, hyperkalemia, hyperuricemia, hypochloremia, hypokalemia, hyponatremia, hypovolemia, metabolic alkalosis, weight loss

Nursing Considerations

- Use cautiously in patients with impaired hepatic function because hydrochlorothiazide may alter fluid and electrolyte balance and lead to hepatic coma.
- Also use cautiously in patients with systemic lupus erythematosus because hydrochlorothiazide may activate or worsne it.
- Monitor blood pressure often to assess effectiveness of lisinopril and hydrochlorothiazide therapy.
- **WARNING** Be aware that the drug may cause severe hypotension with syncope, which may lead to MI or stroke.
- If patient develops hypotension, expect to stop drug temporarily. Immediately place patient in supine position, and prepare to give I.V. normal saline solution, as prescribed. Expect to resume therapy after blood pressure stabilizes.
- **WARNING** Monitor patient closely for angioedema of the face, lips, tongue, glottis, larynx, or limbs. For angioedema of the face and lips, stop drug and give an antihistamine, as prescribed. If tongue, glottis, or larynx is involved, assess patient for airway obstruction, prepare to give epinephrine 1:1,000 (0.3 to 0.5 ml) subcutaneously, and maintain a patent airway.
- Provide hydration, as appropriate, to help prevent hypovolemia.
- Monitor fluid intake and output, daily weight, and serum electrolyte levels (especially potassium) to detect volume depletion or electrolyte imbalance.
- Watch for increased BUN and serum creatinine levels, especially in patients with impaired renal function, because drug may cause acute renal failure. If increases are significant or persistent, notify prescriber immediately.
- Monitor blood glucose level often in diabetic patients, and expect to increase antidiabetic dosage, as needed and ordered.
- Check WBC count periodically, especially in patients with collagen-vascular disease, to detect neutropenia and agranulocytosis. Although they aren't known to occur with lisinopril, they have occurred with captropril, another ACE inhibitor.
- Assess liver enzymes periodically, and monitor patient for jaundice because hepatic failure, although rare, has occurred with other ACE inhibitors. If liver enzymes develop marked elevation or patient develops jaundice, notify prescriber and expect to stop lisinopril and hydrochlorothiazide.

PATIENT TEACHING
- Advise patient to take drug in the morning or early evening to avoid the need to urinate during the night.

- Teach patient to monitor her blood pressure and to report consistently elevated measurements to prescriber.
- Direct patient to weigh herself at the same time each day wearing the same amount of clothing and to notify prescriber if she gains more than 2 lb (0.9 kg) per day or 5 lb (2.3 kg) per week.
- To reduce the risk of dehydration and hypotension, advise patient to avoid exercise in hot weather and alcohol use. Also instruct her to notify prescriber if she experiences prolonged diarrhea, nausea, or vomiting.
- Caution patient to avoid potentially hazardous activities until drug's CNS effects are known.
- Explain the importance of regular exercise, proper diet, and other lifestyle changes in controlling hypertension.
- **WARNING** Strongly urge patient to contact prescriber before using potassium supplements or OTC salt substitutes, which may contain potassium. These products increase the risk of hyperkalemia.
- Advise female patient to notify prescriber immediately if she is or could be pregnant. Lisinopril and hydrochlorothiazide will need to be replaced with another antihypertensive that's safe to use during the second and third trimesters of pregnancy.
- Warn patient with gout that drug may precipitate an acute gout attack.

losartan potassium and hydrochlorothiazide
Hyzaar

Class and Category
Chemical: Angiotensin II receptor antagonist (losartan), benothiadiazide (hydrochlorothiazide)
Therapeutic: Antihypertensive (losartan, hydrochlorothiazide), diuretic (hydrochlorothiazide)
Pregnancy category: C (first trimester), D (second and third trimesters)

Indications and Dosages
▶ *To treat hypertension uncontrolled by losartan or hydrochlorothiazide alone; to treat hypertension in a patient whose blood pressure was controlled with 25 mg hydrochlorothiazide but who developed hypokalemia as a result*
TABLETS
Adults. *Initial:* 50 mg losartan and 12.5 mg hydrochlorothiazide

(1 tablet) daily. After 3 wk, increased as needed to 100 mg losartan and 25 mg hydrochlorothiazide (1 tablet) daily.

▶ *To treat hypertension in patients with left ventricular hypertrophy when losartan alone is ineffective*

TABLETS

Adults. *Initial:* 50 mg losartan and 12.5 mg hydrochlorothiazide (1 tablet) daily; increased, as needed, to 100 mg losartan and 12.5 mg hydrochlorothiazide (1 tablet) daily and then to 100 mg losartan and 25 mg hydrochlorothiazide (1 tablet) daily, if needed.

Mechanism of Action

Losartan blocks the effects of angiotensin II (a potent vasoconstrictor that's part of the renin-angiotensin-aldosterone system) by blocking its binding to angiotensin I receptors in vascular smooth muscles, adrenal glands, and other tissues. This action halts angiotensin II's negative feedback on renin secretion. Thus, circulating renin and angiotensin II levels rise and vascular resistance declines, reducing blood pressure.

Hydrochlorothiazide promotes movement of sodium, chloride, and water from blood in peritubular capillaries into the nephron's distal convoluted tubule. Initially, it may decrease extracellular fluid volume, plasma volume, and cardiac output, which helps explain blood pressure reduction. It also may reduce blood pressure by dilating arteries. After several weeks, extracellular fluid volume, plasma volume, and cardiac output return to normal, and peripheral vascular resistance remains decreased.

Contraindications

Anuria; hypersensitivity to losartan, hydrochlorothiazide, other sulfonamide-derived drugs, or their components

Interactions

DRUGS

losartan and hydrochlorothiazide

antihypertensives, diuretics: Increased antihypertensive effects
indomethacin, NSAIDs, smpathomimetics: Possibly decreased antihypertensive effects, increased risk of renal failure

losartan component

cyclosporine, potassium-sparing diuretics, potassium supplements: Increased risk of hyperkalemia

hydrochlorothiazide component

amantadine: Possibly increased blood amantadine level and risk of toxicity

amiodarone: Increased risk of arrhythmias from hypokalemia
amphotericin B, corticosteroids: Intensified electrolyte depletion, especially hypokalemia
antihypertensives: Increased antihypertensive effects
barbiturates, opioids: May potentiate orthostatic hypotension
calcium: Possibly increased serum calcium level
cholestyramine, colestipol resins: Reduced GI absorption of hydrochlorothiazide
diazoxide: Increased antihypertensive and hyperglycemic effects of hydrochlorothiazide
diflunisal: Possibly increased blood hydrochlorothiazide level
digoxin: Increased risk of digitalis toxicity from hypokalemia
dopamine: Possibly increased diuretic effects of both drugs
insulin, oral antidiabetics: Possibly increased blood glucose level
lithium: Decreased lithium clearance, increased risk of lithium toxicity
neuromuscular blockers: Possibly enhanced neuromuscular blockade from hypokalemia
nondepolarizing skeletal muscle relaxants (such as tubocurarine): Possibly increased responsiveness to the muscle relaxant
pressor amines (such as norepinephrine): Possibly decreased response to pressor amines
oral anticoagulants: Possibly decreased anticoagulant effects
vitamin D: Increased risk of hypercalcemia
FOODS
losartan component
high-potassium diet, potassium-containing salt substitutes: Increased risk of hyperkalemia

Adverse Reactions
CNS: Asthenia, depression, dizziness, drowsiness, fatigue, headache, insomnia, paresthesia, vertigo, weakness
CV: Angina pectoris, atrial fibrillation, bradycardia, edema, extrasystole, hypertriglyceridemia, hypotension, orthostatic hypotension, palpitations, tachycardia, vasculitis
EENT: Blurred vision, dry mouth, pharyngitis, rhinitis, sinusitis
ENDO: Hyperglycemia
GI: Abdominal cramps or pain, anorexia, constipation, diarrhea, hepatitis, indigestion, jaundice, nausea, vomiting
GU: Decreased libido, impotence, interstitial nephritis, nocturia, polyuria, renal failure, UTI
HEME: Agranulocytosis, aplastic and hemolytic anemia, leukopenia, neutropenia, thrombocytopenia

MS: Back or leg pain, muscle spasms and weakness, rhabdomyolysis

RESP: Bronchitis, dry cough, upper respiratory tract infection

SKIN: Alopecia, exfoliative dermatitis, photosensitivity, purpura, rash, urticaria

Other: Anaphylaxis, angioedema, dehydration, hypercalcemia, hyperkalemia, hyperuricemia, hypochloremia, hypokalemia, hyponatremia, hypovolemia, metabolic alkalosis, weight loss

Nursing Considerations

- Use cautiously in patients with impaired hepatic function because hydrochlorothiazide may alter fluid and electrolyte balance and lead to hepatic coma.
- Also use cautiously in patients with systemic lupus erythematosus because hydrochlorothiazide may activate or worsen it.
- If patient has known or suspected hypovolemia, expect to correct it with I.V. normal saline solution, as prescribed, before starting losartan and hydrochlorothiazide therapy.
- Monitor blood pressure often to assess effectiveness of losartan and hydrochlorothiazide therapy.
- If patient develops hypotension, expect to stop drug temporarily. Immediately place patient in supine position, and prepare to give I.V. normal saline solution, as prescribed. Expect to resume therapy after blood pressure stabilizes.
- Provide hydration, as appropriate, to help prevent hypovolemia.
- Monitor fluid intake and output, daily weight, and serum electrolyte levels (especially potassium) to detect volume depletion or electrolyte imbalance.
- Watch for increased BUN and serum creatinine levels, especially in patients with impaired renal function, because drug may cause acute renal failure. If increases are significant or persistent, notify prescriber immediately.
- Monitor blood glucose level often in diabetic patients, and expect to increase antidiabetic dosage, as needed and ordered.

PATIENT TEACHING

- Advise patient to take drug in the morning or early evening to avoid the need to urinate during the night.
- Teach patient to monitor her blood pressure and to report consistently elevated measurements to prescriber.
- **WARNING** Strongly urge patient to contact prescriber before using potassium supplements or OTC salt substitutes, which may contain potassium. These products increase the risk of hyperkalemia.

- Direct patient to weigh herself at the same time each day wearing the same amount of clothing and to notify prescriber if she gains more than 2 lb (0.9 kg) per day or 5 lb (2.3 kg) per week.
- **WARNING** Monitor patient closely for angioedema of the face, lips, tongue, glottis, larynx, or limbs. For angioedema of the face and lips, stop drug and give an antihistamine, as prescribed. If tongue, glottis, or larynx is involved, assess patient for airway obstruction, prepare to give epinephrine 1:1,000 (0.3 to 0.5 ml) subcutaneously, and maintain a patent airway.
- To reduce the risk of dehydration and hypotension, advise patient to avoid exercise in hot weather and to avoid alcohol. Also instruct her to notify prescriber if she has prolonged diarrhea, nausea, or vomiting.
- Caution patient to avoid potentially hazardous activities until drug's CNS effects are known.
- Explain the importance of regular exercise, proper diet, and other lifestyle changes in controlling hypertension.
- Advise female patient to notify prescriber immediately if she is or could be pregnant; losartan and hydrochlorothiazide will need to be replaced with another antihypertensive that's safe to use during the second and third trimesters of pregnancy.

methyldopa and hydrochlorothiazide
Aldoril 15, Aldoril 25, Aldoril D30, Aldoril D50

Class and Category
Chemical: 3,4-dihdroxyphenylalainine (DOPA) analogue (methyldopa), benothiadiazide (hydrochlorothiazide)
Therapeutic: Antihypertensive (methyldopa, hydrochlorothiazide), diuretic (hydrochlorothiazide)
Pregnancy category: C

Indications and Dosages
▶ *To treat hypertension uncontrolled by methyldopa or hydrochlorothiazide alone*
TABLETS
Adults. 250 mg methyldopa and 15 mg hydrochlorothiazide (1 Aldoril 15 tablet) b.i.d. or t.i.d. Or, 250 mg methyldopa and 25 mg hydrochlorothiazide (1 Aldoril 25 tablet) b.i.d. Increased, as needed, to 500 mg methyldopa and 30 mg hydrochlorothiazide (1 Aldoril D30 tablet) daily or 500 mg methyldopa and 50 mg hydrochlorothiazide (1 Aldoril D50 tablet) daily.

Mechanism of Action
Methyldopa is decarboxylated in the body to produce alpha-methylnorepinephrine, a metabolite that stimulates central inhibitory alpha-adrenergic receptors. This action may reduce blood pressure by decreasing sympathetic stimulation of the heart and peripheral vascular system.

Hydrochlorothiazide promotes movement of sodium, chloride, and water from blood in peritubular capillaries into the nephron's distal convoluted tubule. Initially, it may decrease extracellular fluid volume, plasma volume, and cardiac output, which helps explain blood pressure reduction. It also may reduce blood pressure by dilating arteries. After several weeks, extracellular fluid volume, plasma volume, and cardiac output return to normal, and peripheral vascular resistance remains decreased.

Contraindications
Active hepatic disease; anuria; hypersensitivity to methyldopa, hydrochlorothiazide, other sulfonamide-derived drugs, or their components; impaired hepatic function from previous methyldopa therapy; use within 14 days of MAO inhibitor therapy

Interactions
DRUGS
methyldopa and hydrochlorothiazide
diuretics, other antihypertensives: Increased antihypertensive effects
lithium: Decreased lithium clearance and increased risk of toxicity
NSAIDs, sympathomimetics: Decreased antihypertensive effects, increased risk of renal failure
methyldopa component
appetite suppressants, tricyclic antidepressants: Possibly decreased therapeutic effects of methyldopa
central anesthetics: Possibly need for reduced anesthetic dosage
CNS depressants: Possibly increased CNS depression
haloperidol: Increased risk of adverse CNS effects
levodopa: Possibly decreased therapeutic effects of levodopa and increased risk of adverse CNS effects
MAO inhibitors: Possibly hallucinations, headaches, hyperexcitability, and severe hypertension
oral anticoagulants: Possibly decreased effects of anticoagulants
hydrochlorothiazide component
amantadine: Possibly increased blood level and risk of toxicity of amantadine
amiodarone: Increased risk of arrhythmias from hypokalemia

amphotericin B, corticosteroids: Intensified electrolyte depletion, especially hypokalemia
barbiturates, opioids: May potentiate orthostatic hypotension
calcium: Possibly increased serum calcium level
cholestyramine, colestipol resins: Reduced GI absorption of hydrochlorothiazide
diazoxide: Increased antihypertensive and hyperglycemic effects of hydrochlorothiazide
diflunisal: Possibly increased blood hydrochlorothiazide level
digoxin: Increased risk of digitalis toxicity from hypokalemia
dopamine: Possibly increased diuretic effects of both drugs
insulin, oral antidiabetics: Possibly increased blood glucose level
neuromuscular blockers: Possibly enhanced neuromuscular blockade from hypokalemia
nondepolarizing skeletal muscle relaxants (such as tubocurarine): Possibly increased responsiveness to the muscle relaxant
pressor amines (such as norepinephrine): Possibly decreased response to pressor amines
oral anticoagulants: Possibly decreased anticoagulant effects
vitamin D: Increased risk of hypercalcemia
ACTIVITIES
methyldopa component
alcohol use: Possibly increased CNS depression

Adverse Reactions

CNS: Decreased concentration, depression, dizziness, drowsiness, fever, headache, insomnia, involuntary motor activity, memory loss (transient), nightmares, paresthesia, parkinsonism, sedation, vertigo, weakness
CV: Angina, bradycardia, edema, heart failure, hypotension, myocarditis, orthostatic hypotension, vasculitis
EENT: Black or sore tongue, blurred vision, dry mouth, nasal congestion
ENDO: Gynecomastia, hyperglycemia
GI: Abdominal cramps, anorexia, constipation, diarrhea, flatulence, hepatic necrosis, hepatitis, indigestion, jaundice, nausea, pancreatitis, vomiting
GU: Decreased libido, impotence, interstitial nephritis, nocturia, polyuria, renal failure
HEME: Agranulocytosis, aplastic and hemolytic anemia, leukopenia, neutropenia, positive Coombs' test, positive tests for ANA and rheumatoid factor, thrombocytopenia
MS: Muscle spasms and weakness

SKIN: Alopecia, eczema, exfoliative dermatitis, photosensitivity, purpura, rash, urticaria

Other: Anaphylaxis, dehydration, hypercalcemia, hyperuricemia, hypochloremia, hypokalemia, hyponatremia, hypovolemia, metabolic alkalosis, weight gain or loss

Nursing Considerations

- Use cautiously in patients with impaired hepatic function because drug may alter fluid and electrolyte balance and lead to hepatic coma.
- Also use cautiously in patients with systemic lupus erythematosus because hydrochlorothiazide may activate or worsen the disease.
- Check patient's CBC results before therapy, as ordered, to establish a baseline and check for asnemia. Monitor CBC periodically during therapy, as ordered, to detect adverse hematologic reactions to the drug.
- Monitor blood pressure often to assess effectiveness of methyldopa and hydrochlorothiazide.
- Provide hydration, as appropriate, to help prevent hypovolemia.
- Monitor fluid intake and output, daily weight, and serum electrolyte levels (especially potassium) to detect volume depletion or electrolyte imbalance.
- Monitor for increased BUN and serum creatinine levels, especially in patients with impaired renal function, because drug may cause acute renal failure. If increases are significant or persistent, notify prescriber immediately.
- Monitor blood glucose level often in diabetic patients, and expect to increase antidiabetic dosage, as needed and prescribed.
- Monitor results of Coombs' test; a positive result after several months of treatment indicates that patient has hemolytic anemia. Expect prescriber to discontinue drug.
- Notify prescriber if patient experiences signs of heart failure (dyspnea, edema, hypertension) or involuntary, rapid, jerky movements.

PATIENT TEACHING
- Advise patient to take methyldopa and hydrochlorothiazide in the morning or early evening to avoid awakening during the night to urinate.
- Teach patient how to monitor her blood pressure and to report consistently elevated measurements to prescriber.

- Tell patient to take drug exactly as prescribed and not to abruptly stop it. Explain that hypertension can return within 48 hours after stopping drug.
- Direct patient to weigh herself at the same time each day wearing the same amount of clothing and to notify prescriber if she gains more than 2 lb (0.9 kg) per day or 5 lb (2.3 kg) per week.
- Instruct patient to eat a diet high in potassium-rich food, including citrus fruits, bananas, tomatoes, and dates.
- To reduce the risk of dehydration and hypotension, advise patient to avoid exercise in hot weather and alcohol use. Also instruct her to notify prescriber if she experiences prolonged diarrhea, nausea, or vomiting.
- Caution patient to avoid potentially hazardous activities until drug's CNS effects are known.
- Explain the importance of regular exercise, proper diet, and other lifestyle changes in controlling hypertension.
- Direct patient to notify prescriber about bruising, chest pain, fever, involuntary jerky movements, prolonged dizziness, rash, and yellow eyes or skin.

metoprolol tartrate and hydrochlorothiazide

Lopressor HCT

Class and Category

Chemical: Beta$_1$-adrenergic antagonist (metoprolol), benothiadiazide (hydrochlorothiazide)
Therapeutic: Antihypertensive, diuretic
Pregnancy category: C

Indications and Dosages

▶ *To manage hypertension*
TABLETS
Adults. Based on previous dosage of metoprolol or hydrochlorthiazide monotherapy, 100 mg to 200 mg metoprolol and 25 mg to 50 mg hydrochlorothiazide once daily or in divided doses.

Contraindications

Acute heart failure; anuria; bradycardia (heart rate less than 45 beats/minute); cardiogenic shock; hypersensitivity to metoprolol, hydrochlorothiazide, other sulfonamide-derived drugs, or their components; second- or third-degree AV block.

Mechanism of Action

Metoprolol helps reduce blood pressure by decreasing release of renin from the kidneys and by antagonizing the effects of neurotransmitters that compete for the beta receptor sites. Also, metoprolol decreases cardiac output and adrenergic activity.

Hydrochlorothiazide promotes movement of sodium, chloride, and water from blood in peritubular capillaries into the nephron's distal convoluted tubule. Initially, it may decrease extracellular fluid volume, plasma volume, and cardiac output, which helps explain blood pressure reduction. It also may reduce blood pressure by dilating arteries. After several weeks, extracellular fluid volume, plasma volume, and cardiac output return to normal, and peripheral vascular resistance remains decreased.

Interactions

DRUGS

metoprolol and hydrochlorothiazide

antihypertensives, diuretics: Increased antihypertensive effect
neuromuscular blockers: Possibly enhanced and prolonged neuromuscular blockade
NSAIDs, sympathomimetics: Possibly decreased antihypertensive effect of hydrochlorothiazide and metoprolol
insulin, oral antidiabetics: Decreased blood glucose control, possibly masking of signs and symptoms of hypoglcemia by metoprolol

metoprolol component

aluminum salts, barbiturates, calcium salts, cholestyramine, colestipol, rifampin, salicylates, sulfinpyrazone: Decreased therapeutic effects of metoprolol
amiodarone, digoxin, diltiazem, verapamil: Increased risk of complete AV block
calcium channel blockers: Increased risk of heart failure and increased therapeutic effects of both drugs
cimetidine: Increased blood metoprolol level
clonidine, diazoxide, guanabenz: Increased risk of hypotension
estrogens: Possibly decreased antihypertensive effect of metoprolol
general anesthetics: Increased risk of hypotension and heart failure
lidocaine: Increased risk of lidocaine toxicity
MAO inhibitors: Increased risk of hypertension
phenothiazines: Possibly increased blood levels of both drugs
propafenone: Increased blood level and half-life of metoprolol
xanthines: Possibly decreased effects of these drugs or metoprolol

hydrochlorothiazide component

amantadine: Possibly increased blood amantadine level and risk of toxicity

amiodarone: Increased risk of arrhythmias from hypokalemia

amphotericin B, corticosteroids: Intensified electrolyte depletion, especially hypokalemia

antihypertensives: Increased antihypertensive effects

barbiturates, opioids: May potentiate orthostatic hypotension

calcium: Possibly increased serum calcium level

cholestyramine, colestipol resins: Reduced GI absorption of hydrochlorothiazide

diazoxide: Increased antihypertensive and hyperglycemic effects of hydrochlorothiazide

diflunisal: Possibly increased blood hydrochlorothiazide level

digoxin: Increased risk of digitalis toxicity from hypokalemia

dopamine: Possibly increased diuretic effects of both drugs

lithium: Decreased lithium clearance and increased risk of toxicity

nondepolarizing skeletal muscle relaxants (such as tubocurarine): Possibly increased responsiveness to the muscle relaxant

pressor amines (such as norepinephrine): Possibly decreased response to pressor amines

oral anticoagulants: Possibly decreased anticoagulant effects

vitamin D: Increased risk of hypercalcemia

FOODS

metoprolol component

all foods: Increased bioavailability of metoprolol

Adverse Reactions

CNS: Anxiety, confusion, depression, dizziness, drowsiness, fatigue, hallucinations, headache, insomnia, lethargy, nightmares, paresthesia, somnolence, vertigo, weakness

CV: Arrhythmias (including AV block and bradycardia), chest pain, edema, heart failure, hypotension, orthostatic hypotension, vasculitis

EENT: Blurred vision, dry mouth, ear ache, nasal congestion, tinnitus

ENDO: Hyperglycemia

GI: Abdominal cramps, anorexia, constipation, diarrhea, indigestion, jaundice, nausea, vomiting

GU: Decreased libido, impotence, interstitial nephritis, nocturia, polyuria, renal failure

HEME: Agranulocytosis, aplastic and hemolytic anemia, leukopenia, neutropenia, thrombocytopenia

MS: Back pain; muscle pain, spasms and weakness; myalgia

RESP: Bronchospasms, dsypnea
SKIN: Alopecia, diaphoresis, exfoliative dermatitis, photosensitivity, purpura, rash, urticaria
Other: Anaphylaxis, dehydration, flulike syndrome, gout, hypercalcemia, hyperuricemia, hypochloremia, hypokalemia, hyponatremia, hypovolemia, metabolic alkalosis, weight loss

Nursing Considerations

- Use cautiously in patients with heart failure controlled by digitalis and diuretics because both digitalis and metoprolol slow AV conduction.
- Use cautiously in patients with impaired hepatic function because hydrochlorothiazide may alter fluid and electrolyte balance and lead to hepatic coma.
- Also use cautiously in patients with systemic lupus erythematosus because hydrochlorothiazide may activate or worsen it.
- Patients with bronchospastic disease are less likely to develop adverse respiratory effects if drug is given in smaller doses three times daily instead of larger doses twice daily.
- Check blood pressure often to assess effectiveness of therapy.
- Provide hydration, as appropriate, to help prevent hypovolemia.
- Patients who take metoprolol and hydrochlorothiazide may be at risk for AV block. If AV block results from depressed AV node conduction, prepare to give appropriate drug, as prescribed, or assist with insertion of a temporary pacemaker.
- Monitor fluid intake and output, daily weight, and serum electrolyte levels (especially potassium) to detect heart failure, volume depletion, or electrolyte imbalance.
- Watch for increased BUN and serum creatinine levels, especially in patients with impaired renal function, because drug may cause acute renal failure. If increases are significant or persistent, notify prescriber immediately.
- Monitor blood glucose level often in diabetic patients, and expect to increase antidiabetic dosage, as needed and ordered.
- **WARNING** Stopping this drug abruptly can cause myocardial ischemia, MI, ventricular arrhythmias, or severe hypertension, especially in patients with cardiac disease, and can cause thyroid storm in patients with hyperthyroidism or thyrotoxicosis. Expect to taper the drug when therapy ends.

PATIENT TEACHING

- Advise patient to take metoprolol and hydrochlorothiazide with food in the morning or early evening to avoid the need to urinate during the night.

- Advise patient to notify prescriber if pulse rate is less than 60 beats/minute or is significantly lower than usual.
- Teach patient to monitor her blood pressure and to report consistently elevated measurements to prescriber.
- Direct patient to weigh herself at the same time each day wearing the same amount of clothing and to notify prescriber if she gains more than 2 lb (0.9 kg) per day or 5 lb (2.3 kg) per week.
- Instruct patient to eat a diet high in potassium-rich foods, such as citrus fruits, bananas, tomatoes, and dates.
- To reduce the risk of dehydration and hypotension, advise patient to avoid exercise in hot weather and to avoid alcohol. Also instruct her to notify prescriber if she has prolonged diarrhea, nausea, or vomiting.
- Caution patient to avoid potentially hazardous activities until drug's CNS effects are known.
- Explain the importance of regular exercise, proper diet, and other lifestyle changes in controlling hypertension.
- Caution patient not tot stop taking metoprolol and hydrochlorothiazide abruptly.
- Alert patient with diabetes that drug may mask a rapid heart beat caused by hypoglycemia and that the only symptom of hypoglycemia may be sweating. Advise her to check her blood glucose level regularly.

moexipril hydrochloride and hydrochlorothiazide
Uniretic

Class and Category
Chemical: Prodrug of moexiprilat (moexipril), benothiadiazide (hydrochlorothiazide)
Therapeutic: Antihypertensive (moexipril, hydrochlorothiazide), diuretic (hydrochlorothiazide)
Pregnancy category: C (first trimester), D (second and third trimesters)

Indications and Dosages
▶ *To treat hypertension uncontrolled by moexipril or hydrochlorothiazide alone*
TABLETS
Adults. *Initial:* Depending on previous dosage of moexipril or hydrochlorothiazide monotherapy, 7.5 mg or 15 mg moexipril and 12.5 mg or 25 mg hydrochlorothiazide (1 or 2 tablets depending

on strength) daily, 1 hr before meal. Dosage increased as needed q 2 to 3 wk. *Maximum:* 30 mg moexipril and 50 mg hydrochlorothiazide daily 1 hr before meal.

▶ *To treat patients with hypertension controlled by hydrochlorothiazide but who develop hypokalemia*

TABLETS

Adults. 3.75 mg moexipril and 6.25 mg hydrochlorothiazide (½ tablet of the 7.5-mg moexipril and 12.5-mg hydrochlorothiazide strength) daily 1 hr before meal

DOSAGE ADJUSTMENT For patients who have an excessive drop in blood pressure while taking 7.5 mg moexipril and 12.5 mg hydrochlorothiazide, dosage reduced to 3.75 mg moexipril and 6.25 mg hydrochlorothiazide daily 1 hr before meal.

Mechanism of Action

Moexipril may reduce blood pressure by affecting the renin-angiotensin-aldosterone system. By inhibiting ACE, moexipril:

- prevents conversion of angiotensin I to angiotensin II, a potent vasoconstrictor that also stimulates adrenal cortex to secrete aldosterone.
- may inhibit renal and vascular production of angiotensin II.
- decreases serum angiotensin II level and increases serum renin activity. This decreases aldosterone secretion, slightly increasing serum potassium level and fluid loss.
- decreases vascular tone and blood pressure
- inhibits aldosterone release, which reduces sodium and water reabsorption and increases their excretion, further reducing blood pressure.

Hydrochlorothiazide promotes movement of sodium, chloride, and water from blood in peritubular capillaries into the nephron's distal convoluted tubule. Initially, it may decrease extracellular fluid volume, plasma volume, and cardiac output, which helps explain blood pressure reduction. It also may reduce blood pressure by dilating arteries. After several weeks, extracellular fluid volume, plasma volume, and cardiac output return to normal, and peripheral vascular resistance remains decreased.

Contraindications

Anuria; history of angioedema with previous ACE inhibitor use; hypersensitivity to moexipril, hydrochlorothiazide, other sulfonamide-derived drugs, or their components

Interactions

DRUGS

moexipril and hydrochlorothiazide

antihypertensives, diuretics: Increased antihypertensive effect
digoxin: Possibly increased blood digoxin level and toxicity
lithium: Increased blood lithium level and risk of toxicity
NSAIDs, sympathomimetics: Possibly reduced antihypertensive effects of moexipril and hydrochlorothiazide and increased risk of renal toxicity

moexipril component

allopurinol, bone marrow depressants (such as amphotericin B and methotrexate), procainamide, systemic corticosteroids: Possibly increased risk of fatal neutropenia or agranulocytosis
antacids: Possibly decreased moexipril bioavailability
cyclosporine, potassium-sparing diuretics, potassium supplements: Increased risk of hyperkalemia
phenothiazines: Increased pharmacologic effects of moexipril

hydrochlorothiazide component

amantadine: Possibly increased blood amantadine level and risk of toxicity
amiodarone: Increased risk of arrhythmias from hypokalemia
amphotericin B, corticosteroids: Intensified electrolyte depletion, especially hypokalemia
barbiturates, opioids: May potentiate orthostatic hypotension
calcium: Possibly increased serum calcium level
cholestyramine, colestipol resins: Reduced GI absorption of hydrochlorothiazide
diazoxide: Increased antihypertensive and hyperglycemic effects of hydrochlorothiazide
diflunisal: Possibly increased blood hydrochlorothiazide level
dopamine: Possibly increased diuretic effects of both drugs
insulin, oral antidiabetics: Possibly increased blood glucose level
neuromuscular blockers: Possibly enhanced neuromuscular blockade from hypokalemia
nondepolarizing skeletal muscle relaxants (such as tubocurarine): Possibly increased responsiveness to the muscle relaxant
pressor amines (such as norepinephrine): Possibly decreased response to pressor amines
oral anticoagulants: Possibly decreased anticoagulant effects
vitamin D: Increased risk of hypercalcemia

FOODS

moexipril component

all foods: Decreased moexipril absorption
potassium-containing salt substitutes: Increased risk of hyperkalemia

ACTIVITIES
moexipril component
alcohol use: Possibly additive hypotensive effect

Adverse Reactions

CNS: Anxiety, chills, confusion, dizziness, drowsiness, fatigue, fever, headache, hypertonia, insomnia, malaise, mood changes, nervousness, paresthesia, sleep disturbance, stroke, syncope, vertigo, weakness

CV: Abnormal ECG, angina, arrhythmias, chest pain, hypotension, MI, orthostatic hypotension, palpitations, periperal edema, vasculitis

EENT: Blurred vision, dry mouth, hoarseness, laryngeal edema, mouth or tongue swelling, pharnygitis, rhinitis, sinusitis, taste perversion, tinnitus

ENDO: Hyperglycemia

GI: Abdominal cramps, distention or pain; anorexia; constipation; diarrhea; dyspepsia; dysphagia; elevated liver function test results; hepatitis; increased appetite; indigestion; jaundice; nausea; vomiting

GU: Azotemia; decreased libido; elevated BUN, serum creatinine and uric acid levels; impotence; interstitial nephritis; nocturia; oliguria; proteinuria; polyuria; pyuria; renal failure or insufficiency; urinary frequency; UTI

HEME: Agranulocytosis, aplastic and hemolytic anemia, bone marrow depression, elevated erythrocyte sedimentation rate, leukocytosis, leukopenia, neutropenia, thrombocytopenia

MS: Arthralgia, back pain, leg heaviness or weakness, muscle spasms and weakness, myalgia, myositis

RESP: Bronchitis, bronchospasm, cough, dyspnea, upper respiratory infection

SKIN: Alopecia, diaphoresis, exfoliative dermatitis, flushing, pallor, pemphigus, photosensitivity, pruritus, purpura, rash, Stevens-Johnson syndrome, urticaria

Other: Anaphylaxis, angioedema, dehydration, flulike syndrome, hypercalcemia, hyperkalemia, hyperuricemia, hypochloremia, hypokalemia, hyponatremia, hypovolemia, increased SGPT, metabolic alkalosis, positive ANA titer, weight loss

Nursing Considerations

- Use cautiously in patients with impaired hepatic function because hydrochlorothiazide may alter fluid and electrolyte balance and lead to hepatic coma.

- Also use cautiously in patients with systemic lupus erythematosus because hydrochlorothiazide may activate or worsen it.
- **WARNING** Contact prescriber if patient is or may be pregnant. Moexipril may cause fetal or neonatal harm or death if taken during the second or third trimester.
- Check blood pressure often to assess effectiveness of moexipril and hydrochlorothiazide therapy.
- Provide hydration, as appropriate, to help prevent hypovolemia.
- Monitor fluid intake and output, daily weight, and serum electrolyte levels (especially potassium) to detect volume depletion or electrolyte imbalance.
- Watch for increased BUN and serum creatinine levels, especially in patients with impaired renal function, because drug may cause acute renal failure. If increases are significant or persistent, notify prescriber immediately.
- **WARNING** Monitor patient closely for angioedema of the face, lips, tongue, glottis, larynx, or limbs. For angioedema of the face and lips, stop drug and give an antihistamine, as prescribed. If tongue, glottis, or larynx is involved, assess patient for airway obstruction, prepare to give epinephrine 1:1,000 (0.3 to 0.5 ml) subcutaneously, and maintain a patent airway.
- Monitor blood glucose level often in diabetic patients, and expect to increase antidiabetic dosage, as needed and ordered.

PATIENT TEACHING

- Advise patient to take moexipril and hydrochlorothiazide in the morning or early evening 1 hour before a meal to avoid the need to urinate during the night.
- Teach patient to monitor her blood pressure and to report consistently elevated measurements to prescriber.
- Urge female patient to notify prescriber immediately if she is or could be pregnant.
- **WARNING** Instruct patient to stop taking drug and seek immediate medical attention for hoarseness; swelling of tongue, glottis, larynx, face, or feet; or sudden difficulty swallowing or breathing.
- Caution patient not to stop drug without consulting prescriber, even if she feels better.
- Direct patient to weigh herself at the same time each day wearing the same amount of clothing and to notify prescriber if she gains more than 2 lb (0.9 kg) per day or 5 lb (2.3 kg) per week.
- Urge patient to avoid potassium supplements and potassium-containing salt substitutes unless prescriber allows them.

- To reduce the risk of dehydration and hypotension, advise patient to avoid exercise in hot weather and to avoid alcohol. Also instruct her to notify prescriber if she has prolonged diarrhea, nausea, or vomiting.
- Caution patient to avoid potentially hazardous activities until drug's CNS effects are known.
- Tell patient to report evidence of infection (such as chills, fever, and sore throat) as well as diarrhea, nausea, or vomiting, which may lead to dehydration-induced hypotension.
- Explain the importance of regular exercise, proper diet, and other lifestyle changes in controlling hypertension.

nadolol and bendroflumethiazide
Corzide

Class and Category
Chemical: Nonselective beta blocker (nadolol), thiazide (bendroflumethiazide)
Therapeutic: Antihypertensive (nadolol, bendroflumethiazide), diuretic (bendroflumethiazide)
Pregnancy category: C

Indications and Dosages
▶ *To treat hypertension*
TABLETS
Adults. *Initial:* 40 mg nadolol and 5 mg bendroflumethiazide (1 tablet) daily. Increased, as needed, to 80 mg nadolol and 5 mg bendroflumethiazide (1 tablet) daily.
DOSAGE ADJUSTMENT For patients with a creatinine clearance of 31 to 50 ml/min/1.73 m^2, dosage interval increased to q 36 hours. For patients with a creatinine clearance of 30 ml/min/1.73 m^2 or less, combination therapy with a thiazide diuretic such as bendroflumethiazide isn't recommended.

Contraindications
Anuria; asthma; bronchospasm; cardiogenic shock; heart failure; hypersensitivity to nadolol, bendroflumethiazide, other beta blockers or sulfonamide-derived drugs, or their components; second- or third-degree AV block; severe COPD; sinus bradycardia

Interactions
DRUGS
nadolol and bendroflumethiazide
amiodarone: Additive depressant effects on conduction, negative

> ## Mechanism of Action
> Nadolol causes competitive antagonism of catecholamines at peripheral adrenergic neuron sites, leading to decreased cardiac output. It has a central effect leading to reduced tonic-sympathetic nerve outflow to the periphery, and it suppresses renin secretion by blocking beta-adrenergic receptors responsible for renin release from the kidneys. Combined, these effects work together to lower blood pressure.
>
> Bendroflumethiazide promotes movement of sodium, chloride, and water from blood in peritubular capillaries into the nephron's distal convoluted tubule. Initially, it may decrease extracellular fluid volume, plasma volume, and cardiac output, which helps explain blood pressure reduction. It also may reduce blood pressure by dilating arteries. After several weeks, extracellular fluid volume and plasma volume return to near normal, cardiac output returns to normal, and peripheral vascular resistance remains decreased.

inotropic effects, and increased risk of arrhythmias from hypokalemia

antihypertensives, diuretics: Increased antihypertensive effects

insulin, oral antidiabetics: Possible increased blood glucose level

neuromuscular blockers: Possibly enhanced neuromuscular blockade from hypokalemia

NSAIDs: Decreased hypotensive effects

sympathomimetics: Possibly mutual inhibition of therapeutic effects

nadolol component

allergen immunotherapy, allergenic extracts for skin testing: Increased risk of serious systemic adverse reactions or anaphylaxis

anesthetics (general): Increased risk of hypotension and myocardial depression

beta blockers: Additive beta blockade effects

calcium channel blockers: Increased risk of bradycardia

catecholamine-depleting drugs (such as reserpine): Increased catecholamine-blocking action which may result in hypotension, marked bradycardia, vertigo, syncopal attacks, or orthostatic hypotension

cimetidine: Possibly interference with nadolol clearance, resulting in elevated plasma levels

clonidine, guanabenz: Impaired blood pressure control

diazoxide, nitroglycerin: Increased risk of hypotension

estrogens: Decreased antihypertensive effect of nadolol

fentanyl, fentanyl derivatives: Possibly increased risk of initial bradycardia after induction of fentanyl or a derivative (with long-term nadolol use)

insulin, oral antidiabetics: Possibly impaired recovery from hypoglycemia, masking of signs of hypoglycemia
lidocaine: Decreased lidocaine clearance; increased risk of toxicity
phenothiazines: Increased blood levels of both drugs
xanthines: Possibly mutual inhibition of therapeutic effects
bendroflumethiazide component
amantadine: Possibly increased blood amantadine level and risk of toxicity
amiodarone: Increased risk of arrhythmias from hypokalemia
amphotericin B, corticosteroids: Intensified electrolyte depletion, especially hypokalemia
antihypertensives: Increased antihypertensive effects
barbiturates, opioids: May potentiate orthostatic hypotension
calcium: Possibly increased serum calcium level
cholestyramine, colestipol resins: Reduced GI absorption of bendroflumethiazide
diazoxide: Increased antihypertensive and hyperglycemic effects of bendroflumethiazide
diflunisal: Possibly increased blood bendroflumethiazide level
digoxin: Increased risk of digitalis toxicity from hypokalemia
dopamine: Possibly increased diuretic effects of both drugs
insulin, oral antidiabetics: Possibly increased blood glucose level
lithium: Decreased lithium clearance and increased risk of toxicity
MAO inhibitors: Enhanced antihypertensive effect
methenamine: Possibly decreased effectiveness of methenamine
neuromuscular blockers: Possibly enhanced neuromuscular blockade from hypokalemia
nondepolarizing skeletal muscle relaxants (such as tubocurarine): Possibly increased responsiveness to the muscle relaxant
pressor amines (such as norepinephrine): Possibly decreased response to pressor amines
oral anticoagulants: Possibly decreased anticoagulant effects
vitamin D: Increased risk of hypercalcemia
ACTIVITIES
bendroflumethiazide component
alcohol use: Possibly potentiated orthostatic hypotension

Adverse Reactions

CNS: Anxiety, depression, dizziness, drowsiness, fatigue, headache, insomnia, paresthesia, syncope, vertigo, weakness, yawning
CV: Bradycardia, chest pain, edema, heart block, heart failure, hypotension, orthostatic hypotension, vasculitis, ventricular arrhythmias

EENT: Blurred vision, dry mouth, nasal congestion, taste perversion

ENDO: Hyperglycemia

GI: Abdominal cramps, anorexia, constipation, diarrhea, dyspepsia, elevated liver function test results, hepatic necrosis, hepatitis, indigestion, jaundice, nausea, vomiting

GU: Decreased libido, ejaculation failure, impotence, interstitial nephritis, nocturia, polyuria, renal failure

HEME: Agranulocytosis, aplastic and hemolytic anemia, leukopenia, neutropenia, thrombocytopenia

MS: Muscle spasms and weakness

RESP: Cough, dyspnea, wheezing

SKIN: Alopecia, exfoliative dermatitis, photosensitivity, pruritus, purpura, rash, scalp tingling, urticaria

Other: Anaphylaxis, dehydration, hypercalcemia, hyperuricemia, hypochloremia, hypokalemia, hyponatremia, hypovolemia, metabolic alkalosis, weight loss

Nursing Considerations

- Use cautiously in patients with impaired hepatic function because bendroflumethiazide may alter fluid and electrolyte balance and lead to hepatic coma.
- Also use cautiously in patients with systemic lupus erythematosus because bendroflumethiazide may activate or worsen it.
- Monitor blood pressure often to assess effectiveness of nadolol and bendroflumethiazide therapy.
- Anticipate that nadolol may worsen psoriasis and, in patients with myasthenia gravis, it may worsen muscle weakness and diplopia.
- Provide hydration, as appropriate, to help prevent hypovolemia.
- Monitor fluid intake and output, daily weight, and serum electrolyte levels (especially potassium) to detect volume depletion or electrolyte imbalance.
- Watch for increased BUN and serum creatinine levels, especially in patients with impaired renal function, because drug may cause acute renal failure. If increases are significant or persistent, notify prescriber immediately.
- Monitor blood glucose level often in diabetic patients, and expect to increase antidiabetic dosage, as needed and ordered.
- **WARNING** Withdraw drug gradually over 2 weeks, or as ordered, to avoid MI caused by unopposed beta stimulation or thyroid storm caused by underlying hyperthyroidism. Expect drug to mask tachycardia caused by hyperthyroidism.

PATIENT TEACHING
- Advise patient to take nadolol and bendroflumethiazide in the morning or early evening to avoid the need to urinate during the night.
- Teach patient how to monitor her blood pressure and take her pulse. Tell her to report consistent abnormalities to prescriber.
- Caution patient not to stop drug abruptly or change dosage.
- Direct patient to weigh herself at the same time each day wearing the same amount of clothing and to notify prescriber if she gains more than 2 lb (0.9 kg) per day or 5 lb (2.3 kg) per week.
- Instruct patient to eat a diet high in potassium-rich foods, such as citrus fruits, bananas, tomatoes, and dates.
- To reduce the risk of dehydration and hypotension, advise patient to avoid exercise in hot weather and to avoid alcohol. Also instruct her to notify prescriber if she has prolonged diarrhea, nausea, or vomiting.
- Caution patient to avoid potentially hazardous activities until drug's CNS effects are known.
- Explain the importance of regular exercise, proper diet, and other lifestyle changes in controlling hypertension.
- Advise diabetic patient to monitor blood glucose level closely; drug may alter control and mask some signs of hypoglycemia.
- Instruct patient to notify prescriber about shortness of breath.

niacin extended-release and lovastatin
Advicor

Class and Category
Chemical: B complex vitamin (niacin), mevinic acid derivative (lovastatin)
Therapeutic: Antihyperlipidemic (niacin, lovastatin)
Pregnancy category: X

Indications and Dosages
▶ *To treat primary hypercholesterolemia (heterozygous familial and nonfamilial) and mixed dyslipidemia when monotherapy with niacin or lovastatin has failed*
TABLETS
Adults. *Initial:* 500 mg niacin and 20 mg lovastatin (1 tablet) daily h.s. Dosage increased as needed, q 4 wk, first to 1,000 mg niacin and 20 mg lovastatin (1 tablet) daily h.s. and then to 1,500 mg niacin and 40 mg lovastatin (1 tablet containing

500 mg niacin and 20 mg lovastatin and 1 tablet containing 1,000 mg niacin and 20 mg lovastatin) daily h.s. and finally to 2,000 mg niacin and 40 mg lovastatin (2 tablets) daily h.s. *Maximum:* 2,000 mg niacin and 40 mg lovastatin.

Mechanism of Action

Niacin lowers serum cholesterol and triglyceride levels by inhibiting synthesis of very-low-density lipoproteins, which are needed to form low-density lipoproteins, the primary carrier of blood cholesterol.

Lovastatin interferes with the hepatic enzyme hydroxymethylglutaryl-coenzyme A reductase. By doing so, lovastatin reduces formation of mevalonic acid (a cholesterol precursor), thus interrupting the pathway by which cholesterol is synthesized. When the cholesterol level declines in hepatic cells, LDLs are consumed, which also reduces the amount of circulating total cholesterol. The decrease in LDLs may result in a decreased level of apolipoprotein B, which is found in each LDL particle.

Contraindications

Active peptic ulcer disease; arterial bleeding; breastfeeding; hepatic impairment (significant or unexplained); hypersensitivity to lovastatin, niacin, niacinamide, or their components; pregnancy

Interactions

DRUGS

niacin and lovastatin

bile acid sequestrants (cholestyramine, colestipol): Decreased niacin and lovastatin bioavailability and effectiveness

amiodarone, clarithromycin, cyclosporine, erythromycin, fibric acid derivatives, gemfibrozil and other fibrates, immunosuppressants, itraconazole, ketoconazole, nefazodone, protease inhibitors, verapamil: Increased risk of severe myopathy or rhabdomyolysis

niacin component

chenodiol, ursodiol: Decreased antihyperlipidemic effects of niacin

ganglionic blocking and vasoactive antihypertensives: Potentiated antihypertensive effects and possible postural hypotension

nutritional supplements containing large doses of niacin or related compounds, such as nicotinamide; vitamins: Possibly potentiated adverse effects of niacin

lovastatin component

isradipine: Increased hepatic clearance of lovastatin

itraconazole, ketoconazole: Increased blood lovastatin level *oral anticoagulants:* Possibly increased anticoagulant effect and risk of bleeding

FOODS

niacin component
hot drinks: Increased risk of flushing and pruritus

lovastatin component
all foods: Increased lovastatin absorption
grapefruit juice (more than 1 quart daily): Increased risk of myopathy or rhabdomyolysis

ACTIVITIES

niacin component
alcohol use: Increased risk of flushing and pruritus

lovastatin component
alcohol use: Increased blood lovastatin level

Adverse Reactions

CNS: Asthenia, chills, dizziness, fatigue, headache, insomnia, syncope

CV: Arrhythmias, edema, palpitations, peripheral vasodilation, tachycardia

EENT: Blurred vision, cataracts, dry eyes, pharyngitis, rhinitis, sinusitis

ENDO: Hyperglycemia

GI: Abdominal cramps and pain, cholestasis, constipation, diarrhea, dyspepsia, elevated liver function test results, epigastric pain, flatulence, hepatotoxicity, indigestion, nausea, vomiting

MS: Arthritis, back pain, myalgia, myopathy, myositis, rhabdomyolysis

RESP: Cough, shortness of breath, upper respiratory tract infection

SKIN: Dermatomyositis, diaphoresis, dry skin, erythema multiforme, flushing, pruritus, rash, sensation of warmth, Stevens-Johnson syndrome, toxic epidermal necrolysis

Other: Anaphylaxis, angioedema, flulike syndrome, hyperuricemia

Nursing Considerations

• Use cautiously in patients who consume substantial quantities of alcohol or have a history of liver disease because active liver disease and unexplained transaminase elevations contraindicate use of the niacin and lovastatin combination.

• Also use cautiously in patients with unstable angina or who are in the acute phase of MI, particularly if they take vasoactive drugs such as nitrates, calcium channel blockers, or adrenergic blockers because of increased risk of vasodilation.

- Give niacin and lovastatin at bedtime after a low-fat snack to minimize stomach upset and 1 hour before or 4 hours after giving a bile acid sequestrant, cholestyramine, or colestipol.
- **WARNING** Expect to monitor liver function tests every 6 months during therapy or as indicated. Monitor patient for evidence of hepatotoxicity or cholestasis, including darkening of urine, gray stools, loss of appetite, severe stomach pain, and yellow eyes or skin. If present, notify prescriber. Expect drug to be discontinued if serum transaminase level rises to three times the upper limit of normal or if patient has evidence of hepatic dysfunction.
- Monitor patient for flushing, a reaction to niacin caused by dilation of peripheral cutaneous blood vessels, which increases blood flow and causes redness, mainly in the face, neck, and chest. Expect patient to develop tolerance to this effect after 2 weeks of therapy. Notify prescriber about persistent flushing; effects may be controlled with aspirin, as prescribed, taken before each niacin and lovastatin dose.
- Assess patients with peptic ulcer disease for possible worsening of symptoms because nicotinic acid can stimulate histamine release, leading to increased gastric acid production.
- Watch patients with or predisposed to gout for worsening of symptoms because drug can cause hyperuricemia when given in high doses.
- **WARNING** Monitor patient for myopathy and rhabdomyolysis, characterized by unexplained muscle pain, tenderness, or weakness, especially early in therapy or during periods of dosage increases. Be aware that a CK level more than 10 times the upper limit of normal in a patient with unexplained muscle symptoms indicates myopathy. Notifiy prescriber immediately, and be prepared to discontinue therapy if myopathy or rhabdomyolysis is suspected or present.
- Monitor patients with diabetes mellitus for altered glucose control because high doses of niacin may cause hyperglycemia.
- Monitor CBC, especially in patients with thrombocytopenia or coagulopathy and in those who are on anticoagulant therapy, because niacin may promote slight decreases in platelet counts or increased prothrombin times.
- Be prepared to temporarily stop niacin and lovastatin therapy, as ordered, for a few days before elective major surgery or when any major acute medical or surgical condition occurs.

PATIENT TEACHING
• Advise patient not to break, crush, or chew tablets but to swallow them whole.
• Tell patient to take drug at bedtime after a low-fat snack to minimize stomach upset.
• To minimize flushing, urge patient to avoid hot drinks around the time she takes a dose. Explain that she may experience skin flushing, mainly in the face, neck, and chest, but that she may develop tolerance to this effect after 2 weeks of therapy. Advise her to notify prescriber about persistent or intolerable flushing because prescriber may adjust dosage or recommend that patient take aspirin before each dose to control flushing.
• Instruct patient to avoid activities requiring mental alertness, such as driving or operating machinery, until full effects of drug are known because vasodilatory response to niacin may be dramatic at start of therapy.
• Emphasize importance of following a standard low-cholesterol diet during therapy.
• Tell patient to report muscle aches, pains, tenderness, or weakness; severe GI distress; and vision changes promptly.
• Urge patient to avoid consuming alcohol or more than 1 quart of grapefruit juice daily while taking drug.
• Stress the importance of periodic eye examinations during therapy because lovastatin has caused optic nerve degeneration in animals, and similar effects have occurred in patients taking other statin drugs.
• Teach female patient of childbearing age appropriate contraceptive methods. Tell her to report suspected pregnancy immediately because drug may harm fetus and will need to be stopped.
• Tell patient to consult prescriber before taking vitamins or nutritional supplements containing niacin or nicotinamide.

olmesartan medoxomil and hydrochlorothiazide
Benicar HCT

Class and Category
Chemical: AT1 subtype angiotensin II receptor antagonist (olmesartan, benothiadiazide (hydrochlorothiazide)
Therapeutic: Antihypertensive (olmesartan, hydrochlorothiazide), diuretic (hydrochlorothiazide)
Pregnancy category: C (first trimester), D (second and third trimesters)

Indications and Dosages

▶ *To manage hypertension when olmesartan or hydrochlorothiazide alone has failed*

TABLETS

Adults who aren't taking hydrochlorothiazide. *Initial:* 40 mg olmesartan and 12.5 mg hydrochlorothiazide (1 tablet) daily, increased in 2 to 4 wk to 40 mg olmesartan and 25 mg hydrochlorothiazide (1 tablet) daily, if needed.

Adults who aren't taking olmesartan. *Initial:* 20 mg olmesartan and 12.5 mg hydrochlorothiazide (1 tablet) daily, increased q 2 to 4 wk to 40 mg olmesartan and 25 mg hydrochlorothiazide (1 tablet) daily, if needed.

Mechanism of Action

Olmesartan blocks binding of angiotensin II to receptor sites in many tissues, including vascular smooth muscle and adrenal glands. Angiotensin II is a potent vasoconstrictor that also stimulates the adrenal cortex to secrete aldosterone. The inhibiting effects of angiotensin II reduce blood pressure.

Hydrochlorothiazide promotes movement of sodium, chloride, and water from blood in peritubular capillaries into the nephron's distal convoluted tubule. Initially, it may decrease extracellular fluid volume, plasma volume, and cardiac output, which helps explain blood pressure reduction. It also may reduce blood pressure by dilating arteries. After several weeks, extracellular fluid volume, plasma volume, and cardiac output return to normal, and peripheral vascular resistance remains decreased.

Contraindications

Anuria; hypersensitivity to olmesartan, hydrochlorothiazide, other sulfonamide-derived drugs, or their components; pregnancy; renal failure

Interactions

DRUGS

olmesartan component

potassium-sparing diuretics: Increased risk of hyperkalemia

hydrochlorothiazide component

amantadine: Possibly increased blood amantadine level and risk of toxicity

amiodarone: Increased risk of arrhythmias from hypokalemia

amphotericin B, corticosteroids: Intensified electrolyte depletion, especially hypokalemia

antihypertensives: Increased antihypertensive effects

barbiturates, opioids: May potentiate orthostatic hypotension
calcium: Possibly increased serum calcium level
cholestyramine, colestipol resins: Reduced GI absorption of hydrochlorothiazide
diazoxide: Increased antihypertensive and hyperglycemic effects of hydrochlorothiazide
diflunisal: Possibly increased blood hydrochlorothiazide level
digoxin: Increased risk of digitalis toxicity from hypokalemia
dopamine: Possibly increased diuretic effects of both drugs
insulin, oral antidiabetics: Possibly increased blood glucose level
lithium: Decreased lithium clearance and increased risk of toxicity
neuromuscular blockers: Possibly increased neuromuscular blockade from hypokalemia
nondepolarizing skeletal muscle relaxants (such as tubocurarine): Possibly increased responsiveness to the muscle relaxant
NSAIDs: Decreased diuretic effect of hydrochlorothiazide and increased risk of renal failure
pressor amines (such as norepinephrine): Possibly decreased response to pressor amines
oral anticoagulants: Possibly decreased anticoagulant effects
sympathomimetics: Possibly decreased antihypertensive effect of hydrochlorothiazide
vitamin D: Increased risk of hypercalcemia

Adverse Reactions

CNS: Asthenia, dizziness, headache, vertigo
CV: Chest pain, hypercholesterolemia, hyperlipemia, increased liver enzymes, orthostatic hypotension, peripheral edema, tachycardia
ENDO: Hyperglycemia
GI: Abdominal pain, diarrhea, dyspepsia, gastroenteritis, nausea, vomiting
GU: Acute renal failure, elevated BUN and serum creatinine levels, hematuria, interstitial nephritis, renal failure, urinary tract infection
MS: Arthralgia, arthritis, back pain, muscle spasm, myalgia
RESP: Cough, upper respiratory tract infection
SKIN: Alopecia, pruritus, rash,urticaria
Other: Angioedema, hypercalcemia, hyperkalemia, hyperuricemia, hypokalemia, hypomagnesemia

Nursing Considerations

• Use cautiously in patients with impaired hepatic function because hydrochlorothiazide may alter fluid and electrolyte balance and lead to hepatic coma.

- Also use cautiously in patients with systemic lupus erythematosus because hydrochlorothiazide may activate or worsen it.
- Monitor blood pressure often to assess effectiveness of olmesartan and hydrochlorothiazide therapy.
- Provide hydration, as appropriate, to help prevent hypovolemia.
- Monitor fluid intake and output, daily weight, blood pressure, and serum electrolyte levels (especially potassium) to detect volume depletion or electrolyte imbalance.
- **WARNING** Monitor patients who are volume- or sodium-depleted closely because symptomatic hypotension may occur when therapy starts. If hypotension occurs, place patient in supine position and, if needed, give an intravenous infusion of normal saline, as prescribed. Expect to resume drug therapy after blood pressure stabilizes.
- Watch for increased BUN and serum creatinine levels, especially in patients with impaired renal function, because drug may cause acute renal failure. If increases are significant or persistent, notify prescriber immediately.
- Be aware that loop diuretics are preferred to thiazide diuretics in patients with a creatinine clearance greater than 30 ml/min/ 1.73 m^2; expect olmesartan and hydrochlorothiazide to be stopped in patients who develop significant renal impairment during therapy.
- Monitor blood glucose level often in diabetic patients, and expect to increase antidiabetic dosage, as needed and ordered.

PATIENT TEACHING
- Advise patient to take olmesartan and hydrochlorothiazide in the morning or early evening to avoid the need to urinate during the night.
- Instruct patient to take drug with food or milk if adverse GI reactions occur.
- Teach patient to monitor her blood pressure and to report consistently elevated measurements to prescriber.
- Direct patient to weigh herself at the same time each day wearing the same amount of clothing and to notify the prescriber if she gains more than 2 lb (0.9 kg) per day or 5 lb (2.3 kg) per week.
- Instruct patient to eat a diet high in potassium-rich foods, such as citrus fruits, bananas, tomatoes, and dates.
- To reduce the risk of dehydration and hypotension, advise patient to avoid exercise in hot weather and to avoid alcohol.

Also instruct her to notify prescriber if she has prolonged diarrhea, nausea, or vomiting.
• Caution patient to avoid potentially hazardous activities until drug's CNS effects are known.
• Explain the importance of regular exercise, proper diet, and other lifestyle changes in controlling hypertension.
• Advise female patient to notify prescriber immediately about known or suspected pregnancy because olmesartan and hydrochlorothiazide will need to be replaced with another antihypertensive that's safe to use during the second and third trimesters of pregnancy.

prazosin hydrochloride and polythiazide
Minizide

Class and Category
Chemical: Quinazoline derivative (prazosin), benothiadiazide (polythiazide)
Therapeutic: Antihypertensive (prazosin, polythiazide), diuretic (polythiazide)
Pregnancy category: C

Indications and Dosages
▶ *To treat hypertension*
CAPSULES
Adults. *Initial:* 1 mg prazosin and 0.5 mg polythiazide (1 tablet) b.i.d. or t.i.d., increased as needed. *Maximum:* 5 mg prazosin and 0.5 mg polythiazide b.i.d. or t.i.d.

Mechanism of Action
Prazosin selectively and competitively inhibits alpha$_1$-adrenergic receptors. This action promotes peripheral arterial and venous dilation and reduces peripheral vascular resistance, thereby lowering blood pressure.

Polythiazide promotes movement of sodium, chloride, and water from blood in peritubular capillaries into the nephron's distal convoluted tubule. Initially, it may decrease extracellular fluid volume, plasma volume, and cardiac output, which helps explain blood pressure reduction. It also may reduce blood pressure by dilating arteries. After several weeks, extracellular fluid volume, plasma volume, and cardiac output return to normal, and peripheral vascular resistance remains decreased to account for lowering of blood pressure.

Contraindications
Angina; anuria; hypersensitivity to prazosin, polythiazide, other quinazolines or sulfonamide-derived drugs, or their components

Interactions
DRUGS
prazosin and polythiazide
antihypertensives, diuretics: Increased antihypertensive effects
NSAIDs, sympathomimetics: Decreased effectiveness of prazosin
prazosin component
beta blockers: Increased risk of hypotension and syncope
dopamine: Antagonized peripheral vasoconstrictive effect of dopamine (with high doses)
ephedrine: Decreased vasopressor response to ephedrine
epinephrine: Possibly severe hypotension and tachycardia
metaraminol: Decreased vasopressor effect of metaraminol
methoxamine, phenylephrine: Possibly decreased vasopressor effect and shortened duration of action of these drugs
sildenafil, tadalafil, vardenafil: Increased risk of hypotension
polythiazide component
amantadine: Possibly increased blood level and risk of toxicity of amantadine
amiodarone: Increased risk of arrhythmias from hypokalemia
amphotericin B, corticosteroids: Intensified electrolyte depletion, especially hypokalemia
barbiturates, opioids: May potentiate orthostatic hypotension
calcium: Possibly increased serum calcium level
cholestyramine, colestipol resins: Reduced GI absorption of polythiazide
diazoxide: Increased antihypertensive and hyperglycemic effects of polythiazide
diflunisal: Possibly increased blood polythiazide level
digoxin: Increased risk of digitalis toxicity from hypokalemia
dopamine: Possibly increased diuretic effects of both drugs
insulin, oral antidiabetics: Possibly increased blood glucose level
lithium: Decreased lithium clearance and increased risk of toxicity
neuromuscular blockers: Possibly increased neuromuscular blockade from hypokalemia
nondepolarizing skeletal muscle relaxants (such as tubocurarine): Possibly increased responsiveness to the muscle relaxant
pressor amines (such as norepinephrine): Possibly decreased response to pressor amines
oral anticoagulants: Possibly decreased anticoagulant effects

vitamin D: Increased risk of hypercalcemia

Adverse Reactions

CNS: Dizziness, drowsiness, fatigue, headache, insomnia, malaise, nervousness, paresthesia, syncope, vertigo, weakness
CV: Angina, edema, hypotension, orthostatic hypotension, palpitations, vasculitis
EENT: Blurred vision, dry mouth
ENDO: Hyperglycemia
GI: Abdominal cramps, anorexia, constipation, diarrhea, indigestion, jaundice, nausea, vomiting
GU: Decreased libido, impotence, interstitial nephritis, nocturia, polyuria, renal failure, urinary frequency or incontinence
HEME: Agranulocytosis, aplastic and hemolytic anemia, leukopenia, neutropenia, thrombocytopenia
MS: Muscle spasms and weakness
SKIN: Alopecia, exfoliative dermatitis, photosensitivity, priapism, purpura, rash, urticaria
Other: Anaphylaxis, dehydration, gout, hypercalcemia, hyperuricemia, hypochloremia, hypokalemia, hyponatremia, hypovolemia, metabolic alkalosis, weight loss

Nursing Considerations

- Use cautiously in patients with impaired hepatic function because polythiazide may alter fluid and electrolyte balance and cause hepatic coma.
- Also use cautiously in patients with systemic lupus erythematosus because polythiazide may activate or worsen it.
- Use cautiously in patients with renal impairment because of increased sensitivity to prazocin, in those with angina pectoris because drug may induce or aggravate angina, in those with narcolepsy because prazosin may worsen cataplexy, and in elderly patients because of their increased risk of hypotension.
- Monitor patient closely for the first 90 minutes of first dose because syncope may occur. If so, place patient in recumbent position and treat supportively until blood pressure normalizes.
- Check blood pressure often to assess effectiveness of prazosin and polythiazide therapy.
- Provide hydration, as appropriate, to help prevent hypovolemia.
- Monitor fluid intake and output, daily weight, and serum electrolyte levels (especially potassium) to detect volume depletion or electrolyte imbalance.
- Watch for increased BUN and serum creatinine levels, especially in patients with impaired renal function, because drug may

cause acute renal failure. If increases are significant or persistent, notify prescriber immediately.
• Monitor blood glucose level often in diabetic patients, and expect to increase antidiabetic dosage, as needed and ordered.

PATIENT TEACHING
• Teach patient to monitor her blood pressure and to report consistently elevated measurements to prescriber.
• Direct patient to weigh herself at the same time each day wearing the same amount of clothing and to notify the prescriber if
she gains more than 2 lb (0.9 kg) per day or 5 lb (2.3 kg) per
week.
• Instruct patient to eat a diet high in potassium-rich foods, such
as citrus fruits, bananas, tomatoes, and dates.
• To reduce the risk of dehydration and hypotension, advise patient to avoid exercise in hot weather and to avoid alcohol.
Also instruct her to notify prescriber if she has prolonged diarrhea, nausea, or vomiting.
• Caution patient to avoid potentially hazardous activities until
drug's CNS effects are known.
• Suggest rising slowly from a lying or sitting position to minimize the effects of orthostatic hypotension.
• Advise patient to notify prescriber immediately about adverse
reactions, especially dizziness and fainting.
• Instruct patient not to take any drugs, including OTC preparations, without first consulting prescriber to avoid serious interactions.
• Warn patient that drug may precipitate gout and to report toe
pain to prescriber.
• Explain the importance of regular exercise, proper diet, and
other lifestyle changes in controlling hypertension.

propranolol hydrochloride and hydrochlorothiazide

Inderide, Inderide LA

Class and Category

Chemical: Beta-adrenergic blocker (propranolol), benothiadiazide
(hydrochlorothiazide)
Therapeutic: Antihypertensisve (propranolol, hydrochlorothiazide),
diuretic (hydrochlorothiazide)
Pregnancy category: C

Indications and Dosages

▶ *To treat hypertension*
TABLETS
Adults. *Initial:* 40 mg propranolol and 25 mg hydrochlorothiazide (1 tablet) b.i.d., increased as needed to 80 mg propranolol and 25 mg hydrochlorothiazide (1 tablet) b.i.d., as needed.
E.R. CAPSULES
Adults. 80 to 160 mg propranolol and 50 mg hydrochlorothiazide (1 capsule containing 50 mg hydrochlorothiazide and 80, 120, or 160 mg propranolol) daily.

Mechanism of Action

Propranolol competes with adrenergic neurotransmitters for binding at sympathetic receptor sites. Beta$_1$-receptor blockade decreases resting and exercise heart rate and cardiac output and decreases systolic and diastolic blood pressure.

Hydrochlorothiazide promotes movement of sodium, chloride, and water from blood in peritubular capillaries into the nephron's distal convoluted tubule. Initially, it may decrease extracellular fluid volume, plasma volume, and cardiac output, which helps explain blood pressure reduction. It also may reduce blood pressure by dilating arteries. After several weeks, extracellular fluid volume, plasma volume, and cardiac output return to normal, and peripheral vascular resistance remains decreased.

Contraindications

Anuria; asthma including acute bronchospasm; cardiogenic shock; greater than first-degree AV block; heart failure (unless secondary to tachyarrhythmia that's responsive to propranolol); hypersensitivity to propranolol, hydrochlorothiazide, other sulfonamide-derived drugs, or their components; pulmonary edema; sinus bradycardia

Interactions

DRUGS

propranolol and hydrochlorothiazide
amiodarone: Additive depressant effects on conduction, negative inotropic effects, and increased risk of arrhythmias from hypokalemia
antihypertensives, diuretics: Increased antihypertensive effects
insulin, oral antidiabetics: Possibly increased blood glucose level
neuromuscular blockers: Possibly enhanced neuromuscular blockade from hypokalemia

NSAIDs: Decreased hypotensive effects
sympathomimetics: Possibly mutual inhibition of therapeutic effects
propranolol component
allergen immunotherapy, allergenic extracts for skin testing: Increased
risk of serious systemic adverse reactions or anaphylaxis
aluminum hydroxide: Decreased intestinal absorption of propranolol
anesthetics (hydrocarbon inhalation): Increased risk of myocardial depression and hypotension
beta blockers: Additive beta-blockade effects
calcium channel blockers: Possibly depressed myocardial contractility
or atrioventricular conduction
catecholamine-depleting drugs (such as reserpine): Increased
catecholamine-blocking action which may result in hypotension,
marked bradycardia, vertigo, syncopal attacks, or orthostatic hypotension
chlorpromazine: Increased plasma levels of both drugs
cimetidine: Possibly interference with propranolol clearance, resulting in elevated plasma levels
estrogens: Decreased antihypertensive effect of propranolol
fentanyl, fentanyl derivatives: Possibly increased risk of initial bradycardia after induction of fentanyl or a derivative (with long-term
propranolol use)
glucagon: Possibly blunted hyperglycemic response
haloperidol: Increased risk of hypotension and cardiac arrest
lidocaine: Decreased lidocaine clearance, increased risk of lidocaine
toxicity
MAO inhibitors: Increased risk of significant hypertension
phenothiazines: Increased blood levels of both drugs
phenytoin, phenobarbitone, rifampin: Additive cardiac depressant effects (with parenteral phenytoin), accelerated propranolol clearance
propafenone: Increased blood level and half-life of propranolol
thyroxine: Lowered T_3 level
xanthines: Possibly mutual inhibition of therapeutic effects
hydrochlorothiazide component
amantadine: Possibly increased blood amantadine level and risk of
toxicity
amphotericin B, corticosteroids: Intensified electrolyte depletion, especially hypokalemia
barbiturates, opioids: May potentiate orthostatic hypotension
calcium: Possibly increased serum calcium level
cholestyramine, colestipol resins: Reduced GI absorption of hydrochlorothiazide

diazoxide: Increased antihypertensive and hyperglycemic effects of hydrochlorothiazide
diflunisal: Possibly increased blood hydrochlorothiazide level
digoxin: Increased risk of digitalis toxicity from hypokalemia
dopamine: Possibly increased diuretic effects of both drugs
lithium: Decreased lithium clearance and increased risk of toxicity
nondepolarizing skeletal muscle relaxants (such as tubocurarine): Possibly increased responsiveness to the muscle relaxant
pressor amines (such as norepinephrine): Possibly decreased response to pressor amines
oral anticoagulants: Possibly decreased anticoagulant effects
vitamin D: Increased risk of hypercalcemia
ACTIVITIES
propranolol component
alcohol use: Slowed rate of propranolol absorption
nicotine chewing gum, smoking cessation, smoking deterrents: Increased therapeutic effects of propranolol

Adverse Reactions

CNS: Anxiety, depression, dizziness, drowsiness, fatigue, headache, insomnia, lethargy, nervousness, paresthesia, vertigo, weakness
CV: AV conduction disorders, cold extremities, heart failure, hypotension, orthostatic hypotension, sinus bradycardia, vasculitis
EENT: Blurred vision, dry mouth, nasal congestion
ENDO: Hyperglycemia
GI: Abdominal cramps or pain, anorexia, constipation, diarrhea, indigestion, jaundice, nausea, vomiting
GU: Decreased libido, impotence, interstitial nephritis, nocturia, polyuria, renal failure
HEME: Agranulocytosis, aplastic and hemolytic anemia, leukopenia, neutropenia, thrombocytopenia
MS: Muscle spasms and weakness
RESP: Bronchospasm, dyspnea, wheezing
SKIN: Alopecia, erythema multiforme, exfoliative dermatitis, photosensitivity, purpura, rash, Stevens-Johnson syndrome, toxic epidermal necrolysis, urticaria
Other: Anaphylaxis, dehydration, hypercalcemia, hyperuricemia, hypochloremia, hypokalemia, hyponatremia, hypovolemia, metabolic alkalosis, weight loss

Nursing Considerations

• Use cautiously in patients with impaired hepatic function because hydrochlorothiazide may alter fluid and electrolyte balance and lead to hepatic coma.

- Also use cautiously in patients with systemic lupus erythematosus because hydrochlorothiazide may activate or worsen it.
- Monitor blood pressure, apical and radial pulses, respiration, and circulation in limbs before and during therapy to assess effectiveness and detect adverse reactions of therapy.
- Monitor patient closely for hypersensitivity reactions. If patient develops a rash, urticaria, or has trouble breathing, notify prescriber and withhold drug, as ordered. Be aware that patient may be unresponsive to doses of epinephrine usually given to treat allergic reaction.
- Provide adequate hydration, as appropriate, to help prevent hypovolemia.
- Monitor fluid intake and output, daily weight, and serum electrolyte levels (especially potassium) to detect volume depletion or electrolyte imbalance.
- Because propranolol's negative inotropic effect can depress cardiac output, monitor cardiac output in patients with heart failure, particularly those with severely compromised left ventricular dysfunction.
- Be aware that propranolol can mask tachycardia that occurs in hyperthyroidism. Abrupt withdrawal in patients with hyperthyroidism or thyrotoxicosis can precipitate thyroid storm.
- Watch for increased BUN and serum creatinine levels, especially in patients with impaired renal function, because drug may cause acute renal failure. If increases are significant or persistent, notify prescriber immediately.
- Monitor blood glucose level often in diabetic patients. Propranolol may prolong and mask signs of hypoglycemia (especially tachycardia, palpitations, and tremor), but it doesn't suppress diaphoresis or hypertensive response to hypoglycemia. Propranolol and hydrochlorothiazide also may increase blood glucose level. Notify prescriber if hyperglycemia occurs, and expect to increase antidiabetic dosage, as needed and ordered.
- **WARNING** Be aware that stopping propranolol and hydrochlorothiazide abruptly may cause myocardial ischemia, MI, ventricular arrhythmias, or severe hypertension, particularly in patients with cardiac disease.

PATIENT TEACHING
- Teach patient to monitor her blood pressure and take her pulse. Tell her to report consistent abnormalities to prescriber.
- Direct patient to weigh herself at the same time each day wearing the same amount of clothing and to notify prescriber if she gains more than 2 lb (0.9 kg) per day or 5 lb (2.3 kg) per week.

- Instruct patient to eat a diet high in potassium-rich foods, such as citrus fruits, bananas, tomatoes, and dates.
- To reduce the risk of dehydration and hypotension, advise patient to avoid exercise in hot weather and alcohol use. Also instruct her to notify prescriber if she experiences prolonged diarrhea, nausea, or vomiting.
- Caution patient to avoid potentially hazardous activities until drug's CNS effects are known.
- Explain the importance of regular exercise, proper diet, and other lifestyle changes in controlling hypertension.
- Caution patient not to change dosage without consulting prescriber and not to stop taking drug abruptly.
- Advise patient to notify prescriber immediately if she experiences shortness of breath.
- Advise patient to consult prescriber before taking OTC drugs, especially cold remedies.
- Tell smoker to notify prescriber immediately if she stops smoking because smoking cessation may decrease propranolol metabolism, calling for dosage adjustments.
- Advise diabetic patient to monitor blood glucose levels closely as drug may alter control and mask some signs of hypoglycemia.

quinapril and hydrochlorothiazide
Accuretic

Class and Category
Chemical: Ethylester of quinaprilat (quinapril), benothiadiazine (hydrochlorothiazide)
Therapeutic: Antihypertensive, diuretic
Pregnancy category: C (first trimester), D (second and third trimesters)

Indications and Dosages
▶ *To treat hypertension uncontrolled with quinapril alone; to treat hypertension in patients adequately controlled with hydrochlorothiazide alone but who develop significant potassium loss*
TABLETS
Adults. *Initial:* 10 mg quinapril and 12.5 mg hydrochlorothiazide (1 tablet) or 20 mg quinapril and 12.5 mg hydrochlorothiaizide (1 tablet) daily. Increased as needed q 2 to 3 wk. *Maximum:* 20 mg quinapril and 25 mg hydrochlorothiaizide daily.

Mechanism of Action

Quinapril may reduce blood pressure by affecting the renin-angiotensin-aldosterone system. By inhibiting ACE, quinapril:

- prevents conversion of angiotensin I to angiotensin II, a potent vasoconstrictor that also stimulates adrenal cortex to secrete aldosterone.
- may inhibit renal and vascular production of angiotensin II.
- decreases serum angiotensin II level and increases serum renin activity. This decreases aldosterone secretion, slightly increasing serum potassium level.
- decreases vascular tone and blood pressure.
- inhibits aldosterone release, which reduces sodium and water reabsorption and increases their excretion, further reducing blood pressure.

Hydrochlorothiazide promotes movement of sodium, chloride, and water from blood in peritubular capillaries into the nephron's distal convoluted tubule. Initially, it may decrease extracellular fluid volume, plasma volume, and cardiac output, which helps explain blood pressure reduction. It also may reduce blood pressure by dilating arteries. After several weeks, extracellular fluid volume, plasma volume, and cardiac output return to normal, and peripheral vascular resistance remains decreased.

Contraindications

Anuria; hereditary or idiopathic angioedema; history of angioedema from previous ACE inhibitor; hypersensitivity to quinapril, hydrochlorothiazide, other sulfonamide-derived drugs, or their components

Interactions

DRUGS

quinapril and hydrochlorothiaizide

antihypertensives, diuretics: Additive hypotensive effects
lithium: Increased blood lithium level and lithium toxicity
NSAIDs, sympathomimetics: Possibly reduced antihypertensive effects of quinapril and hydrochlorizide and increased risk of renal toxicity

quinapril component

allopurinol, bone marrow depressants (such as amphotericin B and methotrexate), procainamide, systemic corticosteroids: Possibly increased risk of fatal neutropenia or agranulocytosis
CNS depressants: Additive hypotensive effects
cyclosporine, potassium-sparing diuretics, potassium supplements: Increased risk of hyperkalemia

tetracyclines: Reduced tetracycline absorption
hydrochlorothiazide component
amantadine: Possibly increased blood amantadine level and risk of toxicity
amiodarone: Increased risk of arrhythmias from hypokalemia
amphotericin B, corticosteroids: Intensified electrolyte depletion, especially hypokalemia
antihypertensives: Increased antihypertensive effects
barbiturates, opioids: May potentiate orthostatic hypotension
calcium: Possibly increased serum calcium level
cholestyramine, colestipol resins: Reduced GI absorption of hydrochlorothiazide
diazoxide: Increased antihypertensive and hyperglycemic effects of hydrochlorothiazide
diflunisal: Possibly increased blood hydrochlorothiazide level
digoxin: Increased risk of digitalis toxicity from hypokalemia
dopamine: Possibly increased diuretic effects of both drugs
insulin, oral antidiabetics: Possibly increased blood glucose level
lithium: Decreased lithium clearance and increased risk of toxicity
neuromuscular blockers: Possibly enhanced neuromuscular blockade from hypokalemia
nondepolarizing skeletal muscle relaxants (such as tubocurarine): Possibly increased responsiveness to the muscle relaxant
NSAIDs: Increased risk of renal failure
pressor amines (such as norepinephrine): Possibly decreased response to pressor amines
oral anticoagulants: Possibly decreased anticoagulant effects
sympathomimetics: Possibly decreased antihypertensive effect of hydrochlorothiazide
vitamin D: Increased risk of hypercalcemia
FOODS
quinapril component
potassium-containing salt substitutes: Increased risk of hyperkalemia
ACTIVITIES
quinapril component
alcohol use: Possibly additive hypotensive effect

Adverse Reactions

CNS: Depression, dizziness, drowsiness, fatigue, headache, insomnia, light-headedness, malaise, paresthesia, sleep disturbance, syncope, vertigo, weakness
CV: Chest pain, hypotension, orthostatic hypotension, palpitations, tachycardia, vasculitis

EENT: Amblyopia, blurred vision, dry mouth, loss of taste, pharyngitis
ENDO: Hyperglycemia
GI: Abdominal cramps or pain, anorexia, constipation, diarrhea, indigestion, jaundice, nausea, vomiting
GU: Decreased libido, impotence, interstitial nephritis, nocturia, polyuria, renal failure
HEME: Agranulocytosis, aplastic and hemolytic anemia, leukopenia, neutropenia, thrombocytopenia
MS: Arthralgia, back pain, muscle spasms and weakness, myalgia
RESP: Cough, dyspnea
SKIN: Alopecia, diaphoresis, exfoliative dermatitis, flushing, photosensitivity, pruritus, purpura, rash, urticaria
Other: Anaphylaxis, angioedema, dehydration, hypercalcemia, hyperkalemia, hyperuricemia, hypochloremia, hypokalemia, hypomagnesemia, hyponatremia, hypovolemia, metabolic alkalosis, weight loss

Nursing Considerations

- Use cautiously in patients with impaired hepatic function because hydrochlorothiazide may alter fluid and electrolyte balance and lead to hepatic coma. Quinapril, an ACE inhibitor, may induce a syndrome that starts with cholestatic jaundice and progresses to fulminant hepatic necrosis that may be fatal.
- Also use cautiously in patients with systemic lupus erythematosus because hydrochlorothiazide may activate or worsen it.
- **WARNING** Be aware that patients with heart failure, hyponatremia, or severe volume or sodium depletion; those who've recently received intensive diuresis or an increase in diuretic dosage; and those undergoing dialysis may be at risk of excessive hypotension. Monitor blood pressure often during first 2 weeks of therapy and whenever dosage increases. If excessive hypotension occurs, notify prescriber immediately, place patient in a supine position and, if prescribed, infuse normal saline solution.
- Monitor blood pressure often to assess effectiveness of of quinapril and hydrochlorothiazide therapy.
- **WARNING** Because of the risk of angioedema, be prepared to stop drug and administer emergency measures, including subcutaneous epinephrine 1:1,000 (0.3 to 0.5 ml) if swelling of tongue, glottis, or larynx causes airway obstruction.
- Provide adequate hydration, as appropriate, to help prevent hypovolemia.

- If pregnancy is suspected, notify prescriber immediately; drug will need to be stopped.
- Monitor fluid intake and output, daily weight, and serum electrolyte levels (especially potassium) to detect volume depletion or electrolyte imbalance.
- Watch for increased BUN and serum creatinine levels, especially in patients with impaired renal function, because drug may cause acute renal failure. If increases are significant or persistent, notify prescriber immediately.
- Monitor blood glucose level often in diabetic patients, and expect to increase antidiabetic dosage, as needed and ordered.
- Monitor patient's WBC counts regularly, as ordered, especially in patients with collagen vascular disease or renal disease.

PATIENT TEACHING
- Advise patient to take drug in the morning or early evening to avoid the need to urinate during the night.
- Teach patient to monitor her blood pressure and to report consistently elevated measurements to prescriber.
- Instruct patient to stop drug and tell prescriber immediately if she has swelling of face, eyes, lips, or tongue or trouble breathing.
- Direct patient to weigh herself at the same time each day wearing the same amount of clothing and to notify prescriber if she gains more than 2 lb (0.9 kg) per day or 5 lb (2.3 kg) per week.
- Instruct patient to consult prescriber before using potassium supplements or salt substitutes that contain potassium.
- To reduce the risk of dehydration and hypotension, advise patient to avoid exercise in hot weather and to avoid alcohol. Urge her to report prolonged diarrhea, nausea, or vomiting.
- Explain that drug may cause dizziness and light-headedness, especially during the first few days. Caution patient to avoid potentially hazardous activities until drug's CNS effects are known and to notify prescriber immediately if he faints.
- Inform female patient of childbearing age about risks of taking quinapril and hydrochlorothiazide during pregnancy. Caution her to use effective contraception and to notify prescriber immediately about known or suspected pregnancy.
- Advise patient planning to undergo surgery or anesthesia to inform specialist that she takes quinapril and hydrochlorothiazide.
- Tell patient to notify prescriber about yellowing of the skin or whites of her eyes because drug may need to be stopped.
- Stress importance of notifying prescriber if any indications of infection, such as a sore throat or fever occurs.

- Explain the importance of regular exercise, proper diet, and other lifestyle changes in controlling hypertension.

spironolactone and hydrochlorothiazide
Aldactazide

Class and Category

Chemical: Aldosterone antagonist (spironolactone), benothiadiazide (hydrochlorothiazide)

Therapeutic: Antihypertensive (spironolactone, hydrochlorothiazide), potassium-sparing diuretic (spironolactone, hydrochlorothiazide)

Pregnancy category: C

Indications and Dosages

▶ *To treat hypertension*

TABLETS

Adults. *Initial:* 25 mg spironolactone and 25 mg hydrochlorothiazide (1 tablet) daily, increased as needed to 50 to 100 mg spironolactone and 50 to 100 mg hydrochlorothiazide (number of tablets variable depending on strength used) daily or b.i.d.

▶ *To relieve edema in patients with heart failure, hepatic cirrhosis, or nephrotic syndrome*

TABLETS

Adults. 25 to 200 mg spironolactone and 25 to 200 mg hydrochlorothiazide (number of tablets variable depending on strength used) once daily or in divided doses.

Mechanism of Action

Spironolactone competes with aldosterone for receptors on the walls of distal convoluted tubule cells, thereby preventing sodium and water reabsorption and causing their excretion through the distal convoluted tubules while limiting excretion of potassium and magnesium. Increased urinary excretion of sodium and water reduces blood volume and blood pressure.

Hydrochlorothiazide promotes movement of sodium, chloride, and water from blood in peritubular capillaries into the nephron's distal convoluted tubule. Initially, it may decrease extracellular fluid volume, plasma volume, and cardiac output, which helps explain blood pressure reduction. It also may reduce blood pressure by dilating arteries. After several weeks, extracellular fluid volume, plasma volume, and cardiac output return to normal, and peripheral vascular resistance remains decreased.

Contraindications

Acute renal insufficiency, anuria, hyperkalemia, hypersensitivity to spironolactone, hydrochlorothiazide, other sulfonamide-derived drugs, or their components

Interactions

DRUGS

spironolactone and hydrochlorothiazide

antihypertensives: Possibly potentiated antihypertensive or diuretic effects of spironolactone and hydrochlorothizide

digoxin: Possibly increased half-life of digoxin and increased risk of digitalis toxicity

heparin, oral anticoagulants: Decreased anticoagulant effect of these drugs

lithium: Decreased lithium clearance and increased risk of toxicity

NSAIDs, sympathomimetics: Possibly decreased antihypertensive effect of spironolactone and hydrochlorothiazide

spironolactone component

ACE inhibitors, cyclosporine, potassium-containing drugs, potassium-sparing diuretics, potassium supplements: Increased risk of hyperkalemia

exchange resins (sodium cycle), such as sodium polystyrene sulfonate: Increased risk of hypokalemia and fluid retention

hydrochlorothiazide component

amantadine: Possibly increased blood amantadine level and risk of toxicity

amiodarone: Increased risk of arrhythmias from hypokalemia

amphotericin B, corticosteroids: Intensified electrolyte depletion, especially hypokalemia

barbiturates, opioids: May potentiate orthostatic hypotension

calcium: Possibly increased serum calcium level

cholestyramine, colestipol resins: Reduced GI absorption of hydrochlorothiazide

diazoxide: Increased antihypertensive and hyperglycemic effects of hydrochlorothiazide

diflunisal: Possibly increased blood hydrochlorothiazide level

dopamine: Possibly increased diuretic effects of both drugs

insulin, oral antidiabetics: Possibly increased blood glucose level

neuromuscular blockers: Possibly enhanced neuromuscular blockade from hypokalemia

nondepolarizing skeletal muscle relaxants (such as tubocurarine): Possibly increased responsiveness to the muscle relaxant

pressor amines (such as norepinephrine): Possibly decreased response
to pressor amines
vitamin D: Increased risk of hypercalcemia
FOODS
spironolactone component
low-salt milk, salt substitutes: Increased risk of hyperkalemia

Adverse Reactions

CNS: Dizziness, encephalopathy, fatigue, headache, insomnia,
paresthesia, vertigo, weakness
CV: Hypotension, orthostatic hypotension, vasculitis
EENT: Blurred vision, dry mouth, increased intraocular pressure,
nasal congestion, tinnitus, vision changes
ENDO: Gyncomastia, hyperglycemia
GI: Abdominal cramps or pain, anorexia, constipation, diarrhea,
flatulence, indigestion, jaundice, nausea, vomiting
GU: Decreased libido, impotence, interstitial nephritis, nocturia,
polyuria, renal failure
HEME: Agranulocytosis, aplastic and hemolytic anemia, leuko-
penia, neutropenia, thrombocytopenia
MS: Arthralgia, back and leg pain, muscle spasms and weakness,
myalgia
RESP: Cough, dyspnea
SKIN: Alopecia, exfoliative dermatitis, photosensitivity, purpura,
rash, Stevens-Johnson syndrome, urticaria
Other: Anaphylaxis, dehydration, hypercalcemia, hyperkalemia,
hyperuricemia, hypochloremia, hypokalemia, hypomagnesemia,
hyponatremia, hypovolemia, metabolic alkalosis, weight loss

Nursing Considerations

• Use cautiously in patients with impaired hepatic function because hydrochlorothiazide may alter fluid and electrolyte balance and lead to hepatic coma.
• Also use cautiously in patients with systemic lupus erythematosus because hydrochlorothiazide may activate or worsen it.
• Monitor blood pressure often to assess effectiveness of spironolactone and hydrochlorothiazide.
• Provide hydration, as appropriate, to help prevent hypovolemia.
• Monitor fluid intake and output, daily weight, and serum electrolyte levels (especially potassium) to detect volume depletion
or electrolyte imbalance.
• Watch for increased BUN and serum creatinine levels, especially
in patients with impaired renal function, because drug may

cause acute renal failure. If increases are significant or persistent, notify prescriber immediately.

- Monitor blood glucose level often in diabetic patients, and expect to increase antidiabetic dosage, as needed and ordered.

PATIENT TEACHING

- Advise patient to take spironolactone and hydrochlorothiazide in the morning or early evening to avoid the need to urinate during the night. Tell patient to take drug with meals or milk to minimize stomach upset.
- Teach patient to monitor her blood pressure and to report consistently elevated measurements to prescriber.
- Direct patient to weigh herself at the same time each day wearing the same amount of clothing and to notify prescriber if she gains more than 2 lb (0.9 kg) per day or 5 lb (2.3 kg) per week.
- Instruct patient to eat a diet high in potassium-rich foods, such as citrus fruits, bananas, tomatoes, and dates.
- To reduce the risk of dehydration and hypotension, advise patient to avoid exercise in hot weather and to avoid alcohol. Also instruct her to notify prescriber if she has prolonged diarrhea, nausea, or vomiting.
- Caution patient to avoid potentially hazardous activities until drug's CNS effects are known.
- Explain the importance of regular exercise, proper diet, and other lifestyle changes in controlling hypertension.

trandolapril and verapamil hydrochloride

Tarka

Class and Category

Chemical: Non–sulfhydryl-containing ACE inhibitor (trandolapril), phenylalkylamine derivative (verapamil)
Therapeutic: Antihypertensive
Pregnancy: C (first trimester), D (later trimesters)

Indications and Dosages

▶ *To treat hypertension*

E.R. TABLETS

Adults. *Initial:* 1 mg trandolapril and 240 mg verapamil, 2 mg trandolapril and 180 mg verapamil, 2 mg trandolapril and 240 mg verapamil, or 4 mg trandolapril and 240 mg verapamil daily. *Maximum:* 4 mg trandolapril and 240 mg verapamil.

DOSAGE ADJUSTMENT Patients with hepatic impairment given 30% of normal dosage. Dosage may be reduced in patients with cirrhosis and those with creatinine clearance less than 30 ml/min/1.73 m^2.

Mechanism of Action

Trandolapril is the prodrug for trandolaprilat, which reduces blood pressure by inhibiting conversion of angiotensin I to angiotensin II. Angiotensin II is a potent vasoconstrictor that stimulates the renal cortex to secrete aldosterone. Decreased aldosterone release reduces sodium and water retention and increases their excretion, thereby reducing blood pressure. Trandolapril may also inhibit renal and vascular production of angiotensin II.

Verapamil inhibits calcium entry into coronary and vascular smooth-muscle cells by blocking slow calcium channels in cell membranes. The resulting decrease in intracellular calcium level inhibits smooth-muscle cell contractions and decreases myocardial oxygen demand by relaxing coronary and vascular smooth muscle, reducing peripheral vascular resistance, and decreasing systolic and diastolic blood pressures.

Contraindications

Cardiogenic shock; history of angioedema from previous ACE inhibitor use; hypersensitivity to trandolapril, other ACE inhibitors, verapamil, or their components; hypotension; severe heart failure; severe left ventricular dysfunction; sick sinus syndrome or second- or third-degree AV block (unless artificial pacemaker is in place)

Interactions

DRUGS

trandolapril and verapamil

beta blockers: Increased risk of heart failure, hypotension, and severe bradycardia

carbamazepine, cyclosporine, theophylline: Possibly increased blood levels of these drugs and increased risk of toxicity

digoxin: Increased blood digoxin level and risk of digitalis toxicity

disopyramide, flecainide: Possibly additive negative inotropic effects

diuretics: Increased risk of hypotension

lithium: Increased risk of lithium-induced neurotoxicity

neuromuscular blockers: Prolonged recovery from neuromuscular blockade

potassium-sparing diuretics, potassium supplements: Increased risk of hyperkalemia *quinidine:* Increased risk of quinidine toxicity, increased QT interval, additive negative inotropic effects

verapamil component

anesthetics (inhaled): Enhanced cardiodepressive effects of verapamil

cimetidine: Decreased metabolism and increased blood verapamil level

phenobarbital: Increased verapamil clearance

rifampin: Decreased bioavailability of oral verapamil

FOODS

trandolapril and verapamil

high-potassium diet, potassium-containing salt substitutes: Increased risk of hyperkalemia

verapamil component

all foods: Decreased verapamil bioavailability

Adverse Reactions

CNS: Dizziness, fatigue

CV: AV block, bradycardia, junctional rhythm, orthostatic hypotension

EENT: Dry mouth

GI: Constipation

RESP: Cough

Other: Angioedema

Nursing Considerations

- Be aware that disopyramide and flecainide should not be given within 48 hours before or 24 hours after trandolapril and verapamil because additive negative inotropic effects can result.
- **WARNING** Closely monitor blood pressure during first 2 weeks of therapy and whenever dosage or accompanying diuretic dosage is adjusted, especially in patients with heart failure, hyponatremia, or severe volume or sodium loss. If excessive hypotension occurs, notify prescriber immediately, place patient in supine position, and prepare to infuse I.V. normal saline solution, as prescribed.
- **WARNING** Be alert for signs and symptoms of angioedema. If swelling of tongue, glottis, or larynx causes airway obstruction, notify prescriber and be prepared to stop drug and administer emergency measures, including subcutaneous epinephrine 1:1,000 (0.3 to 0.5 ml).
- Assess patient for bradycardia and hypotension, which may indicate AV block, and notify prescriber if heart rate or blood pressure declines significantly.

- Continue to monitor blood pressure to assess drug's long-term effectiveness.

PATIENT TEACHING
- Instruct patient not to crush or chew E.R. trandolapril and verapamil tablet, but inform her that she may break tablet in half to aid in swallowing.
- Advise patient to take drug with food.
- Direct patient to monitor pulse rate before taking drug and to notify prescriber if pulse rate falls below 50 beats/min or as instructed by prescriber.
- Instruct patient to stop drug and notify prescriber immediately if she has swelling of face, eyes, lips, or tongue or has trouble breathing.
- Explain that drug may cause dizziness and light-headedness, especially during first few days of therapy. Urge patient to avoid potentially hazardous activities until drug's adverse CNS effects are known and to notify prescriber immediately if she faints.
- Inform female patient of childbearing age about risks of taking trandolapril and verapamil during pregnancy, especially during second and third trimesters. Urge her to use effective contraception and to notify prescriber immediately if she is or could be pregnant.
- Advise patient planning to undergo surgery or anesthesia to inform specialist that she takes trandolapril and verapamil.
- Instruct patient to consult prescriber before using potassium supplements or salt substitutes containing potassium.
- Encourage patient to increase dietary fiber intake to prevent constipation. Advise her to notify prescriber if constipation persists.

telmisartan and hydrochlorothiazide
Micardis HCT

Class and Category
Chemical: AT1 angiotensin II receptor antagonist (telmisartan), benothiadiazide (hydrochlorothiazide)
Therapeutic: Antihypertensive (telmisartan, hydrochlorothiazide), diuretic (hydrochlorothiazide)
Pregnancy category: C (first trimester), D (second and third trimesters)

Indications and Dosages
▶ *To treat hypertension uncontrolled by 80 mg telmisartan daily*

TABLETS

Adults. *Initial:* 80 mg telmisartan and 12.5 mg hydrochloroth-iazide (1 tablet) daily. Dosage gradually increased q 2 to 4 wk, as needed. *Maximum:* 160 mg telmisartan and 25 mg hydrochloroth-iazide.

▶ *To treat hypertension uncontrolled by 25 mg hydrochlorothiazide daily*

TABLETS

Adults. *Initial:* 80 mg telmisartan and 12.5 mg hydrochloroth-iazide (1 tablet) daily or 80 mg telmisartan and 25 mg hydro-chlorothiazide (1 tablet) daily. Dosage gradually increased q 2 to 4 wk, as needed. *Maximum:* 160 mg telmisartan and 25 mg hy-drochlorothiazide.

▶ *To treat hypertension for patients adequately controlled by hydro-chlorothiazide alone but who develop significant potassium loss*

TABLETS

Adults. 80 mg telmisartan and 12.5 mg hydrochlorothiazide (1 tablet) daily.

Mechanism of Action

Telmisartan blocks angiotensin II from binding to AT1 receptor sites in many tissues, including vascular smooth muscle and adrenal glands. This inhibits the vasoconstrictive and aldosterone-secreting effects of angiotensin II, which reduces blood pressure.

Hydrochlorothiazide promotes movement of sodium, chloride, and water from blood in peritubular capillaries into the nephron's distal convoluted tubule. Initially, it may decrease extracellular fluid volume, plasma volume, and cardiac output, which helps explain blood pressure reduction. It also may reduce blood pressure by dilating arteries. After several weeks, extracellular fluid volume, plasma volume, and cardiac output return to normal, and pe-ripheral vascular resistance remains decreased.

Contraindications

Anuria; hypersensitivity to telmisartan, hydrochlorothiazide, other sulfonamide-derived drugs, or their components; pregnancy; renal failure

Interactions

DRUGS

telmisartan and hydrochlorothiazide

antihypertensives, diuretics: Increased antihypertensive effects
digoxin: Increased risk of digitalis toxicity

telmisartan component
potassium-sparing diuretics: Increased risk of hyperkalemia
warfarin: Possibly slight decrease in mean warfarin trough level
hydrochlorothiazide component
amantadine: Possibly increased blood amantadine level and risk of toxicity
amiodarone: Increased risk of arrhythmias from hypokalemia
amphotericin B, corticosteroids: Intensified electrolyte depletion, especially hypokalemia
barbiturates, opioids: May potentiate orthostatic hypotension
calcium: Possibly increased serum calcium level
cholestyramine, colestipol resins: Reduced GI absorption of hydrochlorothiazide
diazoxide: Increased antihypertensive and hyperglycemic effects of hydrochlorothiazide
diflunisal: Possibly increased blood hydrochlorothiazide level
dopamine: Possibly increased diuretic effects of both drugs
insulin, oral antidiabetics: Possibly increased blood glucose level
lithium: Decreased lithium clearance and increased risk of toxicity
neuromuscular blockers: Possibly increased neuromuscular blockade from hypokalemia
nondepolarizing skeletal muscle relaxants (such as tubocurarine): Possibly increased responsiveness to the muscle relaxant
NSAIDs: Decreased diuretic effect of hydrochlorothiazide, increased risk of renal failure
pressor amines (such as norepinephrine): Possibly decreased response to pressor amines
oral anticoagulants: Possibly decreased anticoagulant effects
sympathomimetics: Possibly decreased antihypertensive effect of hydrochlorothiazide
vitamin D: Increased risk of hypercalcemia

Adverse Reactions
CNS: Dizziness, fatigue, headache, insomnia, paresthesia, syncope, vertigo, weakness
CV: Chest pain, hypotension, orthostatic hypotension, peripheral edema, vasculitis
EENT: Blurred vision, dry mouth
ENDO: Hyperglycemia
GI: Abdominal cramps, anorexia, constipation, diarrhea, indigestion, jaundice, nausea, vomiting
GU: Decreased libido, impotence, interstitial nephritis, nocturia, polyuria, renal failure

HEME: Agranulocytosis, aplastic and hemolytic anemia, leukopenia, neutropenia, thrombocytopenia
MS: Muscle spasms and weakness
SKIN: Alopecia, exfoliative dermatitis, photosensitivity, purpura, rash, Stevens-Johnson syndrome, urticaria
Other: Anaphylaxis, dehydration, hypercalcemia, hyperuricemia, hypochloremia, hypokalemia, hypomagnesemia, hyponatremia, hypovolemia, metabolic alkalosis, weight loss

Nursing Considerations

- Use cautiously in patients with impaired hepatic function.
- Also use cautiously in patients with systemic lupus erythematosus because hydrochlorothiazide may activate or worsen it.
- Monitor liver function test results, as ordered. Assess for signs of drug toxicity and fluid and electrolyte imbalance in patients with severe hepatic disease because altered fluid and electrolyte balance may lead to hepatic coma.
- Monitor blood pressure often to assess effectiveness of telmisartan and hydrochlorothiazide therapy.
- Provide adequate hydration, as appropriate, to help prevent hypovolemia.
- Monitor fluid intake and output, daily weight, and serum electrolyte levels (especially potassium) to detect volume depletion or electrolyte imbalance.
- Watch for increased BUN and serum creatinine levels, especially in patients with impaired renal function, because drug may cause acute renal failure. If increases are significant or persistent, notify prescriber immediately.
- Monitor blood glucose level often in diabetic patients, and expect to increase antidiabetic dosage, as needed and ordered.

PATIENT TEACHING

- Advise patient to take telmisartan and hydrochlorothiazide in the morning or early evening to avoid the need to urinate during the night.
- Teach patient to monitor her blood pressure and report consistent elevations to prescriber.
- Direct patient to weigh herself at the same time each day wearing the same amount of clothing and to notify prescriber if she gains more than 2 lb (0.9 kg) per day or 5 lb (2.3 kg) per week.
- Instruct patient to eat a diet high in potassium-rich foods, such as citrus fruits, bananas, tomatoes, and dates.
- To reduce the risk of dehydration and hypotension, advise patient to avoid exercise in hot weather and to avoid alcohol.

Also instruct her to notify prescriber if she has prolonged diarrhea, nausea, or vomiting.
• Caution patient to avoid potentially hazardous activities until drug's CNS effects are known.
• Explain the importance of regular exercise, proper diet, and other lifestyle changes in controlling hypertension.
• Advise female patients of childbearing age to notify prescriber immediately about known or suspected pregnancy.

timolol maleate and hydrochlorothiazide
Timolide

Class and Category
Chemical: Beta blocker (timolol), benothiadiazide (hydrochlorothiazide)
Therapeutic: Antihypertensive (timolol, hydrochlorothiazide), diuretic (hydrochlorothiazide)
Pregnancy category: C

Indications and Dosages
▶ *To treat hypertension*
TABLETS
Adults. 10 mg timolol and 25 mg hydrochlorothiazide (1 tablet) b.i.d. or 20 mg timiolol and 50 mg hydrochlorothiazide (2 tablets) daily.

Mechanism of Action
Timolol blocks beta$_1$ and beta$_2$ receptors in vascular smooth muscle and beta1 receptors in the heart. This reduces peripheral vascular resistance and blood pressure.

Hydrochlorothiazide promotes movement of sodium, chloride, and water from blood in peritubular capillaries into the nephron's distal convoluted tubule. Initially, it may decrease extracellular fluid volume, plasma volume, and cardiac output, which helps explain blood pressure reduction. It also may reduce blood pressure by dilating arteries. After several weeks, extracellular fluid volume, plasma volume, and cardiac output return to normal, and peripheral vascular resistance remains decreased.

Contraindications
Acute bronchospasm; anuria; asthma; cardiogenic shock; children; COPD (severe); heart failure; hypersensitivity to timolol, hy-

drochlorothiazide, other beta blockers or sulfonamide-derived drugs, or any of their components; pulmonary edema; second- or third-degree AV block; severe sinus bradycardia

Interactions
DRUGS
timolol and hydrochlorothiazide
amiodarone: Additive depressant effects on conduction, negative inotropic effects, increased risk of arrhythmias from hypokalemia,
antihypertensives, diuretics: Increased antihypertensive effects
insulin, oral antidiabetics: Possibly increased blood glucose level
neuromuscular blockers: Possibly increased neuromuscular blockade from hypokalemia
NSAIDs: Decreased hypotensive effects
sympathomimetics: Possibly mutual inhibition of therapeutic effects
timolol component
allergen immunotherapy, allergenic extracts for skin testing: Increased risk of serious systemic adverse reactions or anaphylaxis
anesthetics (hydrocarbon inhalation): Increased risk of myocardial depression and hypotension
beta blockers: Additive beta-blockade effects
calcium channel blockers: Possibly depressed myocardial contractility or atrioventricular conduction.
catecholamine-depleting drugs (such as reserpine): Increased catecholamine-blocking action which may result in hypotension, marked bradycardia, vertigo, syncopal attacks or orthostatic hypotension
cimetidine: Possibly interference with timolol clearance, causing increased plasma levels
estrogens: Decreased antihypertensive effect of timolol
fentanyl, fentanyl derivatives: Possibly increased risk of initial bradycardia after induction of fentanyl or a derivative (with long-term timolol use)
glucagon: Possibly blunted hyperglycemic response
insulin, oral antidiabetics: Possibly masking of tachycardia in response to hypoglycemia
lidocaine: Decreased lidocaine clearance, increased risk of lidocaine toxicity
MAO inhibitors: Increased risk of significant hypertension
phenothiazines: Increased blood levels of both drugs
phenytoin (parenteral): Additive cardiac depressant effects, accelerated timolol clearance
xanthines: Possibly mutual inhibition of therapeutic effects

hydrochlorothiazide component

amantadine: Possibly increased blood level and risk of toxicity of amantadine

amphotericin B, corticosteroids: Intensified electrolyte depletion, especially hypokalemia

barbiturates, opioids: May potentiate orthostatic hypotension

calcium: Possibly increased serum calcium level

cholestyramine, colestipol resins: Reduced GI absorption of hydrochlorothiazide

diazoxide: Increased antihypertensive and hyperglycemic effects of hydrochlorothiazide

diflunisal: Possibly increased blood hydrochlorothiazide level

digoxin: Increased risk of digitalis toxicity from hypokalemia

dopamine: Possibly increased diuretic effects of both drugs

lithium: Decreased lithium clearance and increased risk of toxicity

nondepolarizing skeletal muscle relaxants (such as tubocurarine): Possibly increased responsiveness to the muscle relaxant

pressor amines (such as norepinephrine): Possibly decreased response to pressor amines

oral anticoagulants: Possibly decreased anticoagulant effects

vitamin D: Increased risk of hypercalcemia

Adverse Reactions

CNS: Asthenia, CVA, decreased concentration, depression, dizziness, fatigue, hallucinations, headache, insomnia, nervousness, nightmares, paresthesia, syncope, vertigo, weakness

CV: Angina, arrhythmias, bradycardia, cardiac arrest, chest pain, edema, hypotension, orthostatic hypotension, palpitations, Raynaud's phenomenon, vasodilation, vasculitis

EENT: Blurred vision, diplopia, dry eyes or mouth, eye irritation, ptosis, tinnitus, vision changes

ENDO: Hyperglycemia, hypoglycemia

GI: Abdominal cramps or pain, anorexia, constipation, diarrhea, hepatomegaly, indigestion, jaundice, nausea, vomiting

GU: Decreased libido, impotence, interstitial nephritis, nocturia, polyuria, renal failure

HEME: Agranulocytosis, aplastic and hemolytic anemia, leukopenia, neutropenia, thrombocytopenia

MS: Arthralgia, muscle spasms and weakness

RESP: Bronchospasm, cough, crackles, dyspnea

SKIN: Alopecia, diaphoresis, exfoliative dermatitis, hyperpigmentation, photosensitivity, pruritus, psoriasis flare up, purpura, rash, urticaria

Other: Anaphylaxis, dehydration, hypercalcemia, hyperuricemia, hypochloremia, hypokalemia, hyponatremia, hypovolemia, metabolic alkalosis, weight loss

Nursing Considerations

- Use cautiously in patients with impaired hepatic function because hydrochlorothiazide may alter fluid and electrolyte balance and lead to hepatic coma.
- Also use cautiously in patients with systemic lupus erythematosus because hydrochlorothiazide may activate or worsen it.
- Monitor blood pressure often to assess effectiveness of therapy. Expect varied effectiveness in elderly patients; they may be less sensitive to drug's antihypertensive effect or more sensitive because of reduced drug clearance.
- **WARNING** Be aware that timolol and hydrochlorothiazide shouldn't be stopped abruptly because this may produce MI, myocardial ischemia, severe hypertension, or ventricular arrhythmias, particularly in patient with cardiovascular disease.
- Provide adequate hydration, as appropriate, to help prevent hypovolemia.
- Monitor fluid intake and output, daily weight, and serum electrolyte levels (especially potassium) to detect volume depletion or electrolyte imbalance.
- Watch for increased BUN and serum creatinine levels, especially in patients with impaired renal function, because drug may cause acute renal failure. If increases are significant or persistent, notify prescriber immediately.
- Be aware that timolol may mask signs and symptoms of acute hypoglycemia or prolong hypoglycemia. Monitor blood glucose level often in diabetic patients, and expect to increase antidiabetic dosage, as needed and ordered.
- Know that timolol may mask certain signs of hyperthyroidism, such as tachycardia. Monitor patient closely.
- Watch for impaired circulation in elderly patients with age-related peripheral vascular disease or patients with Raynaud's phenomenon. Alpha stimulation may worsen symptoms in such patients. Elderly patients also are at increased risk for beta-blocker-induced hypothermia.
- If patient develops a serious skin reaction, notify prescriber.

PATIENT TEACHING

- Advise patient to take timolol and hydrochlorothiazide in the morning or early evening to avoid the need to urinate during the night.

- Teach patient to monitor her blood pressure and pulse. Tell her to report consistent abnormalities to prescriber.
- Direct patient to weigh herself at the same time each day wearing the same amount of clothing and to notify prescriber if she gains more than 2 lb (0.9 kg) per day or 5 lb (2.3 kg) per week.
- Instruct patient to eat a diet high in potassium-rich foods, such as citrus fruits, bananas, tomatoes, and dates.
- To reduce the risk of dehydration and hypotension, advise patient to avoid exercise in hot weather and to avoid alcohol. Also instruct her to notify prescriber if she has prolonged diarrhea, nausea, or vomiting.
- Caution patient to avoid potentially hazardous activities until drug's CNS effects are known.
- Explain the importance of regular exercise, proper diet, and other lifestyle changes in controlling hypertension.
- Caution patient not to change dosage without consulting prescriber and not to stop taking drug abruptly.
- Advise patient to notify prescriber immediately if she experiences chest pain, fainting, light-headedness, or shortness of breath, which may indicate a need for dosage adjustment.
- Advise patient to consult prescriber before taking OTC drugs, especially cold remedies.
- Advise diabetic patient to monitor blood glucose level closely because drug may alter control and mask some signs of hypoglycemia.
- Warn patient with psoriasis about possible flare-ups.

valsartan and hydrochlorothiazide
Diovan HCT

Class and Category
Chemical: Nonpeptide tetrazole derivative (valsartan), benothiadiazide (hydrochlorothiazide)
Therapeutic: Antihypertensive (valsartan, hydrochlorothiazide), diuretic (hydrochlorothiazide)
Pregnancy category: C (first trimester), D (second and third trimesters)

Indications and Dosages
▶   *To treat hypertension in patients uncontrolled by valsartan or hydrochlorothiazide alone; to treat patients adequately controlled by 25 mg hydrochlorothiazide but who develop significant potassium*

TABLETS

Adults. *Initial:* 80 to 160 mg valsartan and 12.5 mg hydrochlorothiazide (1 tablet contaning 12.5 mg hydrochlorothiazide and either 80 or 160 mg valsartan) daily. Dosage may be increased, as needed, after 3 to 4 wk to 160 mg valsartan and 25 mg hydrochlorothiazide (1 tablet) daily.

Contraindications

Anuria; hypersensitivity to valsartan, hydrochlorothiazide, other sulfonamide-derived drugs, or their components; pregnancy; renal failure

---

Mechanism of Action

Valsartan blocks the hormone angiotensin II from binding to the receptor sites in vascular smooth muscle, adrenal glands, and other tissues. This action inhibits angiotensin II's vasoconstrictive and aldosterone-secreting effects, thereby reducing blood pressure.

Hydrochlorothiazide promotes movement of sodium, chloride, and water from blood in peritubular capillaries into the nephron's distal convoluted tubule. Initially, it may decrease extracellular fluid volume, plasma volume, and cardiac output, which helps explain blood pressure reduction. It also may reduce blood pressure by dilating arteries. After several weeks, extracellular fluid volume, plasma volume, and cardiac output return to normal, and peripheral vascular resistance remains decreased.

Interactions

DRUGS

valsartan and hydrochlorothiazide

antihypertensives, diuretics: Increased antihypertensive effects

valsartan component

potassium salts, potassium-sparing diuretics: Possibly hyperkalemia

hydrochlorothiazide component

amantadine: Possibly increased blood amantadine level and risk of toxicity

amiodarone: Increased risk of arrhythmias from hypokalemia

amphotericin B, corticosteroids: Intensified electrolyte depletion, especially hypokalemia

barbiturates, opioids: May potentiate orthostatic hypotension

calcium: Possibly increased serum calcium level

cholestyramine, colestipol resins: Reduced GI absorption of hydrochlorothiazide

diazoxide: Increased antihypertensive and hyperglycemic effects of hydrochlorothiazide
diflunisal: Possibly increased blood hydrochlorothiazide level
digoxin: Increased risk of digitalis toxicity from hypokalemia
dopamine: Possibly increased diuretic effects of both drugs
insulin, oral antidiabetics: Possibly increased blood glucose level
lithium: Decreased lithium clearance and increased risk of toxicity
neuromuscular blockers: Possibly increased neuromuscular blockade from hypokalemia
nondepolarizing skeletal muscle relaxants (such as tubocurarine): Possibly increased responsiveness to the muscle relaxant
NSAIDs: Decreased diuretic effect of hydrochlorothiazide and increased risk of renal failure
pressor amines (such as norepinephrine): Possibly decreased response to pressor amines
oral anticoagulants: Possibly decreased anticoagulant effects
sympathomimetics: Possibly decreased antihypertensive effect of hydrochlorothiazide
vitamin D: Increased risk of hypercalcemia
FOODS
valsartan component
potassium-containing salt substitutes: Possibly hyperkalemia

Adverse Reactions

CNS: Dizziness, fatigue, headache, insomnia, paresthesia, vertigo, weakness
CV: Edema, hypotension, orthostatic hypotension, vasculitis
EENT: Blurred vision, dry mouth, pharyngitis, rhinitis, sinusitis
ENDO: Hyperglycemia
GI: Abdominal cramps or pain, anorexia, constipation, diarrhea, indigestion, jaundice, nausea, vomiting
GU: Decreased libido, impotence, interstitial nephritis, nocturia, polyuria, renal failure
HEME: Agranulocytosis, aplastic and hemolytic anemia, leukopenia, neutropenia, thrombocytopenia
MS: Arthralgia, muscle spasms and weakness
RESP: Cough, upper respiratory tract infection
SKIN: Alopecia, exfoliative dermatitis, photosensitivity, purpura, rash, Stevens Johnson syndrome, urticaria
Other: Anaphylaxis, dehydration, hypercalcemia, hyperkalemia, hyperuricemia, hypochloremia, hypokalemia, hypomagnesemia, hyponatremia, hypovolemia, metabolic alkalosis, viral infection, weight loss

Nursing Considerations

- Use cautiously in patients with impaired hepatic function because hydrochlorothiazide may alter fluid and electrolyte balance and lead to hepatic coma.
- Also use cautiously in patients with systemic lupus erythematosus because hydrochlorothiazide may activate or worsen it.
- Monitor blood pressure often to assess drug effectiveness.
- Provide hydration, as appropriate, to help prevent hypovolemia.
- Monitor fluid intake and output, daily weight, and serum electrolyte levels (especially potassium) to detect volume depletion or electrolyte imbalance.
- Watch for increased BUN and serum creatinine levels, especially in patients with impaired renal function, because drug may cause acute renal failure. If increases are significant or persistent, notify prescriber immediately.
- Monitor blood glucose level often in diabetic patients, and expect to increase antidiabetic dosage, as needed and ordered.
- Check patient's CBC routinely, as ordered, for abnormalities. If they are significant or persistent, notify prescriber immediately.

PATIENT TEACHING

- Advise patient to take drug in the morning or early evening to avoid the need to urinate during the night.
- Teach patient to monitor her blood pressure and to report consistently elevated measurements to prescriber.
- Alert patient that full effects of drug may take up to 4 weeks.
- Direct patient to weigh herself at the same time each day wearing the same amount of clothing and to notify prescriber if she gains more than 2 lb (0.9 kg) per day or 5 lb (2.3 kg) per week.
- **WARNING** Strongly urge patient to contact prescriber before using potassium supplements or OTC salt substitutes, which may contain potassium and increase the risk of hyperkalemia.
- Instruct female patient of childbearing age to use reliable birth control during therapy and to notify prescriber immediately about known or suspected pregnancy.
- To reduce the risk of dehydration and hypotension, advise patient to avoid exercise in hot weather and to avoid alcohol. Also instruct her to notify prescriber if she has prolonged diarrhea, nausea, or vomiting.
- Caution patient to avoid potentially hazardous activities until drug's CNS effects are known.
- Explain the importance of regular exercise, proper diet, and other lifestyle changes in controlling hypertension.

Central Nervous System Drugs

acetaminophen, caffeine, and butalbital

Americet, Esgic, Esgic Plus, Fioricet, Margesic, Medigesic, Repan

Class and Category

Chemical: Acetamide (acetaminophen), xanthine derivative (caffeine), barbiturate (butalbital)

Therapeutic: Analgesic (acetaminophen), CNS stimulant (caffeine), muscle relaxant (butalbital)

Pregnancy category: C

Indications and Dosages

▶ *To relieve tension or muscle contraction headache*

CAPSULES, TABLETS

Adults. 325 mg acetaminophen, 40 mg caffeine, and 50 mg butalbital (1 tablet or capsule) to 650 mg acetaminophen, 80 mg caffeine, and 100 mg butalbital (2 tablets or capsules) q 4 hr, as needed, not to exceed 4,000 mg acetaminophen daily. Or, 500 mg acetaminophen, 40 mg caffeine, and 50 mg butalbital (1 tablet or capsule) or 1,000 mg acetaminophen, 80 mg caffeine, and 100 mg butalbital (2 tablets or capsules) q 4 hr, as needed, not to exceed 4,000 mg acetaminophen daily.

Mechanism of Action

Acetaminophen inhibits the enzyme cyclooxygenase, blocking prostaglandin production and disrupting peripheral pain impulse generation.

Caffeine is a potent, competitive inhibitor of phosphodiesterase, an enzyme that degrades c3'5' AMP. Increased cAMP mediates most of its actions, including CNS stimulation to counteract the sedative properties of butalbital and cerebral vasoconstriction to relieve headache caused by increased blood volume from vasodilation.

Butalbital inhibits upward conduction of nerve impulses to the reticular formation of the brain, thereby disrupting impulse transmission to the cortex. This action depresses the CNS, producing drowsiness, hypnosis, and sedation.

Contraindications

History of barbiturate addiction; hypersensitivity to butalbital, acetaminophen, caffeine, other barbitrates or their components; porphyria; severe hepatic impairment; significant respiratory depression

Interactions

DRUGS

acetaminophen, caffeine, and butalbital

CNS depressants, general anesthetics, opioids, tranquilizers: Additive CNS effects

acetaminophen component

barbiturates (except butalbital or primidone), carbamazepine, hydantoins, isoniazid, rifampin, sulfinpyrazone: Decreased therapeutic effects and increased hepatotoxic effects of acetaminophen

lamotrigine, loop diuretics: Possibly decreased therapeutic effects of these drugs

oral contraceptives: Decreased effectiveness of acetaminophen

probenecid: Possibly increased therapeutic effects of acetaminophen

propranolol: Possibly increased action of acetaminophen

zidovudine: Possibly decreased effects of zidovudine

caffeine component

aspirin: Increased GI absorption of aspirin

beta-adrenergic agonists: Possibly enhanced cardiac inotropic effects of beta-adrenergic agonists

cimetidine, contraceptives (oral), disulfiram, fluoroquinolones: Decreased hepatic metabolism of caffeine resulting in increased caffeine effect

clozapine: Possibly increased clozapine level and adverse reactions

lithium: Increased renal clearance of lithium

mexiletine: Decreased caffeine elimination resulting in increased caffeine effect

phenytoin: Increased caffeine clearance, resulting in decreased caffeine effect

theophylline: Reduced theophylline clearance with ingestion of more than 120 mg caffeine daily

butalbital component

adrenocorticoids, anticoagulants (oral), tricyclic antidepressants: Decreased effectiveness of these drugs

disulfiram: Possibly increased risk of barbiturate (butalbital) toxicity

ketamine anesthesia: Increased risk of profound respiratory depression

MAO inhibitors: Increased CNS effects of butalbital
ACTIVITIES
acetaminophen, caffeine, and butalbital
alcohol use: Additive CNS effect; increased risk of hepatotoxicity
caffeine component
smoking: Increased caffeine clearance resulting in decreased caffeine effect

Adverse Reactions

CNS: Anxiety, confusion, depression, dizziness, drowsiness, excitement, headache, insomnia, intoxicated feeling, irritability, lethargy light-headedness, nervousness, restlessness, tremor, twitching, vertigo
CV: Extrasystoles, orthostatic hypotension, palpitations, tachycardia
EENT: Epistaxis, laryngospasm, rhinitis, salivation, tinnitis
ENDO: Alterations in blood glucose level
GI: Abdominal pain, anorexia, constipation, diarrhea, flatulence, jaundice, hepatotoxicity, nausea, vomiting
HEME: Agranulocytosis, hemolytic anemia, leukopenia, neutropenia, pancytopenia, thrombocytopenia
RESP: Apnea, bronchospasm, respiratory depression, shortness of breath
SKIN: Erythema multiforme, exfoliative dermatitis, rash, toxic epidermal necrolysis, urticaria
Other: Angioedema, anaphylaxis, physical and psychological dependence

Nursing Considerations

- Before and during long-term therapy, monitor patient's liver function test results, including AST, ALT, and bilirubin levels, as ordered.
- Evaluate patient for therapeutic response, including reports of decreased pain and body movements that would indicate pain relief has occurred.
- Monitor renal function in patient on long-term therapy.
- Take safety precautions, as needed.
- Monitor patient for CNS depression.
- Monitor patient's respiratory depth, effort, and rate. Notify prescriber immediately if respiratory rate drops below 10 breaths/ minute.
- **WARNING** Assess patient for evidence of physical and psychological dependence.

PATIENT TEACHING
- Instruct patient to take drug with food or after meals to minimize stomach upset.
- Instruct patient to take acetaminophen, caffeine, and butalbital exactly as prescribed and not to adjust dose or frequency without consulting prescriber.
- Instruct patient to notify prescriber about worsening or breakthrough pain.
- Advise patient to notify prescriber if he becomes short of breath or has difficulty breathing.
- Advise patient to avoid potentially hazardous activities until drug's CNS effects are known.
- Caution patient to avoid alcohol or other CNS depressants while taking drug. Also tell patient to contact prescriber before taking other prescription or OTC drugs because they may contain acetaminophen and lead to toxicity.
- Encourage patient to get up slowly from a sitting or lying position.
- To prevent constipation, encourage patient to consume plenty of fluids and high-fiber foods, if not contraindicated by another condition.
- Teach patient to recognize signs of hepatotoxicity, such as bleeding, easy bruising, and chronic overdose.

acetaminophen and codeine phosphate
Aceta with Codeine, Capital with Codeine, Tylenol with Codeine No. 2, Tylenol with Codeine No. 3, Tylenol with Codeine No. 4, Tylenol with Codeine Elixir

Class, Category, and Schedule
Chemical: Acetamide (acetaminophen), phenanthrene derivative (codeine)
Therapeutic: Analgesic (acetaminophen, codeine)
Pregnancy category: C
Controlled substance: Schedule III (tablets), V (oral solution and elixir)

Indications and Dosages
▶ *To relieve mild to moderately severe pain*
ORAL SOLUTION, ORAL SUSPENSION, TABLETS
Adults. 15 to 60 mg codeine and 300 to 1,000 mg acetaminophen (number of tablets or ml dependent on strength) q 4 hr, as

needed. *Maximum:* 360 mg codeine and 4,000 mg acetaminophen in 24 hr.

> ## Mechanism of Action
> Acetaminophen inhibits the enzyme cyclooxygenase, thereby blocking prostaglandin production and interfering with pain impulse generation in the peripheral nervous system.
>   Codeine may produce analgesia through partial metabolism to the opioid, morphine. Opioids bind and interact with opiate receptors in the CNS, altering the perception of and emotional response to pain and causing generalized CNS depression.

Contraindications

Hypersensitivity to acetaminophen, codeine, other opioids, or their components; significant respiratory depression; upper airway obstruction

Interactions

DRUGS

acetaminophen component

barbiturates, carbamazepine, hydantoins, isoniazid, rifampin, sulfinpyrazone: Decreased therapeutic effects and increased hepatotoxic effects of acetaminophen

lamotrigine, loop diuretics: Possibly decreased therapeutic effects of these drugs

oral contraceptives: Decreased effectiveness of acetaminophen

probenecid: Possibly increased therapeutic effects of acetaminophen

propranolol: Possibly increased action of acetaminophen

zidovudine: Possibly decreased effects of zidovudine

codeine component

anticholinergics: Increased risk of paralytic ileus

antihypertensives, diuretics: Potentiated hypotensive effects

buprenorphine: Decreased effectiveness of codeine

CNS depressants: Additive CNS effects

hydroxyzine: Increased codeine analgesic effect; increased CNS depressant and hypotensive effects

MAO inhibitors: Increased risk of unpredictable, severe, and sometimes fatal reactions

metoclopramide: Antagonized effect of metoclopramide on GI motility

naloxone: Antagonized codeine analgesic effect

naltrexone: Precipitated withdrawal symptoms in codeine-dependent patients

neuromuscular blockers: Additive respiratory depressant effects

opioids: Additive CNS and respiratory depressant effects and hypotensive effects

paregoric: Increased risk of severe constipation

ACTIVITIES

acetaminophen and codeine

alcohol use: Additive CNS effects of codeine, increased risk of hepatotoxicity with acetaminophen

Adverse Reactions

CNS: Coma, delirium, depression, disorientation, dizziness, drowsiness, euphoria, hallucinations, headache, lack of coordination, lethargy light-headedness, mental and physical impairment, mood changes, restlessness, sedation, seizures, tremor

CV: Bradycardia, heart block, orthostatic hypotension, palpitations, tachycardia

EENT: Altered taste, blurred vision, diplopia, dry mouth, laryngeal edema, laryngospasm, miosis

ENDO: Alterations in serum blood glucose level

GI: Abdominal cramps and pain, anorexia, constipation, flatulence, gastroesophageal reflux, jaundice, hepatotoxicity, ileus, indigestion, nausea, vomiting

GU: Decreased libido, difficult ejaculation, dysuria, impotence, oliguria, ureteral spasm, urinary incontinence, urine retention

HEME: Hemolytic anemia, leukopenia, neutropenia, pancytopenia, thrombocytopenia

RESP: Apnea, bronchoconstriction, bronchospasm, depressed cough reflex, respiratory depression

SKIN: Diaphoresis, flushing, pallor, pruritus, rash, urticaria

Other: Angioedema, anaphylaxis, physical and psychological dependence

Nursing Considerations

- Use cautiously in patients with head trauma intracranial lesions because codeine can cause exaggerated respiratory depression.
- Use cautiously in elderly and debilitated patients as well as patients with severe renal or hepatic dysfunction, gallbladder disease, respiratory impairment, cardiac arrhythmias, inflammatory disorders of the GI tract, hypothyroidism, Addison's disease, prostatic hypertrophy or urethral stricture, coagulation disorders, or acute abdominal conditions.

- Before and during long-term therapy, monitor patient's liver function test results, including AST, ALT, and bilirubin levels, as ordered.
- Evaluate patient for therapeutic response, including reports of decreased pain and body movements that would indicate pain relief has occurred.
- Monitor renal function in a patient on long-term therapy. Keep in mind that blood or albumin in urine may indicate nephritis or renal failure. Also monitor urine output; decreasing output may signal urine retention or decreased renal function.
- Take safety precautions, as needed.
- Monitor patient for evidence of CNS depression.
- Assess patient's respiratory depth, effort and rate. Notify prescriber immediately if respiratory rate drops below 10 breaths/minute.
- **WARNING** Assess patient for evidence of physical and psychological dependence.

PATIENT TEACHING
- Instruct patient to take acetaminophen and codeine with food or after meals to minimize stomach upset.
- Instruct patient to take acetaminophen and codeine exactly as prescribed and not to adjust dose or frequency without consulting prescriber.
- Advise patient to only use manufacturer's dosage cup for liquid acetaminophen and codeine.
- Instruct patient to notify prescriber about worsening or breakthrough pain.
- Advise patient to notify prescriber if he becomes short of breath or has difficulty breathing.
- Advise patient to avoid potentially hazardous activities until drug's CNS effects are known.
- Caution patient to avoid alcohol or other CNS depressants while taking acetaminophen and codeine; also to contact prescriber before taking other prescription or OTC drugs as they may contain acetaminophen and lead to toxicity.
- Advise the patient to get up slowly from a sitting or lying position.
- To prevent constipation, encourage patient to consume plenty of fluids and high-fiber foods, if not contraindicated.
- Teach patient to recognize signs of hepatotoxicity, such as bleeding, easy bruising, and chronic overdose.

acetaminophen and hydrocodone bitartrate

Allay, Anexsia, Anolor DH 5, Bancap-HC, Co-Gesic, Dolacet, Dolagesic, Duocet, Hycomed, Hyco-Pap, Hydrocet, Hydrogesic, Lorcet-HD, Lorcet Plus, Lortab, Margesic-H, Oncet, Panacet, Panlor, Polygesic, Stagesic, T-Gesic, Ugesic, Vanacet, Vendone, Vicodin, Vicodin ES, Zydone

Class, Category, and Schedule

Chemical: Opioid and phenanthrene derivative (hydrocodone), para-aminophenol derivative (acetaminophen)
Therapeutic: Analgesic
Pregnancy category: C
Controlled substance: Schedule III

Indications and Dosages

▶ *To treat moderate to severe back pain and pain from arthralgia, cancer, dental procedures, headache, and myalgia*

CAPSULES

Adults. 1 capsule (500 mg acetaminophen and 5 mg hydrocodone) q 4 to 6 hr, p.r.n. Or, 2 capsules (1,000 mg acetaminophen and 10 mg hydrocodone) q 6 hr, p.r.n. *Maximum:* 8 capsules (4,000 mg acetaminophen and 40 mg hydrocodone)/24 hr.

ORAL SOLUTION

Adults. 5 to 15 ml (167 mg acetaminophen and 2.5 mg hydrocodone/5 ml) q 4 to 6 hr, p.r.n., for up to 6 days.

TABLETS

Adults. 1 or 2 tablets (500 mg acetaminophen and 2.5 mg hydrocodone/tablet) q 4 to 6 hr, p.r.n. Or, 1 tablet (500 mg acetaminophen and 5 mg hydrocodone) q 4 to 6 hr, p.r.n., up to 2 tablets q 6 hr, p.r.n. Or, 1 tablet (650 mg acetaminophen and 7.5 mg hydrocodone) q 4 to 6 hr, p.r.n., up to 2 tablets q 6 hr, p.r.n. Or, 1 tablet (750 mg acetaminophen and 7.5 mg hydrocodone) q 4 to 6 hr, p.r.n. Or, 1 tablet (650 mg acetaminophen and 10 mg hydrocodone) q 4 to 6 hr, p.r.n. *Maximum:* 4,000 mg acetaminophen and 40 mg hydrocodone daily.

Contraindications

Acute asthma; hypersensitivity to acetaminophen, aspirin, hydrocodone, opioids, NSAIDs, or their components; respiratory depression; upper airway obstruction

Mechanism of Action

Acetaminophen increases the pain threshold at the CNS level by inhibiting cyclooxygenase, an enzyme involved in prostaglandin synthesis. Prostaglandins, important mediators in the inflammatory response, cause local vasodilation with swelling and pain. They also play a role in pain transmission from the periphery to the spinal cord. With the inhibition of cyclooxygenase and prostaglandin synthesis, inflammatory symptoms subside.

Hydrocodone exerts a synergistic analgesic effect through two mechanisms of action. Hydrocodone, a mu opiate-receptor agonist, alters the perception of pain at the spinal cord and higher CNS levels by blocking the release of inhibitory neurotransmitters, such as gamma-aminobutyric acid and acetylcholine. It also alters the emotional response to pain.

Interactions

DRUGS

anticholinergics: Increased risk of ileus, severe constipation, and urine retention

antidiarrheals (antiperistaltic): Increased risk of CNS depression and severe constipation

barbiturate anesthetics: Possibly increased respiratory and CNS depression

chlorpromazine, thioridazine: Increased risk of adverse and toxic effects of hydrocodone

CNS depressants: Increased risk of CNS and respiratory depression and hypotension

diuretics, other antihypertensives: Increased risk of hypotension

MAO inhibitors (such as furazolidone, phenelzine, procarbazine, selegiline, tranylcypromine) within 14 days of taking acetaminophen and hydrocodone: Increased risk of adverse CNS effects

metoclopramide: Possibly antagonized effect of metoclopramide on GI motility

naloxone: Possibly withdrawal symptoms in physically dependent patients

naltrexone: Possibly prolonged respiratory depression or cardiac arrest

opioid analgesics: Risk of increased CNS and respiratory depression and hypotension

ACTIVITIES

alcohol use: Increased risk of CNS depression

Adverse Reactions

CNS: Confusion, dizziness, drowsiness, euphoria, headache, lethargy, restlessness, sedation, syncope
CV: Hypotension, orthostatic hypotension, tachycardia
EENT: Dry mouth, laryngeal edema, laryngospasm, vision changes
GI: Anorexia, constipation, nausea, vomiting
GU: Dysuria, urine retention
RESP: Atelectasis, bronchospasm, respiratory depression, wheezing
SKIN: Diaphoresis, flushing, pruritus, rash, urticaria
Other: Physical and psychological dependence

Nursing Considerations

• Expect prolonged use of acetaminophen and hydrocodone to produce physical and psychological dependence; physical dependence may cause withdrawal symptoms when therapy stops.
• Assess elderly patients for adverse reactions; they're especially sensitive to drug and are at increased risk for constipation.
• **WARNING** Monitor patient for signs of overdose, such as blurred vision; cold, clammy skin; confusion; dizziness; dyspnea; headache; hearing loss; malaise; mental or mood changes; nausea; respiratory depression; sinus bradycardia; tinnitus; and vomiting. Notify prescriber immediately if they develop.

PATIENT TEACHING
• Inform patient that hydrocodone and acetaminophen may cause dizziness and drowsiness.
• Advise patient to avoid potentially hazardous activities until drug's CNS effects are known.
• Caution patient not to take more than prescribed dosage because of risk of dependence.
• Urge patient to avoid using alcohol during drug therapy.
• Advise patient to change position slowly to minimize effects of orthostatic hypotension.
• If patient reports dry mouth, suggest that she use sugarless candy or gum or ice chips.

amphetamine and dextroamphetamine
Adderall, Adderall XR

Class, Category, and Schedule
Chemical: Phenylisopropylamine

Therapeutic: CNS stimulant
Pregnancy category: C
Controlled substance: Schedule II

Indications and Dosages

▶ *To treat attention deficit hyperactivity disorder (ADHD)*

E.R. CAPSULES

Adults. 20 mg daily.

Adolescents ages 13 to 18. *Initial:* 10 mg daily. Dosage increased to 20 mg/day after 1 wk if needed.

Children age 6 and over. *Initial:* 5 or 10 mg daily. Dosage increased by 5 or 10 mg/day q wk until desired response occurs. *Maximum:* 30 mg/day.

TABLETS

Children age 6 and over. *Initial:* 5 mg daily or b.i.d. Increased by 5 mg/day q wk until desired response occurs. *Maximum:* 40 mg/day.

Children ages 3 to 6. *Initial:* 2.5 mg daily. Dosage increased by 2.5 mg/day q wk until desired response occurs. *Maximum:* 40 mg/day.

▶ *To treat narcolepsy*

TABLETS

Adults and children age 12 and over. *Initial:* 10 mg daily. Dosage increased by 10 mg/day q wk until desired response occurs. *Maximum:* 60 mg/day for adults.

Children ages 6 to 12. *Initial:* 5 mg daily. Dosage increased by 5 mg/day q wk until desired response occurs. *Maximum:* 40 mg/day.

Mechanism of Action

Amphetamine and dextroamphetamine may produce its CNS stimulant effects by facilitating the release of norepinephrine at adrenergic nerve terminals and blocking its reuptake and by directly stimulating alpha and beta receptors in the peripheral nervous system. The drug also causes the release and blocks the reuptake of dopamine in limbic regions of the brain.

The main action of amphetamine and dextroamphetamine appears to be in the cerebral cortex and, possibly, the reticular activating system. Also, dextroamphetamine may stimulate inhibitory autoreceptors in the brain. These actions decrease drowsiness, fatigue, and motor restlessness and increase mental alertness. Peripheral actions include increased blood pressure, mild bronchodilation, and respiratory stimulation.

Contraindications
Advanced arteriosclerosis; agitation; glaucoma; history of drug abuse; hypersensitivity to amphetamine, dextroamphetamine, or any of their components; hyperthyroidism; MAO inhibitor therapy within 14 days; moderate to severe hypertension; symptomatic CV disease; structural cardiac abnormalities

Interactions
DRUGS

anesthetics (inhaled): Increased risk of severe ventricular arrhythmias

antacids that contain calcium or magnesium, carbonic anhydrase inhibitors, citrates, sodium bicarbonate: Increased effects of amphetamine

antihypertensives, diuretics: Possibly decreased hypotensive effects

beta blockers: Increased risk of hypertension, excessive bradycardia, possibly heart block

CNS stimulants: Additive CNS stimulation

digoxin, levodopa: Possibly arrhythmias

ethosuximide, phenobarbital, phenytoin: Delayed intestinal absorption of these drugs

glutamic acid hydrochloride, urinary acidifiers (such as ammonium chloride and sodium acid phosphate): Increased excretion and decreased blood level and effects of amphetamine and dextroamphetamine

haloperidol, loxapine, molindone, phenothiazines, pimozide, thioxanthenes: Reduced antipsychotic efficacy of these drugs; inhibited CNS stimulant effects of amphetamine and dextroamphetamine

MAO inhibitors: Potentiated effects of amphetamine, possibly hypertensive crisis

meperidine: Increased analgesia

metrizamide: Increased risk of seizures

norepinephrine: Possibly increased adrenergic effect of norepinephrine

propoxyphene: Increased CNS stimulation, risk of fatal seizures

sympathomimetics: Increased CV effects of both drugs

thyroid replacement drugs: Enhanced effects of both drugs

tricyclic antidepressants: Possibly increased CV effects

FOODS

ascorbic acid, fruit juices: Decreased absorption and effects of amphetamine and dextroamphetamine

Adverse Reactions
CNS: Agitation, anxiety, depression, dizziness, drowsiness, emotional lability, fatigue, fever, headache, insomnia, irritability, light-

headedness, mania, motor tics, nervousness, psychosis, seizures, stroke, tremor
CV: Arrhythmias, hypertension, MI, sudden death, tachycardia
EENT: Accommodation abnormality, blurred vision, dry mouth, taste perversion
GI: Abdominal pain, anorexia, constipation, diarrhea, indigestion, nausea, vomiting
GU: Decreased libido, UTI
RESP: Dyspnea
SKIN: Diaphoresis, rash, Stevens-Johnson syndrome, toxic epidermal necrolysis
Other: Angioedema, anaphylaxis, infection, weight loss

Nursing Considerations

- Keep in mind that, when signs and symptoms of ADHD occur with acute stress reactions or structural cardiac abnormalities, amphetamines usually aren't indicated because these conditions may worsen or sudden death may occur.
- Monitor pulse rate and blood pressure in patients who have hypertension, even mild hypertension, because drug may increase blood pressure and cause arrhythmias, including tachycardia. Report abnormal findings to prescriber.
- **WARNING** If patient suddenly stops taking drug after long-term, high-dose therapy, watch for withdrawal signs and symptoms, such as abdominal pain, depression, fatigue, nausea, tremor, vomiting, and weakness. Anticipate restarting drug and gradually tapering dosage, as prescribed.
- Monitor growth and development in children because drug may adversely affect growth.
- Administer first dose of tablet form when patient awakens and additional doses at 4- to 6-hour intervals. Administer E.R. capsule form when patient awakens.
- If patient currently takes divided doses of tablet form, know that he may be switched to E.R. capsule form at the same daily dose to be taken once in the morning.
- Assess patient for potential drug dependence, drug-seeking behavior, or drug tolerance. Be alert for signs and symptoms of long-term amphetamine abuse characterized by hyperactivity, irritability, marked insomnia, personality changes, and severe dermatoses.
- Assess patient with history of Tourette syndrome, motor or vocal tics, or psychological disorders for exacerbation of these conditions during amphetamine therapy.

PATIENT TEACHING
- Advise patient to take amphetamine and dextroamphetamine with food or after a meal because anorexia may occur.
- Advise patient not to take drug with acidic fruit juice because it may decrease drug absorption.
- Tell patient or caregiver that E.R. capsules may be taken whole or opened and sprinkled on applesauce, then swallowed immediately without chewing.
- Stress the importance of taking drug exactly as prescribed because misuse may cause serious adverse cardiovascular reactions, including sudden death.
- Urge patient to avoid potentially hazardous activities until he knows how drug affects him.
- Inform patient of abuse potential of drug, and stress the importance of not altering dosage unless prescribed.
- Inform parents or caregivers that child may be placed on drug-free weekend and holiday schedule, as prescribed, if signs and symptoms of ADHD are controlled.
- Monitor children and adolescents for first-time evidence of psychotic or manic symptoms. If they appear, notify prescriber and expect drug therapy to be stopped.

aspirin, caffeine, and dihydrocodeine bitartrate
Synalgos-DC

Class, Category, and Schedule
Chemical: Salicylate (aspirin), xanthine derivative (caffeine), opioid agonist (dihydrocodeine)
Therapeutic: Analagesic (aspirin, dihydrocodeine), CNS stimulant (caffeine)
Pregnancy category: D
Controlled substance: Schedule III

Indications and Dosages
▶ *To relieve moderate to moderately severe pain*
CAPSULES
Adults. 712.8 mg aspirin, 60 mg caffeine, and 32 mg dihydrocodeine (2 capsules) q 4 hr, p.r.n.

Contraindications
Allergy to tartrazine dye; asthma; bleeding problems such as hemophilia; children under age 16 who have a viral illness; hyper-

sensitivity to aspirin, dihydrocodeine, NSAIDs, other opioids, or their components; peptic ulcer disease; respiratory depression; severe vitamin K deficiency; upper airway obstruction

---

Mechanism of Action

Aspirin blocks the activity of cyclooxygenase, the enzyme necessary for prostaglandin synthesis. By preventing prostaglandin synthesis, pain is relieved because prostaglandins play a role in pain transmission from the periphery to the spinal cord.

Caffeine is a potent, competitive inhibitor of phosphodiesterase, an enzyme that degrades c3'5' AMP. Increased cAMP mediates most of its actions, including CNS stimulation to counteract the sedative properties of dihydrocodeine.

Dihydrocodeine may produce analgesia through partial metabolism to the opioid, morphine. Opioids bind and interact with opiate receptors in the CNS, altering the perception of and emotional response to pain and causing generalized CNS depression.

Interactions

DRUGS

aspirin, caffeine, and dihydrocodeine
CNS depressants: Additive CNS effects
aspirin component
ACE inhibitors: Decreased antihypertensive effect
activated charcoal: Decreased aspirin absorption
antacids, urine alkalinizers: Decreased aspirin effectiveness
anticoagulants: Increased risk of bleeding; prolonged bleeding time
carbonic anhydrase inhibitors: Salicylism
corticosteroids: Increased excretion and decreased blood level of aspirin
heparin: Increased risk of bleeding
loop diuretics: Possibly decreased effectiveness of loop diuretics
methotrexate: Increased blood level and decreased excretion of methotrexate, causing toxicity
nizatidine: Increased blood aspirin level
NSAIDs: Possibly decreased blood NSAID level and increased risk of adverse GI effects
probenecid, sulfinpyrazone: Decreased effectiveness in treating gout
urine acidifiers, such as ammonium chloride and ascorbic acid: Decreased aspirin excretion
vancomycin: Increased risk of ototoxicity

caffeine component
aspirin: Increased GI absorption of aspirin
beta-adrenergic agonists: Possibly enhanced cardiac inotropic effects of beta-adrenergic agonists
cimetidine, contraceptives (oral), disulfiram, fluoroquinolones: Decreased hepatic metabolism of caffeine and increased caffeine effect
clozapine: Possibly increased clozapine levels resulting in increased incidence of clozapine induced adverse reactions
lithium: Enhanced renal clearance of lithium
mexiletine: Decreased caffeine elimination resulting in increased caffeine effect
phenytoin: Increased caffeine clearance and decreased caffeine effect
theophylline: Reduced theophylline clearance with ingestion of more than 120 mg caffeine daily

dihydrocodeine component
anticholinergics, paregoric: Increased risk of severe constipation
antihypertensives, diuretics: Potentiated hypotensive effects
buprenorphine: Decreased effectiveness of codeine
hydroxyzine: Increased codeine analgesic effect; increased CNS depressant and hypotensive effects
MAO inhibitors: Increased risk of unpredictable, severe, and sometimes fatal reactions
metoclopramide: Antagonized effect of metoclopramide on GI motility
naloxone: Antagonized dihydrocodeine analgesic effect
naltrexone: Precipitated withdrawal symptoms in dihydrocodeine-dependent patients
neuromuscular blockers: Additive respiratory depressant effects
opioids: Additive CNS and respiratory depressant effects and hypotensive effects

ACTIVITIES
aspirin, caffeine, and dihydrocodeine
alcohol use: Additive CNS effects
aspirin component
alcohol use: Increased risk of ulcers
caffeine component
smoking: Increased caffeine clearance resulting in decreased caffeine effect

Adverse Reactions

CNS: Coma, confusion, CNS depression, delirium, depression, disorientation, dizziness, drowsiness, euphoria, hallucinations, headache, lack of coordination

CV: Bradycardia, orthostatic hypotension, palpitations, tachycardia

EENT: Altered taste, blurred vision, diplopia, dry mouth, hearing loss, laryngeal edema, laryngospasm, miosis, tinnitus

GI: Abnormal cramps and pain, anorexia, constipation, diarrhea, flatulence, GI bleeding, gastroesophageal reflux, heartburn, hepatotoxicity, ileus, indigestion, nausea, stomach pain, vomiting

GU: Decreased libido, difficult ejaculation, dysuria, impotence, oliguria, ureteral spasm, urinary incontinence, urine retention

HEME: Decreased blood iron level, hemolytic anemia, leukopenia, prolonged bleeding time, shortened life span of RBCs, thrombocytopenia

RESP: Apnea, bronchoconstriction, bronchospasm, depressed cough reflex, respiratory depression

SKIN: Diaphoresis, ecchymosis, flushing, pallor, pruritus, rash, urticaria

Other: Anaphylaxis, angioedema, physical and psychological dependence, Reye's syndrome

Nursing Considerations

- Use cautiously in patients with head trauma or intracranial lesions because dihydrocodeine can cause an exaggerated respiratory depression and aspirin can increase the risk of bleeding.
- Use cautiously in elderly and debilitated patients as well as patients with severe renal or hepatic dysfunction, gallbladder disease, respiratory impairment, cardiac arrhythmias, inflammatory disorders of the GI tract, hypothyroidism, Addison's disease, prostatic hypertrophy or urethral stricture, coagulation disorders or acute abdominal conditions.
- Evaluate patient for therapeutic response, including report of decreased pain and body movements that would indicate pain relief has occurred.
- Take safety precautions, as needed.
- Monitor patient for CNS depression.
- Monitor patient's respiratory depth, effort and rate. Notify prescriber immediately if respiratory rate drops below 10 breaths/minute.
- **WARNING** Monitor patient closely for allergic reaction. Be aware that anaphylactic shock and other severe allergic reactions can occur without a history of allergy.
- **WARNING** Assess patient for evidence of physical and psy-

chological dependence.
- Monitor urine output; decreasing output may signal urine retention or renal failure.

PATIENT TEACHING
- Instruct patient to take aspirin, caffeine, and dihyrdocodeine with food or after meals to minimize stomach upset.
- Instruct patient to take drug exactly as prescribed and not to adjust dose or frequency without consulting prescriber.
- Instruct patient to notify prescriber about worsening or breakthrough pain.
- Advise patient to notify prescriber if he becomes short of breath or has difficulty breathing.
- Tell patient to consult prescriber before taking drug with any prescription drug for blood disorder, diabetes, gout, or arthritis.
- Advise patient to avoid potentially hazardous activities until drug's CNS effects are known.
- Caution patient to avoid alcohol or other CNS depressants while taking the drug.
- Advise patient to get up slowly from a sitting or lying position.
- To prevent constipation, urge patient to consume plenty of fluids and high-fiber foods, if not contraindicated.

aspirin and codeine phosphate
Empirin with Codeine No. 2, Empirin with Codeine No. 3, Empirin with Codeine No. 4

Class, Category, and Schedule
Chemical: Salicylate (aspirin), phenanthrene derivative (codeine)
Therapeutic: Analgesic (aspirin, codeine)
Pregnancy category: C
Controlled substance: Schedule III

Indications and Dosages
▶ *To relieve mild, moderate, and moderate to severe pain*
TABLETS
Adults. 325 mg aspirin and 15 mg, 30 mg, or 60 mg codeine to 650 mg aspirin and 30 mg, 60 mg, or 120 mg codeine q 4 hr, p.r.n.

Contraindications
Allergy to tartrazine dye; anticoagulant therapy; asthma; bleeding problems such as hemophilia; children under age 16 who have a viral illness; hypersensitivity to aspirin, codeine, NSAIDs, other

opioids, or their components; peptic ulcer disease; respiratory depression; severe vitamin K deficiency; upper airway obstruction

---

Mechanism of Action

Aspirin blocks the activity of cyclooxygenase, the enzyme needed for prostaglandin synthesis. Prostaglandins play a role in pain transmission from the periphery to the spinal cord. By preventing their synthesis, pain is relieved.

Codeine may produce analgesia through partial metabolism to the opioid, morphine. Opioids bind and interact with opiate receptors in the CNS, altering the perception of and emotional response to pain and causing generalized CNS depression.

Interactions

DRUGS

aspirin and codeine

penicillins, sulfonamides: Increased blood levels of penicillins and sulfonamides

aspirin component

ACE inhibitors: Decreased antihypertensive effect

activated charcoal: Decreased aspirin absorption

antacids, urine alkalinizers: Decreased aspirin effectiveness

anticoagulants: Increased risk of bleeding; prolonged bleeding time

carbonic anhydrase inhibitors: Salicylism

corticosteroids: Increased excretion and decreased blood level of aspirin

heparin: Increased risk of bleeding

insulin, oral antidiabetics: Increased risk of hypoglycemia

loop diuretics: Possibly decreased effectiveness of loop diuretics

methotrexate: Increased blood level and decreased excretion of methotrexate, causing toxicity

nizatidine: Increased blood aspirin level

NSAIDs: Possibly decreased blood NSAID level and increased risk of adverse GI effects

probenecid, sulfinpyrazone: Decreased effectiveness in treating gout

urine acidifiers, such as ammonium chloride and ascorbic acid: Decreased aspirin excretion

vancomycin: Increased risk of ototoxicity

codeine component

anticholinergics, paregoric: Increased risk of severe constipation

antihypertensives, diuretics: Potentiated hypotensive effects

buprenorphine: Decreased effectiveness of codeine

CNS depressants: Additive CNS effects

hydroxyzine: Increased codeine analgesic effect; increased CNS depressant and hypotensive effects
MAO inhibitors: Increased risk of unpredictable, severe, and sometimes fatal reactions
metoclopramide: Antagonized effect of metoclopramide on GI motility
naloxone: Antagonized codeine analgesic effect
naltrexone: Precipitated withdrawal symptoms in codeine-dependent patients
neuromuscular blockers: Additive respiratory depressant effects
opioids: Additive CNS and respiratory depressant effects and hypotensive effects
ACTIVITIES
aspirin component
alcohol use: Increased risk of ulcers
codeine component
alcohol use: Additive CNS effects

Adverse Reactions

CNS: Coma, confusion, CNS depression, delirium, depression, disorientation, dizziness, drowsiness, euphoria, hallucinations, headache, lack of coordination, lethargy, light-headedness, mental and physical impairment, mood changes, restlessness, sedation, seizures, tremor
CV: Bradycardia, heart block, orthostatic hypotension, palpitations, tachycardia
EENT: Altered taste, blurred vision, diplopia, dry mouth, hearing loss, laryngeal edema, laryngospasm, miosis, tinnitus
GI: Abdominal cramps and pain, anorexia, constipation, diarrhea, flatulence, GI bleeding, gastroesophageal reflux, heartburn, hepatotoxicity, ileus, indigestion, nausea, vomiting
GU: Decreased libido, difficult ejaculation, dysuria, impotence, nephrotoxicity, oliguria, ureteral spasm, urinary incontinence, urine retention
HEME: Decreased blood iron level, hemolytic anemia, leukopenia, prolonged bleeding time, shortened life span of RBCs, thrombocytopenia
MS: Muscle rigidity
RESP: Apnea, bronchoconstriction, bronchospasm, depressed cough reflex, respiratory depression
SKIN: Diaphoresis, ecchymosis, flushing, pallor, pruritus, rash, urticaria
Other: Anaphylaxis, angioedema, physical and psychological dependence, Reye's syndrome

Nursing Considerations

- Use cautiously in patients with head trauma or intracranial lesions because codeine can cause an exaggerated respiratory depression and aspirin can increase the risk of bleeding.
- Use cautiously in elderly and debilitated patients as well as patients with severe renal or hepatic dysfunction, gallbladder disease, respiratory impairment, cardiac arrhythmias, inflammatory disorders of the GI tract, hypothyroidism, Addison's disease, prostatic hypertrophy or urethral stricture, coagulation disorders or acute abdominal conditions.
- Evaluate paptient for therapeutic response, including report of decreased pain and body movements that would indicate pain relief has occurred.
- Take safety precautions, as needed.
- Monitor patient for CNS depression.
- Monitor respiratory depth, effort and rate. Notify prescriber immediately if respiratory rate drops below 10 breaths/minute.
- **WARNING** Monitor patient closely for allergic reaction. Be aware that anaphylactic shock and other severe allergic reactions can occur without a history of allergy.
- **WARNING** Assess patient for evidence of physical and psychological dependence.
- Monitor urine output; decreasing output may signal urine retention and renal failure.

PATIENT TEACHING

- Instruct patient to take aspirin and codeine with food or after meals to minimize stomach upset.
- Instruct patient to take drug exactly as prescribed and not to adjust dose or frequency without consulting prescriber.
- Instruct patient to notify prescriber about worsening or breakthrough pain.
- Advise patient to notify prescriber if he becomes short of breath or has difficulty breathing.
- Tell patient to consult prescriber before taking drug with any prescription drug for blood disorder, diabetes, gout, or arthritis.
- Advise patient to avoid potentially hazardous activities until drug's CNS effects are known.
- Caution patient to avoid alcohol or other CNS depressants while taking aspirin and codeine.
- Advise patient to get up slowly from a sitting or lying position.
- To prevent constipation, encourage patient to consume plenty of fluids and high-fiber foods, if not contraindicated.

buprenorphine hydrochloride and naloxone hydrochloride

Suboxone

Class, Category, and Schedule

Chemical: Opioid as a thebaine derivative (buprenorphine), thebaine derivative (naloxone)

Therapeutic: Opioid analgesic (buprenorphine), opioid antagonist (naloxone)

Pregnancy category: C

Controlled substance: Schedule III

Indications and Dosages

▶ *To treat opioid dependence*

S.L. TABLETS

Adults. 12 to 16 mg buprenorphine and 3 to 4 mg naloxone (6 to 8 tablets of 2-mg/0.5-mg strength or 2 tablets of 8-mg/2-mg strength for highest dose) as a single dose daily.

Mechanism of Action

Buprenorphine may bind with CNS receptors to alter the perception of and emotional response to pain. Buprenorphine may act by displacing opioid agonists from their binding sites and competitively inhibiting their actions.

Naloxone briefly and competitively antagonizes mu, kappa, and sigma receptors in the CNS, thus reversing the analgesia, hypotension, respiratory depression, and sedation caused by most opioids. Mu receptors are responsible for analgesia, euphoria, miosis, and respiratory depression. Kappa receptors are responsible for analgesia and sedation. Sigma receptors control dysphoria and other delusional states.

Contraindications

Hypersensitivity to buprenorphine, naloxone, or their components

Interactions

DRUGS

buprenorphine and naloxone

antidepressants, benzodiazepines, sedatives, tranquilizers: Increased risk of serious overdose

buprenorphine component

azole antifungals, such as ketoconazole; macrolide antibiotics, such as erythromycin; HIV protease inhibitors, such as indinavir, ritonavir and saquinavir: Possibly increased plasma levels of buprenorphine

CNS depressants, MAO inhibitors: Additive hypotensive and respiratory and CNS depressant effects of these drugs

opioid analgesics: Reduced therapeutic effects if buprenorphine is given before another opioid analgesic

naloxone component

opioid analgesics: Reversal of the analgesic and adverse effects of these drugs; possibly withdrawal symptoms in opioid-dependent patients

ACTIVITIES

buprenorphine and naloxone

alcohol use: Increased risk of serious overdose

Adverse Reactions

CNS: Anxiety, asthenia, chills, depression, dizziness, excitement, fever, headache, insomnia, irritability, nervousness, sedation, somnolence, tremors, vertigo

CV: Hypertension, hypotension, vasodilation, ventricular fibrillation or tachycardia

EENT: Excessive tearing, miosis, pharyngitis, rhinitis

GI: Abdominal pain, constipation, diarrhea, dyspepsia, nausea, vomiting

MS: Back pain

RESP: Bronchospasm, hypoventilation, increased cough, pulmonary edema

SKIN: Diaphoresis, pruritus, rash, urticaria

Other: Anaphylaxis, angioedema, flu syndrome, generalized pain, infection, withdrawal syndrome

Nursing Considerations

- Use buprenorphine and naloxone cautiously in patients with compromised respiratory function, severe hepatic or renal impairment, myxedema, hypothyroidism, adrenal insufficiency, CNS depression, coma, toxic psychosis, prostatic hypertrophy, urethral stricture, acute alcoholism, alcohol withdrawal syndrome, kyphoscoliosis, or biliary tract dysfunction.
- Because buprenorphine can increase cerebrospinal fluid (CSF) pressure, use cautiously in patients with head injury, intracranial lesions, or other conditions that could increase CSF pressure.
- Obtain results of liver function studies, as ordered, before starting buprenorphine and naloxone therapy and then periodically throughout treatment because drug may contribute to the development of a hepatic abnormality. Expect patient with hepatic

dysfunction to have increased circulating blood buprenorphine and naloxone levels, which may increase incidence and severity of adverse reactions.

- Frequently monitor vital signs and response to drug, and take safety precautions, especially after giving first dose.
- **WARNING** Monitor patient for withdrawal symptoms, especially when giving buprenorphine and naloxone to opioid-dependent patient. Symptoms may include abdominal cramps, anorexia, anxiety, backache, bone or joint pain, confusion, depression, diaphoresis, dysphoria, erythema, fear, fever, irritability, labile blood pressure and pulse, lacrimation, muscle spasms, myalgia, mydriasis, nasal congestion, nausea, opioid craving, piloerection, restlessness, rhinorrhea, sensation of crawling skin, sleep disturbances, tremor, uneasiness, vomiting and yawning.

PATIENT TEACHING

- Tell patient, if prescribed, that he will receive only the buprenorphine component of the drug for 1 or 2 days and then be given the combination drug for maintenance therapy.
- Instruct patient to place the S.L. tablet under his tongue until it dissolves. Caution him not to swallow the tablet because it will be less effective. If patient is prescribed more than two tablets per dose, tell him to place all the tablets under his tongue at the same time if they will fit. If not, advise him to place two tablets at a time under his tongue until full dose of tablets has dissolved.
- **WARNING** Warn patient to avoid other CNS depressants, such as alcohol or other opioids, while taking buprenorphine and naloxone because severe respiratory depression may occur.
- Instruct patient to rise slowly from a lying or sitting position to reduce dizziness.
- Advise patient to avoid potentially hazardous activities until drug's CNS effects are known.
- Emphasize importance of wearing a medical alert item that in the event of an emergency, the emergency health team will know he is physically dependent on opioids and is being treated with buprenorphine and naloxone.
- Instruct patient to inform all prescribers that he takes buprenorphine and naloxone before taking any new prescriptions and to avoid OTC drugs that affect the nervous system to avoid potential overdose.

butalbital, acetaminophen, caffeine, and codeine phosphate

Fioricet with Codeine, Phrenilin with Caffeine and Codeine

Class, Category, and Schedule

Chemical: Barbiturate (butalbital), acetamide (acetaminophen), xanthine derivative (caffeine), phenanthrene derivative (codeine)
Therapeutic: Muscle relaxant (butalbital), analgesic (acetaminophen, codeine), CNS stimulant (caffeine)
Pregnancy category: C
Controlled substance: Schedule III

Indications and Dosages

▶ *To relieve tension or muscle contraction headache*

CAPSULES

Adults. 50 mg butalbital, 325 mg acetaminophen, 40 mg caffeine, and 30 mg codeine (1 capsule) to 100 mg butalbital, 650 mg acetaminophen, 80 mg caffeine, and 60 mg codeine (2 capsules) q 4 hr, as needed. *Maximum:* 300 mg butalbital, 1,950 mg acetaminophen, 240 mg caffeine, and 180 mg codeine in 24 hr.

Contraindications

History of barbiturate addiction; hypersensitivity to butalbital, other barbiturates, acetaminophen, caffeine, codeine, other opioids, or their components; porphyria; significant respiratory depression; upper airway obstruction

Mechanism of Action

Butalbital inhibits upward conduction of nerve impulses to the reticular formation of the brain, thereby disrupting impulse transmission to the cortex. This action depresses the CNS, producing drowsiness, hypnosis, and sedation.

Acetaminophen inhibits the enzyme cyclooxygenase, blocking prostaglandin production and disrupting peripheral pain impulse generation.

Caffeine is a potent, competitive inhibitor of phosphodiesterase, an enzyme that degrades c3'5' AMP. Increased cAMP mediates most of its actions, including CNS stimulation to counteract the sedative properties of butalbital and codeine and cerebral vasoconstriction to relieve headache caused by increased blood volume from vasodilation.

Codeine may produce analgesia through partial metabolism to the opioid, morphine. Opioids bind and interact with opiate receptors in the CNS, altering the perception of and emotional response to pain and causing generalized CNS depression.

Interactions

DRUGS

butalbital, acetaminophen, caffeine, and codeine

CNS depressants, general anesthetics, opioids, tranquilizers: Additive CNS effects

butalbital component

adrenocorticoids, oral anticoagulants, tricyclic antidepressants: Decreased effectiveness of these drugs

disulfiram: Possibly increased risk of barbiturate (butalbital) toxicity

ketamine anesthesia: Increased risk of profound respiratory depression

MAO inhibitors: Increased CNS effects of butalbital

acetaminophen component

anticholinergics: Decreased onset of action of acetaminophen

barbiturates (except butalbital or primidone), carbamazepine, hydantoins, isoniazid, rifampin, sulfinpyrazone: Decreased therapeutic effects and increased hepatotoxic effects of acetaminophen

lamotrigine, loop diuretics: Possibly decreased therapeutic effects of these drugs

oral contraceptives: Decreased effectiveness of acetaminophen

probenecid: Possibly increased therapeutic effects of acetaminophen

propranolol: Possibly increased action of acetaminophen

zidovudine: Possibly decreased effects of zidovudine

caffeine component

aspirin: Increased GI absorption of aspirin

beta-adrenergic agonists: Possibly enhanced cardiac inotropic effects of beta-adrenergic agonists

cimetidine, contraceptives (oral), disulfiram, fluoroquinolones: Decreased hepatic metabolism of caffeine resulting in increased caffeine effect

clozapine: Possibly increased clozapine levels resulting in increased incidence of clozapine induced adverse reactions

lithium: Increased renal clearance of lithium

mexiletine: Decreased caffeine elimination resulting in increased caffeine effect

phenytoin: Increased caffeine clearance resulting in decreased caffeine effect

theophylline: Reduced theophylline clearance with ingestion of more than 120 mg caffeine daily

codeine component

anticholinergics: Increased risk of paralytic ileus

antihypertensives, diuretics: Potentiated hypotensive effects
buprenorphine: Decreased effectiveness of codeine
hydroxyzine: Increased codeine analgesic effect; increased CNS depressant and hypotensive effects
MAO inhibitors: Increased risk of unpredictable, severe, and sometimes fatal reactions
metoclopramide: Antagonized effect of metoclopramide on GI motility
naloxone: Antagonized codeine analgesic effect
naltrexone: Precipitated withdrawal symptoms in codeine-dependent patients
neuromuscular blockers: Additive respiratory depressant effects
opioids: Additive CNS and respiratory depressant effects and hypotensive effects
paregoric: Increased risk of severe constipation
ACTIVITIES
butalbital, acetaminophen, caffeine, and codeine
alcohol use: Additive CNS effect; increased risk of hepatotoxicity
caffeine component
smoking: Increased caffeine clearance resulting in decreased caffeine effect

Adverse Reactions

CNS: Anxiety, coma, confusion, delirium, depression, disorientation, dizziness, drowsiness, euphoria, excitement, hallucinations, headache, insomnia, intoxicated feeling, irritability, lack of coordination, lethargy light-headedness, mental and physical impairment, mood changes, nervousness, restlessness, sedation, seizures, tremor, twitching, vertigo
CV: Bradycardia, orthostatic hypotension, palpitations, tachycardia
EENT: Altered taste, blurred vision, diplopia, dry mouth, epistaxis, laryngeal edema, laryngospasm, miosis, salivation
ENDO: Altered blood glucose level
GI: Abdominal cramps and pain, anorexia, constipation, flatulence, gastroesophageal reflux, jaundice, hepatotoxicity, ileus, indigestion, nausea, vomiting
GU: Decreased libido, difficult ejaculation, dysuria, impotence, nephrotoxicity, oliguria, ureteral spasm, urinary incontinence, urine retention
HEME: Agranulocytosis, hemolytic anemia, leukopenia, neutropenia, pancytopenia, thrombocytopenia
MS: Muscle rigidity

RESP: Apnea, bronchoconstriction, bronchospasm, depressed cough reflex, respiratory depression, shortness of breath
SKIN: Diaphoresis, erythema multiforme, exfoliative dermatitis, flushing, pallor, pruritus, rash, toxic epidermal necrolysis, urticaria
Other: Angioedema, anaphylaxis, physical and psychological dependence

Nursing Considerations

- Use cautiously in patients with head trauma or intracranial lesions because codeine can cause an exaggerated respiratory depression.
- Use cautiously in elderly and debilitated patients as well as patients with severe renal or hepatic dysfunction, gallbladder disease, respiratory impairment, cardiac arrhythmias, inflammatory disorders of the GI tract, hypothyroidism, Addison's disease, prostatic hypertrophy or urethral stricture, coagulation disorders, or acute abdominal conditions.
- Before and during long-term therapy, monitor liver function test results, including AST, ALT, and bilirubin levels, as ordered.
- Evaluate patient for therapeutic response, including report of decreased pain that would indicate pain relief has occurred.
- Monitor renal function in patient on long-term therapy. Keep in mind that blood or albumin in urine may indicate nephritis and decreased urine output, renal failure. Expect to reduce dosage for patients with renal dysfunction.
- Take safety precautions, as needed.
- Monitor patient for CNS depression.
- Monitor patient's respiratory depth, effort and rate. Notify prescriber immediately if respiratory rate drops below 10 breaths/minute.
- **WARNING** Assess patient for evidence of physical and psychological dependence.
- Monitor urine output; decreasing output may signal urine retention or renal failure.

PATIENT TEACHING
- Instruct patient to take drug with food or after meals to minimize stomach upset.
- Instruct patient to take butalbital, acetaminophen, caffeine, and codeine exactly as prescribed and not to adjust dose or frequency without consulting prescriber.
- Instruct patient to notify prescriber about worsening or breakthrough pain.

- Advise patient to notify prescriber if he becomes short of breath or has difficulty breathing.
- Advise patient to avoid potentially hazardous activities until drug's CNS effects are known.
- Caution patient to avoid alcohol or other CNS depressants while taking drug. Also to contact prescriber before taking other prescription or OTC drugs as they may contain acetaminophen and lead to toxicity.
- Advise patient to get up slowly from a sitting or lying position.
- To prevent constipation, encourage patient to consume plenty of fluids and high-fiber foods, if not contraindicated by another condition.
- Teach patient to recognize signs of hepatotoxicity, such as bleeding, easy bruising, and chronic overdose.

butalbital, aspirin, and caffeine
Fiorinal, Fortabs

Class, Category, and Schedule
Chemical: Barbiturate (butalbital), salicylate (aspirin), and xanthine derivative (caffeine)
Therapeutic: Muscle relaxant (butalbital), analgesic (aspirin), CNS stimulant (caffeine)
Pregnancy category: C
Controlled substance: Schedule III

Indications and Dosages
▶ *To relieve tension or muscle contraction headache*
CAPSULES
Adults. 50 mg butalbital, 325 mg aspirin, and 40 mg caffeine (1 capsule) to 100 mg butalbital, 650 mg aspirin, and 80 mg caffeine (2 capsules) q 4 hr, as needed. *Maximum:* 300 mg butalbital; 1,950 mg aspirin; and 240 mg caffeine in 24 hr.

Contraindications
Allergy to tartrazine dye; bleeding problems such as hemophilia; children under age 16 with a viral illness; history of barbiturate addiction; hypersensitivity to butalbital, other barbiturates, aspirin, caffeine, or their components; nephritis; peptic ulcer disease; porphyria; severe respiratory impairment; severe vitamin K deficiency; triad syndrome of angioedema, asthma, and nasal polyps

Mechanism of Action

Butalbital inhibits upward conduction of nerve impulses to the reticular formation of the brain, thereby disrupting impulse transmission to the cortex. This action depresses the CNS, producing drowsiness, hypnosis, and sedation.

Aspirin blocks the activity of cyclooxygenase, the enzyme necessary for prostaglandin synthesis. By preventing prostaglandin synthesis, pain is relieved because prostaglandins play a role in pain transmission from the periphery to the spinal cord.

Caffeine is a potent, competitive inhibitor of phosphodiesterase, an enzyme that degrades c3'5' AMP. Increased cAMP mediates most of its action, including CNS stimulation to counteract the sedative properities of butalbital.

Interactions

DRUGS

butalbital component

adrenocorticoids, oral anticoagulants, tricyclic antidepressants: Decreased effectiveness of these drugs

CNS depressants: Increased CNS depressant effects

disulfiram: Possibly increased risk of barbiturate (butalbital) toxicity

ketamine anesthesia: Risk of profound respiratory depression

MAO inhibitors: Increased CNS effects of butalbital

aspirin component

ACE inhibitors: Decreased antihypertensive effect

activated charcoal: Decreased aspirin absorption

antacids, urine alkalinizers: Decreased aspirin effectiveness

anticoagulants: Increased risk of bleeding; prolonged bleeding time

carbonic anhydrase inhibitors: Salicylism

corticosteroids: Increased excretion and decreased aspirin level

heparin: Increased risk of bleeding

loop diuretics: Possibly decreased effectiveness of loop diuretics

methotrexate: Increased blood level and decreased excretion of methotrexate, causing toxicity

nizatidine: Increased blood aspirin level

NSAIDs: Possibly decreased blood NSAID level and increased risk of adverse GI effects

oral antidiabetics and insulin: Increased risk of hypoglycemia

probenecid, sulfinpyrazone: Decreased effectiveness in treating gout

urine acidifiers, such as ammonium chloride and ascorbic acid: Decreased aspirin excretion

vancomycin: Increased risk of ototoxicity

caffeine component
aspirin: Increased GI absorption of aspirin
beta-adrenergic agonists: Possibly enhanced cardiac inotropic effects of beta-adrenergic agonists
cimetidine, contraceptives (oral), disulfiram, fluoroquinolones: Decreased hepatic metabolism of caffeine and increased caffeine effect
clozapine: Possibly increased clozapine levels resulting in increased incidence of clozapine induced adverse reactions
lithium: Enhanced renal clearance of lithium
mexiletine: Decreased caffeine elimination resulting in increased caffeine effect
phenytoin: Increased caffeine clearance resulting in decreased caffeine effect
theophylline: Reduced theophylline clearance with ingestion of more than 120 mg caffeine daily
ACTIVITIES
butalbital component
alcohol use: Increased CNS depression
aspirin component
alcohol use: Increased risk of ulcers
caffeine component
smoking: Increased caffeine clearance resulting in decreased caffeine effect

Adverse Reactions

CNS: Anxiety, clumsiness, confusion, CNS depression, dizziness, drowsiness, hangover, headache, insomnia, irritability, lethargy, light-headedness, nervousness, nightmares, paradoxical stimulation, syncope
CV: Hypotension
EENT: Hearing loss, laryngospasm, tinnitus
GI: Anorexia, constipation, diarrhea, flatulence, GI bleeding, heartburn, hepatotoxicity, jaundice, nausea, stomach pain, vomiting
HEME: Agranulocytosis, bone marrow suppression, decreased blood iron level, hemolytic anemia, leukopenia, megaloblastic anemia, prolonged bleeding time, shortened life span of RBCs, thrombocytopenia
MS: Arthralgia, muscle weakness
RESP: Apnea, bronchospasm, respiratory depression
SKIN: Ecchymosis, erythema multiforme, rash, toxic epidermal necrolysis, urticaria
Other: Angioedema, drug dependence, Reye's syndrome, weight loss

Nursing Considerations

- Use cautiously in patients with head trauma or intracranial lesions because aspirin can increase the risk of bleeding.
- Use cautiously in elderly and debilitated patients as well as patients with severe renal or hepatic dysfunction, gallbladder disease, respiratory impairment, cardiac arrhythmias, inflammatory disorders of the GI tract, hypothyroidism, Addison's disease, prostatic hypertrophy or urethral stricture, coagulation disorders or acute abdominal conditions.
- Evaluate patient for therapeutic response, including report of decreased pain that would indicate pain relief has occurred.
- Take safety precautions, as needed.
- Monitor patient for CNS depression.
- Monitor patient's respiratory depth, effort and rate. Notify prescriber immediately if rate drops below 10 breaths/minute.
- **WARNING** Monitor patient closely for allergic reaction. Be aware that anaphylactic shock and other severe allergic reactions can occur without a history of allergy.
- **WARNING** Assess patient for evidence of physical and psychological dependence.
- Monitor urine output; decreasing output may signal urine retention or renal failure.

PATIENT TEACHING

- Instruct patient to take butalbital, aspirin, and caffeine with food or after meals to minimize stomach upset.
- Instruct patient to take drug exactly as prescribed and not to adjust dose or frequency without consulting prescriber because drug can be habit forming.
- Instruct patient to notify prescriber about worsening or breakthrough pain.
- Advise patient to notify prescriber if he becomes short of breath or has difficulty breathing.
- Tell patient to consult prescriber before taking drug with any prescription drug for blood disorder, diabetes, gout, or arthritis.
- Advise patient to avoid potentially hazardous activities until drug's CNS effects are known.
- Caution patient to avoid alcohol or other CNS depressants while taking drug.
- Advise patient to get up slowly from a sitting or lying position.
- To prevent constipation, encourage patient to consume plenty of fluids and high-fiber foods, if not contraindicated by another condition.

butalbital, aspirin, caffeine, and codeine phosphate

Fiorinal with Codeine, Fiortal

Class, Category, and Schedule

Chemical: Barbiturate (butalbital) salicylate (aspirin), xanthine derivative (caffeine), phenanthrene derivative (codeine)
Therapeutic: Muscle relaxant (butalbital), analgesic (aspirin, codeine), CNS stimulant (caffeine)
Pregnancy category: C
Controlled substance: Schedule III

Indications and Dosages

▶ *To relieve tension or muscle contraction headache*
CAPSULES
Adults. 50 mg butalbital, 325 mg aspirin, 40 mg caffeine, and 30 mg codeine (1 capsule) to 100 mg butalbital, 650 mg aspirin, 80 mg caffeine, and 60 mg codeine (2 capsules) q 4 hr, as needed. *Maximum:* 300 mg butalbital; 1,950 mg aspirin; 240 mg caffeine; 180 mg codeine in 24 hr.

Mechanism of Action

Butalbital inhibits upward conduction of nerve impulses to the reticular formation of the brain, thereby disrupting impulse transmission to the cortex. This action depresses the CNS, producing drowsiness, hypnosis, and sedation.

Aspirin blocks the activity of cyclooxygenase, the enzyme necessary for prostaglandin synthesis. By preventing prostaglandin synthesis, pain is relieved because prostaglandins play a role in pain transmission from the periphery to the spinal cord.

Caffeine is a potent, competitive inhibitor of phosphodiesterase, an enzyme that degrades c3'5' AMP. Increased cAMP mediates most of its action, including CNS stimulation to counteract the sedative properties of butalbital and codeine and cerebral vasoconstriction to relieve headache caused by increased blood volume from vasodilation.

Codeine may produce analgesia through partial metabolism to the opioid, morphine. Opioids bind and interact with opiate receptors in the CNS, altering the perception of and emotional response to pain and causing generalized CNS depression.

Contraindications

Allergy to tartrazine dye; asthma; bleeding problems such as hemophilia; children under age 16 with a viral illness; history of barbiturate addiction; hypersensitivity to aspirin, butalbital, other barbiturates, caffeine, codeine, other opioids, NSAIDs, or their components; nephritis; peptic ulcer disease; porphyria; respiratory depression; severe vitamin K deficiency; triad syndrome of angioedema, asthma, and nasal polyps; upper airway obstruction

Interactions

DRUGS

butalbital component

adrenocorticoids, oral anticoagulants, tricyclic antidepressants: Decreased effectiveness of these drugs

CNS depressants: Increased CNS depressant effects

disulfiram: Possibly increased risk of barbiturate (butalbital) toxicity

ketamine anesthesia: Increased risk of profound respiratory depression

MAO inhibitors: Increased CNS effects of butalbital

aspirin component

ACE inhibitors: Decreased antihypertensive effect

activated charcoal: Decreased aspirin absorption

antacids, urine alkalinizers: Decreased aspirin effectiveness

anticoagulants: Increased risk of bleeding; prolonged bleeding time

carbonic anhydrase inhibitors: Salicylism

corticosteroids: Increased excretion and decreased blood level of aspirin

heparin: Increased risk of bleeding

loop diuretics: Possibly decreased effectiveness of loop diuretics

methotrexate: Increased blood level and decreased excretion of methotrexate, causing toxicity

nizatidine: Increased blood aspirin level

NSAIDs: Possibly decreased blood NSAID level and increased risk of adverse GI effects

oral antidiabetics and insulin: Increased risk of hypoglycemia

probenecid, sulfinpyrazone: Decreased effectiveness in treating gout

urine acidifiers, such as ammonium chloride and ascorbic acid: Decreased aspirin excretion

vancomycin: Increased risk of ototoxicity

caffeine component

aspirin: Increased GI absorption of aspirin

beta-adrenergic agonists: Possibly enhanced cardiac inotropic effects of beta-adrenergic agonists

cimetidine, contraceptives (oral), disulfiram, fluoroquinolones: Decreased hepatic metabolism of caffeine resulting in increased caffeine effect

clozapine: Possibly increased clozapine levels resulting in increased incidence of clozapine induced adverse reactions

lithium: Enhanced renal clearance of lithium

mexiletine: Decreased caffeine elimination resulting in increased caffeine effect

phenytoin: Increased caffeine clearance resulting in decreased caffeine effect

theophylline: Reduced theophylline clearance with ingestion of more than 120 mg caffeine daily

codeine component

anticholinergics, paregoric: Increased risk of severe constipation

antihypertensives, diuretics: Potentiated hypotensive effects

buprenorphine: Decreased effectiveness of codeine

CNS depressants: Additive CNS effects

hydroxyzine: Increased codeine analgesic effect; increased CNS depressant and hypotensive effects

MAO inhibitors: Increased risk of unpredictable, severe, and sometimes fatal reactions

metoclopramide: Antagonized effect of metoclopramide on GI motility

naloxone: Antagonized codeine analgesic effect

naltrexone: Precipitated withdrawal symptoms in codeine-dependent patients

neuromuscular blockers: Additive respiratory depressant effects

opioids: Additive CNS and respiratory depressant effects and hypotensive effects

ACTIVITIES

butalbital component

alcohol use: Increased CNS depression

aspirin component

alcohol use: Increased risk of ulcers

caffeine component

smoking: Increased caffeine clearance and decreased caffeine effect

codeine component

alcohol use: Additive CNS effects

Adverse Reactions

CNS: Anxiety, clumsiness, coma, confusion, CNS depression, delirium, disorientation, dizziness, drowsiness, euphoria, hallucinations, hangover, headache, insomnia, irritability, lack of coordination, lethargy, light-headedness, mental and physical impairment, mood changes, nervousness, nightmares, paradoxical stimulation, restlessness, sedation, seizures, syncope

CV: Bradycardia, orthostatic hypotension, palpitations, tachycardia

EENT: Altered taste, blurred vision, diplopia, dry mouth, hearing loss, laryngeal edema, laryngospasm, miosis, tinnitus

GI: Abdominal cramps and pain, anorexia, constipation, diarrhea, flatulence, gastroesphageal reflux, GI bleeding, heartburn, hepatotoxicity, ileus, indigestion, jaundice, nausea, stomach pain, vomiting

GU: Decreased libido, difficult ejaculation, dysuria, impotence, oliguria, ureteral spasm, urinary incontinence, urine retention

HEME: Agranulocytosis, bone marrow suppression, decreased blood iron level, hemolytic anemia, leukopenia, megaloblastic anemia, prolonged bleeding time, shortened life span of RBCs, thrombocytopenia

MS: Arthralgia, muscle weakness

RESP: Apnea, bronchospasm, respiratory depression

SKIN: Diaphoresis, ecchymosis, erythema multiforme, flushing, pallor, pruritus, rash, toxic epidermal necrolysis, urticaria

Other: Anaphylaxis, angioedema, physical and psychological dependence, Reye's syndrome, weight loss

Nursing Considerations

- Use cautiously in patients with head trauma or intracranial lesions because codeine can cause an exaggerated respiratory depression and aspirin can increase the risk of bleeding.
- Use cautiously in elderly and debilitated patients as well as patients with severe renal or hepatic dysfunction, gallbladder disease, respiratory impairment, cardiac arrhythmias, inflammatory disorders of the GI tract, hypothyroidism, Addison's disease, prostatic hypertrophy or urethral stricture, coagulation disorders or acute abdominal conditions.
- Evaluate patient for therapeutic response, including report of decreased pain that would indicate pain relief has occurred.
- Take safety precautions, as needed.
- Monitor patient for CNS depression.
- Monitor respiratory depth, effort and rate. Notify prescriber immediately if respiratory rate drops below 10 breaths/minute.
- **WARNING** Monitor patient closely for allergic reaction. Be aware that anaphylactic shock and other severe allergic reactions can occur without a history of allergy.
- **WARNING** Assess patient for evidence of physical and psy-

chological dependence.
• Monitor urine output; decreasing output may signal urine retention or renal failure.

PATIENT TEACHING
• Instruct patient to take butalbital, aspirin, caffeine, and codeine with food or after meals to minimize stomach upset.
• Instruct patient to take drug exactly as prescribed and not to adjust dose or frequency without consulting prescriber because drug can be habit forming.
• Instruct patient to notify prescriber about worsening or breakthrough pain.
• Advise patient to notify prescriber if he becomes short of breath or has difficulty breathing.
• Tell patient to consult prescriber before taking drug with any prescription drug for blood disorder, diabetes, gout, or arthritis.
• Advise patient to avoid potentially hazardous activities until drug's CNS effects are known.
• Caution patient to avoid alcohol or other CNS depressants while taking drug.
• Advise patient to get up slowly from a sitting or lying position.
• To prevent constipation, encourage patient to consume plenty of fluids and high-fiber foods, if not contraindicated by another condition.

carisoprodol, aspirin, and codeine phosphate
Soma Compound with Codeine

Class, Category, and Schedule
Chemical: Dicarbamate (carisoprodol), salicylate (aspirin), phenanthrene derivative (codeine)
Therapeutic: Skeletal muscle relaxant (carisoprodol), analgesic (aspirin, codeine)
Pregnancy category: NR (carisoprodol C, aspirin D, codeine C)
Controlled substance: Schedule III

Indications and Dosages
▶ *To treat acute painful musculoskeletal conditions*
TABLETS
Adults. 200 mg carisoprodol, 325 mg aspirin and 16 mg codeine (1 tablet) or 400 mg carisoprodol, 650 mg aspirin and 32 mg codeine (2 tablets) q.i.d.

Mechanism of Action

Carisoprodol blocks interneuronal activity in the descending reticular formation and spinal cord, producing muscle relaxation and sedation

Aspirin blocks the activity of cyclooxygenase, the enzyme necessary for prostaglandin synthesis. By preventing prostaglandin synthesis, pain is relieved because prostaglandins play a role in pain transmission from the periphery to the spinal cord.

Codeine may produce analgesia through partial metabolism to the opioid, morphine. Opioids bind and interact with opiate receptors in the CNS, altering the perception of and emotional response to pain and causing generalized CNS depression.

Contraindications

Allergy to tartrazine dye; asthma; bleeding problems such as hemophilia; children under age 16 with a viral illness; hypersensitivity to carisoprodol, aspirin, codeine, other opioids, NSAIDs, or their components; intermittent porphyria; peptic ulcer disease; respiratory depression; severe vitamin K deficiency; upper airway obstruction

Interactions

DRUGS

carisoprodol component

CNS depressants, psychotropic drugs: Additive CNS depression

aspirin component

ACE inhibitors: Decreased antihypertensive effect

activated charcoal: Decreased aspirin absorption

antacids, urine alkalinizers: Decreased aspirin effectiveness

anticoagulants: Increased risk of bleeding; prolonged bleeding time

carbonic anhydrase inhibitors: Salicylism

corticosteroids: Increased excretion and decreased blood level of aspirin

heparin: Increased risk of bleeding

loop diuretics: Possibly decreased effectiveness of loop diuretics

methotrexate: Increased blood level and decreased excretion of methotrexate, causing toxicity

nizatidine: Increased blood aspirin level

NSAIDs: Possibly decreased blood NSAID level and increased risk of adverse GI effects

probenecid, sulfinpyrazone: Decreased effectiveness in treating gout

urine acidifiers, such as ammonium chloride and ascorbic acid: Decreased aspirin excretion

vancomycin: Increased risk of ototoxicity
codeine component
anticholinergics, paregoric: Increased risk of severe constipation
antihypertensives, diuretics: Potentiated hypotensive effects
buprenorphine: Decreased effectiveness of codeine
CNS depressants: Additive CNS effects
hydroxyzine: Increased codeine analgesic effect; increased CNS depressant and hypotensive effects
MAO inhibitors: Increased risk of unpredictable, severe, and sometimes fatal reactions
metoclopramide: Antagonized effect of metoclopramide on GI motility
naloxone: Antagonized codeine analgesic effect
naltrexone: Precipitated withdrawal symptoms in codeine-dependent patients
neuromuscular blockers: Additive respiratory depressant effects
opioids: Additive CNS and respiratory depressant effects and hypotensive effects
ACTIVITIES
carisoprodol, aspirin, and codeine
alcohol use: Additive CNS effects and increased risk of adverse GI effects

Adverse Reactions
CNS: Agitation, ataxia, coma, confusion, CNS depression, delirium, depression, disorientation, dizziness, drowsiness, euphoria, fever, hallucinations, headache, insomnia, irritability, lack of coordination, syncope, tremor, vertigo
CV: Bradycardia, orthostatic hypotension, palpitations, tachycardia
EENT: Altered taste, blurred vision, diplopia, dry mouth, hearing loss, laryngeal edema, laryngospasm, miosis, tinnitus, transient vision loss
GI: Abnormal cramps and pain, anorexia, constipation, diarrhea, epigastric discomfort, flatulence, GI bleeding, gastroesophageal reflux, heartburn, hepatotoxicity, hiccups, ileus, indigestion, nausea, stomach pain, vomiting
GU: Decreased libido, difficult ejaculation, dysuria, impotence, oliguria, ureteral spasm, urinary incontinence, urine retention
HEME: Decreased blood iron level, eosinophilia, hemolytic anemia, leukopenia, prolonged bleeding time, shortened life span of RBCs, thrombocytopenia
MS: Muscle rigidity

RESP: Apnea, bronchoconstriction, bronchospasm, depressed cough reflex, respiratory depression
SKIN: Diaphoresis, ecchymosis, erythema multiforme, flushing, pallor, pruritus, rash, urticaria
Other: Anaphylaxis, angioedema, physical and psychological dependence, Reye's syndrome

Nursing Considerations

- Use cautiously in patients with drug addiction.
- Use cautiously in patients with head trauma or intracranial lesions because codeine can cause an exaggerated respiratory depression and aspirin can increase the risk of bleeding.
- Use cautiously in elderly and debilitated patients as well as patients with severe renal or hepatic dysfunction, gallbladder disease, respiratory impairment, cardiac arrhythmias, inflammatory disorders of the GI tract, hypothyroidism, Addison's disease, prostatic hypertrophy or urethral stricture, coagulation disorders or acute abdominal conditions.
- Evaluate patient for therapeutic response, including report of decreased pain and body movements that would indicate pain relief has occurred.
- Take safety precautions, as needed.
- Monitor patient for CNS depression.
- Monitor respiratory depth, effort and rate. Notify prescriber immediately if respiratory rate drops below 10 breaths/minute.
- **WARNING** Monitor patient closely for allergic reaction. Be aware that anaphylactic shock and other severe allergic reactions can occur without a history of allergy.
- **WARNING** Assess patient for evidence of physical and psychological dependence.
- Monitor urine output; decreasing output may signal urine retention or renal failure.
- Expect prescriber to taper therapy rather than stopping it abruptly to avoid withdrawal symptoms.

PATIENT TEACHING
- Instruct patient to take carisoprodol, aspirin and codeine with food or after meals to minimize stomach upset.
- Instruct patient to take carisoprodol, aspirin, and codeine exactly as prescribed and not to adjust dose or frequency without consulting prescriber. Tell patient not to abruptly stop taking the drug to prevent withdrawal symptoms. Instead, expect prescriber to taper therapy when no longer needed.

- Instruct patient to notify prescriber about worsening or break-through pain.
- Advise patient to notify prescriber if he becomes short of breath or has difficulty breathing.
- Tell patient to consult prescriber before taking drug with any prescription drug for blood disorder, diabetes, gout, or arthritis.
- Advise patient to avoid potentially hazardous activities until drug's CNS effects are known.
- Caution patient to avoid alcohol or other CNS depressants while taking carisoprodol, aspirin and codeine.
- Advise patient to get up slowly from a sitting or lying position.
- To prevent constipation, encourage patient to consume plenty of fluids and high-fiber foods, if not contraindicated.
- Inform patient that saliva, urine, and sweat may appear darker (red, brown, or black) because of the carisoprodol of the drug and reassure him that the color change is harmless.

chlordiazepoxide and amitriptyline hydrochloride
Limbitrol, Limbitrol DS 10-25

Class, Category, and Schedule
Chemical: Benzodiazepine (chlordiazepoxide), tertiary amine (amitriptyline)
Therapeutic: Antianxiety (chlordiazepoxide), antidepressant (amitriptyline)
Pregnancy category: D
Controlled substance: Schedule IV

Indications and Dosages
▶ *To treat depression with moderate to severe anxiety*
TABLETS
Adults. *Initial:* 10 mg chlordiazepoxide and 25 mg amitriptyline (1 tablet) t.i.d. or q.i.d. *Maintenance:* Increase as needed to six times daily or decrease to twice daily or once daily at bedtime, as needed.

Contraindications
During acute recovery phrase after MI; hypersensitivity to chlordiazepoxide, other benzodiazepines, amitriptyline, other tricyclic antidepressants, or their components; use within 14 days of MAO inhibitor therapy

Mechanism of Action

Chlordiazepoxide may potentiate the effects of gamma-aminobutyric acid (GABA) and other inhibitory neurotransmitters by binding to specific benzodiazepine receptors in the limbic and cortical areas of the CNS. By binding to these receptors, chlordiazepoxide increases GABA's inhibitory effects and blocks cortical and limbic arousal, which helps control emotional behavior.

Amitriptyline blocks serotonin and norepinephrine reuptake by adrenergic nerves. By doing so, it raises serotonin and norepinephrine levels at nerve synapses. This action may elevate mood and reduce depression.

Interactions

DRUGS

chlordiazepoxide and amitriptyline

cimetidine, disulfiram, fluoxetine, fluvoxamine, haloperidol, H$_2$-receptor antagonists, isoniazid, ketoconazole, methylphenidate, metoprolol, oral contraceptives, paroxetine, phenothiazines, propoxyphene, propranolol, sertraline, valproic acid: Increased blood chlordiazepoxide or amitriptyline levels

chlordiazepoxide component

antacids: Altered rate of chlordiazepoxide absorption

CNS depressants: Increased CNS effects

digoxin: Increased blood digoxin level and risk of digitalis toxicity

levodopa: Decreased efficacy of levodopa's antiparkinsonian effects

neuromuscular blockers: Potentiated, counteracted, or diminished effects of neuromuscular blockers

phenytoin: Possibly increased phenytoin toxicity

probenecid: Shortened onset of action or prolonged effect of chlordiazepoxide

rifampin: Decreased chlordiazepoxide effect

theophyllines: Antagonized sedative effects of chlordiazepoxide

amitriptyline component

anticholinergics, epinephrine, norepinephrine: Increased effects of these drugs

barbiturates: Decreased serum amitriptyline level

carbamazepine: Decreased serum amitriptyline level and increased serum carbamazepine level, which increases therapeutic and toxic effects of carbamazepine

cisapride: Possibly prolonged QT interval and increased risk for arrhythmias

clonidine, guanethidine, other antihypertensives: Decreased antihypertensive effects

dicumarol: Increased anticoagulant effect od dicumarol
levodopa: Decreased levodopa absorption; sympathetic hyperactivity, sinus tachycardia, hypertension, agitation
MAO inhibitors: Possibly seizures and death
thyroid replacement drugs: Arrhythmias and increased antidepressant effects
ACTIVITIES
chlordiazepoxide and amitriptyline
alcohol use: Increased CNS effects
amitriptyline component
smoking: Decreased amitriptyline effects

Adverse Reactions

CNS: Anxiety, ataxia, coma, confusion, chills, delusions, depression, disorientation, drowsiness, extrapyramidal reactions, fatigue, fever, headache, insomnia, nightmares, peripheral neuropathy, tremor
CV: Arrhythmias (including prolonged AV conduction, heart block, and tachycardia), cardiomyopathy, hypertension, MI, ECG changes, orthostatic hypotension, palpitations, tachycardia
EENT: Abnormal taste, black tongue, blurred vision, dry mouth, nasal congestion, tinnitus
ENDO: Gynecomastia, increased or decreased blood glucose level, increased prolactin level, syndrome of inappropriate antidiuretic hormone secretion
GI: Abdominal cramps, constipation, diarrhea, flatulence, hepatic dysfunction, ileus, increased appetite, jaundice, nausea, vomiting
GU: Impotence, libido changes, menstrual irregularities, testicular swelling, urinary hesitancy, urine retention
HEME: Agranulocytosis, bone marrow depression, eosinophilia, leukopenia, thrombocytopenia
SKIN: Alopecia, flushing, photosensitivity, purpura
Other: Physical and psychological dependence, weight gain

Nursing Considerations

• Use chlordiazepoxide and amitriptyline cautiously in patients with renal or hepatic impairment, porphyria, or thyroid disorders.
• Because amitriptyline has atropine-like effects, use caution when giving it to a patient with a history of seizures, urine retention, or angle-closure glaucoma.
• **WARNING** Don't give an MAO inhibitor within 14 days of chlordiazepoxide and amitriptyline therapy because of the risk of seizures and death.

- Closely monitor patient with a cardiovascular disorder because amitriptyline may cause arrhythmias, such as sinus tachycardia.
- Monitor blood pressure and assess patient for changes.
- Stay alert for behavior changes, such as hallucinations and decreased interest in personal appearance. Be aware that psychosis may develop in schizophrenic patients and symptoms may increase in paranoid patients.
- **WARNING** Be aware that prolonged use of therapeutic doses can lead to dependence.
- Avoid abrupt withdrawal of drug after prolonged therapy; otherwise, nausea, headache, vertigo, and nightmares may occur.
- Monitor patient being treated for depression with chlordiazepoxide and amitriptyline closely for suicidal tendencies, especially at beginning of therapy and during dosage adjustments as depression may temporarily worsen during these times.
- Monitor patient's blood counts and liver function test results during therapy. Notify prescriber of any abnormalities.

PATIENT TEACHING
- Instruct patient to take drug exactly as prescribed.
- Advise patient to avoid performing hazardous activities until CNS effects of drug are known.
- Instruct patient to avoid using alcohol or OTC drugs that contain alcohol during chlordiazepoxide and amitriptyline therapy because alcohol enhances the drug's CNS depressant effects.
- Warn patient not to take antacids with drug.
- Caution patient not to abruptly stop taking drug because withdrawal symptoms may occur.
- Inform female patients of childbearing age to report planned or suspected pregnancy immediately because drug may cause congenital abnormalities and will need to be stopped.
- Instruct patient to avoid direct sunlight as much as possible and to use sunscreen, protective clothing and sunglasses when exposure to sunlight can not be avoided.

choline salicylate and magnesium salicylate

Tricosal, Trilisate

Class and Category

Chemical: Salicylate
Therapeutic: Analgesic, anti-inflammatory, antipyretic
Pregnancy category: C (first trimester), NR (later trimesters)

Indications and Dosages

▶ *To treat osteoarthritis, rheumatoid arthritis, and acute painful shoulder*
LIQUID, TABLETS
Adults. 1,500 mg b.i.d. or 3,000 mg h.s.
Children weighing more than 37 kg (81 lb). 2,250 mg/day in equally divided doses b.i.d.
Children weighing 37 kg or less. 50 mg/kg/day in equally divided doses b.i.d.
▶ *To treat mild to moderate pain, reduce fever*
LIQUID, TABLETS
Adults. 2,000 to 3,000 mg/day in equally divided doses b.i.d.
DOSAGE ADJUSTMENT Dosage reduced to 750 mg t.i.d. for elderly patients.

Mechanism of Action

Block the activity of cyclooxygenase, the enzyme needed for prostaglandin synthesis. As mediators in the inflammatory process, prostaglandins cause local vasodilation with swelling and pain. They also play a role in pain transmission from the periphery to the spinal cord. By blocking cyclooxygenase and inhibiting prostaglandins, this NSAID decreases inflammatory symptoms and relieves pain. It acts on the heat-regulating center in the hypothalamus and causes peripheral vasodilation, sweating, and heat loss.

Contraindications

Hypersensitivity to nonacetylated salicylates

Interactions

DRUGS
antacids: Increased salicylate clearance and decreased blood level
carbonic anhydrase inhibitors, phenytoin, valproic acid: Decreased blood levels and therapeutic effects of these drugs
corticosteroids: Decreased blood salicylate level, increased salicylate dosage requirements
insulin, sulfonylureas: Increased hypoglycemic response
methotrexate: Increased therapeutic and toxic effects of methotrexate, especially when given in chemotherapeutic doses
oral anticoagulants: Increased blood level of unbound anticoagulant and risk of bleeding
salicylate-containing products: Increased plasma salicylate level, possibly to toxic level
uricosuric drugs: Decreased uricosuric drug efficacy

Adverse Reactions
CNS: Dizziness, drowsiness, headache, lethargy, light-headedness
EENT: Hearing loss, tinnitus
GI: Constipation, diarrhea, epigastric pain, heartburn, indigestion, nausea, vomiting
HEME: Easy bruising, unusual bleeding

Nursing Considerations
- Use these salicylates cautiously in patients with gastritis, hepatic or renal dysfunction, or peptic ulcer disease.
- Don't give salicylates to children or adolescents with chickenpox or flu symptoms because of the risk of Reye's syndrome.
- **WARNING** During high-dose or long-term therapy, monitor for signs of salicylate intoxication, such as headache, dizziness, tinnitus, hearing loss, confusion, drowsiness, diaphoresis, vomiting, diarrhea, and hyperventilation. CNS disturbance, electrolyte imbalance, respiratory acidosis, hyperthermia, and dehydration also may occur. If intoxication occurs, prepare to induce vomiting, administer gastric lavage, and give activated charcoal, as ordered. In extreme cases, prepare patient for peritoneal dialysis or hemodialysis.

PATIENT TEACHING
- Tell patient to store drug at room temperature, away from heat, light, and moisture.
- Instruct patient to take drug with food or after meals with a full glass of water.
- Tell patient to take a missed dose as soon as he remembers but to avoid double-dosing.
- Advise patient that optimal effects may take 2 to 3 weeks.
- Teach patient to recognize and immediately report signs of salicylate toxicity.
- Explain that drug is closely related to aspirin. Advise against taking aspirin-containing OTC remedies during therapy.

diclofenac sodium and misoprostol
Arthrotec

Class and Category
Chemical: Phenylacetic acid derivative (diclofenac), prostaglandin E1 analogue (misoprostol)
Therapeutic: Analgesic (diclofenac), antiulcer, gastric antisecretory (misoprostol)

Pregnancy category: X

Indications and Dosages

▶ *To treat signs and symptoms of osteoarthritis in patients at high risk of developing NSAID-induced gastric and duodenal ulcers and their complications*

TABLETS

Adults. 50 mg diclofenac and 200 mcg misoprostol (1 tablet) b.i.d. or t.i.d. Or, 75 mg diclofenac and 200 mcg misoprostol (1 tablet) b.i.d.

▶ *To treat signs and symptoms of rheumatoid arthritis in patients at high risk of developing NSAID-induced gastric and duodenal ulcers and their complications*

TABLETS

Adults. 50 mg diclofenac and 200 mcg misoprostol (1 tablet) b.i.d. to q.i.d. Or, 75 mg diclofenac and 200 mcg misoprostol (1 tablet) b.i.d.

Mechanism of Action

Diclofenac blocks the activity of cyclooxygenase, the enzyme needed to synthesize prostaglandins, which mediate the inflammatory response and cause local vasodilation, swelling, and pain. By blocking cyclooxygenase and inhibiting prostaglandins, diclofenac reduces inflammatory symptoms. This mechanism also relieves pain because prostaglandins promote pain transmission from the periphery to the spinal cord.

Misoprostol may protect the stomach from NSAID-induced mucosal damage by increasing gastric mucus production and mucosal bicarbonate secretion. Misoprostol also inhibits gastric acid secretion caused by such stimuli as food, coffee, and histamine.

Contraindications

History of asthma, urticaria, or other allergic-type reactions following aspirin or other NSAIDs use; hepatic porphyria; hypersensitivity to diclofenac, misoprostol, other prostaglandins, or their components; pregnancy; severe renal impairment; treatment of peri-operative pain during coronary artery bypass graft surgery

Interactions

DRUGS

diclofenac and misoprostol

antacids: Reduced bioavailability of misoprostol acid; delay absorption of diclofenac

diclofenac component

ACE inhibitors, antihypertensives: Decreased antihypertensive effects
acetaminophen: Increased risk of adverse renal effects with long-term concurrent use
anticoagulants, thrombolytics: Prolonged PT, increased risk of bleeding
aspirin, other NSAIDs, salicylates: Increased GI irritability and bleeding, decreased diclofenac effectiveness
beta blockers: Impaired antihypertensive effects
cefamandole, cefoperazone, cefotetan, plicamycin, valproic acid: Increased risk of hypoprothrombinemia
cimetidine: Altered blood diclofenac level
colchicines, corticotropin (long-term use), glucocorticoids, potassium supplements: Increased GI irritability and bleeding
cyclosporine, gold compounds, nephrotoxic drugs: Increased risk of nephrotoxicity
digoxin: Increased serum digoxin level
insulin, oral antidiabetics: Decreased effects of these drugs
lithium: Increased risk of lithium toxicity
loop diuretics: Decreased loop diuretic effectiveness
methotrexate: Increased risk of methotrexate toxicity
phenytoin: Increased blood phenytoin level
potassium-sparing diuretics: Increased risk of hyperkalemia
probenecid: Increased diclofenac toxicity

misoprostol component
magnesium-containing antacids: Increased misoprostol-induced diarrhea
ACTIVITIES
diclofenac component
alcohol use: Increased risk of GI irritability and bleeding

Adverse Reactions

CNS: Aseptic meningitis, coma, CVA, dizziness, drowsiness, headache, paranoia, psychotic reaction, syncope
CV: Bradycardia and other arrhythmias, congestive heart failure, edema, hypertension, hypotension, MI, palpitations, phlebitis, seizures, thrombosis, vasculitis, vertigo
EENT: Glaucoma, hearing loss, laryngeal and pharyngeal edema, tinnitus
ENDO: Alterations in blood glucose level
GI: Abdominal pain, constipation, diarrhea, dyspepsia, dysphasia, elevated liver function test results, enteritis, esophageal ulceration, flatulence, gastritis, GI bleeding or ulceration, hepatic por-

phyria, hepatitis, hepatotoxicity, indigestion, intestinal perforation, jaundice, nausea, pancreatitis, peptic ulcer, vomiting

GU: Dysmenorrhea, hypermenorrhea, interstitial nephritis, menstrual irregularities, nephritic syndrome, papillary necrosis, renal failure, vaginal bleeding

HEME: Agranulocytosis, aplastic and hemolytic anemia, eosinophilia, increased coagulation time, leukopenia, leukocytosis, pancytopenia, thrombocytopenia

RESP: Asthma, dyspnea, pneumonia, pulmonary embolism, respiratory depression

SKIN: Exfoliative dermatitis, pruritus, rash, Stevens-Johnson Syndrome, toxic epidermal necrolysis, urticaria

Other: Anaphylaxis, angioedema, hyperuricemia, hyponatremia, lymphadenopathy, sepsis

Nursing Considerations

- **WARNING** Ask patient if she is or may be pregnant. If so, notify prescriber because misoprostol may cause uterine bleeding, contractions, and spontaneous abortion as well as teratogenic effects in the fetus.
- Use diclofenac and misoprostol cautiously in patients with cerebrovascular disease, coronary artery disease, congestive heart failure, or uncontrolled epilepsy because of the risk of severe complications.
- Also use diclofenac and misoprostol cautiously in patients with inflammatory bowel disease because drug may worsen intestinal inflammation and cause diarrhea. If diarrhea causes severe dehydration, drug may need to be stopped.
- Rehydrate patient who is seriously dehydrated before initiating diclofenac and misoprostol therapy because drug may cause serious adverse renal effects in patients with dehydration.
- Monitor liver function test results and serum uric acid level. Liver enzyme elevations usually occur within 2 months of starting diclofenac and misoprostol therapy. If abnormal liver test results persist or worsen, if patient exhibits signs and symptoms consistent with liver disease, or if systemic manifestations such as eosinophilia or rash occur, discontinue drug immediately and notify prescriber.
- Monitor renal function in patients on long-term diclofenac and misoprostol therapy because they are at increased risk for renal papillary necrosis and other renal injury and in patients with existing renal disease, heart failure, liver dysfuction, those tak-

ing diuretics and ACE inhibitors, and the elderly. Notify prescriber if abnormalities develop and expect to discontinue drug.

- Be aware that although rare, aseptic meningitis with fever and coma has occurred in patients taking diclofenac, especially patients who have systemic lupus and related connective tissue disease. Notify prescriber immediately if patients develops fever and CNS dysfunction.
- Report weight gain of more than 1 kg (2 lb) in 24 hours, which suggests fluid retention.
- Report signs of bleeding, such as petechiae, ecchymoses, bleeding gums, melena, and cloudy or bloody urine. Monitor patient for signs of GI irritation and ulceration, especially if patient has predisposing conditions, such as a history of GI bleeding, takes an oral corticosteroid or anticoagulant, smokes, is an alcoholic, is over age 60, has poor general health, or tests positive for *Helicobacter pylori.*
- Monitor blood pressure during diclofenac and misoprostol therapy because hypertension may occur or worsen during therapy.
- If patient takes a potassium-sparing diuretic, check for elevated serum potassium level, as ordered.
- Monitor patient's hemoglobin and hematocrit, as ordered, if receiving prolonged drug therapy because drug may cause anemia

PATIENT TEACHING

- Instruct patient to take drug with food to minimize GI distress.
- To decrease risk of esophageal ulceration, instruct patient not to lie down for 15 to 30 minutes after taking drug.
- **WARNING** Caution female patient about the risk of taking diclofenac and misoprostol during pregnancy, and urge her to use reliable contraception during therapy. Urge her to notify prescriber immediately if she is or might be pregnant.
- Inform patient that diarrhea is dose-related and usually resolves after 8 days. Instruct her to avoid magnesium-containing antacids because they may worsen diarrhea and to contact prescriber if diarrhea persists longer than 8 days.
- Urge female patient to notify prescriber immediately about postmenopausal bleeding; she may need diagnostic tests to rule out a gynecologic disorder.
- Warn patient to avoid potentially hazardous activities until drug's CNS effects are known.
- Instruct patient to notify prescriber if she experiences ringing or buzzing in the ears, impaired hearing, dizziness, or GI distress or bleeding.

- Advise patient to consult prescriber before taking aspirin or other OTC analgesics or ingesting alcohol.
- Inform patient that drug increases the risk of inflammation, bleeding, ulceration, and perforation of the stomach and intestines, possibly without warning. If patient feels suddenly ill, she should seek medical attention.
- Warn patient of the possibility of hepatic injury. Instruct patient to notify prescriber if she experiences signs and symptoms of hepatotoxicity such as nausea, fatigue, lethargy, pruritus, jaundice, right upper quadrant tenderness, and flulike symptoms.

ergoloid mesylates
(dihydrogenated ergot alkaloids)
Gerimal, Hydergine, Hydergine LC

Class and Category
Chemical: Dihydrogenated ergot alkaloid derivative
Therapeutic: Antidementia adjunct, cerebral metabolic enhancer
Pregnancy category: Not rated

Indications and Dosages
▶ *To treat age-related decline in mental capacity*
CAPSULES, ORAL SOLUTION, S.L. TABLETS, TABLETS
Adults. 1 to 2 mg t.i.d.

Mechanism of Action
May increase cerebral metabolism, blood flow, and oxygen uptake. These actions may increase neurotransmitter levels.

Contraindications
Acute or chronic psychosis, hypersensitivity to ergoloid mesylates or their components

Interactions
DRUGS
delavirdine, efavirenz, indinavir, nelfinavir, saquinavir: Increased risk of ergotism (blurred vision, dizziness, and headache)
dopamine: Increased risk of gangrene

Adverse Reactions
CNS: Dizziness, headache, light-headedness, syncope
CV: Bradycardia, orthostatic hypotension

EENT: Blurred vision, nasal congestion, tongue soreness (with S.L. tablets)
GI: Abdominal cramps, anorexia, nausea, vomiting
SKIN: Flushing, rash

Nursing Considerations

- Expect ergoloid mesylates to be prescribed only after a pathophysiologic cause for mental decline has been ruled out.
- Measure blood pressure and pulse rate and rhythm before therapy begins and monitor them frequently during therapy.
- If bradycardia or hypotension develops, expect to discontinue drug permanently.

PATIENT TEACHING

- Stress the importance of adhering to prescribed dosage and schedule.
- Teach caregiver to place S.L. tablet under patient's tongue and withhold food, fluids, and cigarettes until tablet dissolves.
- Instruct patient not to swallow S.L. tablets.
- Advise caregiver to skip a missed dose and resume the regular dosing schedule. Warn against doubling the dose, and urge caregiver to notify prescriber if patient misses two or more doses in a row.
- Instruct caregiver to store drug in a tightly closed, light-resistant container.
- Inform caregiver and family that drug may take 3 to 4 weeks to produce its effects.
- Stress the importance of follow-up care.

fluoxetine hydrochloride and olanzapine

Symbyax

Class and Category

Chemical: Thienobenzodiazepine derivative (olanzapine) and selective serotonin reuptake inhibitor (fluoxetine)
Therapeutic: Antipsychotic
Pregnancy category: C

Indications and Dosages

▶ *To treat depression associated with bipolar disorder*
CAPSULES
Adults. *Initial:* 6 mg olanzapine and 25 mg fluoxetine daily in the evening and then dosage increased as needed. *Maximum:* 12 mg olanzapine and 50 mg fluoxetine.

Mechanism of Action

May activate monoaminergic neural system's serotonin, norepinephrine, and dopamine release in the prefrontal cortex to increase antidepressant effect.

Contraindications

Hypersensitivity to olanzapine, fluoxetine, or other selective serotonin reuptake inhibitors or their components; use within 14 days of MAO inhibitor therapy or within 5 weeks of thioridazine therapy

Interactions

DRUGS

almotriptan: Increased risk of weakness, hyperreflexia, and incoordination

alprazolam, diazepam: Possibly prolonged half-life of these drugs

anticholinergics: Increased anticholinergic effects, altered thermoregulation

antihypertensives: Increased effects of both drugs

aspirin, NSAIDS, warfarin: Increased risk of bleeding

astemizole: Increased risk of serious arrhythmias

buspirone: Decreased buspirone effects

carbamazepine, omeprazole, rifampin: Increased olanzapine clearance

clozapine, fluphenazine, haloperidol, maprotiline, trazodone: Increased risk of adverse effects

CNS depressants: Additive CNS depression, potentiated orthostatic hypotension

diazepam: Increased CNS depressant effects

fluvoxamine: Decreased olanzapine clearance

levodopa: Decreased levodopa efficacy

lithium: Increased or decreased blood lithium level

MAO inhibitors: Possibly life-threatening adverse effects

phenytoin: Increased blood phenytoin level and risk of toxicity

pimozide: Possibly bradycardia

serotonergics (such as amphetamines and other psychostimulants, antidepressants, and dopamine agonists): Serotonin syndrome

thioridazine: Increased risk of serious ventricular arrhythmias

tricyclic antidepressants: Increased risk of adverse effects, including seizures

tryptophan: Increased risk of central and peripheral toxicity

ACTIVITIES

alcohol use: Additive CNS depression, potentiated orthostatic hypotension *smoking:* Decreased blood olanzapine level

Adverse Reactions

CNS: Amnesia, asthenia, chills, fever, hyperkinesia, migraine, neuroleptic malignant syndrome, personality changes, seizures, serotonin syndrome, sleep disturbance, somnolence, speech alteration, tardive dyskinesia, tremor

CV: Bradycardia, chest pain, edema, hypertension, orthostatic hypotension, tachycardia, vasodilation

EENT: Abnormal vision, amblyopia, dry mouth, ear pain, increased salivation, otitis media, pharyngitis, taste perversion, tinnitus

ENDO: Breast pain, hyperglycemia, increased prolactin level, menorrhagia

GI: Diarrhea, elevated liver function test results, increased appetite, thirst

GU: Abnormal ejaculation, anorgasmia, decreased libido, impotence, urinary frequency or incontinence, UTI

MS: Arthralgia, muscle twitching, neck pain or rigidity,

RESP: Bronchitis, dyspnea

SKIN: Ecchymosis, photosensitivity, rash, urticaria

Other: Anaphylaxis, angioedema, hyponatremia, infection, weight gain or loss

Nursing Considerations

- Use with caution in patients with cardiovascular or cerebrovascular disease or conditions that would predispose patients to hypotension because of olanzapine and fluoxetine's potential to cause orthostatic hypotension.
- Be aware that the olanzapine component in this combination drug should not be used in patients with dementia-related psychosis because of an increased risk of cerebrovascular adverse effects.
- Monitor patient's blood glucose level routinely because drug may increase risk of developing hyperglycemia.
- Monitor patient closely for neuroleptic malignant syndrome (hyperthermia, muscle rigidity, altered level of consciousness, irregular pulse or blood pressure, tachycardia, diaphoresis, and arrhythmias), a rare but potentially fatal adverse effect.
- Monitor hepatic function, as ordered, in patients with hepatic disease because olanzapine and fluoxetine combination can elevate hepatic enzyme levels.

PATIENT TEACHING
* Advise patient to avoid exercise in hot weather to reduce the risk of dehydration and hypotension. Also instruct him to notify prescriber about prolonged diarrhea, nausea, or vomiting.
* Caution patient to avoid potentially hazardous activities until drug's CNS effects are known.
* Instruct patient to change position slowly to minimize effects of orthostatic hypotension.
* Caution patient to avoid using aspirin or NSAIDs while taking olanzapine and fluoxetine because concomitant use can increase the risk of bleeding.
* Advise patient to avoid alcohol and smoking during therapy because of increased risk of adverse effects.
* Instruct patient to notify prescriber about a rash or hives.

hydrocodone bitartrate and aspirin
Damason-P, Lortab ASA, Panasal 5/500

Class, Category, and Schedule
Chemical: Opioid and phenanthrene derivative (hydrocodone), salicylate (aspirin)
Therapeutic: Analgesic (hydrocodone, aspirin)
Pregnancy category: NR (hydrocodone C, aspirin D)
Controlled substance: Schedule III

Indications and Dosages
▶ *To relieve moderate to severe pain*
TABLETS
Adults. 5 mg hydrocodone and 500 mg aspirin (1 tablet) to 10 mg hydrocodone and 1,000 mg aspirin (2 tablets) q 4 to 6 hr, as needed.

Mechanism of Action
Hydrocodone exerts a synergistic analgesic effect through two mechanisms of action. Hydrocodone, a mu opiate-receptor agonist, alters the perception of pain at the spinal cord and higher CNS levels by blocking the release of inhibitory neurotransmitters, such as gamma-aminobutyric acid and acetylcholine. It also alters the emotional response to pain.

Aspirin blocks cyclooxygenase, the enzyme needed for prostaglandin synthesis. Prostaglandins play a role in pain transmission from the periphery to the spinal cord.

Contraindications

Allergy to tartrazine dye; asthma; bleeding problems such as hemophilia; children under age 16 with a viral illness; hypersensitivity to aspirin, hydrocodone, other opioids, NSAIDs, or their components; peptic ulcer disease; respiratory depression; severe vitamin K deficiency; upper airway obstruction

Interactions

DRUGS

hydrocodone and aspirin

penicillins, sulfonamides: Increased blood levels of penicillins and sulfonamides

hydrocodone component

anticholinergics, paregoric: Increased risk of severe constipation
antihypertensives, diuretics: Potentiated hypotensive effects
buprenorphine: Decreased effectiveness of codeine
CNS depressants: Additive CNS effects
hydroxyzine: Increased codeine analgesic effect; increased CNS depressant and hypotensive effects
MAO inhibitors: Increased risk of unpredictable, severe, and sometimes fatal reactions
metoclopramide: Antagonized effect of metoclopramide on GI motility
naloxone: Antagonized hydrocodone analgesic effect
naltrexone: Precipitated withdrawal symptoms in hydrocodone-dependent patients
neuromuscular blockers: Additive respiratory depressant effects
opioids: Additive CNS and respiratory depressant effects and hypotensive effects

aspirin component

ACE inhibitors: Decreased antihypertensive effect
activated charcoal: Decreased aspirin absorption
antacids, urine alkalinizers: Decreased aspirin effectiveness
anticoagulants: Increased risk of bleeding and prolonged bleeding time
carbonic anhydrase inhibitors: Salicylism
corticosteroids: Increased excretion and decreased blood level of aspirin
heparin: Increased risk of bleeding
loop diuretics: Decreased effectiveness of loop diuretics
methotrexate: Increased blood level and decreased excretion of methotrexate, causing toxicity
nizatidine: Increased blood aspirin level

NSAIDs: Possibly decreased blood NSAID level and increased risk of adverse GI effects

oral antidiabetics, insulin: Increased risk of hypoglycemia

probenecid, sulfinpyrazone: Decreased effectiveness in treating gout

urine acidifiers, such as ammonium chloride and ascorbic acid: Decreased aspirin excretion

vancomycin: Increased risk of ototoxicity

ACTIVITIES

hydrocodone component

alcohol use: Additive CNS effects

aspirin component

alcohol use: Increased risk of ulcers

Adverse Reactions

CNS: Coma, confusion, CNS depression, delirium, depression, disorientation, dizziness, drowsiness, euphoria, hallucinations, headache, lack of coordination

CV: Bradycardia, orthostatic hypotension, palpitations, tachycardia

EENT: Altered taste, blurred vision, diplopia, dry mouth, hearing loss, laryngeal edema, laryngospasm, miosis, tinnitus

GI: Abnormal cramps and pain, anorexia, constipation, diarrhea, flatulence, GI bleeding, gastroesophageal reflux, heartburn, hepatotoxicity, ileus, indigestion, nausea, stomach pain, vomiting

GU: Decreased libido, difficult ejaculation, dysuria, impotence, oliguria, ureteral spasm, urinary incontinence, urine retention

HEME: Decreased blood iron level, hemolytic anemia, leukopenia, prolonged bleeding time, shortened life span of RBCs, thrombocytopenia

RESP: Apnea, bronchoconstriction, bronchospasm, depressed cough reflex, respiratory depression

SKIN: Diaphoresis, ecchymosis, flushing, pallor, pruritus, rash, urticaria

Other: Anaphylaxis, angioedema, physical and psychological dependence, Reye's syndrome

Nursing Considerations

- Use cautiously in patients with head trauma or intracranial lesions because hydrocodone can cause an exaggerated respiratory depression and aspirin can increase the risk of bleeding.
- Use cautiously in elderly and debilitated patients as well as patients with severe renal or hepatic dysfunction, gallbladder disease, respiratory impairment, cardiac arrhythmias, inflammatory disorders of the GI tract, hypothyroidism, Addison's disease,

prostatic hypertrophy or urethral stricture, coagulation disorders or acute abdominal conditions.

- Evaluate patient for therapeutic response, including report of decreased pain and body movements that would indicate pain relief has occurred.
- Take safety precautions, as needed.
- Monitor patient for evidence of CNS depression.
- Monitor respiratory depth, effort and rate. Notify prescriber immediately if respiratory rate drops below 10 breaths/min.
- **WARNING** Monitor patient closely for allergic reaction. Be aware that anaphylactic shock and other severe allergic reactions can occur without a history of allergy.
- **WARNING** Assess patient for evidence of physical and psychological dependence.
- Monitor urine output; decreasing output may signal urine retention or renal failure.

PATIENT TEACHING

- Instruct patient to take hydrocodone and aspirin with food or after meals to minimize stomach upset.
- Instruct patient to take hydrocodone and aspirin exactly as prescribed and not to adjust dose or frequency without consulting prescriber.
- Instruct patient to notify prescriber about worsening or breakthrough pain.
- Advise patient to notify prescriber if he becomes short of breath or has difficulty breathing.
- Tell patient to consult prescriber before taking drug with any prescription drug for blood disorder, diabetes, gout, or arthritis.
- Advise patient to avoid potentially hazardous activities until drug's CNS effects are known.
- Caution patient to avoid alcohol or other CNS depressants while taking aspirin and codeine.
- Advise patient to get up slowly from a sitting or lying position.
- To prevent constipation, encourage patient to consume plenty of fluids and high-fiber foods, if not contraindicated.

hydrocodone and ibuprofen
Vicoprofen

Class, Category, and Schedule
Chemical: Opioid and phenanthrene derivative (hydrocodone), propionic acid derivative (ibuprofen)

Therapeutic: Analgesic
Pregnancy category: C
Controlled substance: Schedule III

Indications and Dosages

▶ *To relieve acute pain*
TABLETS
Adults. 1 tablet (7.5 mg of hydrocodone and 200 mg of ibuprofen) q 4 to 6 hr, p.r.n., for up to 5 days. *Maximum:* 5 tablets (37.5 mg of hydrocodone and 1,000 mg of ibuprofen)/day.

Mechanism of Action

Exerts a synergistic analgesic effect through two mechanisms of action. Hydrocodone, a mu opiate-receptor agonist, alters the perception of pain at the spinal cord and higher CNS levels by blocking the release of inhibitory neurotransmitters, such as gamma-aminobutyric acid and acetylcholine. It also alters the emotional response to pain.

Ibuprofen blocks the activity of cyclooxygenase, the enzyme necessary for prostaglandin synthesis. Prostaglandins, important mediators in the inflammatory response, cause local vasodilation with swelling and pain. They also play a role in pain transmission from the periphery to the spinal cord. With the inhibition of cyclooxygenase and prostaglandin synthesis, inflammatory symptoms subside.

Contraindications

Hypersensitivity to aspirin, hydrocodone, ibuprofen, opioids, other NSAIDs, or their components; respiratory depression; severe asthma; upper airway obstruction

Interactions

DRUGS
ACE inhibitors (such as benazepril, captopril, and enalapril): Possibly decreased therapeutic effects of ACE inhibitors
anticholinergics: Increased risk of ileus
aspirin, corticosteroids, NSAIDs: Possibly increased risk of GI ulceration and hemorrhage
CNS depressants: Increased CNS depression
diuretics: Possibly decreased diuresis, increased risk of renal failure
lithium: Increased blood lithium level, increased risk of lithium toxicity
methotrexate: Increased blood methotrexate level, increased risk of methotrexate toxicity

MAO inhibitors (such as furazolidone, phenelzine, procarbazine, selegiline, tranylcypromine): Increased risk of adverse CNS effects
naloxone: Possibly withdrawal symptoms in physically dependent patients
naltrexone: Possibly prolonged respiratory depression and cardiac arrest
oral anticoagulants: Increased risk of GI bleeding
tricyclic antidepressants: Possibly increased adverse effects of hydrocodone or potentiated antidepressant effects
ACTIVITIES
alcohol use: Possibly increased CNS depression

Adverse Reactions

CNS: Anxiety, confusion, depression, dizziness, euphoria, fatigue, fever, headache, insomnia, irritability, lethargy, nervousness, paresthesia, sedation, slurred speech, somnolence, tremor, weakness
CV: Arrhythmias, peripheral edema, hypotension, orthostatic hypotension, palpitations
EENT: Dry mouth, mouth ulcers, pharyngitis, rhinitis, sinusitis, tinnitus, vision changes
GI: Anorexia, constipation, dysphagia, esophagitis, flatulence, gastritis, gastroenteritis, indigestion, nausea, vomiting
GU: Impotence, urinary frequency, urine retention
RESP: Bronchitis, dyspnea, respiratory depression
SKIN: Diaphoresis, flushing, pruritus, rash, urticaria
Other: Physical and psychological dependence

Nursing Considerations

- Expect to give hydrocodone and ibuprofen for short-term pain relief only (no more than 10 days).
- **WARNING** Monitor for signs of overdose, such as blurred vision; cold, clammy skin; confusion; dizziness; dyspnea; headache; hearing loss; malaise; mental or mood changes; nausea; respiratory depression; sinus bradycardia; tinnitus; and vomiting. Notify prescriber immediately if they develop.

PATIENT TEACHING
- Inform patient that hydrocodone and ibuprofen may cause drowsiness and dizziness.
- Caution patient not to take more than prescribed dosage because of the risk of dependence.
- Urge patient to avoid using alcohol during drug therapy.
- Advise patient to change position slowly to minimize effects of orthostatic hypotension.

levodopa and carbidopa

Apo-Levocarb (CAN), Atamet, Parcopa, Sinemet, Sinemet CR

Class and Category

Chemical: Hydralazine analogue of levodopa (carbidopa), levorotatory isomer of dihydroxyphenylalanine (levodopa)
Therapeutic: Antidyskinetic
Pregnancy category: C

Indications and Dosages

▶ *To relieve symptoms of Parkinson's disease*

E.R. TABLETS

Adults not taking levodopa. *Initial:* 1 tablet of 100 mg levodopa and 25 mg carbidopa b.i.d. or 1 tablet of 200 mg levodopa and 50 mg carbidopa b.i.d. with doses spaced at least 6 hr apart. Dose increased or decreased q 3 days or more, if needed, based on response. *Maintenance:* 400 to 1,600 mg levodopa daily in divided doses q 4 to 8 hr. *Maximum:* 2,400 mg levodopa daily.

Adults taking levodopa regardless of dose. 1 tablet of 100 mg levodopa and 25 mg carbidopa b.i.d. or 1 tablet of 200 mg levodopa and 50 mg carbidopa b.i.d. at least 12 hr after levodopa is stopped. *Maximum:* 2,400 mg levodopa daily.

Adults taking conventional carbidopa-levodopa. If patient takes 300 to 400 mg of levodopa in combination product, regimen switched to 1 E.R. tablet (200 mg levodopa) b.i.d. given 4 to 8 hr apart. If patient takes 500 to 600 mg of levodopa in combination product, regimen switched to 1 E.R. tablet (300 mg levodopa) b.i.d. or t.i.d. given 4 to 8 hr apart. If patient takes 700 to 800 mg of levodopa in combination product, regimen switched to 4 E.R. tablets (800 mg levodopa) daily divided into three doses and given 4 to 8 hr apart. *Maximum:* 2,400 mg levodopa daily.

TABLETS

Adults not taking levodopa. *Initial:* 1 tablet of 100 mg levodopa and 25 mg carbidopa t.i.d., or 1 tablet of 100 mg levodopa and 10 mg carbidopa t.i.d. or q.i.d. Increased by 1 tablet daily or every other day, if needed, up to maximum. *Maximum:* 2,000 mg levodopa and 200 mg carbidopa daily.

Adults taking more than 1,500 mg of levodopa. 1 tablet of 250 mg levodopa and 25 mg carbidopa t.i.d. or q.i.d. at least 12 hr after levodopa stops. *Maximum:* 2,000 mg levodopa and 200 mg carbidopa daily.

Adults taking less than 1,500 mg of levodopa. 1 tablet of 100 mg levodopa and 25 mg carbidopa t.i.d. or q.i.d. or 1 tablet of 100 mg levodopa and 10 mg carbidopa t.i.d. or q.i.d. at least

12 hr after levodopa stops. *Maximum:* 2,000 mg levodopa and 200 mg carbidopa daily.

ORALLY DISINTEGRATING TABLETS

Adults. *Initial:* 1 tablet of 100 mg levodopa and 25 mg carbidopa t.i.d., increased as needed by 1 tablet daily or every other day. Or 1 tablet of 100 mg levodopa and 10 mg carbidopa t.i.d. or q.i.d., increased as needed by 1 tablet daily or every other day. *Maximum:* 8 tablets of 100 mg levodopa and 25 mg carbidopa or 100 mg levodopa and 10 mg carbidopa daily.

Mechanism of Action

Carbidopa inhibits peripheral distribution of levodopa, making more levodopa available to the brain. In extracerebral tissues, levodopa is converted to dopamine and moves to the CNS, where it replenishes dopamine, thus helping to improve muscle control and normalize body movements.

Contraindications

Concurrent MAO inhibitor therapy; history of melanoma; hypersensitivity to carbidopa, levodopa, or their components; narrow-angle glaucoma; suspicious undiagnosed skin lesions

Interactions

DRUGS

antihypertensives: Increased risk of symptomatic orthostatic hypotension

benzodiazepines, droperidol, haloperidol, hydantoin anticonvulsants, loxapine, metoclopramide, metyrosine, molindone, papaverine, phenothiazines, rauwolfia alkaloids, thioxanthenes: Decreased carbidopa-levodopa effects

bromocriptine: Additive levodopa and carbidopa effects

iron salts: Decreased absorption, blood level, and effectiveness of levodopa

MAO inhibitors: Increased risk of severe orthostatic hypotension

methyldopa: Altered antiparkinsonian effects of levodopa, additive toxic CNS effects

pyridoxine: Reversed levodopa effects

tricyclic antidepressants: Increased risk of adverse reactions to levodopa and carbidopa

FOODS

high-protein food: Possibly delayed or reduced drug absorption

Adverse Reactions

CNS: Anxiety, confusion, depression, headache, insomnia, mood or mental changes, nervousness, neuroleptic malignant syndrome, nightmares, tiredness, uncontrolled movements, weakness
CV: Arrhythmias, orthostatic hypotension
EENT: Blurred vision, darkened saliva, dry mouth, eyelid spasm, ptosis
GI: Anorexia, constipation, diarrhea, nausea, vomiting
GU: Darkened urine, dysuria
MS: Muscle twitching
SKIN: Darkened sweat, flushing

Nursing Considerations

- Use drug cautiously in patients with history of psychosis. Monitor all patients for depression and suicidal tendencies.
- Administer cautiously to patients with severe CV or pulmonary disease; bronchial asthma; renal, hepatic, or endocrine disease; history of MI and residual atrial, nodal, or ventricular arrhythmias; or history of peptic ulcer. Monitor patient closely, especially when therapy begins and dosage is adjusted.
- **WARNING** Avoid giving levodopa and carbidopa within 2 weeks of an MAO inhibitor because sudden, extreme hypertension may occur.
- Assess patient for neuroleptic malignant syndrome if drug is stopped or dose reduced, especially if patient also takes a neuroleptic drug. Rare but life-threatening, the syndrome causes altered level of consciousness, autonomic dysfunction, diaphoresis, fever, altered blood pressure, involuntary movement, muscle rigidity, tachycardia, and tachypnea. If these changes occur, notify prescriber immediately.

PATIENT TEACHING

- If patient can't swallow E.R. tablet whole, tell him to break it in half for swallowing but not to crush or chew it.
- If patient takes orally disintegrating form, tell him to gently remove tab from bottle with dry hands, place it on top of his tongue, let it dissolve (which takes seconds), and swallow it with saliva. Explain that no other liquids are needed.
- Remind patient that it may take several weeks or months to feel full drug effects.
- Stress importance of taking levodopa and carbidopa regularly and in exact dose prescribed. Altering the dose or interval may increase the risk of adverse reactions or decrease drug effectiveness.

- Tell patient to notify prescriber if involuntary movements appear or worsen during therapy; dose may need to be adjusted.
- Inform patient being switched from regular to E.R. tablets that effect may be delayed for up to 1 hour after the first morning dose, compared with the effect from the regular tablet. If delay poses a problem, tell patient to notify prescriber.

levodopa, carbidopa, and entacapone
Stalevo

Class and Category
Chemical: Levorotatory isomer of dihydroxyphenylalanine (levodopa), hydralazine analogue of levodopa (carbidopa), catechol-O-methyltransferase (COMT) inhibitor (entacapone)
Therapeutic: Antidyskinetic
Pregnancy category: C

Indications and Dosages
▶ *To treat idiopathic Parkinson's disease*
TABLETS
Adults. Highly individualized and used only as a substitute for patients already stabilized on equivalent doses of levodopa, carbidopa, and entacapone. *Maintenance:* Highly individualized. When less levodopa is needed, strength or frequency of dosage can be decreased; when more levodopa is needed, frequency can be increased or next higher strength can be given. *Maximum:* 1 tablet of equivalent strength (50 mg levodopa, 12.5 mg carbidopa, and 200 mg entacapone; 100 mg levodopa, 25 mg carbidopa, and 200 mg entacapone; or 150 mg levodopa, 37.5 mg carbidopa, and 200 mg entacapone) per dosing interval; 8 tablets daily.

Mechanism of Action
Carbidopa inhibits peripheral distribution of levodopa, making more levodopa available in the brain.

Entacapone inhibits peripheral COMT, the major metabolizing enzyme for levodopa. During levodopa metabolism, COMT produces a levodopa metabolite that reduces levodopa effectiveness. By inhibiting COMT, entacapone increases levodopa level, making more available for diffusion into the CNS.

Levodopa is transported to the CNS, where it replenishes depleted dopamine, which is thought to cause Parkinson's disease, thus helping to improve muscle control and normalize body movements.

Contraindications

Angle-closure glaucoma; history of melanoma; hypersensitivity to levodopa, carbidopa, entacapone, or their components; suspicious, undiagnosed skin lesions; use within 14 days of an MAO inhibitor

Interactions

DRUGS

levodopa, carbidopa, and entacapone

alpha-methyldopa, apomorphine, bitolterol, dobutamine, dopamine, epinephrine, isoetharine, isoproterenol, norepinephrine, other COMT metabolizers: Possibly increased heart rate, arrhythmias, and extreme changes in blood pressure

anti-hypertensives: Possibly symptomatic orthostatic hypotension

iron salts: Possibly reduced bioavailability of carbidopa, levodopa, and entacapone

MAO inhibitors: Possibly inhibited catecholamine metabolism

selegiline: Possibly severe orthostatic hypotension

tricyclic antidepressants: Possibly hypertension and dyskinesia

levodopa component

dopamine D2-receptor antagonists (such as butyrophenones, isoniazid, phenothiazines, and risperidone): Possible reduced effectiveness of levodopa

metoclopramide: Increased bioavailability but decreased effectiveness of levodopa

papaverine, phenytoin: Possible reversed effects of levodopa in Parkinson's disease

entacapone component

ampicillin, cholestyramine, erythromycin, probenecid, rifampin: Possible interference with biliary excretion of entacapone

FOODS

high-protein food: Possibly delayed or reduced drug absorption

Adverse Reactions

CNS: Activation of latent Horner's syndrome, aggravation of Parkinson's disease symptoms, agitation, anxiety, asthenia, ataxia, bradykinetic episodes, confusion, decreased mental acuity, delusions, dementia, depression, disorientation, dizziness, dyskinesia, euphoria, fatigue, gait abnormalities, hallucinations, headache, hyperkinesia, hypokinesia, insomnia, malaise, memory loss, nervousness, neuroleptic malignant syndrome, nightmares, paranoia, paresthesia, peripheral neuropathy, sense of stimulation, somnolence, syncope, tremor increase, trismus

CV: Arrhythmias; chest pain; edema; hypotension, including orthostatic; hypertension; MI; palpitations; phlebitis
EENT: Blepharospasm, blurred vision, darkened saliva, dilated pupils, diplopia, dry mouth, excessive salivation, hoarseness, oculogyric crisis, taste disturbance, tongue burning
ENDO: Hyperglycemia
GI: Abdominal pain, elevated function test results, anorexia, bruxism, constipation, diarrhea, duodenal ulcer, dysphagia, flatulence, gastritis, GI bleeding, GI pain, hiccups, indigestion, nausea, vomiting
GU: Bacteria, blood, glucose, or protein in urine, darkened urine; elevated BUN and serum creatinine levels; elevated uric acid levels; elevated WBC count in urine; increased libido; urinary frequency, incontinence, or retention; UTI
HEME: Agranulocytosis, decreased hemoglobin and hematocrit, hemolytic and nonhemolytic anemia, leukopenia, positive Coombs' test, thrombocytopenia
MS: Back, leg, and shoulder pain; muscle cramps or twitching; rhabdomyolysis
RESP: Abnormal breathing patterns, dyspnea, upper respiratory tract infection
SKIN: Alopecia, bullous lesions, darkened sweat, diaphoresis, flushing, malignant melanoma, pruritus, purpura, rash, urticaria
Other: Angioedema, hot flashes, hypokalemia, weight gain or loss

Nursing Considerations
- Use drug cautiously in patients with past or current psychosis because drug may cause depression and suicidal tendencies.
- Use cautiously in patients with severe CV or pulmonary disease; biliary obstruction; bronchial asthma; or renal, hepatic, or endocrine disease.
- If patient has chronic open-angle glaucoma, make sure intraocular pressure is well controlled because drug may lead to increased intraocular pressure.
- If patient has a history of MI with residual atrial, nodal, or ventricular arrhythmias, expect to make initial dosage adjustment in a facility with intensive cardiac care.
- Monitor patient closely for adverse CNS effects. Such adverse effects as dyskinesia may occur at lower dosages and more quickly with the use of carbidopa, levodopa, and entacapone tablets than when levodopa is used alone. If dyskinesia occurs, notify prescriber and expect to decrease dosage.

• Closely monitor patient with a history of peptic ulcer because drug may increase risk of GI hemorrhage.
• If drug must be stopped, taper it slowly to prevent high fever or severe rigidity.
• Assess for neuroleptic malignant syndrome during dosage reduction or drug discontinuation, especially in a patient who also receives a neuroleptic drug. This uncommon syndrome is life-threatening and causes altered level of consciousness, autonomic dysfunction, diaphoresis, fever, high or low blood pressure, involuntary movement, muscle rigidity, tachycardia, and tachypnea. If these occur, notify prescriber immediately.

PATIENT TEACHING
• To provide uniform drug effect, stress importance of taking carbidopa, levodopa, and entacapone at regular intervals according to the prescribed schedule.
• Advise patient to avoid a high-protein diet and iron salts (such as those found in many multi-vitamin tablets) because protein and iron may delay absorption of the levodopa component of drug and reduce the amount available for the body to use to control the symptoms of Parkinson's disease.
• Alert patient to the possibility of nausea, especially at the beginning of therapy. Tell him that this adverse reaction usually resolves with continued therapy.
• Tell patient to notify prescriber if he's taking any other medication, including OTC and herbal preparations, because of potential drug interactions.
• Inform patient that drug's effect may sometimes appear to wear off at the end of a dosing interval. If this occurs, instruct him to notify his prescriber to determine if a dosage adjustment is needed.
• Caution patient that hallucinations may occur and advise him to avoid potentially hazardous activities until drug's CNS effects are known.
• Advise patient to rise slowly after sitting or lying down to avoid a sudden drop in blood pressure.
• Instruct patient to notify prescriber if dyskinesia occurs.
• Tell patient that body fluids, such as saliva, urine and sweat, may turn a dark color, such as red, brown, or black. Reassure him that this effect is harmless but that fluids may stain clothing.
• Advise female patients of childbearing age to notify prescriber immediately about known or suspected pregnancy because changes to drug therapy may be required.

• Inform patient with diabetes that drug may cause a false-positive result for urinary ketones when a test tape product is used to check for ketonuria and a false-negative result for urine glucose when a glucose-oxidase method is used. Encourage patient to monitor blood glucose levels and seek medical attention if he suspects ketonuria.

meperidine hydrochloride and promethazine hydrochloride

Mepergan, Mepergan Forte

Class, Category, and Schedule

Chemical: Phenylpiperidine derivative opioid (merperidine), phenothiazine derivative (promethazine)

Therapeutic: Analgesic (meperidine), antiemetic (promethazine)

Pregnancy category: C (D for prolonged use or high dose at term)

Controlled substance: Schedule II

Indications and Dosages

▶ *To relieve moderate to severe pain*

CAPSULES

Adults. 50 mg meperidine and 25 mg promethazine (1 capsule) q 4 to 6 hr, as needed.

I.M. INJECTION

Adults. 25 mg meperidine and 25 mg promethazine q 4 to 6 hr, as needed.

Mechanism of Action

Meperidine binds with opiate receptors in the spinal cord and higher levels of the CNS. In this way, meperidine stimulates mu and kappa receptors, which alters the perception of and emotional response to pain.

Promethazine may prevent nausea and vertigo by acting centrally on the medullary chemoreceptive trigger zone and by decreasing vestibular stimulation and labyrinthine function in the inner ear. In addition, it promotes sedation and relieves anxiety by blocking receptor sites within the CNS, directly reducing stimuli to the brain.

Contraindications

Acute asthma, angle-closure glaucoma; benign prostatic hyperplasia; bladder neck obstruction; bone marrow depression; breastfeeding; coma; hypersensitivity or history of idiosyncratic reaction to meperidine, other opioids, promethazine, other phenothiazines, or their components; hypertensive crisis; increased intracranial pressure; pyloroduodenal obstruction; severe respiratory depression; stenosing peptic ulcer; upper respiratory tract obstruction; use of large quantities of CNS depressants or within 14 days of MAO inhibitor therapy

Interactions
DRUGS
meperidine and promethazine
amphetamines, MAO inhibitors: Risk of increased CNS excitation or depression with possibly fatal reactions
anticholinergics: Increased risk of intensified anticholinergic adverse effects
meperidine component
acyclovir, ritonavir: Possibly increased blood meperidine level
alfentanil, CNS depressants, fentanyl, sufentanil: Increased risk of CNS and respiratory depression and hypotension
antidiarrheals (such as loperamide and difenoxin and atropine): Increased risk of severe constipation and increased CNS depression
antihypertensives: Increased risk of hypotension
buprenorphine: Possibly decreased therapeutic effects of meperidine and increased risk of respiratory depression
cimetidine: Reduced clearance and volume of distribution of meperidine
hydroxyzine: Increased risk of CNS depression and hypotension
metoclopramide: Possibly decreased effects of metoclopramide
naloxone, naltrexone: Decreased pharmacologic effects of meperidine
neuromuscular blockers: Increased risk of prolonged respiratory and CNS depression
oral anticoagulants: Possibly increased anticoagulant effect and risk of bleeding
phenytoin: Possibly enhanced hepatic metabolism of meperidine
promethazine component
anticonvulsants: Lowered seizure threshold
appetite suppressants: Possibly antagonized anorectic effect of appetite suppressants
beta blockers: Increased risk of additive hypotensive effects, irreversible retinopathy, arrhythmias, and tardive dyskinesia
bromocriptine: Decreased effectiveness of bromocriptine
CNS depressants: Additive CNS depression

dopamine: Possibly antagonized peripheral vasoconstriction (with high doses of dopamine)

ephedrine, metaraminol, methoxamine: Decreased vasopressor response to these drugs

epinephrine: Blocked alpha-adrenergic effects of epinephrine, increased risk of hypotension

guanadrel, guanethidine: Decreased antihypertensive effects of these drugs

hepatotoxic drugs: Increased risk of hepatotoxicity

hypotension-producing drugs: Possibly severe hypotension with syncope

levodopa: Inhibitied antidyskinetic effects of levodopa

metrizamide: Increased risk of seizures

ototoxic drugs: Possibly masking of some symptoms of ototoxicity, such as dizziness, tinnitus, and vertigo

quinidine: Additive cardiac effects

riboflavin: Increased riboflavin requirements

ACTIVITIES

meperidine and promethazine

alcohol use: Possibly increased CNS and respiratory depression and hypotension

Adverse Reactions

CNS: Akathisia, CNS stimulation, confusion, depression, dizziness, drowsiness, dystonia, euphoria, excitation, fatigue, hallucinations, headache, hysteria, increased intracranial pressure, insomnia, irritability, lack of coordination, malaise, nervousness, neuroleptic malignant syndrome, nightmares, paradoxical stimulation, pseudoparkinsonism, restlessness, sedation, seizures, syncope, tardive dyskinesia, tremor

CV: Bradycardia, hypertension, hypotension, orthostatic hypotension, tachycardia

EENT: Blurred vision; diplopia; dry mouth, nose, and throat; nasal congestion; tinnitus; vision changes

ENDO: Hyperglycemia

GI: Abdominal cramps, pain, or spasms; anorexia; cholestatic jaundice; constipation; ileus; nausea; vomiting

GU: Dysuria, urinary frequency, urine retention

HEME: Agranulocytosis, leukopenia, thrombocytopenia, thrombocytopenic purpura

RESP: Apnea, dyspnea, respiratory arrest or depression, tenacious bronchial secretions, wheezing

SKIN: Dermatitis, diaphoresis, flushing, photosensitivity, rash, urticaria

Other: Angioedema; injection site pain, redness, and swelling; paradoxical reactions; physical and psychological dependence

Nursing Considerations

- Use with extreme caution in patients with acute abdominal conditions, hepatic or renal disorders, hypothyroidism, prostatic hyperplasia, seizures, or supraventricular tachycardia. Be aware that multiple doses are not recommended for these patients.
- Also use cautiously in patients with asthma because of its anticholinergic effects and in patients with seizure disorders or those who use medication that may affect seizure threshold because meperidine and promethazine may lower patient's seizure threshold.
- Know that meperidine and promethazine should not be used longer than 48 hours to manage acute pain.
- Inject I.M. form deep into large muscle mass and rotate sites. Never inject the drug subcutaneously.
- **WARNING** Avoid inadvertent intra-arterial injection of promethazine because it can cause arteriospasm; gangrene may develop from impaired circulation.
- **WARNING** Monitor respiratory function because drug may suppress cough reflex and cause thickening of bronchial secretions, aggravating such conditions as asthma and COPD, and, in rare cases, may depress respirations and induce apnea. Notify prescriber immediately and expect to discontinue drug if respiratory rate falls to less than 12 breaths/minute or if respiratory depth decreases.
- Evaluate for therapeutic response, including report of decreased pain and body movements that would indicate pain relief has occurred.
- Monitor bowel function to detect constipation and assess the need for stool softeners.
- Monitor patient's hematologic status as ordered because promethazine component of drug may cause bone marrow depression, especially when used with other known marrow-toxic agents. Assess patient for signs and symptoms of infection or bleeding.
- **WARNING** Monitor patient for evidence of neuroleptic malignant syndrome, such as fever, hypertension or hypotension, involuntary motor activity, mental changes, muscle rigidity, tachycardia, and tachypnea. Be prepared to provide support-

ive treatment and additional drug therapy as prescribed.
- Assess for signs of physical and psychological dependence and abuse.
- Expect withdrawal symptoms to occur if drug is abruptly stopped after long-term use.
- Be aware that patient shouldn't have intradermal allergen tests within 72 hours of receiving promethazine because drug may significantly alter flare response.

PATIENT TEACHING
- Inform patient that meperidine and promethazine is a controlled substance and is habit forming if taken long-term.
- Advise patient to take drug exactly as prescribed.
- Instruct patient to report constipation, severe nausea, and shortness of breath and to notify prescriber immediately if he experiences involuntary movements and restlessness.
- Instruct patient to notify prescriber about worsening or breakthrough pain
- Advise patient to avoid potentially hazardous activities until drug's CNS effects are known.
- Urge patient to avoid alcohol, OTC drugs, sedatives, and tranquilizers during meperidine and promethazine use unless approved by prescriber.
- Suggest frequent rinsing and use of sugarless gum or hard candy to relieve dry mouth.
- Advise patient to avoid excessive sun exposure and to use sunscreen when outdoors.

meprobamate and aspirin
Equagesic, Micrainin

Class, Category, and Schedule
Chemical: Carbamate derivative (meprobamate), salicylate (aspirin)
Therapeutic: Antianxiety (meprobamate), analgesic (aspirin)
Pregnancy category: X
Controlled substance: Schedule IV

Indications and Dosages
▶ *To relieve pain accompanied by tension or anxiety in patients with musculoskeletal disease.*

TABLETS
Adults. 200 mg meprobamate and 325 mg aspirin (1 tablet) or 400 mg meprobamate and 650 mg aspirin (2 tablets) t.i.d. or q.i.d., as needed

Mechanism of Action

Meprobamate is an anxiolytic that may act at multiple sites in the CNS, including the thalamus and limbic system. Meprobamate inhibits spinal reflexes, causing CNS relaxation. It also has muscle relaxant properties.

Aspirin blocks the activity of cyclooxygenase, the enzyme necessary for prostaglandin synthesis. By preventing prostaglandin synthesis, pain is relieved because prostaglandins play a role in pain transmission from the periphery to the spinal cord.

Contraindications

Acute intermittent porphyria; allergy to tartrazine dye; asthma; bleeding problems such as hemophilia; breastfeeding; children under age 16 with a viral illness; hypersensitivity to meprobamate, aspirin or their components; peptic ulcer disease; pregnancy; triad syndrome of asthma, rhinitis, and nasal polyps

Interactions

DRUGS

meprobamate component

CNS depressants: Increased CNS depression

aspirin component

acetazolamide: Increased serum acetazolamide level and risk of toxicity

ACE inhibitors: Decreased antihypertensive effect

activated charcoal: Decreased aspirin absorption

antacids, urine alkalinizers: Decreased aspirin effectiveness

anticoagulants: Increased risk of bleeding; prolonged bleeding time

beta blockers: Diminished hypotensive effect of beta blockers

carbonic anhydrase inhibitors: Salicylism

corticosteroids: Increased excretion and decreased blood level of aspirin

heparin: Increased risk of bleeding

loop diuretics: Decreased effectiveness of loop diuretics

methotrexate: Increased blood level and decreased excretion of methotrexate, causing toxicity

nizatidine: Increased blood aspirin level

NSAIDs: Possibly decreased blood NSAID level and increased risk of adverse GI effects

oral hypoglycemics: Increased effectiveness of oral hypoglycemics increasing risk of hypoglycemia

phenytoin, valproic acid: Decreased phenytoin level; increased serum valproic acid levels

probenecid, sulfinpyrazone: Decreased effectiveness in treating gout
urine acidifiers, such as ammonium chloride and ascorbic acid: Decreased aspirin excretion
vancomycin: Increased risk of ototoxicity
ACTIVITIES
meprobamate and aspirin
alcohol use: Increased CNS depression; increased risk of ulcers

Adverse Reactions

CNS: Ataxia, confusion, CNS depression, dizziness, drowsiness, euphoria, headache, light-headedness, paradoxical stimulation, paresthesia, slurred speech, syncope, vertigo, weakness
CV: Arrhythmias, including tachycardia; hypotension; palpitations
EENT: Blurred vision, hearing loss, impaired visual accommodation, tinnitus
GI: Diarrhea, GI bleeding, heartburn, hepatotoxicity, nausea, stomach pain, vomiting
GU: Nephrotoxicity
HEME: Decreased blood iron level, hemolytic anemia, leukopenia, prolonged bleeding time, shortened life span of RBCs, thrombocytopenia
SKIN: Ecchymosis, erythematous maculopapular rash, pruritus, Stevens-Johnson syndrome, urticaria
Other: Anaphylaxis, angioedema, physical dependence, Reye's syndrome

Nursing Considerations

- Use cautiously in elderly and debilitated patients as well as patients with severe renal or hepatic dysfunction, seizure disorder, gallbladder disease, respiratory impairment, cardiac arrhythmias, inflammatory disorders of the GI tract, hypothyroidism, Addison's disease, prostatic hypertrophy or urethral stricture, coagulation disorders or acute abdominal conditions.
- Also use drug cautiously in patients with suicidal tendencies or a history of drug dependence or abuse because meprobamate component of drug can lead to physical dependence and abuse.
- Evaluate for therapeutic response, including report of decreased pain and body movements that would indicate pain relief has occurred.
- Observe for signs of chronic drug intoxication, such as ataxia, slurred speech, and vertigo or CNS depression.
- Be aware that meprobamate and aspirin should be used for no longer than 10 days. If drug is used longer, expect to taper dosage gradually when discontinuing because abrupt discontinua-

tion could exacerbate previous symptoms, such as anxiety, or cause withdrawal symptoms, such as confusion, hallucinations, muscle twitching, tremor, and vomiting.

PATIENT TEACHING

- Instruct patient to take meprobamate and aspirin exactly as directed and not to stop taking it abruptly.
- Tell patient to take drug with food or after meals because it may cause GI upset if taken on an empty stomach.
- Instruct patient to notify prescriber about worsening or breakthrough pain.
- Advise patient to consult prescriber before taking drug with any prescription drug for blood disorder, diabetes, gout, or arthritis.
- Advise patient to avoid hazardous activities until drug's CNS effects are known.
- Direct patient to avoid alcohol, sedatives, and other CNS depressants while taking drug.
- Instruct patient to report rash.
- Urge female patients of childbearing age to use effective contraception during drug therapy and to notify prescriber immediately if pregnancy is suspected.

oxycodone and acetaminophen

Endocet, Oxycocet (CAN), Percocet, Percocet-Demi (CAN), Roxicet, Roxilox, Tylox

Class, Category, and Schedule

Chemical: Phenanthrene derivative (oxycodone), aminophenyl derivative (acetaminophen)
Therapeutic: Analgesic
Pregnancy category: Not rated
Controlled substance: Schedule II

Indications and Dosages

▶ *To control moderate to moderately severe pain*

CAPSULES, TABLETS

Adults. 5 mg of oxycodone and 325 to 500 mg of acetaminophen (1 tablet or capsule) q 4 to 6 hr, p.r.n. *Maximum:* 4,000 mg/day of acetaminophen.

ORAL SOLUTION

Adults. 5 mg (5 ml) of oxycodone and 325 mg of acetaminophen q 4 to 6 hr, p.r.n. *Maximum:* 4,000 mg/day of acetaminophen.

Mechanism of Action

Produces a synergistic analgesic effect through two mechanisms of action. Oxycodone, a mu receptor agonist, alters the perception of and emotional response to pain at the spinal cord and higher levels of the CNS by blocking the release of inhibitory neurotransmitters, such as gamma-aminobutyric acid and acetylcholine.

Acetaminophen blocks the activity of cyclooxygenase, an enzyme necessary for prostaglandin synthesis. Prostaglandins, important mediators in the inflammatory response, cause local vasodilation with swelling and pain.

Contraindications

Hypercapnia; hypersensitivity to oxycodone, acetaminophen, or their components; ileus; use within 14 days of MAO inhibitor therapy

Interactions

DRUGS

antacids: Decreased and delayed acetaminophen absorption

antianxiety drugs, benzodiazepines, brompheniramine, carbinoxamine, chlorpheniramine, clemastine, dimenhydrinate, diphenhydramine, doxylamine, general anesthetics, hypnotics, methdilazine, opioid antagonists, phenothiazines, promethazine, sedatives, skeletal muscle relaxants, tramadol, tricyclic antidepressants, trimeprazine: Potentiated respiratory depression from these drugs and oxycodone

anticholinergics: Possibly severe constipation and paralytic ileus

antidiarrheals: Possibly severe constipation and additive CNS depression

antihypertensives: Possibly exaggerated antihypertensive effects and risk of orthostatic hypotension

antineoplastics, immunosuppressants: Risk of masking signs of infection, such as fever and pain

barbiturates: Additive CNS depression

butorphanol, pentazocine: Possibly acute withdrawal symptoms in opioid-dependent patients, decreased analgesic effect

carbamazepine, phenobarbital, phenytoin, primidone, rifampin: Possibly a need for increased oxycodone dosage to achieve analgesia and prevent withdrawal symptoms in opioid-dependent patients; possibly increased risk of acetaminophen-induced hepatotoxicity

cimetidine, ritonavir: Possibly apnea, confusion, disorientation, and seizures from respiratory depression and impaired CNS function, increased risk of acetaminophen-induced hepatotoxicity (ritonavir)

MAO inhibitors: Possibly fatal reactions, including cardiac arrest, coma, respiratory depression, seizures, and severe hypertension
nalbuphine, nalmefene, naloxone, naltrexone: Blocked oxycodone effects, withdrawal symptoms in opioid-dependent patients
verapamil: Increased constipation
warfarin: Increased INR and risk of bleeding
FOODS
all foods: Decreased and delayed acetaminophen absorption
ACTIVITIES
alcohol use: Additive CNS depression; increased risk of acetaminophen-induced hepatotoxicity

Adverse Reactions

CNS: Confusion, dizziness, drowsiness, euphoria, excitation, hallucinations, headache, restlessness, sedation, somnolence
CV: Bradycardia, hypotension, orthostatic hypotension, palpitations
EENT: Blurred vision, dry eyes, lens opacities, miosis
GI: Abdominal pain, constipation, elevated liver function test results, hepatotoxicity, nausea, vomiting
GU: Amenorrhea, decreased libido, erectile dysfunction, oliguria, renal tubular necrosis, urinary hesitancy, urine retention
RESP: Respiratory depression
SKIN: Erythema, flushing, pruritus, urticaria
Other: Drug tolerance, hypoprothrombinemia, physical and psychological dependence, withdrawal symptoms

Nursing Considerations

• **WARNING** Be aware that oxycodone has a high potential for abuse.
• Use drug cautiously in patients with head injury because drug may alter neurologic findings.
• Assess pain level regularly, and give drug as prescribed before pain becomes severe.
• Administer drug with a full glass of water or, to minimize GI distress, with food or milk.
• Adjust dosage to relieve pain as prescribed, keeping in mind the maximum daily dose of acetaminophen. Be prepared to adjust dosage for patient who hasn't previously received opioids until he can tolerate drug's effects.
• Avoid giving drug within 1 to 2 hours of antacids or food because of risk of decreased drug effectiveness.
• Assess for possible respiratory depression or paradoxical excitation during dosage titration.

- Assess for abdominal pain because oxycodone may mask signs and symptoms of underlying GI disorders.
- Increase patient's dietary fiber intake if needed to prevent constipation.
- Anticipate an increased risk of falling during therapy. Institute safety precautions according to facility policy.

PATIENT TEACHING
- Instruct patient not to take oxycodone and acetaminophen more often than prescribed and not to stop taking drug abruptly after long-term use.
- Encourage patient to take drug with a full glass of water and with food, if possible.
- Suggest that patient change position slowly to minimize effects of orthostatic hypotension.
- Instruct patient to avoid alcohol and potentially hazardous activities during therapy.
- Advise patient to notify prescriber about possible signs of toxicity or hypersensitivity, such as excessive light-headedness, extreme dizziness, itching, swelling, and trouble breathing.

oxycodone hydrochloride, oxycodone terephthalate, and aspirin
Endodan, Percodan-Demi, Percodan, Roxiprin

Class, Category, and Schedule
Chemical: Phenanthrene derivative (oxycodone), salicylate (aspirin)
Therapeutic: Anaglesic (oxycodone, aspirin)
Pregnancy category: Not rated (oxycodone C, aspirin D)
Controlled substance: Schedule II

Indications and Dosages
▶ *To manage acute, moderate to moderately severe pain short term*
TABLETS
Adults. 2.25 mg oxycodone hydrodrochloride, 0.19 mg oxycodone terephthalate and 325 mg aspirin (1 tablet) to 4.5 mg oxycodone hydrochloride, 0.38 mg oxycodone terephthalate and 325 mg aspirin (1 tablet) q 4 to 6 hr, as needed.

Contraindications
Allergy to tartrazine dye; asthma; bleeding problems such as hemophilia; children under age 16 with a viral illness; hypercapnia; hypersensitivity to oxycodone, other opioids, aspirin, or their

components; ileus; peptic ulcer disease; respiratory depression; severe vitamin K deficiency; upper airway obstruction; use within 14 days of MAO inhibitor therapy

---

Mechanism of Action

Oxycodone alters the perception of and emotional response to pain at the spinal cord and higher levels of the CNS by blocking the release of inhibitory neurotransmitters, such as gamma-aminobutyric acid and acetylcholine.

Aspirin blocks the activity of cyclooxygenase, the enzyme necessary for prostaglandin synthesis. By preventing prostaglandin synthesis, pain is relieved because prostaglandins play a role in pain transmission from the periphery to the spinal cord.

Interactions
DRUGS

oxycodone component

anticholinergics: Possibly severe constipation and ileus
antidiarrheals: Possibly severe constipation and additive CNS depression
antihypertensives: Possibly exaggerated antihypertensive effects and risk of orthostatic hypotension
butorphanol, pentazocine: Possibly acute withdrawal symptoms in opioid-dependent patients, decreased analgesic effects
CNS depressants: Possibly increased CNS and respiratory depression and orthostatic hypotension
MAO inhibitors: Possibly fatal reactions, including cardiac arrest, coma, respiratory depression, seizures, and severe hypertension
nalbuphine, nalmefene, naloxone, naltrexone: Blocked oxycodone effects, withdrawal symptoms in opioid-dependent patients

aspirin component

ACE inhibitors: Decreased antihypertensive effect
activated charcoal: Decreased aspirin absorption
antacids, urine alkalinizers: Decreased aspirin effectiveness
anticoagulants: Increased risk of bleeding; prolonged bleeding time
carbonic anhydrase inhibitors: Salicylism
corticosteroids: Increased excretion and decreased blood level of aspirin
heparin: Increased risk of bleeding
loop diuretics: Decreased effectiveness of loop diuretics
methotrexate: Increased blood level and decreased excretion of methotrexate, causing toxicity
nizatidine: Increased blood aspirin level

NSAIDs: Possibly decreased blood NSAID level and increased risk of adverse GI effects

probenecid, sulfinpyrazone: Decreased effectiveness in treating gout

urine acidifiers, such as ammonium chloride and ascorbic acid: Decreased aspirin excretion

vancomycin: Increased risk of ototoxicity

ACTIVIITES

oxycodone and aspirin

alcohol use: Additive CNS effects and increased risk of adverse GI effects

Adverse Reactions

CNS: Confusion, CNS depression, dizziness, drowsiness, euphoria, excitation, headache, sedation, somnolence

CV: Braydcardia, chest pain, hypotension, orthostatic hypotension, palpitations, tachycardia

EENT: Blurred vision, dry eyes, hearing loss, lens opacitites, miosis, tinnitus

GI: Constipation, diarrhea, elevated liver function tests results, GI bleeding, heartburn, hepatotoxicity, nausea, stomach pain, vomiting

GU: Amenorrhea, decreased libido, erectile dysfunction, oliguria, urinary hesitancy, urine retention

HEME: Decreased blood iron level, hemolytic anemia, leukopenia, prolonged bleeding time, shortened life span of RBCs, thrombocytopenia

RESP: Apnea, bronchoconstriction, bronchospasm, respiratory depression

SKIN: Ecchymosis, pruritus, rash, urticaria

Other: Anaphylaxis, angioedema, drug tolerance, physical and psychological dependence, Reye's syndrome

Nursing Considerations

- Use with extreme caution in patients with significant chronic obstructive pulmonary disease or cor pulmonale and in patients who have substantially decreased respiratory reserve, hypoxia, or hypercapnia because oxycodone component can depress respiratory drive.
- Use with caution in elderly or debilitated patients and in those with severe impairment of hepatic or renal function, hypothyroidism, Addison's disease, acute alcoholism, convulsive disorders, CNS depression or coma, delirium tremens, kyphoscoliosis associated with respiratory depression, toxic psychosis, prostatic

hypertrophy or urethral stricture because drug can cause hypotension, alter mental state, or depress respirations.

- Monitor patient's blood pressure because opioid analgesics such as the oxycodone-aspirin combination can cause severe hypotension.
- Monitor patients with biliary tract disease including pancreatitis for pain because the drug may cause spasm of the sphincter of Oddi.
- **WARNING** Be aware that oxycodone and aspirin have a high potential for abuse because of the oxycodone component of the drug.
- Assess pain level regularly and give drug as prescribed before pain becomes severe.
- Be prepared to adjust the dosage for a patient who hasn't previously received opioids until he can tolerate drug's effects.
- Assess patient for possible respiratory depression or paradoxical excitation during dosage titration.
- Monitor patient for evidence of CNS depression.
- Assess patient for abdominal pain because oxycodone component of drug may mask signs and symptoms of underlying GI disorders.
- Be aware that aspirin's anti-inflammatory and antipyretic actions may mask signs and symptoms of infection.

PATIENT TEACHING

- Tell patient to take oxycodone and aspirin with food or after meals to reduce GI distress that may occur as a result of the aspirin component of drug. Also to take with a full glass of water and to avoid lying down for 15 to 30 minutes afterward to prevent esophageal irritation.
- Warn patient to take drug only as prescribed and needed because it can become habit-forming.
- Instruct patient to notify prescriber about worsening or breakthrough pain.
- Advise patient to avoid taking another NSAID at the same time, unless directed by prescriber because of increased risk of adverse reactions.
- Tell patient to avoid alcohol and potentially hazardous activities during oxycodone and aspirin therapy.
- Advise patient to notify prescriber about possible signs of toxicity or hypersensitivity, such as excessive light-headedness, extreme dizziness, itching, swelling, and trouble breathing.

oxycodone hydrochloride and ibuprofen
Combunox

Class, Category, and Schedule
Chemical: Phenanthrene derivative (oxycodone), propionic acid derivative (ibuprofen)
Therapeutic: Anaglesic
Pregnancy category: C
Controlled substance: Schedule II

Indications and Dosages
▶ *To manage acute, moderate to severe pain short term*
TABLETS
Adults. 5 mg oxycodone and 400 mg ibuprofen (1 tablet) q 6 hr for no longer than 7 days.

Mechanism of Action
Oxycodone alters the perception of and emotional response to pain at the spinal cord and higher levels of the CNS by blocking the release of inhibitory neurotransmitters, such as gamma-aminobutyric acid and acetylcholine.

Ibuprofen blocks the activity of cyclooxygenase, the enzyme needed to synthesize prostaglandins, which mediate the inflammatory response and cause local vasodilation, swelling, and pain. By blocking cyclooxygenase and inhibiting prostaglandins, this NSAID reduces inflammatory symptoms and relieves pain.

Contraindications
Angioedema; asthma; bronchospasm; hypercapnia; hypersensitivity to oxycodone, other opioids, ibuprofen, other NSAIDs, or their components; paralytic ileus; previously experienced allergic reactions after taking aspirin or other NSAIDs; respiratory depression; use within 14 days of MAO inhibitor therapy

Interactions
DRUGS
oxycodone and ibuprofen
antihypertensives: Possibly exaggerated antihypertensive effects and risk of orthostatic hypotension
oxycodone component
anticholinergics: Possibly severe constipation and ileus
antidiarrheals: Possibly severe constipation and additive CNS depression
butorphanol, pentazocine: Possibly acute withdrawal symptoms in

opioid-dependent patients, decreased analgesic effects

CNS depressants: Possibly increased CNS and respiratory depression and orthostatic hypotension

MAO inhibitors: Possibly fatal reactions, including cardiac arrest, coma, respiratory depression, seizures, and severe hypertension

nalbuphine, nalmefene, naloxone, naltrexone: Blocked oxycodone effects, withdrawal symptoms in opioid-dependent patients

ibuprofen component

ACE inhibitors: Possibly decreased antihypertensive effect of ACE inhibitors

acetaminophen: Possibly increased renal effects with long-term use of both drugs

aspirin, other NSAIDs: Increased risk of bleeding and adverse GI effects

bone marrow depressants: Possibly increased leukopenic and thrombocytopenic effects of bone marrow depressants

cefamandole, cefoperazone, cefotetan: Increased risk of hypoprothrombinemia and bleeding

colchicines, platelet aggregation inhibitors: Increased risk of GI bleeding, hemorrhage, and ulcers

corticosteroids, potassium supplements: Increased risk of adverse GI effects

cyclosporine: Increased risk of nehprotoxicity from both drugs, increased blood cyclosporine level

digoxin: Increased blood digoxin level and risk of digitalis toxicity

diuretics (loop, potassium-sparing, and thiazide): Decreased diuretic and antihypertensive effects

gold compounds, nephrotoxic drugs: Increased risk of adverse renal effects

heparin, oral anticoagulants, thrombolytics: Increased anticoagulant effects, increased risk of hemorrhage

insulin, oral antidiabetics: Possibly increased hypoglycemic effects of these drugs

lithium: Increased blood lithium level

methotrexate: Decreased methotrexate clearance, increased risk of methotrexate toxicity

plicamycin, valproic acid: Increased risk of hypoprothrombinemia and GI bleeding, hemorrhage, and ulcers

probenecid: Possibly increased blood level, effectiveness, and risk of toxicity of ibuprofen

warfarin: Increased risk of serious GI bleeding because of synergistic effects

ACTIVITIES
oxycodone and ibuprofen
alcohol use: Additive CNS effects and increased risk of adverse GI effects

Adverse Reactions
CNS: Abnormal thinking, anxiety, aseptic meningitis, asthenia, chills, dizziness, drowsiness, euphoria, excitation, fever, headache, hyperkinesias, hypertonia, nervousness, sedation, somnolence
CV: Bradycardia, chest pain, fluid retention, heart failure, hypertension, hypotension, left ventricular dysfunction, palpitations, peripheral edema, thrombophlebitis, thromboembolism, vasodilation
EENT: Amblyopia, blurred vision, dry eyes, epistaxis, lens opacities, miosis, stomatitis, taste perversion, tinnitus
GI: Abdominal cramps or pain, anorexia, constipation, diarrhea, distention, dyspepsia, elevated liver function test results, epigastric discomfort, flatulence, gastritis, GI bleeding or ulceration, heartburn, hepatitis, indigestion, nausea, vomiting
GU: Acute renal failure, amenorrhea, cystitis, decreased libido, erectile dysfunction, hematuria, oliguria, urinary frequency or hesitancy, urine retention
HEME: Agranulocytosis, anemia, aplastic anemia, eosinophilia, hemolytic anemia, neutropenia, prolonged bleeding time, thromboctopenia
RESP: Bronchospasm, dyspnea, respiratory depression, wheezing
MS: Arthritis, back pain
SKIN: Blisters, diaphoresis, ecchymosis, erythema multiforme, photosensitivity, pruritus, rash, Stevens-Johnson syndrome, urticaria
Other: Anaphylaxis, angioedema, drug tolerance, flulike symptoms, hypokalemia, infection, physical and psychological dependence, weight gain, withdrawal symptoms

Nursing Considerations
- Use with extreme caution in patients with significant chronic obstructive pulmonary disease or cor pulmonale and in patients who have substantially decreased respiratory reserve, hypoxia, or hypercapnia because oxycodone component can depress respiratory drive.
- Use with caution in elderly or debilitated patients and in those with severe impairment of hepatic or renal function, hypothyroidism, Addison's disease, acute alcoholism, convulsive disorders, CNS depression or coma, delirium tremens, kyphoscoliosis

associated with respiratory depression, toxic psychosis, prostatic hypertrophy or urethral stricture because drug can cause hypotension, alter mental state, or depress respirations.

- Monitor patient's cardiovascular status closely because the use of NSAIDs like the ibuprofen component of drug increases the patient's risk for developing serious cardiovascular adverse effects. Also be aware that opioid analgesics like the oxycodone component of drug can cause severe hypotension.
- Monitor patient closely for gastrointestinal bleeding such as abdominal pain, melena, nausea, vomiting, or rectal bleeding because the ibuprofen component of drug increases the risk for GI bleeding.
- Monitor patients with biliary tract disease including pancreatitis for pain because the drug may cause spasm of the sphincter of Oddi.
- **WARNING** Be aware that oxycodone and ibuprofen have a high potential for abuse
- Assess pain level regularly and give drug as prescribed before pain becomes severe.
- Monitor patient for evidence of CNS depression caused by oxycodone component of drug.
- Be prepared to adjust dosage for patient who hasn't previously received opioids until he can tolerate drug's effects.
- Assess patient for possible respiratory depression or paradoxical excitation during dosage titration.
- Assess patient for abdominal pain because oxycodone component of drug may mask signs and symptoms of underlying GI disorders.
- Be aware that ibuprofen's anti-inflammatory and antipyretic actions may mask signs and symptoms of infection.

PATIENT TEACHING

- Tell patient to take oxycodone and ibuprofen with food or after meals to reduce GI distress that may occur as a result of the ibuprofen component of drug. Also advise to take the drug with a full glass of water and to avoid lying down for 15 to 30 minutes afterward to prevent esophageal irritation.
- Instruct patient not to take oxycodone and ibuprofen more often than prescribed and that drug should not be used longer than 7 days.
- Instruct patient to notify prescriber about worsening or breakthrough pain

- Advise patient to avoid taking another NSAID at the same time, unless directed by prescriber because of increased risk of adverse reactions.
- Tell patient to avoid alcohol, aspirin, and potentially hazardous activities during oxycodone and ibuprofen therapy.
- Advise patient to notify prescriber about possible signs of toxicity or hypersensitivity, such as excessive light-headedness, extreme dizziness, itching, swelling of any body area and trouble breathing.
- Suggest that patient wear sunscreen and protective clothing when outdoors to minimize photosensitivity.

pentazocine hydrochloride and acetaminophen

Talacen

Class, Category, and Schedule

Chemical: Benzaocine (pentazocine), acetamide (acetaminophen)
Therapeutic: Analgesic (pentazocine, acetaminophen)
Pregnancy category: C
Controlled substance: Schedule IV

Indications and Dosages

▶ *To relieve mild to moderate pain*

CAPLETS

Adults. 25 mg pentazocine and 650 mg acetaminophen (1 caplet) q 4 hr, as needed. *Maximum:* 150 mg pentazocine and 3,900 mg acetaminophen q 24 hr.

Mechanism of Action

Pentazocine binds with opioid receptors, primarily kappa and sigma receptors, at many CNS sites to alter the perception of and emotional response to pain.

Acetaminophen inhibits the enzyme cyclooxygenase, thereby blocking prostaglandin production and interfering with pain impulse generation in the peripheral nervous system.

Contraindications

Hypersensitivity to pentazocine, acetaminophen or their components; severe hepatic impairment

Interactions
DRUGS
pentazocine and acetaminophen
anticholinergics: Increased risk of urine retention and severe constipation
pentazocine component
antidiarrheals, antiperistaltics: Increased risk of severe constipation and CNS depression
antihypertensives, diuretics, other hypotension-producing drugs: Additive hypotensive effects
buprenorphine: Increased respiratory depression
CNS depressants: Increased CNS depression, increased risk of habituation
MAO inhibitors: Increased risk of unpredictable, severe, and sometimes fatal adverse reactions
metoclopramide: Antagonized metoclopramide effects on GI motility
naloxone: Antagonized analgesic, CNS, and respiratory depressant effects of pentazocine
naltrexone: Withdrawal symptoms in patients who are physically dependent on pentazocine
neuromuscular blockers: Increased respiratory depression
opioid analgesics: Increased analgesia, CNS depression, and hypotensive effects; possibly withdrawal symptoms
acetaminophen component
barbiturates, carbamazepine, hydantoins, isoniazid, rifampin, sulfinpyrazone: Decreased therapeutic effects and increased hepatotoxic effects of acetaminophen
lamotrigine, loop diuretics: Possibly decreased therapeutic effects of these drugs
oral contraceptives: Decreased effectiveness of acetaminophen
probenecid: Possibly increased therapeutic effects of acetaminophen
propranolol: Possibly increased action of acetaminophen
zidovudine: Possibly decreased effects of zidovudine
ACTIVITIES
pentazocine and acetaminophen
alcohol use: Additive CNS depression and increased risk of habituation (pentazocine); increased risk of hepatotoxicity (acetaminophen)

Adverse Reactions
CNS: Dizziness, drowsiness, euphoria, fatigue, headache, lightheadedness, nervousness, nightmares, restlessness, weakness
CV: Hypotension, tachycardia

EENT: Blurred vision, diplopia, dry mouth, laryngeal edema, larngospasm
ENDO: Hypoglycemic coma
GI: Abdominal pain, constipation, hepatotoxicity, jaundice, nausea, vomiting
GU: Decreased urine output, dysuria, urinary frequency
HEME: Hemolytic anemia, leukopenia, neutropenia, pancytopenia, thrombocytopenia
RESP: Atelectasis, bronchospasm, dyspnea, hypoventilation, wheezing
SKIN: Diaphoresis, facial flushing, pruritus, rash, toxic epidermal necrolysis, urticaria
Other: Angioedema, physical and psychological dependence

Nursing Considerations

- Use combination drug with extreme caution in patients who have a head injury, an intracranial lesion, or increased intracranial pressure because drug may mask neurologic signs and symptoms.
- Use combination drug cautiously in patients who are physically dependent on opioid agonists because drug may prompt withdrawal symptoms; in patients with acute MI because drug's cardiovascular effects can increase cardiac workload; in patients with renal or hepatic dysfunction because drug is metabolized in the liver and excreted in urine; and in patients with respiratory conditions because drug depresses the respiratory system.
- Monitor patient for evidence of CNS depression.
- Before and during long-term therapy, monitor liver function test results, including AST, ALT, and bilirubin levels, as ordered.
- Evaluate for therapeutic response, including report of decreased pain and body movements that would indicate pain relief has occurred.
- Monitor renal function in patient on long-term therapy. Keep in mind that blood or albumin in urine may indicate nephritis; decreased urine output may indicate renal failure.
- Expect to reduce dosage for patients with renal dysfunction.

PATIENT TEACHING
- Instruct patient to take pentazocine and acetaminophen exactly as prescribed and not to increase dosage or frequency without consulting prescriber.
- Caution patient that prolonged use of pentazocine and acetaminophen may result in drug dependence.

- Inform patient about possible dizziness, drowsiness and other adverse CNS effects. Advise her to avoid potentially hazardous activities until drug's CNS effects are known.
- Caution patient not to use alcohol or OTC drugs without consulting prescriber.
- Instruct patient to notify prescriber about worsening or breakthrough pain.
- Advise patient to notify prescriber if she notices signs of an allergic reaction, such as a rash or itching.
- Teach patient to recognize signs of hepatotoxicity, such as bleeding, easy bruising, and malaise, which commonly occurs with chronic overdose.

pentazocine hydrochloride and naloxone hydrochloride
Talwin NX

Class, Category, and Schedule
Chemical: Benzaocine (pentazocine), thebaine derivative (naloxone)
Therapeutic: Analgesic (pentazocine), opioid antagonist (naloxone)
Pregnancy category: C
Controlled substance: Schedule IV

Indications and Dosages
▶ *To relieve mild to moderate pain*
TABLETS
Adults. 50 mg pentazocine and 0.5 mg naloxone (1 tablet) q 3 to 4 hr, increased to 100 mg pentazocine and 1 mg naloxone (2 tablets), as needed. *Maximum:* 600 mg pentazocine and 6 mg naloxone daily.

Mechanism of Action
Pentazocine binds with opioid receptors, primarily kappa and sigma receptors, at many CNS sites to alter the perception of and emotional response to pain.

While naloxone briefly and competitively antagonizes mu, kappa, and sigma receptors in the CNS, thus reversing the analgesia, hypotension, respiratory depression, and sedation caused by most opioids, this effect is negligible in this combination product because oral bioavailability is poor and is used instead to decrease risk of physical dependence on pentazocine.

Contraindications
Hypersensitivity to pentazocine, naloxone, or their components

Interactions
DRUGS
pentazocine component
antidiarrheals, antiperistaltics: Increased risk of severe constipation and CNS depression
antihypertensives, diuretics, other hypotension-producing drugs: Additive hypotensive effects
buprenorphine: Decreased pentazocine effectiveness, increased respiratory depression
CNS depressants: Increased CNS depression, increased risk of habituation
hydroxyzine, other opioid analgesics: Increased analgesia, CNS depression, and hypotensive effects
MAO inhibitors: Increased risk of unpredictable, severe, and sometimes fatal adverse reactions
metoclopramide: Antagonized metoclopramide effects on GI motility
naloxone: Antagonized analgesic, CNS, and respiratory depressant effects of pentazocine
naltrexone: Withdrawal symptoms in patients who are physically dependent on pentazocine
neuromuscular blockers: Increased respiratory depression
naloxone component
butorphanol, nalbuphine, pentazocine: Reversal of these drugs' analgesic and adverse effects
opioid analgesics: Reversal of these drugs' analgesic and adverse effects; possibly withdrawal symptoms in opioid-dependent patients

Adverse Reactions
CNS: Chills, dizziness, drowsiness, excitement, euphoria, fatigue, headache, insomnia, irritability, light-headedness, nervousness, nightmares, paresthesia, restlessness, weakness
CV: Hypertension, hypotension, tachycardia
EENT: Blurred vision, diplopia, dry mouth, laryngeal edema, laryngospasm
GI: Constipation, hepatotoxicity, nausea, vomiting
GU: Decreased urine output, dysuria, urinary frequency, urinary retention
RESP: Atelectasis, bronchospasm, dyspnea, hypoventilation, wheezing
SKIN: Diaphoresis, erythema multiforme, facial flushing, pruri-

tus, rash, Stevens-Johnson syndrome, toxic epidermal necrolysis, urticaria

Other: Angioedema, physical and psychological dependence

Nursing Considerations

- Use with extreme caution in patients who have a head injury, an intracranial lesion, or increased intracranial pressure because drug may mask neurologic signs and symptoms.
- Use drug cautiously in patients who are physically dependent on opioid agonists because drug may prompt withdrawal symptoms and in patients with acute MI because drug's cardiovascular effects can increase cardiac workload.
- Evaluate for therapeutic response, including report of decreased pain and body movements that would indicate pain relief has occurred.

PATIENT TEACHING

- Instruct patient to take pentazocine and naloxone exactly as prescribed and not to increase dosage or frequency without consulting prescriber.
- Caution patient that prolonged use of pentazocine and naloxone may result in drug dependence because pentazocine may overcome naloxone effect with increased doses.
- Inform patient about possible dizziness, drowsiness and other adverse CNS effects. Advise her to avoid potentially hazardous activities until drug's CNS effects are known.
- Caution patient not to use alcohol or OTC drugs without consulting prescriber.
- Instruct patient to notify prescriber about worsening or breakthrough pain.
- Advise patient to notify prescriber if she notices signs of an allergic reaction, such as a rash or itching.

perphenazine and amitriptyline hydrochloride

Etrafon-A, Etrafon Forte, Etrafon 2-10, Triavil, Triavil 2-10, Triavil 2-25, Triavil 4-10, Triavil 4-25

Class and Category

Chemical: Piperazine phenothiazine (perphenazine), tertiary amine (amitriptyline)

Therapeutic: Antipyschotic (perphenazine), antianxiety, antidepressant (amitriptyline)

Pregnancy category: Not rated (perphenazine not rated, amitriptyline D)

Indications and Dosages

▶ *To treat moderate to severe anxiety or agitation and depression associated with chronic disease or when anxiety and depression cannot be clearly differentiated; to treat depression in schizophrenic patients*

TABLETS

Adults. 2 to 4 mg perphenazine and 10 to 50 mg amitriptyline (1 to 2 tablets depending on strength used) t.i.d. or q.i.d.

Mechanism of Action

Perphenazine depresses areas of the brain that governs activity and aggression, including the cerebral cortex, hypothalamus, and limbic system through an unknown mechanism. This action may be responsible for controlling agitation and aggression seen in schizophenia.

Amitriptyline blocks serotonin and norepinephrine reuptake by adrenergic nerves. By doing so, it raises serotonin and norepinephrine levels at nerve synapses. This action may elevate mood and reduce depression.

Contraindications

Blood dysrasias; bone marrow depression; cerebral arteriosclerosis; coma; concurrent use of CNS depressants (large doses); coronary artery disease; during acute recovery phase after MI; hepatic impairment; hypersensitivity to perphenazine, amitriptyline, other phenothiazines or their components; myeloproliferative disorders; severe CNS depression; severe hypertension or hypotension; subcortical brain damage; use of MAO inhibitor therapy within 14 days

Interactions

DRUGS

perphenazine and amitriptyline

anticholinergics: Increased adverse anticholinergic effects

perphenazine component

aluminum- and magnesium-containing antacids, antidiarrheals (adsorbent): Decreased absorption of oral perphenazine

amantadine, antidyskinetics, antihistamines: Increased adverse anticholinergic effects

amphetamines: Decreased therapeutic effects of both drugs

anticonvulsants: Decreased seizure threshold, inhibited metabolism and toxicity of anticonvulsant

antithyroid drugs: Increased risk of agranulocytosis

apomorphine: Additive CNS depression, decreased emetic response to apomorphine if perphenazine is given first

appetite suppressants (except phenmetrazine): Antagonized anorectic effect of appetite suppressants

beta blockers: Increased blood levels of both drugs and risk of arrhythmias, hypotension, irreversible retinopathy, and tardive dyskinesia

bromocriptine: Possibly interference with bromocriptine's effects

CNS depressants: Increased CNS and respiratory depression and hypotensive effects

dopamine: Antagonized peripheral vasoconstriction with high doses of dopamin

ephedrine: Decreased vasopressor response to ephedrine

epinephrine: Blocked alpha-adrenergic effects of epinephrine, possibly causing severe hypotension and tachycardia

hepatotoxic drugs: Increased risk of hepatotoxicity

hypotension-causing drugs: Increased risk of severe orthostatic hypotension

levodopa: Inhibited antidyskinetic effects of levodopa

lithium: Possibly neurotoxicity (disorientation, extrapyramidal symptoms, unconsciousness)

maprotiline, selective serotonin reuptake inhibitors, tricyclic antidepressants: Prolonged and intensified sedative and anticholinergic effects of these drugs or perphenazine

metrizamide: Decreased seizure threshold

opioid analgesics: Increased CNS and respiratory depression, increased risk of orthostatic hypotension and severe constipation

ototoxic drugs, especially antibiotics: Possibly masking of some symptoms of ototoxicity, such as dizziness, tinnitus, and vertigo

probucol, other drugs that prolong the QT interval: Prolonged QT interval, which may increase risk of ventricular tachycardia

thiazide diuretics: Possibly hyponatremia and water intoxication

amitriptyline component

barbiturates: Decreased serum amitriptyline level

carbamazepine: Decreased serum amitriptyline level and increased serum carbamazepine level, which increases therapeutic and toxic effects of carbamazepine

cimetidine, disulfiram, fluoxetine, fluvoxamine, haloperidol, H_2-receptor antagonists, methylphenidate, oral contraceptives, paroxetine, phenothiazines, sertraline: Increased serum amitriptyline level

cisapride: Possibly prolonged QT interval and increased risk for arrhythmias *clonidine, guanethidine, other antihypertensives:* Decreased antihypertensive effects

dicumarol: Increased anticoagulant effect of dicumarol

epinephrine, norepinephrine: Increased effects of these drugs

levodopa: Decreased levodopa absorption; sympathetic hyperactivity, sinus tachycardia, hypertension, agitation

MAO inhibitors: Possibly seizures and death

thyroid replacement drugs: Arrhythmias and increased antidepressant effects

ACTIVITIES

perphenazine component

alcohol use: Increased CNS and respiratory depression, hypotensive effects, and risk of heatstroke

amitriptyline component

smoking: Decreased amitriptyline effects

Adverse Reactions

CNS: Anxiety, ataxia, behavioral changes, cerebral edema, chills, coma, delusions, disorientation, dizziness, drowsiness, extrapyramidal reactions, fatigue, fever, headache, insomnia, neuroleptic malignant syndrome, nightmares, peripheral neuropathy, seizures, syncope, tardive dyskinesia (persistent), tremor

CV: Arrhythmias (including prolonged AV conduction and heart block), bradycardia, cardiac arrest, cardiomyopathy, hypertension, hypotension, MI, nonspecific ECG changes, orthostatic hypotension, palpitations, tachycardia

EENT: Abnormal taste, black tongue, blurred vision, dry mouth, glaucoma, increased salivation, laryngeal edema, miosis, mydraisis, nasal congestion, ocular changes (corneal opacification, retinopathy), tinnitus

ENDO: Decreased libido, galactorrhea, gynecomastia, hyperglycemia, hypoglycemia, syndrome of inappropriate ADH secretion

GI: Abnormal cramps, anorexia, constipation, diarrhea, fecal impaction, flatulence, ileus, increased appetite, nausea, vomiting

GU: Bladder paralysis, ejaculation failure, impotence, libido changes, menstrual irregularities, polyuria, testicular swelling, urinary frequency, urinary hesitancy, urinary incontinence, urine retention

HEME: Agranulocytosis, bone marrow depression, eosinophilia, hemolytic anemia, leukopenia, pancytopenia, thrombocytopenic purpura

RESP: Asthma

SKIN: Alopecia, diaphoresis, eczema, erythema, exfoliative dermatitis, flushing, hyperpigmentation, jaundice, pallor, photosensitivity, pruritus, purpura, urticaria

Other: Anaphylaxis, angioedema, weight gain

Nursing Considerations

- Use cautiously in patient with a history of seizures, urine retention, or angle-closure glaucoma because of amitriptyline component's atropine-like effects.
- Use cautiously in patient with hepatic, pulmonary or renal dysfunction and in elderly patients who are at increased risk for increased plasma concentrations and tardive dyskinesia from perphenazine component of drug.
- **WARNING** Don't give an MAO inhibitor within 14 days of perphenazine and amitriptyline therapy because of the risk of seizures and death.
- Closely monitor patient with cardiovascular disorder because perphenazine and amitriptyline may cause arrhythmias, such as conduction abnormalities or sinus tachycardia.
- Monitor blood pressure and assess patient for hypotension or hypertension.
- Avoid abrupt withdrawal of drug after prolonged therapy; otherwise withdrawal symptoms such as nausea, headache, vertigo, and nightmares may occur.
- Monitor patient being treated for depression with perphenazine and amitriptyline closely for suicidal tendencies, especially when therapy starts or dosage changes; depression may worsen temporarily during these times.
- Monitor patient's blood counts and liver and renal function test results during therapy. Notify prescriber of any abnormalities.
- Monitor temperature frequently and notify prescriber if it rises; a significant increase suggests drug intolerance to the perphenazine component of the drug.
- Stay alert for behavior changes, such as hallucinations and decreased interest in personal appearance. Be aware that psychosis may develop in schizophrenic patients and symptoms may increase in paranoid patients.
- Assess patient regularly to determine effectiveness of perphenazine and amitriptyline therapy.

PATIENT TEACHING

- Instruct patient to take perphenazine exactly as prescribed to ensure optimal effectiveness and minimize adverse reactions.

- Instruct patient to avoid using alcohol, OTC drugs that contain alcohol or to smoke during perphenazine and amitriptyline therapy because of potential adverse effects.
- Urge patient to avoid potentially hazardous activities until drug's CNS effects are known.
- Advise patient to avoid excessive sun exposure and to protect skin when outdoors.
- Instruct patient to notify prescriber about persistent or severe adverse reactions.
- Urge patient to comply with long-term follow up to detect adverse reactions and need for dosage adjustments.

propoxyphene hydrochloride and acetaminophen
E-Lor, Wygesic

propoxyphene napsylate and acetaminophen
Darvocet-N 50, Darvocet-N 100, Propacet 100

Class, Category, and Schedule
Chemical: Synthetic opioid (propoxyphene), acetamide (acetaminophen)
Therapeutic: Analgesic (propoxyphene, acetaminophen)
Pregnancy category: C
Controlled substance: Schedule IV

Indications and Dosages
▶ *To relieve mild to moderate pain*
TABLETS (PROPOXYPHENE HYDROCHLORIDE AND ACETAMINOPHEN)
Adults. 65 mg propoxyphene and 650 mg acetaminophen (1 tablet) q 4 hr, p.r.n.
TABLETS (PROPOXYPHENE NAPSYLATE AND ACETAMINOPHEN)
Adults. 100 mg propoxyphene and 650 mg acetaminophen (1 or 2 tablets depending on strength prescribed) q 4 hr, p.r.n.

Mechanism of Action
Propoxyphene strongly antagonizes mu receptors, blocking release of such inhibitory neurotransmitters as gamma-aminobutyric acid (GABA) and acetylcholine. It also mediates analgesia by changing pain perception at the spinal cord and higher CNS levels and by altering the emotional response to pain.

Acetaminophen acts centrally to increase the pain threshold by inhibiting cyclooxygenase, an enzyme involved in prostaglandin synthesis.

Contraindications

Hypersensitivity to propoxyphene, acetaminophen or their components, respiratory depression, severe asthma, upper airway obstruction, use within 14 days of MAO inhibitor therapy

Interactions

DRUGS

propoxyphene and acetaminophen

anticholinergics: Decreased onset of action of acetaminophen; increased risk of severe constipation and urine retention

carbamazepine: Decreased therapeutic effects and increased hepatotoxic effects of acetaminophen; possibly carbamazepine toxicity from propoxyphene use

propoxyphene component

amphetamines: Possibly fatal seizures (with propoxyphene overdose)

antidiarrheals: Severe constipation, possibly increased CNS depression

antihypertensives: Possibly exaggerated antihypertensive response

buprenorphine: Possibly decreased propoxyphene effectiveness, increased respiratory depression

CNS depressants: Increased CNS and respiratory depression, hypotensive effects, and risk of habituation

hydroxyzine: Increased analgesic, CNS depressant, and hypotensive effects of propoxyphene

MAO inhibitors: Severe, possibly fatal reactions, including hypertensive crisis

metoclopramide: Possibly antagonized effects of metoclopramide on GI motility

naloxone: Antagonized analgesic and CNS and respiratory depressant effects of propoxyphene

naltrexone: Risk of withdrawal symptoms in patients who are dependent on propoxyphene, possibly decreased analgesic effect of propoxyphene

neuromuscular blockers: Additive respiratory depressant effects

opioid analgesics: Additive CNS and respiratory depressant and hypotensive effects

warfarin: Increased anticoagulation effects

acetaminophen component

barbiturates, hydantoins, isoniazid, rifampin, sulfinpyrazone: Decreased therapeutic effects and increased hepatotoxic effects of acetaminophen

lamotrigine, loop diuretics: Possibly decreased therapeutic effects of these drugs
oral contraceptives: Decreased effectiveness of acetaminophen
probenecid: Possibly increased therapeutic effects of acetaminophen
propranolol: Possibly increased action of acetaminophen
zidovudine: Possibly decreased effects of zidovudine
ACTIVITIES
propoxyphene component
alcohol use: Increased CNS and respiratory depression, hypotensive effects, and risk of habituation
nicotine chewing gum, other smoking deterrents, smoking cessation: Decreased effectiveness of propoxyphene

Adverse Reactions

CNS: Dizziness, drowsiness, fatigue, insomnia, light-headedness, malaise, nervousness, sedation, tremor
CV: Orthostatic hypotension, tachycardia
EENT: Blurred vision, diplopia, dry mouth, tinnitus
ENDO: Hypoglycemic coma
GI: Abdominal cramps or pain, anorexia, constipation, jaundice, hepatotoxicity, nausea, vomiting
GU: Decreased urine output
HEME: Hemolytic anemia (with long-term use), leukopenia, neutropenia, pancytopenia, thrombocytopenia
MS: Muscle weakness
RESP: Dyspnea, respiratory depression, wheezing
SKIN: Facial flushing, pruritus, rash, urticaria
Other: Angioedema, psychological dependence

Nursing Considerations

- Use propoxyphene and acetaminophen cautiously in patients with hepatic or renal dysfunction because delayed elimination may occur. Monitor hepatic and renal function test results.
- Monitor patient's response to drug for pain relief.
- **WARNING** Be aware that long-term, high dose propoxyphene and acetaminophen therapy may lead to psychological dependence in some patients. Assess for opioid and alcohol use, which increase the risk of drug abuse or dependence.
- Be aware that abruptly discontinuing drug can result in withdrawal symptoms.
- Know that the dosage of acetaminophen in the combination drug should not exceed 4 g/day to reduce the risk of acetaminophen-induced hepatotoxicity.

PATIENT TEACHING
* Inform patient she may take propoxyphene and acetaminophen with food if she experiences GI distress.
* Instruct patient not to take more than the prescribed amount because drug may be addictive.
* Caution patient to avoid potentially hazardous activities until drug's CNS effects are known.
* Instruct patient to avoid alcohol and other sedatives while taking drug.
* Advise smokers to inform prescriber if they attempt to stop smoking during propoxyphene and acetaminophen therapy because increased drug dosage may be required for effective analgesia.
* Urge patient to notify prescriber immediately if pain isn't relieved or worsens.
* Advise her to contact prescriber before taking other prescription or OTC drugs; they may contain acetaminophen and lead to toxicity.
* Teach patient to recognize signs of hepatotoxicity, such as bleeding, easy bruising, and chronic overdose.

propoxyphene hydrochloride, aspirin, and caffeine
Darvon Compound-65, PC-Cap, Propoxyphene Compound-65
propoxyphene napsylate and aspirin
Darvon-N (CAN)
propoxyphene napsylate, aspirin and caffeine
Darvon-N Compound (CAN)

Class, Category, and Schedule
Chemical: Synthetic opioid (propoxyphene), salicylate (aspirin), xanthine derivative (caffeine)
Therapeutic: Analgesic (propoxyphene, aspirin), CNS stimulant (caffeine)
Pregnancy category: NR
Controlled substance: Schedule IV

Indications and Dosages
▶ *To relieve mild to moderate pain*
CAPSULES (PROPOXYPHENE HYDROCHLORIDE, ASPIRIN AND CAFFEINE)
Adults. 65 mg propoxyphene, 389 mg aspirin, and 32.4 mg caf-

feine (1 capsule) q 4 hr, p.r.n. *Maximum:* 390 mg propoxyphene hydrochloride daily
TABLETS (PROPOXYPHENE HYDROCHLORIDE, ASPIRIN, AND CAFFEINE)
Adults. 65 mg propoxyphene, 375 mg aspirin, and 30 mg caffeine (1 tablet) q 4 hr, p.r.n. *Maximum:* 390 mg propoxyphene hydrochloride daily
CAPSULES (PROPOXYPHENE NAPSYLATE AND ASPIRIN)
Adults. 100 mg propoxyphene and 325 mg aspirin (1 capsule) q 4 hr, p.rn. *Maximum:* 600 mg of propoxyphene napsylate daily.
CAPSULES (PROPOXYPHENE NAPSYLATE, ASPIRIN, AND CAFFEINE)
Adults. 100 mg propoxyphene napsylate, 375 mg aspirin, and 30 mg caffeine (1 capsule) q 4 hr, p.rn. *Maximum:* 600 mg propoxyphene napsylate daily.

Mechanism of Action
Propoxyphene strongly antagonizes mu receptors, blocking the release of such inhibitory neurotransmitters as gamma-aminobutyric acid (GABA) and acetylcholine. It also mediates analgesia by changing pain perception at the spinal cord and higher CNS levels and by altering the emotional response to pain.

Aspirin blocks the activity of cyclooxygenase, the enzyme necessary for prostaglandin synthesis. By preventing prostaglandin synthesis, pain is relieved because prostaglandins play a role in pain transmission from the periphery to the spinal cord.

Caffeine is a competitive, nonselective antagonist of adenosine receptor sites, which results in stimulation of the central nervous system to counteract the sedative properties of propoxyphene.

Contraindications
Allergy to tartrazine dye; asthma; bleeding problems such as hemophilia; hypersensitivity to propoxyphene, aspirin, caffeine or their components; peptic ulcer disease; respiratory depression; upper airway obstruction; use within 14 days of MAO inhibitor therapy

Interactions
DRUGS
propoxyphene component
amphetamines: Possibly fatal seizures (with propoxyphene overdose)
anticholinergics: Increased risk of severe constipation and urine retention

antidiarrheals: Severe constipation, possibly increased CNS depression

antihypertensives: Possibly exaggerated antihypertensive response

buprenorphine: Possibly decreased propoxyphene effectiveness, increased respiratory depression

carbamazepine: Possibly carbamazepine toxicity from propoxyphene use

CNS depressants: Increased CNS and respiratory depression, hypotensive effects, and risk of habituation

hydroxyzine: Increased analgesic, CNS depressant, and hypotensive effects of propoxyphene

MAO inhibitors: Severe, possibly fatal reactions, including hypertensive crisis

metoclopramide: Possibly antagonized effects of metoclopramide on GI motility

naloxone: Antagonized analgesic and CNS and respiratory depressant effects of propoxyphene

naltrexone: Risk of withdrawal symptoms in patients who are dependent on propoxyphene, possibly decreased analgesic effect of propoxyphene

neuromuscular blockers: Additive respiratory depressant effects

opioid analgesics: Additive CNS and respiratory depressant and hypotensive effects

warfarin: Increased anticoagulation effects

aspirin component

ACE inhibitors: Decreased antihypertensive effect

activated charcoal: Decreased aspirin absorption

antacids, urine alkalinizers: Decreased aspirin effectiveness

anticoagulants: Increased risk of bleeding; prolonged bleeding time

carbonic anhydrase inhibitors: Salicylism

corticosteroids: Increased excretion and decreased blood level of aspirin

heparin: Increased risk of bleeding

loop diuretics: Decreased effectiveness of loop diuretics

methotrexate: Increased blood level and decreased excretion of methotrexate, causing toxicity

nizatidine: Increased blood aspirin level

NSAIDs: Possibly decreased blood NSAID level and increased risk of adverse GI effects

probenecid, sulfinpyrazone: Decreased effectiveness in treating gout

urine acidifiers, such as ammonium chloride and ascorbic acid: Decreased aspirin excretion

vancomycin: Increased risk of ototoxicity
caffeine component
aspirin: Increased GI absorption of aspirin
beta-adrenergic agonists: Possibly enhanced cardiac inotropic effects of beta-adrenergic agonists
cimetidine, contraceptives (oral), disulfiram, fluoroquinolones: Decreased hepatic metabolism of caffeine resulting in increased caffeine effect
clozapine: Possibly increased clozapine levels resulting in increased incidence of clozapine induced adverse reactions
lithium: Enhanced renal clearance of lithium
mexiletine: Decreased caffeine elimination resulting in increased caffeine effect
phenytoin: Increased caffeine clearance resulting in decreased caffeine effect
theophylline: Reduced theophylline clearance with ingestion of more than 120 mg caffeine daily
ACTIVITIES
propoxyphene, aspirin and caffeine
alcohol use: Increased risk of ulcers (aspirin, caffeine); increased CNS and respiratory depression, hypotensive effects, and risk of habituation (propoxyphene)
propoxyphene component
nicotine chewing gum, other smoking deterrents, smoking cessation: Decreased effectiveness of propoxyphene

Adverse Reactions

CNS: Confusion, CNS depression, dizziness, drowsiness, fatigue, insomnia, light-headedness, malaise, nervousness, sedation, tremor
CV: Orthostatic hypotension, tachycardia
EENT: Blurred vision, diplopia, dry mouth, hearing loss, tinnitus
ENDO: Hypoglycemic coma
GI: Abdominal cramps or pain, anorexia, constipation, diarrhea, GI bleeding, heartburn, nausea, vomiting
GU: Decreased urine output
HEME: Decreased blood iron level, leukopenia, prolonged bleeding time, shortened life span of RBCs, thrombocytopenia
MS: Muscle weakness
RESP: Dyspnea, respiratory depression, wheezing
SKIN: Ecchymosis, facial flushing, pruritus, rash, urticaria
Other: Angioedema, Reye's syndrome, psychological dependence

Nursing Considerations
• Be aware that drug should not be taken by patients who are suicidal or prone to addiction.
• Use drug cautiously in patients with hepatic or renal dysfunction because delayed elimination may occur. Monitor hepatic and renal function test results.
• Monitor patient's response to drug for pain relief.
• **WARNING** Be aware that long-term, high-dose propoxyphene therapy may lead to psychological dependence in some patients. Assess for opioid and alcohol use, which increase the risk of drug abuse or dependence.
• Be aware that abruptly discontinuing drug can result in withdrawal symptoms.
• Question patient taking drug regularly about presence of tinnitus. This reaction usually occurs when blood aspirin level reaches or exceeds maximum for therapeutic effect.

PATIENT TEACHING
• Tell patient to take drug with food to minimize stomach upset.
• Instruct patient not to take more than the prescribed amount because drug may be addictive.
• Caution patient to avoid potentially hazardous activities until drug's CNS effects are known.
• Instruct patient to avoid alcohol and other sedatives while taking drug.
• Advise smokers to inform prescriber if they attempt to stop smoking during propoxyphene and aspirin or propoxyphene, aspirin and caffeine therapy because increased drug dosage may be required for effective analgesia.
• Urge patient to notify prescriber immediately if pain isn't relieved or worsens.
• Tell patient to consult prescriber before taking drug with any prescription or OTC preparation that may contain aspirin to avoid aspirin overdose.

tramadol hydrochloride and acetaminophen
Ultracet

Class and Category
Chemical: Cyclohexanol (tramadol), aminophenol derivative (acetaminophen)

Therapeutic: Opioid analgesic (tramadol), non-opioid analgesic (acetaminophen)
Pregnancy category: C

Indications and Dosages

▶ *To provide short-term management of acute pain*

TABLETS

Adults. Initial: 75 mg tramadol and 650 mg acetaminophen q 4 to 6 hr, p.r.n. *Maximum:* 300 mg tramadol and 2,600 mg acetaminophen/day for up to 5 days.

DOSAGE ADJUSTMENT Dosing interval increased to 12 hr and maximum dose reduced to 75 mg tramadol and 650 mg acetaminophen/dose in patients with creatinine clearance of less than 30 ml/min/1.73 m^2.

Mechanism of Action

Tramadol binds with mu receptors and inhibits the reuptake of norepinephrine and serotonin, which may account for the drug's analgesic effect.

Acetaminophen blocks the activity of cyclooxygenase, an enzyme needed for prostaglandin synthesis. Prostaglandins are important mediators of the inflammatory response that cause local vasodilation, swelling, and pain.

Contraindications

Acute intoxication with alcohol, centrally acting analgesics, hypnotics, opioids, or psychotropic drugs; hypersensitivity to tramadol, other opioids, acetaminophen, or components of these drugs

Interactions

DRUGS

acetaminophen-containing products: Increased risk of hepatotoxicity
carbamazepine: Increased metabolism of tramadol and increased risk of seizures; possibly significantly reduced analgesic effect of tramadol
CNS depressants: Increased risk of CNS and respiratory depression
CYP 2D6 inhibitors, such as amitriptyline, fluoxetine, and paroxetine: Possibly inhibited tramadol metabolism
digoxin: Possibly digitalis toxicity, although rare
MAO inhibitors, selective serotonin reuptake inhibitors: Increased risk of seizures and serotonin syndrome
neuroleptics, opioids, tricyclic antidepressants: Increased risk of seizures
quinidine: Increased blood tramadol level
warfarin: Possibly elevated PT and altered effects of warfarin

FOODS
any food: Possibly delayed peak plasma time
ACTIVITIES
alcohol use: Increased risk of CNS and respiratory depression

Adverse Reactions
CNS: Dizziness, insomnia, seizures, somnolence
EENT: Dry mouth
GI: Anorexia, constipation, diarrhea, hepatotoxicity, nausea
GU: Prostate disorder
RESP: Respiratory depression
SKIN: Increased sweating, pruritus
Other: Hypersensitivity, physical and psychological dependence

Nursing Considerations
• Be aware that tramadol and acetaminophen shouldn't be given to patients with a history of anaphylactoid reactions to codeine or other opioid analgesics.
• Avoid giving tramadol and acetaminophen to patients with acute abdominal conditions because drug may mask signs and symptoms and disrupt assessment of the abdomen.
• Monitor liver function test results, as appropriate, and notify prescriber of abnormal results. This drug combination isn't recommended for patients with hepatic impairment.
• After patient receives first dose, watch for allergic reactions, including angioedema, bronchospasm, pruritus, Stevens-Johnson syndrome, toxic epidermal necrolysis, and urticaria. Also watch for evidence of anaphylaxis, such as dyspnea and hypotension.
• If patient has respiratory depression, assess respiratory status often, and expect to give a nonopioid analgesic—not tramadol and acetaminophen.
• If patient develops respiratory depression, expect to give naloxone. Watch for seizures, because naloxone may increase this risk. Take seizure precautions.
• Assess respiratory status often if patient has increased intracranial pressure or head injury because of possible increased carbon dioxide retention and CSF pressure, either of which may cause respiratory depression. Also, be aware that tramadol may constrict pupils, obscuring evidence of intracranial complications.
• **WARNING** Watch for seizures in patients with epilepsy, a history of seizures, or an increased risk of seizures, such as those with head injury, metabolic disorders, alcohol or drug withdrawal, or CNS infection.

• Expect to taper dosage rather than stopping drug abruptly to avoid such acute withdrawal symptoms as anxiety, diarrhea, insomnia, nausea, pain, panic attacks, paresthesia, piloerection, rigors, sweating, tremor, and upper respiratory symptoms.
• Because tramadol and acetaminophen may lead to physical and psychological dependence and abuse, assess patient for evidence of dependence or abuse, such as drug-seeking behavior. Be aware that drug shouldn't be used in patients with a history of dependence on other opioids because dependence may recur.

PATIENT TEACHING

• Caution patient that taking more of this drug than prescribed or taking it more often than prescribed can lead to serious adverse reactions, including respiratory depression, seizures, hepatotoxicity, and death.
• Caution patient not to stop drug abruptly.
• Tell patient to avoid potentially hazardous activities until drug's adverse effects are known.
• Warn patient to avoid alcohol while taking tramadol and acetaminophen.
• Warn patient to avoid other drugs that contain tramadol or acetaminophen, including OTC preparations.
• Urge patient to notify prescriber if she becomes pregnant, thinks she might be pregnant, or is trying to become pregnant.

Dermatologic Drugs

benzocaine 14%, butyl aminobenzoate 2%, and tetracaine hydrochloride 2%

Cetacaine

Class and Category

Chemical: Aminobenzoate (benzocaine, butyl aminobenzoate), amethocaine (tetracaine)

Therapeutic: Local anesthetic (benzocaine, butyl aminobenzoate, tetracaine)

Pregnancy category: NR

Indications and Dosages

▶ *To anesthetize all accessible mucous membranes except eyes*

GEL, LIQUID, OINTMENT, SPRAY

Adults. Sprayed or applied with cotton applicator to affected area for 1 second or less at needed time.

Mechanism of Action

Benzocaine, butyl aminobenzoate, and tetracaine act by reversibly blocking nerve conduction to prevent pain perception.

Contraindications

Application to eyes or large denuded or inflamed areas; cholinesterase deficiencies; hypersensitivity to benzocaine, butyl aminobenzoate, tetracaine, or their components

Adverse Reactions

SKIN: Local site reactions such as dehydration of epithelium, edema, erythema, pruritus, rash, urticaria, vesiculation, oozing

Other: Anaphylaxis, methemoglobinemia

Nursing Considerations

• Ask any female patient of childbearing age whether she is or could be pregnant. Notify prescriber before applying benzocaine, butyl aminobenzoate, and tetracaine because drug isn't recommended during early pregnancy.

- Apply directly to the site where pain control is needed. There's no need to dry the area before applying the drug. If applying to the face, avoid contact with patient's eyes.
- Don't spray or apply under dentures or on cotton rolls because doing so increases the risk of an escharotic effect. Never spray or apply for more than 2 seconds because doing so increases the risk of serious, local adverse reactions and may induce methemoglobinemia.
- **WARNING** If application exceeds 2 seconds, notify prescriber and monitor patient for cyanosis. If if occurs, be prepared to provide supportive care and counteract drug with methylene blue, if prescribed.
- In debilitated, elderly, or acutely ill patients, reduce the amount used.
- Assess patient's response, and notify prescriber if it's less than optimal; tolerance varies among patients.

PATIENT TEACHING
- Warn patient to follow application directions exactly to prevent serious local skin reactions at application site.
- Instruct patient to alert prescriber if pain control is inadequate.

benzoyl peroxide 5% and sulfur 2%
Sulfoxyl Lotion Regular
benzoyl peroxide 10% and sulfur 5%
Sulfoxyl Lotion Strong

Class and Category
Chemical: Benzoic acid derivative (benzoyl peroxide), nonmetal element (sulfur)
Therapeutic: Antiacne and keratolyitc (benzoyl peroxide, sulfur)
Pregnancy category: C

Indications and Dosages
▶ *To treat acne vulgaris*
LOTION
Adults and adolescents. Applied to affected areas once daily for 1 wk and then b.i.d. thereafter, as tolerated and needed.

Contraindications
Hypersensitivity to benzoyl peroxide, other benzoic acid derivatives, sulfur, or their components

Mechanism of Action

Benzoyl peroxide exerts antibacterial action against *Propionibacerium acnes*, an anaerobe found in sebaceous follicles and comedones of acne, by releasing active oxygen to cause cell death. It also has some keratolytic effect, which produces comedone lysis and drying and desquamative effects. These contribute to the improvement of acne vulgaris.

Sulfur is thought to also inhibit *Propionibacerium acnes* and the formation of fatty acids through unknown mechanisms. It relieves the plugging and rupturing of follicles, easing the evacuation of comedones and promoting peeling of the skin to reduce acne vulgaris symptoms.

Adverse Reactions
SKIN: Excessive erythema and peeling

Nursing Considerations
• Be aware that benzoyl peroxide 5% and sulfur 2% (Sulfoxyl Lotion Regular) is recommended for use first; if tolerated, patient may be advanced to benzoyl peroxide 10% and sulfur 5% (Sulfoxyl Lotion Strong).

PATIENT TEACHING
• Stress the importance of continuous use to obtain maximum effectiveness of benzoyl peroxide and sulfur lotion.
• Instruct patient to shake container well before applying and to cleanse affected area with a non-medicated soap before application.
• Inform patient that visible improvement may take up to 3 weeks and that maximum improvement may take up to 12 weeks of drug use.
• Tell patient to notify prescriber about excessive erythema and peeling because strength or frequency of benzoyl peroxide and sulfur lotion may need to be decreased.

clindamycin phosphate 1% and benzoyl peroxide 5%

BenzaClin, Duac

Class and Category
Chemical: Lincosamide (clindamycin), benzoic acid derivative (benzoyl peroxide)
Therapeutic: Antiacne, antibiotic (clindamycin, benzoyl peroxide), keratolytic (benzoyl peroxide)

Pregnancy category: C

Indications and Dosages

▶ *To treat acne vulgaris*

GEL

Adults and adolescents. Applied to affected areas b.i.d., morning and evening, after skin has been washed, rinsed with warm water, and patted dry.

Mechanism of Action

Clindamycin inhibits protein synthesis against *Propionibacerium acnes*, an anaerobe found in sebaceous follicles and comedones of acne, by binding to the 50S subunits of bacterial ribosomes and preventing peptide bond formation, which causes bacterial cells to die. This eradicates the bacterial infection present in acne vulgaris.

Benzoyl peroxide exerts antibacterial action against *Propionibacterium acnes* by releasing active oxygen to cause cell death. It also has some keratolytic effect, which produces comedone lysis and drying and desquamative effects. These contribute to the improvement of acne vulgaris.

Contraindications

History of regional enteritis, ulcerative colitis, or antibiotic-related colitis; hypersensitivity to clindamycin, benzoyl peroxide, other benzoic acid derivatives, lincomycin, or their components

Interactions

DRUGS

clindamycin component

erythromycin: Possibly blocked access of clindamycin to its site of action

neuromuscular blockers: Increased neuromuscular blockade

Adverse Reactions

EENT: Mouth ulcerations

GI: Abdominal cramps, diarrhea (including bloody diarrhea), pseudomembranous colitis, severe colitis

GU: Vaginitis

SKIN: Dry or peeling skin, erythema, photosensitivity, pruritus

Nursing Considerations

• Be aware that clindamycin and benzoyl peroxide should be used cautiously in patients using topical acne therapy because of possible cumulative irritation, especially if the patient uses peeling, desquamating, or abrasive agents.

- Don't give drug with products that contain erythromycin because clindamycin and erythromycin may inactivate each other. Notify prescriber if patient is using an erythromycin product.
- When applying drug, avoid contact with patient's eyes and mucous membranes.
- Observe patient for signs of superinfection, such as vaginal itching and sore mouth. If present, notify prescriber.
- **WARNING** Monitor patient closely for diarrhea, which may herald pseudomembranous colitis because clindamycin is absorbed systemically. If diarrhea occurs, notify prescriber and expect to stop topical application of drug. If pseudomembranous colitis occurs, expect to stop drug and possibly administer fluids, electrolytes, protein, and an antibiotic effective against *Clostridium difficile.*

PATIENT TEACHING

- Instruct patient to wash the affected area, rinse with warm water, and gently pat area dry before applying clindamycin and benzolyl peroxide gel.
- Tell patient to apply gel exactly as prescribed and to avoid contact with eyes, inside the nose, mouth, and all mucous membranes.
- Warn patient not to use any other topical acne preparation unless instructed by prescriber.
- Urge patient to minimize exposure to sunlight and to take precautions when outdoors, such as wearing a hat and protective clothing and using a sunscreen that's SPF 15 or higher.
- Tell patient to report adverse reactions to prescriber, especially abdominal cramps, diarrhea, and signs of superinfection, such as vaginal itching or sore mouth.
- Warn patient that drug may bleach hair or colored fabric.
- Tell patient to discard any unused product after 3 months.

clotrimazole 1% and betamethasone dipropionate 0.05%

Lotrisone

Class and Category

Chemical: Imidazole (clotrimazole), corticosteroid (betamethasone)
Therapeutic: Antifungal (clotrimazole), anti-inflammatory (betamethasone)
Pregnancy category: C

Indications and Dosages
▶ *To treat symptomatic inflammatory tinea pedis, tinea cruris, or tinea corporis caused by* Epidermophyton floccosum, Trichophyton mentagrophytes, *or* Trichophyton rubrum
CREAM, LOTION
Adults. Sufficient amount applied to affected skin areas b.i.d. in the morning and evening. *Maximum:* 45 g (cream) or 45 ml (lotion) per week for 2 wk (tinea corporis or cruris) or 4 wk (tinea pedis).

Mechanism of Action
Clotrimazole binds to one of the cytochrome P-450 enzymes inhibiting 14-alpha-demethylation of lanosterol in fungi. This leads to an accumulation of 14-alpha-methysterols and reduced concentrations of ergosterol, a sterol essential for the development of fungal cytoplasmic membrane. Clotrimazole also may affect the electron transport system to inhibit fungal growth.

Betamethasone may decrease the number and activity of cells involved in the inflammatory response, such as mast cells, eosinophils, basophils, lymphocytes, macrophages, and neutrophils.

Contraindications
Hypersensitivity to clotrimazole, betamethasone, other corticosteroids or imidazoles, or their components

Interactions
DRUGS
betamethasone component
other corticosteroids: Increased risk of adverse reactions

Adverse Reactions
CNS: Paresthesia
EENT: Perioral dermatitis
ENDO: Cushing's syndrome, hyperglycemia, hypothalamic-pituitary-adrenal (HPA) axis suppression
SKIN: Acneiform eruptions, allergic contact dermatitis, atrophy or maceration of the skin, blisters, burning, dryness, erythema, folliculitis, hypertrichosis, hypopigmentation, itching, irritation, localized edema, miliaria, peeling, pruritis, rash, secondary infection, stinging, striae, urticaria

Nursing Considerations
• Monitor patient for HPA axis suppression, especially if using clotrimazole and betamethasone cream or lotion over a large

surface, for longer than recommended time (2 weeks for tinea corporis or cruris or 4 weeks for tinea pedis), or with other corticosteroids. If suppression is suspected, contact prescriber and prepare patient for ACTH stimulation, morning plasma cortisol, and urine free-cortisol tests, as ordered. If confirmed, expect to withdraw the drug, reduce the frequency of application, or substitute a less potent corticosteroid, as prescribed.

• Don't use clotrimazole and betamethasone under occlusive dressings because of the increased risk of systemic absorption.

PATIENT TEACHING

• Instruct patient to use clotrimazole and betamethasone cream or lotion exactly as prescribed and for the length of time prescribed, even when symptoms improve.

• Teach patient to wash her hands before and after applying drug.

• Tell patient to shake lotion well before applying and to store container in an upright position.

• Instruct patient to store clotrimazole and betamethasone cream or lotion at room temperature.

• Remind patient that drug is for topical use only and to avoid contact with eyes or mouth during application.

• Instruct patient with groin involvement to use drug sparingly in the groin area and to wear loose-fitting clothes throughout treatment.

• Tell patient not to cover treated area after applying drug unless instructed to do so by prescriber.

• Inform female patients that drug is not for intravaginal use.

• Instruct patient to notify prescriber if symptoms don't improve after 1 week (tinea cruris or tinea corporis) or 2 weeks (tinea pedis).

• Caution patient to avoid anyone with an infection and to avoid re-infecting herself.

• Urge patient to notify prescriber about adverse reactions at application site.

erythromycin 3% and benzoyl peroxide 5%

Benzamycin, Benzamycin Pak

Class and Category

Chemical: Macrolide (erythromycin), benzoic acid derivative (benzoyl peroxide)

Therapeutic: Antiacne, antibotic (erythromycin, benzoyl peroxide)
Pregnancy category: C

Indications and Dosages

▶ *To treat acne vulgaris*
GEL
Adults and adolescents. Applied to affected areas b.i.d., morning and evening, after skin has been washed, rinsed with warm water, and patted gently dry.

Mechanism of Action

Erythromycin inhibits protein synthesis in susceptible organisms by reversibly binding to 50S ribosomal subunits, thereby inhibiting translocation of aminoacyl transfer-RNA and inhibiting polypeptide synthesis. This eradicates the bacterial infection in acne vulgaris.

Benzoyl peroxide exerts antibacterial action against *Propionibacerium acnes*, an anaerobe found in sebaceous follicles and comedones of acne, by releasing active oxygen to cause cell death. It also has some keratolytic effect, which produces comedone lysis and drying and desquamative effects. These contribute to the improvement of acne vulgaris.

Contraindications
Hypersensitivity to erythromycin, benzoyl peroxide, other benzoic acid derivatives, or their components

Interactions
DRUGS
erythromycin component
chloramphenicol, clindamycin, lincomycin: Antagonized actions between both drugs

Adverse Reactions
EENT: Mouth ulcerations
GI: Diarrhea
GU: Vaginitis
SKIN: Application site reaction such as stinging, erythema, and burning; blepharitis; dry skin; photosensitivity; pruritus

Nursing Considerations
• Use erythromycin and benzoyl peroxide cautiously in patients using other topical acne therapy (especially peeling, desquamating, or abrasive agents) because of possible cumulative irritation.

- Don't give drug with any product that contains clindamycin because erythromcyin and clindamycin may inactivate each other. Notify prescriber if patient is using a clindamycin product.
- Avoid contact with eyes and mucous membranes when applying drug.
- Observe patient for signs of superinfection, such as diarrhea, vaginal itching, and sore mouth. If present, notify prescriber.

PATIENT TEACHING
- Instruct patient to wash the affected area, rinse with warm water, and gently pat dry before applying erythromycin and benzoyl peroxide gel.
- Teach patient how to thoroughly mix drug in the palm of her hand immediately before each application. Drug comes in a two-compartment foil pouch.
- Tell patient to apply erythromycin and benzoyl peroxide exactly as prescribed and to avoid contact with eyes, inside the nose, mouth, and all mucous membranes.
- Instruct patient to wash hands thoroughly after mixing and applying drug.
- Caution patient not to apply drug near an open flame and to store it away from heat.
- Warn patient not to use any other topical acne preparation unless instructed by prescriber.
- Instruct patient to minimize exposure to sunlight and to take precautions when outdoors, such as wearing a hat and protective clothing and using a sunscreen of SPF 15 or higher.
- Tell patient to report adverse reactions to prescriber, especially severe skin reactions and signs of superinfection, such as diarrhea, vaginal itching, or sore mouth.
- Warn patient that drug may bleach hair or colored fabric.

fluocinolone acetonide 0.01%, hydroquinone 4%, tretinoin 0.05%
Tri-Luma

Class and Category
Chemical: Florinated corticosteroid (fluocinolone), benzoquinone (hydroquinone), retinoid (tretinoin)
Therapeutic: Anti-inflammatory (fluocinolone), depigmenting agent (hydroquinone), keratolytic (tretinoin)
Pregnancy category: C

Indications and Dosages

▶ *To treat moderate to severe melasma of the face with measures for sun avoidance*

CREAM

Adults. Thin film applied and then gently rubbed into hyperpigmented areas of melasma including about ½ inch of normal-looking skin around each lesion daily, 30 minutes before bedtime.

Mechanism of Action

Absorbed through the skin, fluocinolone binds to intracellular glucocorticoid receptors and suppresses the inflammatory and immune responses by:

• inhibiting neutrophil and monocyte accumulation at the inflammation site and suppressing their phagocytic and bactericidal activity

• stabilizing lysosomal membranes

• suppressing the antigen response of macrophages and helper T cells

• inhibiting synthesis of cellular mediators of the inflammatory response, such as cytokines, interleukins, and prostaglandins

Hydroquinone may interrupt one or more steps in the tyrosine-tyrosinase pathway of melanin synthesis to reduce skin color.

Tretinoin increases the number and activity of fibroblasts in photo-damaged skin, which disperses melanin granules and decreases melanin content to lighten dark spots caused by excessive sun exposure.

Contraindications

Hypersensitivity to fluocinolone, hydroquinone, tretinoin, or their components

Interactions

DRUGS

fluocinolone, hydroquinone and tretinoin

photosensitizers (such as fluoroquinolones, phenothiazines, sulfonamides, tetracyclines, and thiazides): Increased risk of phototoxicity

ACTIVITIES

hair depilatories or waxes; medicated soaps or shampoos; permanent wave solutions; topical products with strong skin-drying effect or high concentrations of alcohol, astringent, spices, or lime: Increased risk of skin dryness or irritation

Adverse Reactions

EENT: Dry mouth

ENDO: Cushing's syndrome, hyperglycemia, hypothalamic-pituitary-adrenal (HPA) axis suppression

SKIN: Acne, allergic contact dermatitis, blistering, burning, crusting, desquamation, dryness, erythema, exogenous ochronosis, hypopigmentation, irritation, localized hyperesthesia or paresthesia, peeling, pruritus, rash, rosacea, swelling, telangiectasia, vesicles

Nursing Considerations

- Monitor patient for HPA axis suppression, especially if using fluocinolone, hydroquinolone, and tretinoin cream with other corticosteroids.
- Contact prescriber if HPA axis suppression is suspected, and prepare patient for ACTH stimulation, morning plasma cortisol, and urine free-cortisol tests, as ordered. If confirmed, expect to withdraw the drug.
- Regularly assess effectiveness of fluocinolone, hydroquinolone, and tretinoin cream in lightening dark spots.
- Discontinue topical fluocinolone, hydroquinolone, and tretinoin and notoify prescriber if serious irritation or a gradual blue-black skin darkening develops at application sites.

PATIENT TEACHING
- Inform patient that results may be seen in as little as 4 weeks, but that drug may need to be used for months or therapy repeated if melasma returns.
- Instruct patient to wash her face with a mild soapless cleanser, pat dry, apply cream to hyperpigmented areas and about ½ inch of normal-looking skin around each lesion, and then lightly and uniformly rub into the skin.
- Tell patient not to cover treated areas with any type of dressing.
- Advise patient to avoid applying excessive amounts of cream to affected areas because doing so may cause marked redness, peeling, or discomfort.
- Caution patient not to get solution into her eyes or on mucous membranes inside her nose or mouth.
- Advise patient to apply a moisturizer after washing her face in the morning, and tell her she may use cosmetics.
- Warn patient to avoid exposing her face to sunlight and ultraviolet light (including sunlamp), to use a daily sunscreen of at least SPF 30, and to wear protective clothing during therapy.
- Tell patient that skin reddening or mild burning sensation may occur. Urge her to notify prescriber if local irritation persists or becomes severe or skin undergoes a gradual blue-black darkening. The drug will need to be discontinued.
- Warn patient that extremes of hot or cold weather may cause discomfort.

• Instruct patient to stop treatment when melasma is resolved.

hydrocortisone acetate 1% and iodoquinol 1%

Hydrocortisone and Iodoquinol 1% Cream, Vytone

Class and Category

Chemical: Glucocorticoid (hydrocortisone), halogenated 8-hydroxyquinoline (iodoquinol)

Therapeutic: Anti-inflammatory (hydrocortisone), antifungal and antibacterial (iodoquinol)

Pregnancy category: C

Indications and Dosages

▶ *To treat chronic and subacute dermatoses*

CREAM

Adults and adolescents. Applied to affected areas t.i.d. or q.i.d.

Mechanism of Action

Absorbed through the skin, hydrocortisone binds to intracellular glucocorticoid receptors and suppresses the inflammatory and immune responses by:

• inhibiting neutrophil and monocyte accumulation at the inflammation site and suppressing their phagocytic and bactericidal activity

• stabilizing lysosomal membranes

• suppressing the antigen response of macrophages and helper T cells

• inhibiting the synthesis of cellular mediators of the inflammatory response, such as cytokines, interleukins, and prostaglandins.

Combined, these actions alleviate inflammation.

   Iodoquinol destroys trace metals on bacterial surfaces essential for bacterial growth. It also has slight antifungal activity, although the exact mechanism is unknown. These actions irradiate underlying bacterial and fungal infections in dermatoses.

Contraindications

Hypersensitivity to hydrocortisone, other corticosteroids, iodoquinol, other 8-hydroxyquinolines, or their components

Adverse Reactions

EENT: Perioral dermatitis

ENDO: Cushing's syndrome, hyperglycemia, hypothalamic-pituitary-adrenal (HPA) axis suppression

SKIN: Allergic contact dermatitis; acneiform eruptions; folliculitis; hypertrichosis; hypopigmentation; localized atrophy, burning, dryness, irritation, maceration, miliaria, pruritus, and striae

Nursing Considerations
• Monitor patient for HPA axis suppression, especially if using topical hydrocortisone and iodoquinol over a large surface, applying occlusive dressings over application sites, or using other corticosteroid products. Also monitor adolescents closely for HPA suppression because they may absorb proportionally larger amounts of drug.
• If HPA suppression is suspected, contact prescriber and prepare patient for ACTH stimulation, morning plasma cortisol, and urine free-cortisol tests, as ordered. If confirmed, expect to withdraw the drug, reduce frequency of application, or substitute a less potent corticosteroid, as prescribed.
• Assess effectiveness of topical hydrocortisone and iodoquinol regularly.
• Notify prescriber and stop topical hydrocortisone and iodoquinol if irritation develops at application sites.
• High iodine content in iodoquinol may alter thyroid function test results; they shouldn't be done until at least 1 month after hydrocortisone and iodoquinol therapy has stopped.

PATIENT TEACHING
• Instruct patient to use topical hydrocortisone and iodoquinol exactly as prescribed.
• Advise patient to keep drug away from her eyes, and remind her that drug is for external use only.
• Tell patient to wash her hands before and after applying drug.
• Instruct patient not to bandage, cover, or wrap affected area unless directed to do so by prescriber.
• Instruct patient to notify prescriber if about local adverse reactions and symptoms that worsen or do not improve.
• Warn patient that cream may alter color of skin and clothing.
• Advise patient to wait at least 1 month before having any thyroid function studies performed.

hydrocortisone acetate 1% and pramoxine hydrochloride 1%
Analpram-HC, Enzone, Epifoam, Pramosone, ProctoCream-HC, ProctoFoam-HC, Zone-A

hydrocortisone acetate 2.5% and pramoxine hydrochloride 1%

Analpram-HC, Enzone, Epifoam, Pramosone, Proctocream HC, ProctoFoam HC, Rectocort HC, Zone-A Forte

Class and Category

Chemical: Glucocortoid (hydrocortisone), unclassified (pramoxine)
Therapeutic: Anti-inflammatory (hydrocortisone), local anesthetic (pramoxine)
Pregnancy category: C

Indications and Dosages

▶ *To relieve inflammation, pruritis, and pain from dermatoses*

CREAM, LOTION, OINTMENT

Adults and children. Thin layer applied to affected area and rubbed in gently t.i.d. or q.i.d.

FOAM

Adults and children. Foam dispensed onto tissue or cloth and gently rubbed into affected area or applicator used to instill foam into the rectum t.i.d. or q.i.d.

Mechanism of Action

Absorbed through the skin, hydrocortisone binds to intracellular glucocorticoid receptors and suppresses the inflammatory and immune responses by:

- inhibiting neutrophil and monocyte accumulation at the inflammation site and suppressing their phagocytic and bactericidal activity
- stabilizing lysosomal membranes
- suppressing the antigen response of macrophages and helper T cells
- inhibiting synthesis of cellular mediators of the inflammatory response, such as cytokines, interleukins, and prostaglandins.

Pramoxine, once absorbed through the skin, provides temporary relief from itching and pain by stabilizing the neuronal membrane of nerve endings it contacts.

Contraindications

Hypersensitivity to hydrocortisone, other corticosteroids, pramoxine or their components

Adverse Reactions

EENT: Perioral dermatitis
ENDO: Cushing's syndrome, hyperglycemia, hypothalamic-pituitary-adrenal (HPA) axis suppression
SKIN: Allergic contact dermatitis; acneiform eruptions; folliculitis;

hypertrichosis; hypopigmentation; localized atrophy, burning, dryness, irritation, maceration, miliaria, pruritus and striae; secondary dermatologic infection

Nursing Considerations

- Monitor patient for HPA axis suppression, especially if using topical hydrocortisone and pramoxine over a large surface, applying occlusive dressings over application sites, or using other corticosteroid products. Also monitor children closely for HPA suppression because they may absorb proportionally larger amounts of drug.
- Contact prescriber if HPA suppression is suspected, and prepare patient for ACTH stimulation, morning plasma cortisol, and urine free-cortisol tests, as ordered. If confirmed, expect to withdraw the drug, reduce frequency of application, or substitute a less potent corticosteroid, as prescribed.
- Assess effectiveness of topical hydrocortisone and pramoxine regularly.
- If irritation develops at application sites, stop topical hydrocortisone and pramoxine and notify prescriber.
- Monitor patient for development of dermatologic infections. If present, notify prescriber and expect to use an appropriate antifungal or antibacterial agent, as prescribed. If infection isn't resolved promptly, expect topical hydrocortisone and pramoxine to be stopped.

PATIENT TEACHING
- Instruct patient to use topical hydrocortisone and pramoxine exactly as prescribed and for no more than 14 days unless instructed by prescriber.
- Advise patient to avoid getting the drug in her eyes, and remind her that drug is for external use only.
- Urge patient to wash her hands before and after applying drug.
- If cream, ointment, or lotion is prescribed, advise patient to use her fingers or a tissue to apply a thin film to the affected area and rub in gently.
- If foam is prescribed, instruct her to shake the container vigorously for 5 to 10 seconds before each use. Tell her to press down on the top several times until foam appears and then dispense it onto a tissue or cloth and gently rub into the affected area. Caution her not to use her fingers to apply the foam and not to inhale its vapors. Tell her to rinse the container and cap after applying the drug.

- If foam is prescribed for rectal use, give patient these instructions: Hold the container upright and gently place the tip of the applicator onto the nose of the container cap. Then pull the applicator plunger past the fill line on the applicator barrel. Holding the container and applicator at eye level, place your index and middle fingers on the arms of the container cap and your thumb beneath container. Support the applicator with your other hand. Prime the container by pressing down firmly on the arms of the cap, and then release. It usually takes one or two pumps for the foam to appear. To fill the applicator, press down firmly on the cap flanges, hold for 1 or 2 seconds, and then release. Wait 5 to 10 seconds to let the foam expand in the applicator. Repeat until the foam reaches the fill line, which may take three or four pumps. Then remove the applicator from the container. Holding the applicator firmly, place your index finger over the plunger. Gently insert the tip of the applicator into your anus. Once it's in place, push the plunger to expel the foam, and then withdraw the applicator. After each use, disassemble the applicator parts, container, and cap, and rinse with warm water.
- Alert patient that foam is flammable, and instruct her not to use it near heat or while smoking.
- Tell patient not to bandage, cover, or wrap affected area unless directed by prescriber. Advise parents of young children not to use tight-fitting diapers or plastic pants if child is being treated in the diapered area.
- Instruct patient to notify prescriber about local adverse reactions and symptoms that worsen or don't improve in 7 days.

lidocaine hydrochloride 3% and hydrocortisone acetate 0.5%

AnaMantle HC, LidaMantle HC

Class and Category

Chemical: Aminoacyamide (lidocaine), glucocorticoid (hydrocortisone)

Therapeutic: Local anesthetic (lidocaine), anti-inflammatory (hydrocortisone)

Pregnancy category: C

Indications and Dosages

▶ *To relieve inflammation, itching, pain and soreness from*

hemorrhoids, anal fissures, pruritus ani, and other anal conditions
CREAM, LOTION
Adults. Thin film applied externally to affected area or 1 applicatorful inserted into rectum b.i.d.

Mechanism of Action
Lidocaine blocks nerve impulses by decreasing the permeability of neuronal membranes to sodium. This action produces local anesthesia.

Hydrocortisone, absorbed through the skin, binds to intracellular glucocorticoid receptors and suppresses inflammatory and immune responses by:
- inhibiting neutrophil and monocyte accumulation at the inflammation site and suppressing their phagocytic and bactericidal activity
- stabilizing lysosomal membranes
- suppressing the antigen response of macrophages and helper T cells
- inhibiting synthesis of cellular mediators of the inflammatory response, such as cytokines, interleukins, and prostaglandins.

Contraindications
Hypersensitivity to lidocaine, other amide anesthetics, hydrocortisone, or their components; presence of tuberculous, fungal, or viral lesions of the skin (herpes simplex, vaccinia, and varicella)

Interactions
DRUGS
lidocaine component
class I antiarrhythmic drugs: Additive and synergistic adverse effects

Adverse Reactions
ENDO: Cushing's syndrome, hyperglycemia, hypothalamic-pituitary-adrenal (HPA) axis suppression
SKIN: Transient blanching, burning, erythema, or stinging at application site

Nursing Considerations
- Use cautiously in patients with impaired liver function, those who are seriously ill or elderly, and those who are taking antiarrhythmic class I drugs.
- Monitor patient for HPA axis suppression, especially if using topical lidocaine and hydrocortisone over a large surface, using for a prolonged period, using occlusive dressings over application sites, or using other corticosteroid products.
- Contact prescriber if HPA suppression is suspected, and prepare patient for ACTH stimulation, morning plasma cortisol, and

urine free cortisol tests, as ordered. If confirmed, expect to withdraw the drug, reduce frequency of application, or substitute a less potent corticosteroid, as prescribed.
- Assess effectiveness of topical lidocaine and hydrocortisone to relieve dermatoses regularly.
- Discontinue use of topical lidocaine and hydrocortisone if irritation develops at application sites and notify prescriber.

PATIENT TEACHING
- Instruct patient to use topical lidocaine and hydrocortisone exactly as prescribed.
- Instruct patient to wash her hands before and after applying drug.
- Instruct patient how to administer lidocaine and hydrocortisone when prescribed for rectal administration. Tell patient, after screwing the applicator tip unto the end of the tube tightly, to squeeze the tube to fill the applicator until a small amount of cream shows and lubricates the end of the tip with cream. Then she should gently insert the applicator tip with attached tube into anal area and continue squeezing the body of the tube as it is moved around the areas of discomfort and lastly around and in the anal opening, if directed to do so by prescriber. Warn patient not to completely insert the applicator and tube into the anus or insert deep into the rectum. When administration is finished, instruct patient to gently remove the applicator and tube from the area and dispose.
- Advise patient to avoid drug contact with her eyes and other mucus membranes such as inside of nose or mouth. If eye contact accidentally occurs, instruct patient to rinse eye immediately with saline or water and protect the eye surface until sensation is restored.
- Tell patient not to bandage, cover or wrap affected area unless directed to do so by prescriber.
- Instruct patient to notify prescriber if any signs of local adverse reactions or infection occurs and if symptoms worsen or do not improve.
- Warn patients with small children that individual tubes are not child resistant and so should be left inside the child-resistant blister unit until ready to use.

lidocaine 2.5% and prilocaine 2.5%
EMLA

Class and Category
Chemical: Acetamide (lidocaine), propanamide (prilocaine)
Therapeutic: Local anesthetics (lidocaine, prilocaine)
Pregnancy category: B

Indications and Dosages
▶ *To provide local analgesia on normal intact skin before minor dermal procedures*

CREAM

Adults and adolescents. 2.5 g (half of 5-g tube) applied at selected site to cover 20 to 25 cm^2 of skin surface at least 1 hour before procedure.

Children ages 7 to 12 weighing more than 20 kg (44 lb). Up to 20 g applied to maximum skin surface of 200 cm^2 for no longer than 4 hr.

Children ages 1 to 7 weighing more than 10 kg (22 lb). Up to 10 g applied to maximum skin surface of 100 cm^2 for no longer than 4 hr.

Children ages 3 months to 12 months weighing more than 5 kg (11 lb). Up to 2 g applied to maximum skin surface of 20 cm^2 for no longer than 4 hr.

Newborns (at least 37 wk gestational age) to age 3 months weighing less than 5 kg. Up to 1 g applied to maximum skin surface of 10 cm^2 for no longer than 1 hr.

▶ *To provide local analgesia on normal intact skin before major dermal procedure*

CREAM

Adults and adolescents. 2 g (slightly less than half of 5-g tube) applied at selected site to cover 10 cm^2 of skin surface at least 2 hr before procedure.

Children ages 7 to 12 weighing more than 20 kg. Up to 20 g applied to maximum skin surface of 200 cm^2 for no longer than 4 hr.

Children ages 1 to 7 weighing more than 10 kg. Up to 10 g applied to maximum skin surface of 100 cm^2 for no longer than 4 hr.

Children ages 3 months to 12 months weighing more than 5 kg. Up to 2 g applied to maximum skin surface of 20 cm^2 for no longer than 4 hr.

Newborns (at least 37 wk gestational age) to age 3 months weighing less than 5 kg. Up to 1 g applied to maximum skin surface of 10 cm^2 for no longer than 1 hr.

▶ *To provide adjunct local analgesia to male genital skin before*

infiltration of local anesthetic
CREAM
Male adults. 1 g/10 cm^2 applied to genital skin 15 minutes before infiltration of local anesthetic.
▶ *To provide local analgesia to female genital mucous membranes*
CREAM
Female adults. 5 to 10 g applied to site for 5 to 10 minutes before procedure or infiltration of local anesthetic.

Mechanism of Action

Lidocaine and prilocaine are released from cream into the epidermal and dermal layers of the skin, where they accumulate in the vicinity of dermal pain receptors and nerve endings. There they inhibit the ionic fluxes needed for initiation and conduction of pain impulses, thus producing local anesthesia.

Contraindications

Congenital or idiopathic methemoglobinemia; hypersensitivity to lidocaine, prilocaine, other local anesthetics of the amide type, or their components; infants under age 12 months who are receiving treatment with methemoglobin-inducing agents

Interactions

DRUGS

lidocaine and prilocaine

acetaminophen, acetanilide, aniline dyes, benzocaine, chloroquine, dapsone, naphthalene, nitrates and nitrites, nitrofurantoin, nitroglycerin, nitroprusside, pamaquine, para-aminosalicylic acid, phenacetin, phenobarbital, phenytoin, primaquine, quinine, sulfonamides: Increased risk for developing methemoglobinemia

Class I antiarrhythmic drugs (such as tocainide and mexiletine): Additive toxic effects and potentially synergistic activity

Adverse Reactions

CNS: Apprehension, confusion, dizziness, drowsiness, euphoria, light-headedness, nervousness, seizures, tremors, unconsciousness
CV: Bradycardia, circulatory collapse, hypotension, shock
EENT: Blurred or double vision, tinnitus
GI: Vomiting
GU: Blistering on foreskin (neonates); burning, edema or erythema of female genital mucous membranes
HEME: Methemoglobinemia
RESP: Bronchospasm, respiratory depression or arrest

SKIN: Alteration of temperature sensation; edema, erythema, pallor, pruritis, purpuric or petechial reactions, rash, or swelling at application site; urticaria
Other: Allergic reaction, angioedema

Nursing Considerations

- Use cautiously in patients who may be more sensitive to absorbed lidocaine and prilocaine, such as those who are acutely ill, debilitated, or elderly; those with a history of drug sensitivities; and those with severe hepatic disease because drug metabolism may be impaired, leading to possibly toxic plasma levels of lidocaine and prilocaine.
- Don't apply more cream or leave it on longer than prescribed because excessive absorption may cause serious adverse reactions, such as methemoglobinemia.
- Wipe off lidocaine and prilocaine cream at the prescribed time, and clean the entire area with an antiseptic solution. Effective skin anesthesia will last at least 1 hour after removal.
- Lidocaine and prilocaine cream shouldn't be used for any condition in which its penetration or migration beyond the tympanic membrane into the middle ear is possible because it may have an ototoxic effect.
- Monitor patients, especially young patients, patients with glucose-6-phosphate dehydrogenase deficiencies, and patients taking drugs linked to drug-induced methemoglobinemia, closely for methemoglobinemia throughout therapy. If suspected, discontinue lidocaine and prilocaine immediately and notify prescriber. Although most patients recover spontaneously after removal of cream, be prepared to give I.V. methylene blue, if needed and prescribed.
- Monitor neonates and infants up to age 3 months for Met-Hb levels before, during, and after application of lidocaine and prilocaine cream, as ordered, provided test results can be obtained quickly.
- **WARNING** Especially when applying cream over large areas and leaving it on longer than 2 hours, monitor patient for systemic adverse effects from drug absorption. Although unlikely, they can be severe and lead to cardiac or respiratory arrest.

PATIENT TEACHING

- Stress importance of applying lidocaine and prilocaine cream carefully and exactly as prescribed.

- Caution patient to avoid getting drug into his eyes. If he does, tell him to immediately wash the affected eye with water or saline solution and protect it until sensation returns.
- Until normal sensation returns, urge patient to avoid inadvertent trauma to the treated area by not scratching, rubbing, or exposing it to extreme hot or cold.
- Advise patient to avoid hazardous activities until CNS effects of drug are known.
- Caution patient or parents to remove drug immediately and to seek emergency medical care if application causes dizziness, excessive sleepiness, or duskiness of face or lips.

mequinol 2% and tretinoin 0.01%
Solage

Class and Category
Chemical: 4-hydroxyanisole (mequinol), retinoid (tretinoin)
Therapeutic: Depigmentor (mequinol, tretinoin)
Pregnancy category: X

Indications and Dosages
▶ *To treat solar lentigines*
SOLUTION
Adults. Applied to affected areas using the applicator tip b.i.d., morning and evening, with at least 8 hr between applications.

Mechanism of Action
Mequinol acts competitively to inhibit formation of melania precursors, which decreases melanin pigmentation in melanocytes and keratinocytes to lighten or irradiate brown spots on the skin caused by prolonged sun exposure.

Tretinoin increases the number and activity of fibroblasts in photo-damaged skin, which disperses melanin granules and decreases melanin content to lighten dark spots on skin.

Contraindications
Hypersensitivity to mequinol, tretinoin, or their components; pregnancy

Interactions
DRUGS
mequinol and tretinoin
photosensitizers (such as fluoroquinolones, phenothiazines, sulfonamides,

tetracyclines, and thiazides): Increased risk of augmented phototoxicity

ACTIVITIES

mequinol and tretinoin

electrolysis; hair depilatories or waxes; medicated soaps or shampoos; permanent wave solutions; topical products with strong skin-drying effect or high concentrations of alcohol, astringents, spices, or lime: Increased risk of skin dryness or irritation

Adverse Reactions

SKIN: Burning sensation, crusting, dermatitis, desquamation, dryness, erythema, halo hypopigmentation, hypopigmentation, irritation, pruritus, rash, stinging, tingling

Nursing Considerations

• Use with extreme caution in patients with eczema because mequinol and tretinoin can be highly irritating when applied to eczematous skin.

• Use mequinol and tretinoin cautiously in patients with a personal or family history of vitiligo because hypopigmentation may occur even in areas not exposed to drug.

• When applying drug, avoid getting solution on surrounding normal-pigmented skin because hypopigmentation may occur.

• Before therapy starts, make sure female patient of childbearing age isn't pregnant. The drug may cause fetal harm.

PATIENT TEACHING

• Warn patient to avoid getting mequinol and tretinoin on surrounding normal-pigmented skin during application and to apply just enough solution to each spot to make it moist.

• Caution patient also to avoid getting drug in her eyes, mouth, paranasal creases, and any mucous membrane. If it does, instruct patient to wash area liberally with water and to notify the prescriber.

• Tell patient to stop applying drug to lesions that have become the same color as surrounding skin.

• Alert patient that drug may need to be used for up to 6 months and that some repigmentation of lesions may occur over time after drug is stopped.

• Tell patient not to shower or bathe the treatment areas for at least 6 hours after applying the drug. If cosmetics are worn, advise patient to wait at least 30 minutes after applying drug before applying cosmetics.

- Explain to patient that using more solution than prescribed will not cause faster or better results and may cause serious adverse reactions.
- Instruct patient to notify prescriber if adverse reactions occur. Dosage frequency or amount applied may need to be decreased or drug may need to be withheld temporarily or permanently.
- Warn female patients of childbearing to use adequate birth control measures during mequinol and tretinoin therapy and to stop the drug and notify the prescriber immediately if pregnancy is suspected.
- Caution patient to wear protective clothing outdoors and to avoid exposing treated areas to sunlight, including sunlamps. If sunburn occurs, instruct patient to notify prescriber and temporarily withhold drug until sunburn is completely gone.
- Alert patient that weather conditions such as wind or cold may be more irritating during mequinol and tretinoin therapy.
- Warn patient that drug solution is flammable; urge her to store it away from heat.
- Advise patient to avoid topical products that contain strong skin-drying effects or high concentrations of alcohol, astringent, spices, or lime; medicated soaps or shampoos; permanent wave solutions; electrolysis; and hair depilatories or waxes during therapy.

neomycin sulfate 0.5%, polymyxin B sulfate, bacitracin zinc, and hydrocortisone acetate 1%

Cortisporin Ointment

Class and Category

Chemical: *Streptomyces fradiae Waksman* derivative (neomycin), *Bacillus polymyxa* derivative (polymyxin B), *Bacillus subtilis* derivative (bacitracin), glucocorticoid (hydrocortisone)
Therapeutic: Antibiotic (neomycin, polymyxin B, bacitracin), anti-inflammatory (hydrocortisone)
Pregnancy category: C

Indications and Dosages

▶ *To treat corticosteroid-responsive dermatoses with secondary infection*
CREAM
Adults. Small quantity applied to affected areas and gently rubbed in, if appropriate, b.i.d. to q.i.d. for no longer than 7 days.

Mechanism of Action

Neomycin is transported into bacterial cells, where it competes with messenger RNA to bind with a specific receptor protein on the 30S ribosomal subunit of DNA. This action causes abnormal, nonfunctioning proteins to form. A lack of functional proteins causes bacterial cells to die.

Polymyxin B binds to cell membrane phospholipids in gram-negative bacteria, increasing cell membrane permeability. Polymyxin B also acts as a cationic detergent, altering the membrane's osmotic barrier and causing essential intracellular metabolites to leak out. Both actions lead to cell death.

Bacitracin interferes with bacterial cell-wall synthesis by binding with isoprenyl pyrophosphate (a lipid-carrying molecule that transports substances out of bacterial cells to help build new cell walls), forming an unusable complex in bacterial cells. This weakens cell walls and causes lysis and death.

Hydrocortisone, absorbed through the skin, binds to intracellular glucocorticoid receptors and suppresses inflammatory and immune responses by:

- inhibiting neutrophil and monocyte accumulation at the inflammation site and suppressing their phagocytic and bactericidal activity
- stabilizing lysosomal membranes
- suppressing the antigen response of macrophages and helper T cells
- inhibiting the synthesis of cellular mediators of the inflammatory response, such as cytokines, interleukins, and prostaglandins.

Contraindications

Hypersensitivity to neomycin, polymyxin B, bacitracin, hydrocortisone, or their components; presence of tuberculous, fungal, or viral lesions of the skin (herpes simplex, vaccinia, and varicella)

Adverse Reactions

EENT: Hearing loss, mouth ulcerations, tinnitus
ENDO: Cushing's syndrome, hyperglycemia, hypothalamic-pituitary-adrenal (HPA) axis suppression
GI: Diarrhea
GU: Nephrotoxicity, vaginitis
SKIN: Allergic contact dermatitis; acneiform eruptions; folliculitis; hypertrichosis; hypopigmentation; localized atrophy, burning, dryness, irritation, maceration, miliaria, pruritus and striae; secondary dermatologic infection

Nursing Considerations

- Because of the neomycin component, ointment shouldn't be used over a wide area of the body or for extended periods of time to avoid nephrotoxicity and ototoxicity. If use is necessary, expect to monitor BUN and serum creatinine levels to assess renal function and patient's hearing before and during topical therapy. If nephrotoxicity or ototoxicity (hearing loss or tinnitus) develops, expect to decrease frequency of dosage or discontinue drug as ordered.

- Watch for HPA axis suppression, especially in patients who use neomycin, polymyxin B, bacitracin, and hydrocortisone ointment for a prolonged period or over a large surface, those who use occlusive dressings over application sites, and those who use other corticosteroid products.
- Contact prescriber if HPA suppression is suspected, and prepare patient for ACTH stimulation, morning plasma cortisol, and urine free-cortisol tests, as ordered. If confirmed, expect to withdraw the drug, reduce frequency of application, or substitute a less potent corticosteroid, as prescribed.
- Assess effectiveness of topical neomycin, polymyxin B, bacitracin, and hydrocortisone regularly.
- If irritation develops at application sites, stop use of topical neomycin, polymyxin B, bacitracin and hydrocortisone and notify prescriber.
- Observe patient for signs of superinfection, such as diarrhea, vaginal itching, and sore mouth. If present, notify prescriber.

PATIENT TEACHING
- Instruct patient to use drug exactly as prescribed and for length of time prescribed.
- Advise patient to avoid getting drug in her eyes, and remind her that drug is for external use only.
- Instruct patient to wash her hands before and after applying drug.
- Instruct patient to notify prescriber if local adverse reactions such as redness, irritation, swelling, or pain persist or increase.
- Tell patient to notify prescriber immediately about diarrhea, mouth sores, or vaginitis, possible early signs of superinfection.

neomycin sulfate 0.5%, polymyxin B sulfate, and hydrocortisone acetate 1%
Cortisporin Cream

Class and Category
Chemical: Streptomyces fradiae Waksman derivative (neomycin), *Bacillus polymyxa* derivative (polymyxin B), glucocorticoid (hydrocortisone)

Therapeutic: Antibiotic (neomycin, polymyxin B), anti-inflammatory (hydrocortisone)
Pregnancy category: C

Indications and Dosages

▶ *To treat corticosteroid-responsive dermatoses with secondary infection*
CREAM
Adults. Small quantity applied to affected areas and gently rubbed in, if appropriate, b.i.d. to q.i.d.

Mechanism of Action

Neomycin is transported into bacterial cells, where it competes with messenger RNA to bind with a specific receptor protein on the 30S ribosomal subunit of DNA. This action causes abnormal, nonfunctioning proteins to form. A lack of functional proteins causes bacterial cells to die.

Polymyxin B binds to cell membrane phospholipids in gram-negative bacteria, increasing the permeability of the cell membrane. Polymyxin B also acts as a cationic detergent, altering the osmotic barrier of the membrane and causing essential intracellular metabolites to leak out. Both actions lead to cell death.

Hydrocortisone, absorbed through the skin, binds to intracellular glucocorticoid receptors and suppresses the inflammatory and immune responses by:
• inhibiting neutrophil and monocyte accumulation at the inflammation site and suppressing their phagocytic and bactericidal activity
• stabilizing lysosomal membranes
• suppressing the antigen response of macrophages and helper T cells
• inhibiting the synthesis of cellular mediators of the inflammatory response, such as cytokines, interleukins, and prostaglandins.

Contraindications

Hypersensitivity to neomycin, polymyxin B or hydrocortisone, and their components; presence of tuberculous, fungal, or viral lesions of the skin (herpes simplex, vaccinia, and varicella)

Adverse Reactions

EENT: Hearing loss, mouth ulcerations, tinnitus
ENDO: Cushing's syndrome, hyperglycemia, hypothalamic-pituitary-adrenal (HPA) axis suppression
GI: Diarrhea
GU: Nephrotoxicity, vaginitis
SKIN: Allergic contact dermatitis; acneiform eruptions; folliculitis; hypertrichosis; hypopigmentation; localized atrophy, burning, dry-

ness, irritation, maceration, miliaria, pruritus and striae; secondary dermatologic infection

Nursing Considerations

- Because of the neomycin component of drug, the cream shouldn't be used over a wide area of the body or for extended periods of time to avoid nephrotoxicity and ototoxicity. If use is necessary, expect to monitor BUN and serum creatinine levels to assess renal function and patient's hearing before and during topical drug therapy. If nephrotoxicity or ototoxicity (hearing loss or tinnitus) develops, expect to decrease frequency of dosage or stop drug, as ordered.
- Watch for HPA axis suppression, especially in patients using neomycin, polymyxin B, and hydrocortisone cream for prolonged period or over a large surface, using occlusive dressings over application sites, or using other corticosteroid products.
- Contact prescriber if HPA suppression is suspected, and prepare patient for ACTH stimulation, morning plasma cortisol, and urine free-cortisol tests, as ordered. If confirmed, expect to withdraw the drug, reduce frequency of application, or substitute a less potent corticosteroid, as prescribed.
- Assess effectiveness of topical neomycin, polymyxin B, and hydrocortisone regularly.
- If irritation develops at application sites, stop drug notify prescriber.
- Observe patient for signs of superinfection, such as diarrhea, vaginal itching, and sore mouth. Notify prescriber, if present.

PATIENT TEACHING
- Instruct patient to use cream exactly as prescribed, for as long as prescribed.
- Advise patient to avoid getting drug in her eyes, and remind her that drug is for external use only.
- Urge patient to wash her hands before and after applying drug.
- Instruct patient to notify prescriber if local adverse reactions such as redness, irritation, swelling, or pain persist or increase.
- Tell patient to notify prescriber immediately about diarrhea, mouth sores, or vaginitis; they may be signs of superinfection.

nystatin and triamcinolone acetonide 0.1%

Mycogen, Mycolog, Mycolog-II, Myconel, Myco-Triacet II, Mytrex, Tri-Statin

Class and Category
Chemical: Amphoteric polyene macrolide (nystatin), glucocorticoid (triamcinolone)
Therapeutic: Antifungal (nystatin), anti-inflammatory (triamcinolone)
Pregnancy category: NR

Indications and Dosages
▶ *To treat skin infection caused by candidiasis*
CREAM, OINTMENT
Adults and children. Applied to affected areas b.i.d., morning and evening.

Mechanism of Action
Nystatin binds to sterols in fungal cell membranes, thereby impairing membrane integrity. As a result, fungal cells lose intracellular potassium and other cellular contents and eventually die.

Triamcinolone, absorbed through the skin, binds to intracellular glucocorticoid receptors and suppresses the inflammatory and immune responses by:
• inhibiting neutrophil and monocyte accumulation at the inflammation site and suppressing their phagocytic and bactericidal activity
• stabilizing lysosomal membranes
• suppressing the antigen response of macrophages and helper T cells
• inhibiting the synthesis of cellular mediators of the inflammatory response, such as cytokines, interleukins, and prostaglandins.

Contraindications
Hypersensitivity to nystatin, triamcinolone, acetonide, other antifungals or steroids, or their components

Adverse Reactions
ENDO: Cushing's syndrome, hyperglycemia, hypothalamic-pituitary-adrenal (HPA) axis suppression
SKIN: Alopecia; blistering; burning; dryness; eruptions resembling acne; excessive discoloring of the skin; excessive hair growth; inflammation around mouth or hair follicles; irritation; itching; peeling; prickly heat; reddish purple lines on skin; secondary infection; severe inflammation, softening, stretching or thinning of skin; stretch marks

Nursing Considerations
• Watch for HPA axis suppression, especially in patients using nystatin and triamcinolone cream or ointment for a prolonged

period or over a large surface, using occlusive dressings over application sites, or using other corticosteroid products because of absorption of triamcinolone.
- Contact prescriber if HPA suppression is suspected, and prepare patient for ACTH stimulation, morning plasma cortisol, and urine free-cortisol tests, as ordered. If confirmed, expect to withdraw the drug, reduce frequency of application or substitute a less potent corticosteroid, as prescribed.
- Assess effectiveness of topical nystatin and triamcinolone regularly.
- Be aware that drug shouldn't be used longer than 25 days.
- If irritation develops at application sites, stop drug and notify prescriber.

PATIENT TEACHING
- Instruct patient to use topical nystatin and triamcinolone cream or ointment exactly as prescribed for length of time prescribed.
- Urge patient to wash her hands before and after applying drug.
- Inform patient that drug shouldn't be used beyond 25 days.
- Advise patient to avoid drug contact with her eyes and remind her that drug is for external use only. Tell her to immediately wash her eye(s) with water and notify prescriber if accidental drug contact occurs with either of her eyes.
- Tell patient or parent not to wrap or bandage the affected areas after applying drug. If patient is being treated in the groin area, advise wearing loose-fitting clothing. Tight-fitting clothing, including diapers or plastic pants for young children, are not recommended because these garments act like airtight dressings and increase the risk of adverse reactions from drug absorption through the skin.
- Instruct patient to notify prescriber if local adverse reactions, such as redness, irritation, swelling, or pain, persist or increase or if condition persists or worsens after 2 to 3 weeks of therapy with nystatin and triamcinolone.

papain and urea 10%
Accuzyme, Ethezyme 830, Gladase, Panafil

Class and Category
Chemical: Carica papaya fruit enzyme (papain), diamide of carbonic acid (urea)
Therapeutic: Debriding agent (papain), denaturant of proteins (urea)

Pregnancy category: NR

Indications and Dosages

▶ *For debridement of necrotic tissue and liquefaction of slough in acute and chronic lesions, such as pressure ulcers, varicose and diabetic ulcers, burns, postoperative wounds, pilonidal cyst wounds, carbuncles, and traumatic or infected wounds*

OINTMENT

Adults. Applied directly to wound and then covered with appropriate dressing once or twice daily.

Mechanism of Action

Papain is the proteolytic enzyme from the fruit of carica papaya, which digests nonviable protein matter when the surrounding pH is 3 to 12.

Urea doubles the action of papain by releasing activators of papain through a solvent action and denaturing nonviable protein matter in lesions. This makes necrotic tissue and slough more susceptible to enzymatic digestion.

Contraindications

Hypersensitivity to papain, urea, or their components

Adverse Reactions

SKIN: Irritation of surrounding area, transient burning on application

Nursing Considerations

- Cleanse wound with prescribed wound cleanser or saline solution before applying drug. Avoid using hydrogen peroxide solution because it may inactivate papain.
- Apply papain and urea ointment directly to wound, cover with an appropriate dressing, and secure the dressing.
- Irrigate the wound at each redressing to remove any accumulation of liquefied necrotic material.
- Avoid contact between drug and the salts of heavy metals, such as lead, silver and mercury, because they can inactivate papain and urea.
- Assess effectiveness of papain and urea regularly.
- If profuse exudate causes skin irritation, increase frequency of dressing changes to reduce discomfort until exudate decreases.

PATIENT TEACHING

- Warn patient that drug may cause a transient burning sensation when applied.

- Show caregiver how to apply papain and urea ointment to wound.
- Teach caregiver how to irrigate wound before reapplying papain and urea ointment. Tell caregiver to use a prescribed cleanser or saline solution to irrigate the wound but not hydrogen peroxide.
- Tell caregiver to keep wound covered with an appropriate dressing between drug applications.

sodium sulfacetamide 10% and sulfur 5%

Rosac Cream, Rosula, Zetacet

Class and Category

Chemical: Sulfonamide (sodium sulfacetamide), nonmetal element (sulfur)

Therapeutic: Antiacne and antibacterial (sodium sulfacetamide), antiacne and keratolytic (sulfur)

Pregnancy category: C

Indications and Dosages

▶ *To treat acne vulgaris, acne rosacea, and seborrheic dermatitis*

CREAM, GEL, LOTION, TOPICAL SUSPENSION

Adults and adolescents. Thin film applied to affected areas once daily to t.i.d.

ACQUEOUS CLEANSER, WASH

Adults and adolescents. Applied to affected areas after wetting skin, massaging into skin gently for 10 to 20 seconds to work into a full lather, and then rinsed off thoroughly and skin patted dry once daily or b.i.d.

Mechanism of Action

Sodium sulfacetamide acts as a competitive antagonist to para-aminobenzoic acid (PABA), which is an essential component in bacterial growth. By disrupting bacterial ability to grow, symptoms of acne, such as pus formation and inflammation, improve.

Sulfur is thought to inhibit growth of *Propionibacerium acnes* and formation of fatty acids through unknown mechanisms that help relieve plugging and rupturing of follicles. By easing the evacuation of comedones and promoting peeling of the skin, it helps eradicate the symptoms of acne and dermatitis.

Contraindications

Hypersensitivity to sodium sulfacetamide, other sulfonamides, sulfur or their components, renal disease

Adverse Reactions

HEME: Acute hemolytic anemia, agranulocytosis, purpura hemorrhagica
SKIN: Contact dermatitis, dry skin, erythema, jaundice, scaling of epidermis
Other: Drug fever

Nursing Considerations

- Observe patient closely for local irritation, such as contact dermatitis or sensitization, during long-term therapy. Notify prescriber and expect to stop therapy.
- **WARNING** Monitor patient for systemic hypersensitivity reactions, such as acute hemolytic anemia, agranulocytosis, and purpura hemorrhagica, especially if applying drug to denuded or abraded skin. Although rare, these toxic reactions may occur because sodium sulfacetamide can induce toxic hypersensitivity reactions in susceptible patients after being absorbed.

PATIENT TEACHING

- Instruct patient to wash the affected area, rinse with warm water, and pat gently dry before applying sodium sulfacetamide and sulfur cream, lotion, or topical suspension.
- If lotion form is prescribed, tell patient to shake container well before using and to lightly massage into skin.
- If wash is prescribed, tell patient to wet application site and apply wash liberally, gently massaging it into skin for 10 to 20 seconds to work into a full lather, and then to rinse the area thoroughly and pat it dry. If dryness occurs at application site, urge him to notify prescriber; rinsing wash off more quickly or using it less often may control the dryness.
- Tell patient to apply drug exactly as prescribed and to avoid getting it in eyes, nose, mouth, and all mucous membranes.

sodium thiosulfate and salicylic acid

Versiclear

Class and Category

Chemical: Sulfate derivative (sodium thiosulfate), salicylate (salicylic acid)

Therapeutic: Antiacne and antifungal (sodium thiosulfate), antiacne and keratolytic (salicylic acid)
Pregnancy category: C

Indications and Dosages

▶ *To treat tinea versicolor (*Malassezia furfur *infection)*
LOTION
Adults. Thin film of lotion applied to affected and susceptible ar-
eas b.i.d.

Mechanism of Action

Sodium thiosulfate damages fungal cells by interfering with a cytochrome
P-450 enzyme needed to convert lanosterol to ergosterol, an essential part of
the fungal cell membrane. Decreased ergosterol synthesis causes increased
cell permeability, which allows cell contents to leak. Sodium thiosulfate also
may lead to fungal cell death by inhibiting fungal respiration under aerobic
conditions. Removing fungal activity alleviates source of acne formation.

   Salicylic acid softens and destroys the stratum corneum by increasing endogenous hydration, probably because of decreased pH, which causes the
cornified epithelium of the skin to swell, soften, and then desquamate. Maceration and desquamation of epidermal tissue reduces the number and
severity of acne lesions.

Contraindications

Hypersensitivity to sodium thiosulfate, salicylic acid or their components

Adverse Reactions

SKIN: Dry or peeling skin, erythema, pruritus

Nursing Considerations

• Monitor effectiveness of sodium thiosulfate and salicylic acid
  therapy to reduce number and severity of acne lesions.
• Notify prescriber if local skin reactions develop; drug may need
  to be stopped.
PATIENT TEACHING
• Tell patient to thoroughly wash, rinse, and dry affected and susceptible areas before applying sodium thiosulfate and salicylic
  acid.
• Caution patient to avoid getting drug on or around eye area.
• To prevent relapse, stress importance of using drug exactly as
  prescribed and not stopping, even after acne improves, until directed by prescriber.

trypsin and balsam peru
Granulderm, Granulex

Class and Category
Chemical: Enzyme (trypsin), *Myroxolon balsamum* derivative (balsam peru)
Therapeutic: Debriding agent (trypsin), circulatory stimulant, odor reducer (balsam peru)
Pregnancy category: NR

Indications and Dosages
▶ *To promote wound healing of varicose ulcers, dehiscent wounds, and decubital ulcers; to promote debridement of eschar; to reduce odor from necrotic wounds*
AEROSOL
Adults. Sprayed rapidly, holding can about 12 inches from affected areas to coat wound completely b.i.d.

Mechanism of Action
Trypsin promotes wound healing by stimulating the vascular bed and improving epithelization by reducing premature epithelial desiccation and cornification. It also digests nonviable protein matter.

Balsam peru stimulates the capillary bed to increase circulation to the wound site, which promotes healing. Its vanilla scent helps to lessen odor from necrotic wounds.

Contraindications
Hypersensitivity to trypsin, balsam peru, or their components; use on fresh arterial clots

Adverse Reactions
SKIN: Transient stinging at application site

Nursing Considerations
• Shake can well before spraying. Hold can upright, about 12 inches from affected area, and spray to cover wound rapidly with trypsin and balsam peru.
• Leave wound unbandaged or apply a wet dressing, as ordered.
• Before reapplication, wash area gently with water to remove residual drug.
• Evaluate effectiveness of drug regularly.
PATIENT TEACHING
• Warn patient that drug may cause temporary stinging when applied to a sensitive area.

- Teach patient or caregiver how to administer drug. Tell him to avoid getting drug in eyes. If it does, tell patient to wash his eyes with water immediately and to notify prescriber.
- Warn patient or caregiver that drug is flammable and should be kept away from fire or open flame.
- Instruct patient or caregiver not to puncture or incinerate the can because it could explode.

alendronate sodium and cholecalciferol

Fosamax Plus D

Class and Category

Chemical: Bisphosphonate (alendronate), vitamin D analogue (cholecalciferol)

Therapeutic: Antiosteoporotic (alendronate), antihypocalcemic (cholecalciferol)

Pregnancy category: C

Indications and Dosages

▶ *To treat postmenopausal osteoporosis; to increase bone mass in men with osteoporosis*

TABLETS

Adults. 70 mg alendronate and 2,800 international units cholecalciferol (1 tablet) q wk.

Mechanism of Action

Alendronate binds to bone hydroxyapatite and reduces the activity of cells that cause bone loss, slows the rate of bone loss after menopause, and increases the amount of bone mass. It may act by inhibiting osteoclast activity on newly formed bone resorption surfaces, which reduces the number of sites where bone is remodeled. Bone formation then exceeds bone resorption at these remodeling sites, and bone mass gradually increases.

Cholecalciferol is the natural precursor of the calcium-regulating hormone calcitriol and is converted to calcitriol in the kidneys under the influence of parathyroid hormone and hypophosphatemia. Calcitriol binds to specific receptors in the intestinal mucosa to increase intestinal absorption of calcium and phosphate and to regulate serum calcium, renal excretion of calcium and phosphate, bone formation, and bone resorption.

Contraindications

Esophageal abnormalities that delay esophageal emptying, such as stricture or achalasia; hypersensitivity to alendronate, cholecalciferol, or their components; hypocalcemia; inability to stand or sit upright for at least 30 minutes

Interactions

DRUGS

alendronate and cholecalciferol

estrogen-progestin combinations: Increased suppression of bone turnover, enhancing effectiveness of alendronate and cholecalciferol

alendronate component

antacids, calcium, iron, multivalent cations: Decreased alendronate absorption

aspirin: Increased risk of GI distress

rantidine (I.V. form): Doubled alendronate bioavailability

cholecalciferol component

anticonvulsants, cimetidine, thiazide diuretics: Increased vitamin D catabolism

cholestyramine, colestipol, mineral oil, olestra, orlistat: Decreased calcitriol absorption

FOODS

alendronate component

any food: Delayed absorption and decreased serum level of alendronate

Adverse Reactions

CNS: Headache

EENT: Episcleritis, localized osteonecrosis of the jaw, oropharyngeal ulceration, scleritis, uveitis

GI: Abdominal distention and pain, constipation, diarrhea, dysphagia, esophageal perforation or ulceration, esophagitis, fever, flatulence, gastric or duodenal ulcers, gastritis, heartburn, indigestion, malaise, melena, nausea, vomiting

MS: Arthralgia; bone, joint, and muscle pain; focal osteomalacia; muscle spasms; myalgia

SKIN: Photosensitivity, pruritus, rash, Stevens-Johnson syndrome, toxic epidermal necrolysis

Other: Angioedema, hypocalcemia

Nursing Considerations

• Be aware that alendronate and cholecalciferol therapy isn't recommended for patients with renal insufficiency and a creatinine clearance less than 35 ml/minute.

- Use alendronate and cholecalciferol cautiously in patients with active upper GI problems such as dysphagia, esophageal diseases, gastritis, duodenitis, or ulcers.
- Monitor serum calcium level before, during, and after treatment. If patient has hypocalcemia or vitamin D deficiency, expect prescriber to order a calcium supplement and vitamin D replacement before therapy begins.
- Monitor serum calcium level, as ordered, and patient for signs and symptoms of hypocalcemia. If present, withhold alendronate and cholecalciferol therapy and notify prescriber.
- Ensure adequate dietary intake of calcium and vitamin D before, during, and after treatment.
- Be aware that alendronate and cholecalciferol shouldn't be used alone to treat vitamin D deficiency. Patients at risk for vitamin D deficiency (such as those who are homebound, chronically ill or over age 70) also should receive vitamin D supplementation, as ordered.
- Expect to give higher doses of vitamin D supplement and to measure 25-hydroxyvitamin D level, as ordered, in patients with GI malabsorption syndromes who receive alendronate and cholecalciferol.
- Check to determine if patient has had a dental examination before starting alendronate and cholecalciferol therapy, especially if patient has cancer; is receiving chemotherapy, head or neck radiation, or corticosteroids; or has poor oral hygiene. The risk of osteonecrosis is higher in these patients and invasive dental procedures and alendronate can worsen osteonecrosis.
- **WARNING** Alendronate may irritate upper GI mucosa, causing such adverse reactions as esophageal ulceration. To help minimize these reactions, have patient take drug with a full glass of water and remain upright for at least 30 minutes.
- If patient receives long-term alendronate and cholecalciferol therapy, be alert for vitamin D toxicity. Early signs and symptoms include bone pain, constipation, dry mouth, headache, metallic taste, myalgia, nausea, somnolence, vomiting, and weakness. Late signs and symptoms include albuminuria, anorexia, arrhythmias, azotemia, conjunctivitis, decreased libido, elevated AST and ALT levels, elevated BUN level, generalized vascular calcification, hypercholesterolemia, hypertension, hyperthermia, irritability, mild acidosis, nephrocalcinosis, nocturia, pancreatitis, photophobia, polydipsia, polyuria, pruritus, rhinorrhea, and weight loss.

PATIENT TEACHING
- Advise patient to take alendronate and cholecaliferol in the morning with a full glass of water. Explain that such beverages as orange juice, coffee, and mineral water reduce alendronate's effects.
- To help reduce esophageal irritation, tell patient not to chew or suck on tablet.
- Instruct patient to wait at least 30 minutes after taking alendronate to eat, drink, or take other drugs. Teach patient to remain upright for 30 minutes after taking alendronate and cholecaliferol and until he has eaten the first food of the day.
- Advise patient that if he misses a dose, he should take 1 tablet on the morning after he remembers and then return to his originally scheduled weekly dose. Tell him never to take 2 tablets on the same day.
- Tell patient to stop taking alendronate and cholecaliferol and to notify prescriber if he develops difficulty swallowing or talking, retrosternal pain, or new or worsening heartburn.
- Warn patient not to take other forms of vitamin D while taking alendronate and cholecalciferol unless otherwise prescribed.
- Advise patient to notify prescriber immediately if he develops evidence of vitamin D toxicity, such as headache, irritability, nausea, photophobia, vomiting, weakness, and weight loss.
- Instruct patient on proper oral hygiene and to notify prescriber before having any invasive dental procedure performed.

17 beta-estradiol and norgestimate

Prefest

Class and Category

Chemical: Estrogen steroid hormone derivative (17 beta-estradiol), progesterone derivative (norgestimate)
Therapeutic: Antiosteoporotic, ovarian hormone replacement (17 beta-estradiol, norgestimate)
Pregnancy category: X

Indications and Dosages

▶ *To treat menopausal symptoms and vaginal and vulvar atrophy in postmenopausal women with an intact uterus; to prevent osteoporosis from estrogen deficiency in postmenopausal women with an intact uterus*
TABLETS
Adult females. 1 mg 17 beta-estradiol (1 tablet) daily for 3 days

followed by 1 mg 17 beta-estradiol and 0.09 mg norgestimate
(1 tablet) for 3 days. Cycle repeated continuously.

Mechanism of Action

Estrogens such as 17 beta-estradiol increase the rate of DNA and RNA synthesis in the cells of female reproductive organs, pituitary gland, hypothalamus, and other target organs. In the hypothalamus, estrogens decrease release of gonadotropin-releasing hormone, which reduces pituitary release of
follicle-stimulating hormone and luteinizing hormone. In women, these hormones are needed for normal GU and other essential body functions. At the
cellular level, estrogens increase cervical secretions, cause endometrial cell
proliferation, and improve uterine tone. Estrogen replacement helps maintain
GU function and reduces vasomotor symptoms when estrogen production declines from menopause, surgical removal of ovaries, or other estrogen deficiency. Estrogen replacement also helps prevent osteoporosis by inhibiting
bone resorption.

Progestins such as norgestimate prolong some positive effects of estrogens
on HDL cholesterol. Norgestimate diffuses freely into target cells of the female reproductive tract, mammary glands, hypothalamus, and pituitary gland
and binds to the progesterone cell receptor. It converts a proliferative endometrium into a secretory one in women with adequate estrogen replacement,
reducing endometrial growth and the risk of endometrial cancer compared
with women who have an intact uterus and take unopposed estrogens.
Norgestimate also decreases nuclear estradiol receptors and suppresses epithelial DNA synthesis in endometrial tissues.

Contraindications

Active thrombophlebitis or thromboembolic disorders; hepatic disorders; hypersensitivity to 17 beta-estradiol, norgestimate, or their
components; jaundice; known or suspected breast cancer or history of breast cancer from estrogen use; known or suspected
estrogen-dependent cancer; pregnancy; undiagnosed abnormal
genital bleeding; vaginal disorders

Interactions

DRUGS

17 beta-estradiol and norgestimate

corticosteroids: Increased therapeutic and toxic effects of corticosteroids

cyclosporine: Increased risk of hepatotoxicity and nephrotoxicity

hepatotoxic drugs, such as isoniazid: Increased risk of hepatitis and
hepatotoxicity

oral antidiabetics: Decreased therapeutic effects of these drugs
thyroid hormones: Decreased effectiveness of thyroid hormones
warfarin: Altered anticoagulant effect

FOODS

17 beta-estradiol component

grapefruit juice: Decreased metabolism and possibly increased adverse effects of 17 beta-estradiol

ACTIVITIES

17 beta-estradiol and norgestimate

smoking: Increased risk of CVA, pulmonary embolism, thrombophlebitis, and transient ischemic attack

Adverse Reactions

CNS: Chorea, CVA, dementia, depression, dizziness, exacerbation of epilepsy, headache, irritability, migraine headache, mood disturbances, nervousness, porphyria

CV: Hypertension, increased triglycerides, MI, peripheral edema, pulmonary embolism, thromboembolism, thrombophlebitis

EENT: Diplopia, intolerance of contact lenses, retinal vascular thrombosis, sinusitis, vision changes or loss

ENDO: Breast enlargement, pain, tenderness, or tumors; endometrial hyperplasia, galactorrhea; gynecomastia; hyperglycemia; nipple discharge

GI: Abdominal cramps or pain, aggravation of hepatic porphyria, anorexia, bloating, constipation, diarrhea, elevated liver function test results, enlargement of hepatic hemangiomas, flatulence, gallbladder obstruction, hepatitis, increased appetite, nausea, pancreatitis, vomiting

GU: Amenorrhea, breakthrough bleeding, cervical erosion, clear vaginal discharge, dysmenorrhea, endometiral or ovarian tumors, increased libido, increased size of uterine leiomyomata, leukorrhea, prolonged or heavy menstrual bleeding, urinary tract infection, vaginitis including vaginal candidiasis

MS: Arthralgias, back or extremity pain, leg cramps

RESP: Bronchitis, exacerbation of asthma, upper respiratory infection

SKIN: Alopecia, application site irritation, chloasma, erythema multiforme or nodosum, hirsutism, jaundice, melasma, pruritus, purpura, rash, urticaria

Other: Anaphylaxis, angioedema, flulike syndrome, folic acid deficiency, hypercalcemia (with bone metastases), hypocalcemia, hyperkalemia, hyponatremia, weight gain or loss

Nursing Considerations

- Use 17 beta-estradiol and norgestimate cautiously in women with asthma, diabetes mellitus, epilepsy, migraine headaches, porphyria, systemic lupus erythematosus, or hepatic hemangiomas because estradiol can worsen these conditions.
- Verify that patient has an intact uterus before starting 17 beta-estradiol and norgestimate therapy. If not, patient doesn't need a product that contains a progestin, such as norgestimate.
- **WARNING** Assess patient for possible contact lens intolerance or changes in vision or visual acuity because estrogens can cause keratoconus. Be prepared to stop therapy immediately, as prescribed, if patient has sudden partial or complete loss of vision or sudden onset of diplopia or migraine.
- Monitor PT in patients taking warfarin. Estrogens such as 17 beta-estradiol increase production of clotting factors VII, VIII, IX, and X and promote platelet aggregation and thus may lead to loss of anticoagulant effect.
- Monitor patient for elevated liver function test results because estrogens and progestins such as 17 beta-estradiol and norgestimate may worsen such conditions as acute intermittent or variegate hepatic porphyria.
- Closely monitor patient's blood pressure. Some patients may have a substantial increase in blood pressure as an indiosyncratic reaction to estrogens such as 17 beta-estradiol. Monitor patients who already have hypertension for increases in blood pressure because estrogens may cause fluid retention. Also monitor patients with asthma, heart disease, migraines, renal disease, or seizure disorder for worsening of these conditions.
- Monitor blood glucose level often in patients who have diabetes mellitus because 17 beta-estradiol may decrease insulin sensitivity and alter glucose tolerance.
- **WARNING** Expect to stop 17 beta-estradiol and norgestimate therapy in any woman who develops signs or symptoms of dementia or cardiovascular disease, such as CVA, MI, pulmonary embolism, or venous thrombosis.
- Be aware that 17 beta-estradiol and norgestimate may worsen mood disorders, including depression. Monitor patient for depression, mood changes, anxiety, fatigue, dizziness, or insomnia.
- **WARNING** Be aware that patients with bone metastasis from breast cancer may develop severe hypercalcemia because estrogens such as 17 beta-estradiol influence calcium and phosphorus metabolism. Watch for toxic effects of increased cal-

cium absorption in patients predisposed to hypercalcemia or nephrolithiasis.

• Assess patient's skin for melasma (tan or brown patches), which may develop on forehead, cheeks, temples, and upper lip. These patches may persist after drug is stopped.

• Monitor thyroid function test results in patients with hypothyroidism because long-term use of 17 beta-estradiol may decrease effectiveness of thyroid therapy.

• Expect to stop 17 beta-estradiol and norgestimate therapy several weeks before patient undergoes major surgery, as prescribed, because prolonged immobilization poses a risk of thromboembolism.

PATIENT TEACHING

• Before therapy starts, inform patient of risks involved in taking 17 beta-estradiol and norgestimate therapy, such as increased risk of cardiovascular disease, breast or endometrial cancer, dementia, gallbladder disease, and vision abnormalities.

• Urge patient to notify prescriber immediately if vaginal bleeding or any other abnormal signs and symptoms occur while taking 17 beta-estradiol and norgestimate.

• Advise patient to avoid smoking while taking an estrogen-progestin product such as 17 beta-estradiol and norgestimate.

• Stress importance of having follow-up visits every 3 to 6 months to determine effectiveness of 17 beta-estradiol and norgestimate in relieving menopausal symptoms and osteoporosis. Also stress importance of having scheduled diagnostic tests to detect adverse reactions.

• Emphasize importance of good dental hygiene and regular dental checkups because an elevated progestin (norgestimate) blood level increases growth of normal oral flora, which may lead to gum tenderness, bleeding, or swelling.

drospirenone and estradiol
Angeliq

Class and Category
Chemical: Synthetic progestin and spironolactone analogue (drospirenone), estrogenic steroid hormone derivative (estradiol)
Therapeutic: Ovarian hormone replacement (drospirenone and estradiol)
Pregnancy category: X

Indications and Dosages

▶ *To treat moderate to severe vasomotor symptoms of menopause; to treat moderate to severe vulvar and vaginal atrophy in menopause*

TABLETS

Adult females. 0.5 mg drospirenone and 1 mg estradiol (1 tablet) daily.

Mechanism of Action

Drospirenone counters estrogenic effects in menopause by decreasing the number of nuclear estradiol receptors and suppressing epithelial DNA synthesis in endometrial tissue. It also is an aldosterone antagonist, which increases excretion of sodium and water.

Estradiol increases the rate of DNA and RNA synthesis in the cells of female reproductive organs, pituitary gland, hypothalamus, and other target organs. In the hypothalamus, estrogens reduce the release of gonadotropin-releasing hormone, which decreases pituitary release of follicle-stimulating hormone and luteinizing hormone. In women, these hormones are required for normal GU and other essential body functions. At the cellular level, estrogens increase cervical secretions, cause endometrial cell proliferation, and improve uterine tone. Estrogen replacement helps maintain GU function and reduces vasomotor symptoms when estrogen production declines from menopause, surgical removal of ovaries, or other estrogen deficiency.

Contraindications

Active deep vein thrombosis, pulmonary embolism, or history of these conditions; adrenal insufficiency; hepatic disorders; hypersensitivity to drospirenone, estradiol, or their components; known or suspected breast cancer or history of breast cancer from estrogen use; known or suspected estrogen-dependent cancer; new or recent (within past year) CVA or MI; hysterectomy; pregnancy; renal insufficiency; undiagnosed abnormal genital bleeding

Interactions

DRUGS

drospirenone component

ACE inhibitors, angiotensin receptor blockers, heparin, NSAIDs, potassium-sparing diuretics, potassium supplements: Increased risk of hyperkalemia

estradiol component

barbiturates, carbamazepine, hydantoins, rifabutin, rifampin: Possibly reduced activity of estradiol

corticosteroids: Increased therapeutic and toxic effects of corticosteroids

cyclosporine: Increased risk of hepatotoxicity and nephrotoxicity

didanosine, lamivudine, zalcitabine: Possibly pancreatitis

clarithromycin, erythromycin, itraconazole, ketoconazole, ritonivir: Decreased metabolism and possible increased adverse effects of estradiol

hepatotoxic drugs (such as isoniazid): Increased risk of hepatitis and hepatotoxicity

oral antidiabetics: Decreased therapeutic effects of these drugs

warfarin: Decreased or increased anticoagulant effect

FOODS

estradiol component

grapefruit juice: Decreased metabolism and possibly increased adverse effects of estradiol

ACTIVITIES

estradiol component

smoking: Increased risk of CVA, pulmonary embolism, thrombophlebitis, and transient ischemic attack

Adverse Reactions

CNS: Chorea, CVA, dementia, depression, dizziness, exacerbation of epilepsy, headache, irritability, migraine headache, mood disturbances, nervousness, porphyria

CV: Hypertension, increased triglycerides, MI, peripheral edema, pulmonary embolism, thromboembolism, thrombophlebitis

EENT: Diplopia, intolerance of contact lenses, retinal vascular thrombosis, sinusitis, vision changes or loss

ENDO: Breast enlargement, pain, tenderness, or tumors; endometrial hyperplasia, galactorrhea; gynecomastia; hyperglycemia; nipple discharge

GI: Abdominal cramps or pain, anorexia, bloating, constipation, diarrhea, elevated liver function test results, enlargement of hepatic hemangiomas, gallbladder obstruction, hepatitis, increased appetite, nausea, pancreatitis, vomiting

GU: Amenorrhea, breakthrough bleeding, cervical erosion, clear vaginal discharge, dysmenorrhea, endometiral or ovarian tumors, increased libido, leukorrhea, prolonged or heavy menstrual bleeding, vaginal candidiasis

MS: Arthralgias, back or extremity pain, leg cramps

RESP: Exacerbation of asthma, upper respiratory infection

SKIN: Alopecia, chloasma, erythema multiforme or nodosum, hirsutism, jaundice, melasma, pruritus, purpura, rash, urticaria

Other: Anaphylaxis, angioedema, flulike syndrome, folic acid deficiency, hypercalcemia (with bone metastases), hypocalcemia, hyperkalemia, hyponatremia, weight gain or loss

Nursing Considerations

- Use drospirenone and estradiol cautiously in women with asthma, diabetes mellitus, epilepsy, migraine headaches, porphyria, systemic lupus erythematosus, and hepatic hemangiomas because estrogens may worsen these conditions.
- Give drospirenone and estradiol with or immediately after food to decrease nausea.
- **WARNING** Assess patient for possible contact lens intolerance or changes in vision or visual acuity because estrogens can cause keratoconus. Be prepared to stop therapy immediately, as prescribed, if patient has sudden partial or complete loss of vision or sudden onset of diplopia or migraine.
- Monitor PT in patients taking warfarin. Estrogens increase production of clotting factors VII, VIII, IX, and X and promote platelet aggregation and thus may cause loss of anticoagulant effect.
- Monitor patient for elevated liver function test results because estrogens and progestins may worsen such conditions as acute intermittent or variegate hepatic porphyria.
- Monitor patient's electrolyte levels as ordered, especially early in therapy, because drospirenone has antialdosterone activity, which may increase serum potassium and decrease serum sodium levels in high-risk patients.
- Closely monitor patient's blood pressure. Some patients may have a substantial increase in blood pressure as an indiosyncratic reaction to estrogen. Monitor patients who already have hypertension for increased blood pressure because estrogens may cause fluid retention. Also monitor patients with asthma, heart disease, migraines, renal disease, or seizure disorder for exacerbation of these conditions.
- Monitor blood glucose level often in patients who have diabetes mellitus because estrogens may decrease insulin sensitivity and alter glucose tolerance.
- Expect to stop drospirenone and estradiol in any woman who develops signs or symptoms of cardiovascular disease, such as CVA, MI, pulmonary embolism, or venous thrombosis.
- Be aware that drospirenone and estradiol may worsen mood disorders, including depression. Monitor patient for depression, mood changes, anxiety, fatigue, dizziness, or insomnia.

- **WARNING** Be aware that patients with breast cancer and bone metastasis may develop severe hypercalcemia because estrogens influence calcium and phosphorus metabolism. Watch for toxic effects of increased calcium absorption in patients predisposed to hypercalcemia or nephrolithiasis.
- Assess skin for melasma (tan or brown patches), which may develop on forehead, cheeks, temples, and upper lip. These patches may persist after drug is stopped.
- Monitor thyroid function test results in patients with hypothyroidism because long-term use of estradiol may decrease effectiveness of thyroid therapy.
- Expect to stop drospirenone and estradiol therapy several weeks before patient undergoes major surgery, as prescribed, because prolonged immobilization poses a risk of thromboembolism.

PATIENT TEACHING

- Before therapy starts, inform patient of the risks of estrogen-progestin therapy, such as increased risk of cardiovascular disease, breast or endometrial cancer, dementia, gallbladder disease, and vision abnormalities.
- Inform patient that a cyclic regimen of drospirenone and estradiol may cause monthly withdrawal bleeding.
- Instruct patient to avoid eating large quantities of foods high in potassium (such as bananas, oranges, or spinach) or using salt substitutes that contain potassium.
- Instruct patient to report any abnormal signs and symptoms to prescriber.
- Stress importance of having follow-up visits every 3 to 6 months to determine effectiveness of drospirenone and estradiol in relieving menopausal symptoms and having scheduled diagnostic tests to detect adverse reactions.

estradiol and levonorgestrel

Climara Pro

Class and Category

Chemical: Estrogenic steroid hormone derivative (estradiol), progesterone steroid hormone derivative (levonorgestrel),
Therapeutic: Ovarian hormone replacement (estradiol, levonorgestrel)
Pregnancy category: X

Indications and Dosages

▶ *To treat moderate to severe vasomotor symptoms of menopause in women who have an intact uterus*

PATCH

Adult females. 1 patch (4.4 mg estradiol and 1.39 mg levonorgestrel) applied weekly to lower abdomen, which delivers 0.045 mg estradiol and 0.015 mg levonorgestrel daily.

Mechanism of Action

Estrogens like estradiol increases the rate of DNA and RNA synthesis in the cells of female reproductive organs, pituitary gland, hypothalamus, and other target organs. In the hypothalamus, estrogens reduce the release of gonadotropin-releasing hormone, which decreases pituitary release of follicle-stimulating hormone and luteinizing hormone. In women, these hormones are required for normal GU and other essential body functions. At the cellular level, estrogens increase cervical secretions, cause endometrial cell proliferation, and improve uterine tone. Estrogen replacement helps maintain GU function and reduces vasomotor symptoms when estrogen production declines as a result of menopause, surgical removal of ovaries, or other estrogen deficiency states.

Levonorgestrel inhibits gonadotropin production resulting in retardation of follicular growth and inhibition of ovulation. It also counteracts the proliferative effects of estrogens on the endometrium.

Contraindications

Active deep vein thrombosis, pulmonary embolism, or history of these conditions; adrenal insufficiency; hepatic disorders; hypersensitivity to estradiol, levonorgestrel, or their components; known or suspected breast cancer or history of breast cancer from estrogen use; known or suspected estrogen-dependent cancer, new or recent (within past year) CVA or MI; hysterectomy; pregnancy; renal insufficiency; undiagnosed abnormal genital bleeding

Interactions

DRUGS

estradiol and levonorgestrel

barbiturates, carbamazepine, phenytoin, rifabutin, rifampin: Possibly reduced activity of estradiol and levonorgestrel

estradiol component

corticosteroids: Increased therapeutic and toxic effects of corticosteroids

hepatotoxic drugs (such as isoniazid): Increased risk of hepatitis and hepatotoxicity
oral antidiabetics: Decreased therapeutic effects of these drugs
warfarin: Decreased anticoagulant effect
FOODS
estradiol component
grapefruit juice: Decreased metabolism and possibly increased adverse effects of estradiol
ACTIVITIES
estradiol component
smoking: Increased risk of CVA, pulmonary embolism, thrombophlebitis, and transient ischemic attack

Adverse Reactions

CNS: Chorea, CVA, dementia, depression, dizziness, exacerbation of epilepsy, headache, irritability, migraine headache, mood disturbances, nervousness, porphyria
CV: Hypertension, increased triglycerides, MI, peripheral edema, pulmonary embolism, thromboembolism, thrombophlebitis
EENT: Diplopia, intolerance of contact lenses, retinal vascular thrombosis, sinusitis, vision changes or loss
ENDO: Breast enlargement, pain, tenderness, or tumors; endometrial hyperplasia, fibrocystic breast changes; galactorrhea; hyperglycemia; nipple discharge
GI: Abdominal cramps or pain, aggravation of porphyria, anorexia, bloating, cholestatic jaundice, constipation, diarrhea, elevated liver function test results, enlargement of hepatic hemangiomas, flatulence, gallbladder obstruction, hepatitis, increased appetite or incidence of gallbladder disease, nausea, pancreatitis, vomiting
GU: Amenorrhea, breakthrough bleeding, cervical erosion, clear vaginal discharge, dysmenorrhea, endometiral or ovarian tumors, increased libido, increased size of uterine leiomyomata, leukorrhea, prolonged or heavy menstrual bleeding, urinary tract infection, vaginitis including vaginal candidiasis
MS: Arthralgias, back or extremity pain, leg cramps
RESP: Bronchitis, exacerbation of asthma, upper respiratory infection
SKIN: Alopecia, application site irritation, chloasma, erythema multiforme or nodosum, hirsutism, jaundice, melasma, pruritus, purpura, rash, urticaria
Other: Anaphylaxis, angioedema, flulike syndrome, folic acid de-

ficiency, hypercalcemia (with bone metastases), hypocalcemia, hyperkalemia, hyponatremia, weight gain or loss

Nursing Considerations

- Use estradiol and levonorgestrel cautiously in women with asthma, diabetes mellitus, epilepsy, migraine headaches, porphyria, systemic lupus erythematosus, and hepatic hemangiomas because estrogens may worsen these conditions.
- Women using continuous estrogen or combination estrogen-progestin therapy should complete the current cycle of therapy before starting estradiol and levonorgestrel. Those not using continuous estrogen or combination estrogen-progestin therapy may start estradiol and levonorgestrel immediately.
- Verify that patient has an intact uterus before starting estradiol and levonorgestrel. If not, she doesn't need a product that contains a progestin such as levonorgestrel.
- **WARNING** Assess patient for possible contact lens intolerance or changes in vision or visual acuity because estrogens can cause keratoconus. Be prepared to stop therapy immediately, as prescribed, if patient has sudden partial or complete loss of vision or sudden onset of diplopia or migraine.
- Monitor PT in patients taking warfarin. Estrogens increase production of clotting factors VII, VIII, IX, and X and promote platelet aggregation and thus may cause loss of anticoagulant effect.
- Watch for elevated liver function test results because estrogens and progestins may worsen such conditions as acute intermittent or variegate hepatic porphyria.
- Closely monitor patient's blood pressure. Some patients may have a substantial increase in blood pressure as an indiosyncratic reaction to estrogen. Monitor patients who already have hypertension for increased blood pressure because estrogens may cause fluid retention. Also monitor patients with asthma, heart disease, migraines, renal disease, or seizure disorder for worsening of these conditions.
- Monitor blood glucose level often in patients who have diabetes mellitus because estrogens may decrease insulin sensitivity and alter glucose tolerance.
- **WARNING** Expect to stop estradiol and levonorgestrel in any woman who develops signs or symptoms of dementia or cardiovascular disease, such as CVA, MI, pulmonary embolism, or venous thrombosis.

- Be aware that estradiol and levonorgestrel may worsen mood disorders, including depression. Monitor patient for depression, mood changes, anxiety, fatigue, dizziness, or insomnia.
- **WARNING** Be aware that patients with breast cancer and bone metastasis may develop severe hypercalcemia because estrogens influence calcium and phosphorus metabolism. Watch for toxic effects of increased calcium absorption in patients predisposed to hypercalcemia or nephrolithiasis.
- Assess skin for melasma (tan or brown patches), which may develop on forehead, cheeks, temples, and upper lip. These patches may persist after drug is stopped.
- Monitor thyroid function test results in patients with hypothyroidism because long-term use of estradiol may decrease effectiveness of thyroid therapy.
- Expect to stop estradiol and levonorgestrel therapy several weeks before patient undergoes major surgery, as prescribed, because prolonged immobilization poses a risk of thromboembolism.

PATIENT TEACHING

- Before therapy starts, inform patient of the risks of estrogen-progestin therapy, such as increased risk of cardiovascular disease, breast or endometrial cancer, dementia, gallbladder disease, and vision abnormalities.
- Instruct patient to select application site on lower abdomen but not to use a site that's oily, scarred, irritated, or at the waistline.
- Teach patient how to apply the transdermal patch. Tell patient to remove one side of the protective liner, being careful not to touch the adhesive part of the patch, and immediately apply to a smooth area of skin. She should then remove the second side of the protective liner and press the patch firmly in place for at least 10 seconds, ensuring good contact, especially at the edges.
- Caution patient never to apply patch on or near the breasts.
- Instruct patient to apply a new patch once a week, rotating sites in the lower abdomen after carefully and gently removing the previous patch. If any adhesive remains on the skin, instruct patient to let the area dry for 15 minutes and then gently rub it with an oil-based cream or lotion to remove the adhesive residue. Tell her to fold the used patch carefully in half so that it sticks to itself before discarding it.
- Tell patient that if patch is dislodged, it can be reapplied to another area of the lower abdomen or a new patch applied, keeping the original treatment schedule.

- Stress importance of wearing only one patch at a time.
- Caution patient to avoid exposing patch to sun for long periods.
- Urge patient to notify prescriber immediately about vaginal bleeding or any other abnormal signs and symptoms while using estradiol and levonorgestrel.
- Advise patient to avoid smoking while using an estrogen-progestin product such as estradiol and levonorgestrel.
- Stress importance of having follow-up visits every 3 to 6 months to determine effectiveness of estradiol and levonorges-trel at relieving menopausal symptoms. Also stress need to have scheduled diagnostic tests to detect adverse reactions.
- Emphasize importance of good dental hygiene and regular dental checkups because an elevated progestin blood level increases the growth of normal oral flora, which may lead to gum tenderness, bleeding, or swelling.

estradiol and norethindrone acetate
Activella, CombiPatch

Class and Category
Chemical: Estrogen derivative (estradiol), steroid hormone (norethindrone)
Therapeutic: Antiosteoporotic agent, ovarian hormone replacement
Pregnancy category: X

Indications and Dosages
▶ *To treat estrogen deficiency caused by hypogonadism, oophorectomy, or primary ovarian failure in patients with an intact uterus*
TRANSDERMAL (COMBIPATCH)
Adult females. For continuous combined regimen in women who don't want to resume menses: 9-cm² CombiPatch (0.05 mg estradiol and 0.14 mg norethindrone acetate daily) worn continuously on lower abdomen; may be increased to 16-cm² Combi-Patch (0.05 mg estradiol and 0.25 mg norethindrone acetate daily), as prescribed, if a larger progestin dose is desired. New patch is applied twice weekly (q 3 to 4 days) during a 28-day cycle.

For continuous sequential regimen in combination with transdermal estradiol-only system: Vivelle (0.05 mg daily) estradiol transdermal system is worn for the first 14 days of a 28-day cycle, replaced twice weekly according to product directions. For the remaining 14 days of the 28-day cycle, 9-cm² CombiPatch

(0.05 mg estradiol and 0.14 mg norethindrone acetate daily) is worn on the lower abdomen; may be increased to 16-cm^2 Combi-Patch (0.05 mg estradiol and 0.25-mg norethindrone acetate daily), as prescribed, if a larger progestin dose is desired. Combi-Patch should be replaced twice weekly (q 3 to 4 days) during this period in the cycle.

▶ *To treat menopausal symptoms and prevent osteoporosis from estrogen deficiency in postmenopausal women with an intact uterus*

TABLETS (ACTIVELLA)

Adult females. 1 tablet (1 mg estradiol and 0.5 mg norethindrone acetate) daily.

TRANSDERMAL (COMBIPATCH)

Adult females. For continuous combined regimen in women who don't want to resume menses: 9-cm^2 CombiPatch (0.05 mg estradiol and 0.14 mg norethindrone acetate daily) worn continuously on lower abdomen; may be increased to 16-cm^2 Combi-Patch (0.05 mg estradiol and 0.25 mg norethindrone acetate daily), as prescribed, if a larger progestin dose is desired. New patch is applied twice weekly (q 3 to 4 days) during a 28-day cycle.

For continuous sequential regimen in combination with transdermal estradiol-only system: Vivelle (0.05 mg daily) estradiol transdermal system is worn for the first 14 days of a 28-day cycle, replaced twice weekly according to product directions. For the remaining 14 days of the 28-day cycle, 9-cm^2 CombiPatch (0.05 mg estradiol and 0.14 mg norethindrone acetate daily) is worn on the lower abdomen; may be increased to 16-cm^2 Combi-Patch (0.05 mg estradiol and 0.25-mg norethindrone acetate daily), as prescribed, if a larger progestin dose is desired. Combi-Patch should be replaced twice weekly (q 3 to 4 days) during this period in the cycle.

Contraindications

Active deep vein thrombosis, pulmonary embolism, or history of these conditions; endometrial hyperplasia; hepatic disorders; hypersensitivity to estradiol, norethindrone, or their components; jaundice; known or suspected breast cancer or history of breast cancer from estrogen use; known or suspected estrogen-dependent cancer; new or recent (within past year) CVA or MI; pregnancy; undiagnosed abnormal genital bleeding; vaginal disorders

Mechanism of Action

Estradiol increases the rate of DNA and RNA synthesis in the cells of female reproductive organs, pituitary gland, hypothalamus, and other target organs. In the hypothalamus, estrogens decrease release of gonadotropin-releasing hormone, which reduces pituitary release of follicle-stimulating hormone and luteinizing hormone. In women, these hormones are required for normal GU and other essential body functions. At the cellular level, estrogens increase cervical secretions, cause endometrial cell proliferation, and improve uterine tone. Estrogen replacement helps maintain GU function and reduces vasomotor symptoms when estrogen production declines from menopause, removal of ovaries, or estrogen deficiency. Estrogen replacement also helps prevent osteoporosis by inhibiting bone resorption.

Norethindrone is a progestin. Progestins prolong some positive effects of estrogens on high-density lipoprotein cholesterol. Norethindrone diffuses freely into target cells of the female reproductive tract, mammary glands, hypothalamus, and pituitary gland and binds to the progesterone cell receptor. It converts a proliferative endometrium into a secretory one in women with adequate estrogen replacement, reducing endometrial growth and the risk of endometrial cancer compared with women who have an intact uterus and take unopposed estrogens. Norethindrone also decreases nuclear estradiol receptors and suppresses epithelial DNA synthesis in endometrial tissues.

Interactions

DRUGS

estradiol and norethindrone

aminocaproic acid: Possibly an increase in hypercoagulability caused by aminocaproic acid

barbiturates, carbamazepine, hydantoins, rifabutin, rifampin: Possibly reduced activity of estradiol and norethindrone

bromocriptine: Possibly decreased bromocriptine effects

calcium: Possibly increased calcium absorption

corticosteroids: Increased therapeutic and toxic effects of corticosteroids

cyclosporine: Increased risk of hepatotoxicity and nephrotoxicity

didanosine, lamivudine, zalcitabine: Possibly pancreatitis

hepatotoxic drugs (such as isoniazid): Increased risk of hepatitis and hepatotoxicity

oral antidiabetics: Decreased therapeutic effects of these drugs

somatrem, somatropin: Possibly accelerated epiphyseal maturation

tamoxifen: Possibly decreased therapeutic effects of tamoxifen

vitamin C: Decreased metabolism and possibly increased adverse effects of estradiol and norethindrone
warfarin: Decreased anticoagulant effect
FOODS
estradiol and norethindrone
grapefruit juice: Decreased metabolism and possibly increased adverse effects of estradiol and norethindrone
ACTIVITIES
estradiol and norethindrone
smoking: Increased risk of CVA, pulmonary embolism, thrombophlebitis, and transient ischemic attack

Adverse Reactions

CNS: CVA, dementia, depression, dizziness, headache, irritability, migraine headache, mood swings, worsening of epilepsy
CV: Deep and superficial venous thrombosis, hypertension, hypertriglyceridemia, MI, peripheral edema, pulmonary embolism, thromboembolism, thrombophlebitis
EENT: Intolerance of contact lenses, retinal vascular thrombosis, vision changes
ENDO: Breast enlargement, pain, tenderness, or tumors; gynecomastia; hyperglycemia; nipple discharge
GI: Abdominal cramps or pain, anorexia, constipation, diarrhea, elevated liver function test results, enlargement of hepatic hemangiomas, gallbladder obstruction, hepatitis, increased appetite, nausea, pancreatitis, vomiting
GU: Amenorrhea, breakthrough bleeding, cervical erosion, clear vaginal discharge, decreased libido (males), dysmenorrhea, endometrial hyperplasia or cancer, impotence, increased libido (females), ovarian cancer, prolonged or heavy menstrual bleeding, testicular atrophy, vaginal candidiasis
MS: Leg cramps
SKIN: Acne, alopecia, hirsutism, jaundice, melasma, oily skin, purpura, rash, seborrhea, urticaria
Other: Anaphylaxis, folic acid deficiency, hypercalcemia (in metastatic bone disease), hypocalcemia, weight gain

Nursing Considerations

- **WARNING** Be aware that patients with breast cancer and bone metastasis may develop severe hypercalcemia because estrogens influence calcium and phosphorus metabolism. Watch for toxic effects of increased calcium absorption in patients predisposed to hypercalcemia or nephrolithiasis.
- **WARNING** Assess patient for contact lens intolerance or

changes in vision or visual acuity because estrogens can cause keratoconus. Be prepared to stop drug immediately, as prescribed, if patient has sudden partial or complete loss of vision or sudden onset of diplopia, migraine, or proptosis.

- Monitor PT in patients receiving warfarin for loss of anticoagulant effect because estrogens increase production of clotting factors VII, VIII, IX, and X and promote platelet aggregation.
- Watch for elevated liver function test results because estrogen and progestins may worsen such conditions as acute intermittent or variegate hepatic porphyria.
- Closely monitor patient's blood pressure. Some patients may have a substantial increase in blood pressure as an idiosyncratic reaction to estrogen. Monitor patients who already have hypertension for increases in blood pressure because estrogens may cause fluid retention. Also monitor patients with asthma, heart disease, migraines, renal disease, or seizure disorder for worsening of these conditions.
- Watch for peripheral edema or mild weight gain because estrogens can cause sodium and fluid retention.
- Check triglyceride levels routinely because, in patients with hypertriglyceridemia, estrogen may increase serum triglyceride level enough to cause pancreatitis and other complications.
- Monitor blood glucose level often in patients who have diabetes mellitus because conjugated estrogens may decrease insulin sensitivity and alter glucose tolerance.
- Be aware that exogenous estradiol and norethindrone may worsen mood disorders, including depression. Monitor patient for anxiety, depression, dizziness, fatigue, insomnia, or mood changes. If significant depression occurs, expect to stop hormone replacement therapy.
- Assess skin for melasma (tan or brown patches), which may develop on forehead, cheeks, temples, and upper lip. These patches may persist after drug is stopped.
- Expect to stop estrogen combination therapy in any woman with evidence of dementia, cancer, or cardiovascular disease, such as CVA, MI pulmonary embolism, or venous thrombosis.
- Expect to stop estrogen therapy several weeks before major surgery, as prescribed, because prolonged immobilization increases the risk of thromboembolism.

PATIENT TEACHING
- Before therapy starts, explain the risks of estrogen-progestin therapy, such as increased risk of breast, endometrial, or ovar-

ian cancer; cardiovascular disease; gallbladder disease; and vision abnormalities.

• Teach patient proper application and use of CombiPatch. Instruct her to tear pouch open, rather than cutting it with scissors, and to remove stiff protective liner covering adhesive without touching adhesive. Tell her not to cut or trim the patch. Advise her to apply patch to a clean, dry, hairless part of lower abdomen. Caution her not to apply patch to breasts; to injured, irritated, callused, or scarred areas; or to areas where it may not adhere properly, such as the waistline.

• Advise patient to rotate application sites at least weekly and to remove old patch before applying new one. If patch falls off, instruct her to reapply it to another area or to apply a new patch and continue the original treatment schedule. Caution her not to expose patch to sun for prolonged periods. Explain that she may bathe while wearing the patch.

• Advise patient taking estradiol and norethindrone not to smoke because smoking increases the risk of deep vein thrombosis, MI, and other thromboembolic disorders.

• Explain that estradiol and norethindrone may cause monthly withdrawal bleeding.

• Advise patient receiving estradiol treatment to have an annual pelvic examination, including a Papanicolaou smear, to screen for cervical dysplasia.

estrogens (conjugated) and medroxyprogesterone
Premphase, Prempro

Class and Category
Chemical: Estrogen steroid hormone derivative (conjugated estrogens), progesterone steroid hormone derivative (medroxyprogesterone)
Therapeutic: Antiosteoporotic, ovarian hormone replacement (conjugated estrogens, medroxyprogesterone)
Pregnancy category: X

Indications and Dosages
▶ *To treat moderate to severe vasomotor menopausal symptoms and vaginal and vulvar atrophy*
TABLETS (PREMPRO)
Adult females. 0.3 mg conjugated estrogens and 1.5 mg

medroxyprogesterone (1 tablet) daily. Increased to 0.625 mg conjugated estrogens and 5 mg medroxyprogesterone (1 tablet) daily as needed.

TABLETS (PREMPHASE)

Adult females. 0.625 mg conjugated estrogen (1 tablet) daily on days 1 through day 14 and 0.625 mg conjugated estrogens and 5 mg medroxyprogesterone (1 tablet) on days 15 through 28. Cycle repeated q 28 days.

▶ *To prevent postmenopausal osteoporosis*

TABLETS (PREMPRO)

Adult females. 0.3 mg conjugated estrogens and 1.5 mg medroxyprogesterone (1 tablet) daily. Increased to 0.625 mg conjugated estrogens and 5 mg medroxyprogesterone (1 tablet) daily as needed.

TABLETS (PREMPHASE)

Adult females. 0.625 mg conjugated estrogen (1 tablet) daily on days 1 through 14. Then 0.625 mg conjugated estrogens and 5 mg medroxyprogesterone (1 tablet) on days 15 through 28.

Mechanism of Action

Conjugated estrogens increase DNA and RNA synthesis in the cells of female reproductive organs, hypothalamus, pituitary glands, and other target organs. In the hypothalamus, estrogens reduce release of gonadotropin-releasing hormone, which decreases pituitary release of follicle-stimulating hormone and luteinizing hormone. In women, these hormones are required for normal GU and other essential body functions. At the cellular level, estrogens increase cervical secretions, cause endometrial cell proliferation, and increase uterine tone. Estrogen replacement helps maintain GU function and reduce vasomotor symptoms when estrogen production declines from menopause, surgical removal of ovaries, or other estrogen deficiency states. Estrogen replacement also helps prevent osteoporosis by inhibiting bone resorption so that resorption doesn't exceed bone formation.

Medroxyprogesterone, a progestin, may achieve its beneficial effect on the endometrium in part by decreasing nuclear estrogen receptors and suppression of epithelial DNA synthesis in endometrial tissue.

Contraindications

Abnormal or undiagnosed vaginal bleeding; breast, endometrial, or estrogen-dependent cancer; hypersensitivity to conjugated estrogens, medroxyprogesterone, other progestins, peanuts or their components; pregnancy; thromboembolic disorders

Interactions

DRUGS

conjugated estrogens and medroxyprogesterone

barbiturates, carbamazepine, hydantoins, rifabutin, rifampin: Possibly reduced activity of estrogen and medroxyprogesterone

conjugated estrogens component

corticosteroids: Increased therapeutic and toxic effects of corticosteroids

cyclosporine: Increased risk of hepatotoxicity and nephrotoxicity

oral antidiabetics: Decreased therapeutic effects of these drugs

warfarin: Decreased anticoagulant effect

medroxyprogesterone component

aminoglutethimide: Possibly increased hepatic metabolism of medroxyprogesterone, decreasing its therapeutic effects

ACTIVITIES

conjugated estrogens component

smoking: Increased risk of CVA, pulmonary embolism, thrombophlebitis, and transient ischemic attack

Adverse Reactions

CNS: Anxiety, chorea, CVA, dementia, depression, dizziness, exacerbation of epilepsy, fatigue, fever, headache, insomnia, irritability, migraine headache, mood disturbances, nervousness, somnolence

CV: Edema, increased triglycerides, MI, peripheral edema, hypertension, thromboembolism, thrombophlebitis

EENT: Diplopia, intolerance of contact lenses, neuro-ocular lesions, optic neuritis, retinal vascular thrombosis, vision change or loss

ENDO: Breast enlargement, pain, tenderness, or tumors; fibrocystic breast changes; galactorrhea; hyperglycemia; nipple discharge

GI: Abdominal cramps or pain, aggravation of porphyria, anorexia, bloating, cholestatic jaundice, constipation, diarrhea, enlargment of hepatic hemangiomas, gallbladder obstruction, hepatitis, increased or decreased appetite, increased incidence of gallbladder disease, nausea, pancreatitis, vomiting

GU: Amenorrhea, breakthrough bleeding, change in cervical erosion, change in amount of cervical secretions, clear vaginal discharge, cystitislike syndrome, changes in libido, dysmenorrhea, endometrial hyperplasia, increase in size of uterine leiomyomata, premenstruallike syndrome, prolonged or heavy menstrual bleeding, vaginal candidiasis

MS: Backache
RESP: Exacerbation of asthma, pulmonary embolism
SKIN: Acne, alopecia, chloasma, erythema multiforme, erythema nodosum, hemorrhagic eruption, hirsutism, jaundice, melasma, oily skin, purpura, pruritus, rash, seborrhea, urticaria
Other: Anaphylaxis, angioedema, folic acid deficiency, hypercalcemia (in metastatic bone disease), hypocalcemia, weight gain or loss

Nursing Considerations

- Use conjugated estrogens and medroxyprogesterone cautiously in patients with severe hypocalcemia because a sudden increase in serum calcium level may cause adverse effects.
- Monitor serum calcium level in patients with breast cancer and bone metastasis for severe hypercalcemia because conjugated estrogens influence calcium and phosphorus metabolism.
- Assess for peripheral edema, a sign of fluid retention, and evaluate patient's fluid intake and output, watching for positive fluid balance.
- Assess hypertensive patients for increases in blood pressure because conjugated estrogens may cause fluid retention.
- Monitor patients with asthma, diabetes mellitus, endometriosis, heart disease, renal disease, migraine headaches, seizure disorder, or lupus erythematosus for worsening of these conditions.
- **WARNING** Assess patient for possible contact lens intolerance or changes in vision or visual acuity because estrogens can cause keratoconus. Be prepared to stop drug immediately, as prescribed, if patient has sudden partial or complete loss of vision or sudden onset of diplopia or migraine.
- If patient takes warfarin, assess PT for loss of anticoagulant effects because conjugated estrogens increase production of clotting factors and promote platelet aggregation.
- Monitor blood glucose level often in patients who have diabetes mellitus because conjugated estrogens may decrease insulin sensitivity and alter glucose tolerance.
- Assess skin for melasma (tan or brown patches), which may develop on forehead, cheeks, temples, and upper lip. These patches may persist after drug is stopped.
- **WARNING** Expect to stop conjugated estrogens and medroxyprogesterone in any woman with cardiovascular disease, such as CVA, MI, pulmonary embolism, or venous thrombosis or dementia.

- Assess patient for evidence of depression, such as changes in mental status, affect, and mood.
- Watch for elevated liver function test values because conjugated estrogen and medroxyprogesterone may worsen such conditions as acute intermittent or variegate hepatic porphyria.
- Expect to stop therapy during periods of immobilization, 4 weeks before elective surgery, and if jaundice develops.

PATIENT TEACHING
- Before therapy starts, explain the risks of conjugated estrogens and medoxyprogesterone, such as an increased risk of cardiovascular disease, breast or endometrial cancer, dementia, and gallbladder disease.
- Urge patient to immediately report breakthrough bleeding.
- Instruct patient to perform monthly breast self-examination and comply with all prescribed follow-up examinations, especially endometrial tests, because conjugated estrogens increase the risk of breast and endometrial cancer.
- Encourage patient to stay active to reduce the risk of thrombophlebitis.
- Warn women that long-term use may increase risk of heart disease, stroke, dementia, and breast or endometrial cancer.
- Urge patient to avoid smoking while using conjugated estrogens and medroxyprogesterone.
- Emphasize importance of good dental hygiene and regular dental checkups because an elevated progestin level increases growth of normal oral flora, which may lead to gum tenderness, bleeding, or swelling.

estrogens (esterified) and methyltestosterone
Estratest, Estratest H.S.

Class and Category
Chemical: Sodium salts of sulfate esters of estrogenic substances (esterified estrogens), synthetic androgen (methyltestosterone)
Therapeutic: Hormone replacement (esterified estrogens, methyltestosterone)
Pregnancy category: X

Indications and Dosages
▶ *To treat moderate to severe vasomotor symptoms of menopause in patients who haven't responded to estrogen alone*

TABLETS
Adult females. 0.625 mg to 1.25 mg esterified estrogens and
1.25 to 2.5 mg methyltestosterone (1 or 2 tablets Estratest H.S.,
1 tablet Estratest) daily for 21 days, followed by 7 days without
therapy. Cycle repeated as often as needed.

Mechanism of Action

Esterified estrogens increase DNA and RNA synthesis in the cells of female
reproductive organs, pituitary gland, hypothalamus, and other target organs.
In the hypothalamus, estrogens reduce release of gonadotropin-releasing hormone, which reduces pituitary release of follicle-stimulating hormone and
luteinizing hormone. In women, these hormones are required for normal GU
and other essential body functions. At the cellular level, estrogens increase
cervical secretions, cause endometrial cell proliferation, and improve uterine
tone. Estrogen replacement helps maintain GU function and reduces vasomotor symptoms when estrogen production declines from menopause, surgical
removal of ovaries, or other estrogen deficiency.

Methyltestosterone is a synthetic form of testosterone. Testosterone first
undergoes hydrolysis to the active form, free testosterone in the liver. Free
testosterone is further converted into two of the major active metabolites,
DHT and estradiol. Thus, testosterone can produce estrogenic effects as a result of its conversion to estradiol to help maintain GU function and reduce
vasomotor symptoms when estrogen production declines from menopause,
surgical removal of ovaries, or other estrogen deficiency.

Contraindications

Active thrombophlebitis or thromboembolic disorders; breastfeeding; hypersensitivity to estrogens, methyltestosterone, or their
components; known or suspected breast cancer (except in select
patients being treated for metastatic disease); known or suspected
estrogen-dependent cancer; pregnancy; severe liver damage; undiagnosed abnormal genital bleeding

Interactions
DRUGS
esterified estrogens and methyltestosterone
oral antidiabetics: Decreased or increased therapeutic effects of
these drugs with risk of hyperglycemia or hypoglycemia
warfarin: Altered anticoagulant effect
esterified estrogens component
barbiturates, carbamazepine, hydantoins, rifabutin, rifampin: Possibly
reduced activity of esterified estrogens

clarithromycin, erythromycin, intraconazole, ketoconazole, ritonivir: Possibly increased plasma estrogen concentration

hepatotoxic drugs (such as isoniazid): Increased risk of hepatitis and hepatotoxicity

methyltestosterone component

cyclosporine: Possibly increased risk of nephrotoxicity

estradiol, estrogens: Enhanced estrogenic effects

oxyphenbutazone: Increased serum oxyphenbutazone levels

FOODS

esterified estrogens component

grapefruit juice: Decreased metabolism and possibly increased adverse effects of esterified estrogens

ACTIVITIES

esterified estrogens and methyltestosterone

smoking: Increased risk of CVA, pulmonary embolism, thrombophlebitis, and transient ischemic attack

Adverse Reactions

CNS: Anxiety, chorea, CVA, dementia, depression, dizziness, exacerbation of epilepsy, generalized parasthesia, headache, irritability, migraine headache, mood disturbances, nervousness

CV: Edema, elevated cholesterol and triglyceride levels, hypertension, MI, peripheral edema, thromboembolism, thrombophlebitis

EENT: Diplopia, intolerance of contact lenses, retinal vascular thrombosis, steepening of corneal curvature, vision changes or loss

ENDO: Breast enlargement, pain, tenderness or tumors; fibrocystic breast changes; galactorrhea; hypercalcemia; hyperglycemia; hypocalcemia; hypoglycemia; nipple discharge; virilization

GI: Abdominal cramps or pain, aggravation of porphyria, anorexia, bloating, cholestatic jaundice, constipation, diarrhea, elevated liver function test results, gallbladder obstruction, hepatitis including increased appetite, jaundice, nausea, pancreatitis, vomiting

GU: Alteration in amount of cervical secretions, amenorrhea, breakthrough bleeding, cervical erosion, changes in cervical ectropion, clear vaginal discharge, cystitis-like syndrome, dysmenorrhea, changes in libido, increased size of uterine leiomyomata, ovarian cancer, prolonged or heavy menstrual bleeding, vaginitis including vaginal candidiasis

HEME: Polycythemia

MS: Arthralgias, leg cramps

RESP: Exacerbation of asthma, pulmonary embolism

SKIN: Acne, alopecia, chloasma, erythema multiforme or no-dosum, hemorrhagic eruption, hirsutism, jaundice, melasma, oily skin, pruritis, purpura, rash, seborrhea, urticaria
Other: Anaphylaxis, angioedema, fluid and electrolyte imbalance, folic acid deficiency, weight gain or loss

Nursing Considerations

- Use cautiously in patients with mild to moderate hepatic dysfunction because estrogens such as esterified estrogens are poorly metabolized in patients with hepatic dysfunction. Do not administer the drug to patients with severe hepatic dysfunction.
- Also use cautiously in patients with renal insufficiency or patients with metabolic bone diseases because estrogens influence the metabolism of calcium and phosphorus.
- **WARNING** Be aware that patients with breast cancer and bone metastasis may develop severe hypercalcemia because esterified estrogens influence calcium and phosphorus metabolism and methyltestosterone stimulates osteolysis. Watch for toxic effects of increased calcium levels in patients predisposed to hypercalcemia or nephrolithiasis.
- Monitor PT in patients receiving warfarin for altered anticoagulant effect because estrogens increase production of clotting factors VII, VIII, IX, and X and promote platelet aggregation.
- Watch for elevated liver function test results because esterified estrogens and methyltestosterone may worsen such conditions as acute intermittent or variegate hepatic porphyria as well as cause peliosis hepatis, cholestatic hepatitis, and hepatocellular carcinoma. If jaundice develops, stop drug and notify prescriber.
- **WARNING** Assess patient for possible contact lens intolerance or changes in vision or visual acuity because estrogens can cause keratoconus. Be prepared to stop drug immediately, as prescribed, if patient has sudden partial or complete loss of vision or sudden onset of diplopia or migraine.
- Closely monitor patient's blood pressure. Some patients may have a substantial increase in blood pressure as an indiosyncratic reaction to estrogens. Monitor patients who already have hypertension for increases in blood pressure because estrogens may cause fluid retention. Also monitor patients with asthma, heart disease, migraines, renal disease, or seizure disorder for exacerbation of these conditions.
- Watch for peripheral edema or mild weight gain because esterified estrogens and methyltestosterone can cause sodium and fluid retention.

- Monitor blood glucose level often in patients with diabetes mellitus because estrogens may decrease insulin sensitivity and alter glucose tolerance.
- **WARNING** Expect to stop esterified estrogens and methyltestosterone therapy in any woman who develops signs or symptoms of cardiovascular disease, such as CVA, MI, pulmonary embolism, or venous thrombosis.
- Be aware that exogenous estrogens may worsen mood disorders, including depression. Monitor patient for depression, mood changes, anxiety, fatigue, dizziness, or insomnia.
- Assess skin for melasma (tan or brown patches), which may develop on forehead, cheeks, temples, and upper lip. These patches may persist after drug is stopped.
- Monitor thyroid function test results in patients with hypothyroidism because long-term use of esterified estrogens may decrease effectiveness of thyroid therapy.
- Expect to stop esterified estrogens and methyltestosterone therapy several weeks before patient undergoes major surgery, as prescribed, because prolonged immobilization poses a risk of thromboembolism.

PATIENT TEACHING
- Before therapy starts, inform patient of risks involved in esterified estrogens and methyltestosterone therapy, such as increased risk of cardiovascular disease, breast or endometrial cancer, dementia, gallbladder disease, and vision abnormalities.
- Inform patient receiving esterified estrogens and methyltestosterone that she should have an annual physical examination including a pelvic examination to screen for adverse effects such as cervical dysplasia.
- Inform patient that a cyclic combination regimen of esterified estrogens and methyltestosterone may cause monthly withdrawal bleeding.
- Instruct patient to notify prescriber if masculine changes appear, such as a deepening of the voice or facial hair growth.
- Also tell patient to notify prescriber of any unusual signs and symptoms because combination drug can cause serious adverse effects.
- Urge patient taking esterified estrogens and methyltestosterone not to smoke because smoking increases the risk of deep vein thrombosis, heart attack, and other thromboemolic disorders.

ethinyl estradiol and norethindrone
Femhrt

Class and Category
Chemical: Estrogen steroid hormone derivative (ethinyl estradiol), progesterone derivative (norethindrone)
Therapeutic: Antiosteoporotic, ovarian hormone replacement (ethinyl estradiol, norethindrone)
Pregnancy category: X

Indications and Dosages
▶ *To treat moderate to severe vasomotor symptoms of menopause; to prevent osteoporosis from estrogen deficiency in postmenopausal women with an intact uterus*
TABLETS
Adult females. 0.05 mg ethinyl estradiol and 1 mg norethindrone (1 tablet) daily.

Mechanism of Action
Ethinyl estradiol is an estrogen that increases DNA and RNA synthesis in the cells of female reproductive organs, pituitary gland, hypothalamus, and other target organs. In the hypothalamus, estrogens decrease the release of gonadotropin-releasing hormone, which reduces pituitary release of follicle-stimulating hormone and luteinizing hormone. In women, these hormones are required for normal GU and other essential body functions. At the cellular level, estrogens increase cervical secretions, cause endometrial cell proliferation, and improve uterine tone. Estrogen replacement helps maintain GU function and reduces vasomotor symptoms when estrogen production declines from menopause, surgical removal of ovaries, or other estrogen deficiency. Estrogen replacement also helps prevent osteoporosis by inhibiting bone resorption.

Norethindrone is a progestin. Progestins prolong some of the positive effects of estrogens on HDL cholesterol. Norethindrone diffuses freely into target cells of the female reproductive tract, mammary glands, hypothalamus, and pituitary gland and binds to the progesterone cell receptor. It converts a proliferative endometrium into a secretory one in women with adequate estrogen replacement, reducing endometrial growth and the risk of endometrial cancer compared with women who have an intact uterus and take unopposed estrogens. Norethindrone also decreases nuclear estradiol receptors and suppresses epithelial DNA synthesis in endometrial tissues.

Contraindications

Thrombophlebitis, thromboembolic disorders, or a history of them; hypersensitivity to ethinyl estradiol, norethindrone, or their components; known or suspected breast cancer or history of breast cancer from estrogen use; known or suspected estrogen-dependent cancer; pregnancy; undiagnosed abnormal genital bleeding

Interactions

DRUGS

ethinyl estradiol and norethindrone

corticosteroids: Increased therapeutic and toxic effects of corticosteroids

cyclosporine: Increased risk of hepatotoxicity and nephrotoxicity

hepatotoxic drugs (such as isoniazid): Increased risk of hepatitis and hepatotoxicity

oral antidiabetics: Decreased therapeutic effects of these drugs

thyroid hormones: Decreased effectiveness of thyroid hormones

warfarin: Altered anticoagulant effect

ethinyl estradiol component

vitamin C: Decreased metabolism and possibly increased adverse effects of ethinyl estradiol

FOODS

ethinyl estradiol component

grapefruit juice: Decreased metabolism and possibly increased adverse effects of ethinyl estradiol

ACTIVITIES

ethinyl estradiol and norethindrone

smoking: Increased risk of CVA, pulmonary embolism, thrombophlebitis, and transient ischemic attack

Adverse Reactions

CNS: Chorea, CVA, dementia, depression, dizziness, exacerbation of epilepsy, headache, irritability, migraine headache, mood disturbances, nervousness, porphyria

CV: Hypertension, increased triglycerides, MI, peripheral edema, pulmonary embolism, thromboembolism, thrombophlebitis

EENT: Diplopia, intolerance of contact lenses, retinal vascular thrombosis, sinusitis, vision changes or loss

ENDO: Breast enlargement, pain, tenderness, or tumors; endometrial hyperplasia; galactorrhea; hyperglycemia; nipple discharge

GI: Abdominal cramps or pain, aggravation of hepatic porphyria, anorexia, bloating, constipation, diarrhea, elevated liver function test results, enlargement of hepatic hemangiomas, flatulence, gallbladder obstruction, hepatitis, increased appetite, nausea, pancreatitis, vomiting

GU: Amenorrhea, breakthrough bleeding, cervical erosion, clear vaginal discharge, dysmenorrhea, endometrial or ovarian tumors, increased libido, increased size of uterine leiomyomata, leukorrhea, prolonged or heavy menstrual bleeding, urinary tract infection, vaginitis including vaginal candidiasis

MS: Arthralgias, back or extremity pain, leg cramps

RESP: Bronchitis, exacerbation of asthma, upper respiratory infection

SKIN: Alopecia, application site irritation, chloasma, erythema multiforme or nodosum, hirsutism, jaundice, melasma, pruritus, purpura, rash, urticaria

Other: Anaphylaxis, angioedema, flulike syndrome, folic acid deficiency, hypercalcemia (with bone metastases), hypocalcemia, hyperkalemia, hyponatremia, weight gain or loss

Nursing Considerations

- Use ethinyl estradiol and norethindrone cautiously in women with asthma, diabetes mellitus, epilepsy, migraine headaches, porphyria, systemic lupus erythematosus, and hepatic hemangiomas because ethinyl estradiol can worsen these conditions.
- Verify that patient has an intact uterus before starting ethinyl estradiol and norethindrone therapy. If not, she doesn't need a product that contains a progestin such as norethindrone.
- **WARNING** Assess patient for contact lens intolerance or changes in vision or acuity because estrogens such as ethinyl estradiol can cause keratoconus. Be prepared to stop drug immediately, as prescribed, if patient has sudden partial or complete loss of vision or sudden onset of diplopia or migraine.
- Monitor PT in patients taking warfarin for loss of anticoagulant effect because ethinyl estradiol can increase clotting factors VII, VIII, IX, and X and promote platelet aggregation.
- Watch for elevated liver function test results because ethinyl estradiol and norethindrone may worsen such conditions as acute intermittent or variegate hepatic porphyria.
- Closely monitor patient's blood pressure. Some patients may have a substantial increase in blood pressure as an indiosyncratic reaction to estrogens such as ethinyl estradiol. Monitor patients who already have hypertension for increases in blood pressure because estrogens may cause fluid retention. Also

monitor patients with asthma, heart disease, migraines, renal disease, or seizure disorder for worsening of these conditions.

- Monitor blood glucose level often in patients wiht diabetes mellitus because estrogens such as ethinyl estradiol may decrease insulin sensitivity and alter glucose tolerance.
- **WARNING** Expect to stop ethinyl estradiol and norethindrone in any woman who develops evidence of dementia, cardiovascular disease, such as CVA, MI, pulmonary embolism, or venous thrombosis.
- Be aware that ethinyl estradiol and norethindrone may worsen mood disorders, including depression. Monitor patient for depression, mood changes, anxiety, fatigue, dizziness, or insomnia.
- **WARNING** Be aware that patients with breast cancer and bone metastasis may develop severe hypercalcemia because estrogens influence calcium and phosphorus metabolism. Watch for toxic effects of increased calcium absorption in patients predisposed to hypercalcemia or nephrolithiasis.
- Assess skin for melasma (tan or brown patches), which may develop on forehead, cheeks, temples, and upper lip. These patches may persist after combination drug is stopped.
- Monitor thyroid function test results in patients with hypothyroidism because long-term use of ethinyl estradiol may decrease effectiveness of thyroid therapy.
- Expect to stop ethinyl estradiol and norethindrone therapy several weeks before patient undergoes major surgery, as prescribed, because prolonged immobilization poses a risk of thromboembolism.

PATIENT TEACHING
- Before therapy starts, inform patient about risks of taking ethinyl estradiol and norethindrone, such as increased risk of cardiovascular disease, breast or endometrial cancer, dementia, gallbladder disease, and vision abnormalities.
- Urge patient to notify prescriber immediately about vaginal bleeding or any other abnormal signs and symptoms during ethinyl estradiol and norethindrone therapy.
- Caution patient to avoid smoking while using an estrogen-progestin product like ethinyl estradiol and norethindrone.
- Stress importance of keeping follow-up visits every 3 to 6 months to determine effectiveness of ethinyl estradiol and norethindrone at relieving menopausal symptoms and osteoporosis as well as having scheduled diagnostic tests to detect adverse reactions.

• Emphasize importance of good dental hygiene and regular dental checkups because an elevated progestin (norethindrone) blood level increases growth of normal oral flora, which may lead to gum tenderness, bleeding, or swelling.

glipizide and metformin hydrochloride
Metaglip

Class and Category
Chemical: Sulfonylurea (glipizide), dimethylbiguanide (metformin)
Therapeutic: Antidiabetic
Pregnancy category: C

Indications and Dosages
▶ *To reduce blood glucose level as initial therapy in patients with type 2 diabetes mellitus*
TABLETS
Adults. *Initial:* If fasting blood glucose is 280 to 320 mg/dl, give 2.5 mg glipizide and 250 mg metformin daily with morning meal or 2.5 mg glipizide and 500 mg metformin b.i.d. with morning and evening meals. Dosage increased by initial dosage strength q 2 wk, as needed. *Maximum:* 10 mg glipizde and 1,000 mg metformin, or 10 mg glipizide and 2,000 mg metformin daily in divided doses if initial fasting glucose level is 280 to 320 mg/dl.
▶ *To reduce blood glucose level in patients with type 2 diabetes mellitus who aren't adequately controlled with either a sulfonylurea or metformin*
TABLETS
Adults. *Initial:* 2.5 mg glipizide and 500 mg metformin or 5 mg glipizide and 500 mg metformin b.i.d. with morning and evening meals. Dosage increased by no more than 5 mg glipizide and 500 mg metformin as needed. *Maximum:* 20 mg glipizide and 2,000 mg metformin daily.
DOSAGE ADJUSTMENT For patients taking glipizide or another sulfonylurea, metformin, or a combination of these drugs, expect initial dosage of combination drug to be equal to or less than that currently being taken individually.

Contraindications
Acute or chronic metabolic acidosis; diabetic coma; heart failure requiring drug treatment; hypersensitivity to glipizide, metformin, or their components; ketoacidosis; pregnancy; renal disease or dysfunction (serum creatinine level 1.5 mg/dl or more in men or 1.4 mg/dl or more in women or abnormal creatinine clearance)

Mechanism of Action

Glipizide and metformin hydrochloride work in complementary ways to improve glucose control. Glipizide stimulates insulin release from beta cells in the pancreas. It also increases peripheral tissue sensitivity to insulin, either by enhancing insulin binding to cellular receptors or by increasing the number of insulin receptors.

Metformin may promote storage of excess glucose as glycogen in the liver, thus reducing glucose production. It also may improve glucose use by skeletal muscle and adipose tissue by facilitating glucose transport, increasing insulin receptors, and making them more sensitive to insulin.

Interactions

DRUGS

glipizide and metformin hydrochloride

calcium channel blockers, corticosteroids, diuretics, estrogens, isoniazid, nicotinic acid, oral contraceptives, phenothiazine, phenytoin, sympathomimetics, thiazide diuretics, thyroid hormones: Possibly hyperglycemia or hypoglycemia when these drugs are withdrawn
vitamin B$_{12}$: Probably decreased vitamin B$_{12}$ absorption

glipizide component

ACE inhibitors, anabolic steroids, androgens, azole antifungals, bromocriptine, chloramphenicol, disopyramide, fibric acid derivatives, guanethidine, H$_2$-receptor antagonists, insulin, magnesium salts, MAO inhibitors, methyldopa, octreotide, oral anticoagulants, oxyphenbutazone, phenylbutazone, probenecid, quinidine, salicylates, sulfonamides, tetracycline, theophylline, tricyclic antidepressants, urinary acidifiers: Increased risk of hypoglycemia
asparaginase, calcium channel blockers, cholestyramine, clonidine, corticosteroids, danazol, diazoxide, estrogen, glucagons, hydantoins, isoniazid, lithium, morphine, nicotinic acid, oral contraceptives, phenothiazines, rifabutin, rifampin, sympathomimetics, thiazide diuretics, thyroid drugs, urinary alkalinizers: Increased risk of hyperglycemia
beta blockers: Possibly hyperglycemia or masking of hypoglycemia
cardiac glycosides: Increased risk of digitalis toxicity
pentamidine: Initially hypoglycemia and then hyperglycemia if beta cell damage occurs

metformin component

calcium channel blockers, corticosteroids, estrogens, hormonal contraceptives, isoniazid, nicotinic acid, phenothiazines, phenytoin, sympathomimetics, thiazide and other diuretics, thyroid drugs: Possibly hyperglycemia *clofibrate, MAO inhibitors, probenecid, propranolol, rifabutin, rifampin, salicylates, sulfonamides, sulfonylureas:* Increased risk of hypoglycemia

cationic drugs (such as amiloride, cimetidine, digoxin, morphine, procainamide, quinidine, quinine, ranitidine, triamterene, trimethoprim, vancomycin) nifedipine: Increased blood metformin level

ACTIVITIES

metformin component

alcohol use: Possibly increased risk of hypoglycemia; possibly potentiated lactate metabolism by metformin

Adverse Reactions

CNS: Dizziness, headache
CV: Hypertension
ENDO: Hypoglycemia
GI: Abdominal pain, diarrhea, nausea, vomiting
GU: UTI
MS: Pain
RESP: Upper respiratory tract infection

Nursing Considerations

- **WARNING** Monitor renal function, as ordered, before starting glipizide and metformin therapy and at least annually thereafter because renal impairment can result in tissue hypoperfusion and hypoxemia, leading to lactic acidosis.
- **WARNING** Monitor patient closely for signs and symptoms of lactic acidosis or ketoacidosis (changes in level of consciousness, fruity breath, Kussmaul's respirations, restlessness), especially during new onset of illness or trauma. If acidosis or ketoacidosis is suspected, obtain blood samples to evaluate serum electrolyte, ketone, glucose, possibly blood pH, lactate, pyruvate, and metformin levels, as ordered. If acidosis is confirmed, expect to stop drug immediately and provide corrective care, as prescribed.
- Expect to stop drug, as ordered, if patient develops cardiovascular collapse, acute heart failure, acute MI, or other conditions that include hypoxemia, or if patient develops hepatic insufficiency, because lactic acidosis may develop.
- **WARNING** Monitor patients—especially those who are malnourished or debilitated; those with renal, pituitary or adrenal insufficiency; and those with alcohol intoxication—for hypoglycemia because the drug increases the risk.
- Monitor vitamin B_{12} levels at least every 2 to 3 years in patients with inadequate vitamin B_{12} or calcium intake or absorp-

tion because prolonged drug use may result in decreased vitamin B_{12} response.

- Know that drug should be temporarily withheld for any surgical procedure that requires restricted intake of food and fluids and should not be restarted until the patient is able to eat and drink and renal function is normal.

- Expect to stop glipizide and metformin for 48 hours before and after radiographic tests involving I.V. administration of iodinated contrast materials because iodinated media increase the risk of renal failure and lactic acidosis during drug therapy. Check patient's renal function before restarting glipizide and metform 48 hours after radiographic tests are completed, as ordered.

- Monitor patient's blood glucose level to determine response to drug. Expect to monitor glycosylated hemoglobin level every 3 to 6 months, as ordered, to evaluate long-term blood glucose control.

- Monitor blood glucose level often to detect hyperglycemia and to assess the need for supplemental insulin during circumstances of increased stress, such as infection, surgery, or trauma.

- Arrange for instruction about diabetes and consultation with a dietitian or certified diabetes educator, if possible.

PATIENT TEACHING

- Instruct patient to take glipizide and metformin with morning meal if taking once a day or morning and evening meals if taking twice a day. Caution against skipping meals after taking drug.

- Advise patient not to skip doses, stop therapy, or take OTC drugs without first consulting prescriber because of a risk of hyperglycemia.

- Advise patient to report evidence of hypoglycemia (anxiety, confusion, dizziness, excessive sweating, headache, nausea), and teach him how to respond to hypoglycemia if it occurs.

- Tell patient to stop drug and notify prescriber immediately if he develops an increased respiratory rate unexplained by exercise or other activities, myalgia, malaise, unusual somnolence, or other nonspecific symptoms.

- Instruct patient to carry identification indicating that he has diabetes.

- Caution patient to avoid alcohol because it increases the risk of hypoglycemia.

- Tell patient to inform all prescribers that he is taking glipizide and metformin.

glyburide and metformin hydrochloride
Glucovance

Class and Category
Chemical: Sulfonylurea (glyburide), dimethylbiguanide (metformin)
Therapeutic: Antidiabetic
Pregnancy category: B

Indications and Dosages
▶ *To reduce blood glucose level as initial therapy in patients with type 2 diabetes mellitus or in those receiving glyburide and metformin combination therapy who need addition of a thiazolidinedione*
TABLETS
Adults. *Initial:* 1.25 mg glyburide and 250 mg metformin daily or b.i.d. Dosage increased by 1.25 mg glyburide and 250 mg metformin daily q 2 wk as needed.
▶ *To reduce blood glucose level in patients with type 2 diabetes mellitus who aren't adequately controlled by a sulfonylurea or metformin alone*
TABLETS
Adults. *Initial:* 2.5 mg glyburide and 500 mg metformin or 5 mg glyburide and 500 mg metformin b.i.d. Dosage increased, as prescribed, by 5 mg glyburide and 500 mg metformin daily. *Maximum:* 20 mg glyburide and 2,000 mg metformin daily.
DOSAGE ADJUSTMENT For patients currently receiving glyburide or another sulfonylurea, metformin, or a combination of these drugs, expect initial dosage to be equal to or less than that currently being taken. For patients receiving a combination of glyburide and metformin who also need a thiazolidinedione, expect dosage of glyburide and metformin combination to be unchanged when the thiazolidinedione is added.

Mechanism of Action
Glyburide and metformin work in complementary ways to improve glucose control. Glyburide stimulates insulin release from beta cells in the pancreas. It also increases peripheral tissue sensitivity to insulin either by enhancing insulin binding to cellular receptors or by increasing the number of insulin receptors.

Metformin hydrochloride may promote the storage of excess glucose as glycogen in the liver, thus reducing glucose production. Metformin also may improve glucose use by skeletal muscle and adipose tissue by facilitating glucose transport across cell membranes. It also may increase the number of insulin receptors on cell membranes and make them more sensitive to insulin.

Contraindications

Acute or chronic metabolic acidosis; diabetes complicated by pregnancy; diabetic coma; heart failure requiring drug treatment; hypersensitivity to glyburide, metformin, biguanides, sulfonylureas, or their components; ketoacidosis; renal disease or dysfunction (serum creatinine level of 1.5 mg/dl or more in men or 1.4 mg/dl or more in women); type 1 diabetes

Interactions

DRUGS

glyburide and metformin hydrochloride

calcium channel blockers, corticosteroids, diuretics, estrogens, hormonal contraceptives, isoniazid, nicotinic acid, phenothiazine, phenytoin, sympathomimetics, thiazide diuretics, thyroid hormones: Possibly hyperglycemia; possibly hypoglycemia when these drugs are withdrawn

vitamin B_{12}: Probably decreased vitamin B_{12} absorption

glyburide component

beta blockers, chloramphenicol, highly protein-bound drugs, MAO inhibitors, NSAIDs, oral anticoagulants, probenecid, salicylates, sulfonamides: Potentiated hypoglycemic action of glyburide; possibly hyperglycemia when these drugs are withdrawn

ciprofloxacin: Potentiated hypoglycemic action of glyburide

miconazole (oral): Possibly severe hypoglycemia

metformin hydrochloride component

cimetidine: Increased blood metformin level and possibly increased risk of hypoglycemia

furosemide: Increased blood metformin level and decreased blood furosemide level

nifedipine: Enhanced metformin absorption

FOODS

metformin hydrochloride component

all foods: Delayed and reduced metformin absorption

ACTIVITIES

metformin hydrochloride component

alcohol use: Altered blood glucose control (usually hyperglycemia); possibly potentiated effect of metformin on lactate metabolism

Adverse Reactions

CNS: Headache
ENDO: Hypoglycemia
GI: Abdominal pain, diarrhea, indigestion, nausea, vomiting
HEME: Megaloblastic anemia, thrombocytopenia
RESP: Upper respiratory tract infection

Other: Lactic acidosis

Nursing Considerations

- Administer glyburide and metformin as a single dose before first meal of the day. If patient takes more than 10 mg of glyburide daily or if severe GI distress occurs, expect to divide dose and give b.i.d. before morning and evening meals.
- **WARNING** Monitor renal function, as ordered, before beginning therapy and at least annually thereafter because significant renal impairment can result in tissue hypoperfusion and hypoxemia, leading to lactic acidosis.
- **WARNING** Expect to stop glyburide and metformin for 48 hours before and after radiographic tests involving I.V. administration of iodinated contrast materials because iodinated media increase the risk of renal failure and lactic acidosis during drug therapy.
- **WARNING** Monitor malnourished or debilitated patients; those with renal, hepatic, pituitary, or adrenal insufficiency; and those who are also prescribed a thiazolidinedione because they're at increased risk for hypoglycemia. Expect to monitor vitamin B_{12} blood levels at least every 2 to 3 years in patients with inadequate vitamin B_{12} or calcium intake or absorption because prolonged drug use may result in decreased vitamin B_{12} absorption.
- Monitor fasting blood glucose level to determine patient's response to drug. Expect to monitor glycosylated hemoglobin (HbA_{1c}) level every 3 to 6 months, as ordered, to evaluate long-term blood glucose control.
- Monitor blood glucose level often to detect hyperglycemia and to assess the need for supplemental insulin during circumstances of increased stress, such as infection, surgery, and trauma.
- When patient switches from insulin to glyburide and metformin, expect to increase frequency of blood glucose monitoring to t.i.d. before meals.
- In pregnant women, expect to stop drug at least 2 weeks before expected delivery date, as prescribed, to avoid profound hypoglycemia in neonate.
- Arrange for diabetes teaching and consultation with a dietitian or certified diabetes educator, if possible.

PATIENT TEACHING

- Instruct patient to take glyburide and metformin with morning meal if taking once a day, or with morning and evening meals

if taking twice a day. Caution him not to skip meal after taking
drug.

• Advise patient not to skip doses, stop drug, or take OTC drugs
without asking prescriber because hyperglycemia may result.

• Inform patient that most common adverse effects are minor, including diarrhea, nausea, and upset stomach, and typically occur during first few weeks of therapy; explain that taking drug
with meals reduces these effects.

• Teach patient how to monitor his blood glucose level and when
to notify prescriber.

• Advise patient to expect laboratory monitoring of HbA_{1c} level
every 3 months until blood glucose level is controlled.

• Instruct patient to report signs of hypoglycemia, such as anxiety, confusion, dizziness, excessive sweating, headache, and
nausea.

• Advise patient to carry identification showing that he has diabetes, and suggest carrying candy to treat mild hypoglycemia.

• Teach patient about exercise, diet, signs of hyperglycemia and
hypoglycemia, hygiene, foot care, and ways to avoid infection.

• Urge patient to notify prescriber if he develops easy bruising,
unusual bleeding, fever, hypoglycemia or hyperglycemia, rash,
or sore throat because drug may need to be stopped.

• Advise patient to avoid alcohol because it increases the risk of
hypoglycemia.

• Inform pregnant patient that she may be taken off glyburide
and metformin and switched to insulin therapy, as prescribed,
at least 2 weeks before expected delivery date.

70% insulin aspart protamine suspension and 30% insulin aspart injection

NovoLog Mix70/30

Class and Category

Chemical: Human insulin analogue (insulin aspart protamine suspension, insulin aspart injection)

Therapeutic: Antidiabetic (insulin aspart protamine suspension, insulin aspart injection)

Pregnancy category: C

Indications and Dosages

▶ *To control hyperglycemia in patients with diabetes mellitus*

S.C. INJECTION
Adults. Dosage highly individualized based on patient's metabolic needs, eating habits, and other lifestyle variables. Injected b.i.d. within 15 minutes of breakfast and dinner.
DOSAGE ADJUSTMENT Dosage reduced in patients with renal impairment and possibly those with hepatic impairment

---

Mechanism of Action
Insulin aspart protamine suspension and insulin aspart injection bind to insulin receptors in muscle and other tissues (except the brain) causing rapid intracellular transport of glucose and amino acids, promoting anabolism, and inhibiting protein catabolism. In the liver, insulin promotes the uptake and storage of glucose in the form of glycogen, inhibits gluconeogenesis, and promotes conversion of excess glucose into fat. All of these actions contribute to lowering blood glucose levels.

Contraindications
Episodes of hypoglycemia, diabetic coma, diabetic ketoacidosis, hyperosmolar hyperglycemic state, hypersensitivity to insulin aspart or its components

Interactions
DRUGS
insulin aspart protamine suspension and insulin aspart injection
anabolic steroids, baclofen, beta blockers, clonidine, corticosteroids, danazol, diuretics, estrogens, hormonal contraceptives, isoniazid, lithium salts, phenothiazines, some lipid-lowering drugs (such as niacin), somatropin, sympathomimetics, thyroid hormone: Possibly increased risk of hyperglycemia
ACE inhibitors, androgens, beta blockers, clonidine, disopyramide, fibrates, fluoxetine, inhibitors of pancreatic function (such as octreotide), lithium salts, MAO inhibitors, oral antidiabetics, propoxyphene, salicylates, sulfa antibiotics: Increased risk of hypoglycemia
beta blockers, clonidine, guanethidine, reserpine: Possibly masked symptoms of hypoglycemia
pentamidine: Possibly hypoglycemia, sometimes followed by hyperglycemia
ACTIVITIES
insulin aspart protamine suspension and insulin aspart injection
alcohol use: Possibly increased or decreased blood glucose–lowering effect of insulin

Adverse Reactions

ENDO: Hypoglycemia, insulin resistance
SKIN: Injection site reaction, such as redness, swelling, or pruritus; lipodystrophy; whole body pruritus or rash
Other: Anaphylaxis, hypokalemia, weight gain

Nursing Considerations

• Give insulin aspart protamine suspension and insulin aspart injection by subcutaneous injection, never intravenously. Rotate injection site within selected anatomical site.
• Be aware that 1 unit of insulin aspart protamine suspension and insulin aspart injection has the same glucose-lowering effect as 1 unit of regular human insulin, but its effect is more rapid and of shorter duration.
• **WARNING** Monitor patient closely for hypoglycemia, the most common adverse effect of insulin therapy. Evidence includes sudden fatigue or weakness, irritability, shakiness, trouble concentrating, diaphoresis, headache, or change in mental status that may progress to coma, seizure, or neurologic impairment if treatment is delayed. Know that early warning symptoms may be different or less pronounced under certain conditions, such as the patient having been diabetic for a long time, presence of diabetic neuropathy, or use of beta blockers. More intensified diabetes control also increases risk of hypoglycemia.
• If hypoglycemia is suspected, obtain blood glucose level to confirm, and treat according to severity.
• For mild hypoglycemia, give 10 to 15 grams of a fast-acting carbohydrate such as 4 ounces of orange juice, 6 ounces of regular soda, 6 to 8 ounces of skim or 1% milk, 2 large lumps or teaspoons of sugar, 5 to 7 Lifesavers, or 2 to 5 glucose tablets. Wait 15 minutes; then retest patient's blood glucose level. If it's still low, treat again. If the patient's next meal or snack is more than 30 minutes away, also provide a follow-up snack. Determine the cause of hypoglycemia to prevent future episodes, if possible, and notify prescriber to determine next insulin dose.
• For severe hypoglycemia, expect to give subcutaneous or intramuscular glucagon or concentrated intravenous glucose, as ordered. If glucagon is given, keep patient's head turned to the side and elevated because vomiting may occur. If patient doesn't respond within 5 to 20 minutes, repeat glucagon injection. Once the patient is awake enough to swallow, provide some clear liquids such as regular non-cola soda followed by a

substantial snack, such as a roll with peanut butter or half of a cheese sandwich. Determine the cause of hypoglycemia to prevent future episodes, if possible, and notify prescriber to determine next insulin dose.

• Monitor patient's blood glucose level and glycosylated hemoglobin level, as ordered to determine insulin dosage needs.

• Inspect patient's injection site regularly for adverse reactions, such as localized redness, swelling, pruritus, or lipodystrophy.

• Monitor patient's serum potassium level because hypokalemia may occur with insulin use, especially in patients with autonomic neuropathy, patients who are fasting (always check with prescriber before administering insulin in a patient who is fasting), or patients who are using potassium-lowering drugs or taking drugs known to alter serum potassium level.

PATIENT TEACHING

• Tell patient that insulin aspart protamine suspension and insulin aspart injection needs to be resuspended immediately before use. To resuspend, tell patient to roll the vial, cartridge, or prefilled pen syringe between the palms of his hands 10 times. In addition, if the patient is using the prefilled cartridge or pen syringe form, tell him he must then turn the cartridge or syringe upside down so the glass ball moves from one end of the delivery system to the other, and keep turning it at least 10 times to ensure solution becomes uniformly white and cloudy. If needed, instruct patient to repeat rolling and turning procedure until the insulin solution is uniformly white and cloudy.

• Teach patient how to measure insulin dosage and use a standard insulin syringe, the NovoLog Mix 70/30 FlexPen, or PenFill cartridge compatible delivery device prescribed. Inform patient that drug comes mixed as a 70% insulin aspart protamine suspension and 30% insulin aspart injection solution and shouldn't be mixed with any other insulin.

• Instruct patient how to administer insulin subcutaneously. Review anatomical sites for injection (abdomen [best site for absorption], thigh, upper arm) and stress importance of rotating injection sites within selected area. Alert patient that the rate of insulin absorption and consequently its onset of action can be affected by exercise and by changing the injection site. Urge patient to follow guidelines provided by the prescriber.

• Caution patient only to use insulin aspart protamine suspension and insulin aspart injection if it appears uniformly cloudy after resuspension and not to use after its expiration date.

- Tell patient to keep spare insulin vials, cartridges, or pens in the refrigerator. Remind him that unrefrigerated vials must be used within 28 days of removing from the refrigerator and unrefrigerated prefilled cartridges and pens must be used within 14 days. Tell patient to keep the prefilled cartridge or pen currently in use at room temperature but as cool as possible.
- Caution patient to protect unrefrigerated insulin from direct heat and light.
- Instruct patient to measure insulin dosage carefully and inject it within 15 minutes of eating breakfast and dinner.
- Stress importance of following a regular meal plan and exercise program, monitoring his blood glucose level regularly, and testing glycosylated hemoglobin periodically.
- Explain signs and symptoms and proper management of hypoglycemia and hyperglycemia. Tell patient to notify prescriber episodes are frequent, severe, or difficult to bring under control.
- Stress importance of keeping follow-up appointments to determine effectiveness of prescribed insulin therapy and monitor for diabetes complications.
- Tell female patients to alert the prescriber if they become pregnant or intend to become pregnant because their insulin dosage will need to be adjusted.
- Advise patient to notify prescriber about changes in physical activity or meal plan because insulin dosage will need adjustment.
- Tell patient to notify prescriber about illness, emotional disturbance, or other stress because the insulin dosage may need to be adjusted.
- Advise patient to obtain and wear medical identification indicating that he takes insulin.
- Encourage family members to learn about signs and symptoms of hypoglycemia and how to administer glucagon in an emergency.

70% insulin isophane (human) suspension and 30% insulin (human) injection

Humulin 70/30, Novolin 70/30

50% human insulin isophane suspension and 50% human insulin injection

Humulin 50/50

Class and Category

Chemical: Human insulin analogue (human insulin isophane suspension, human insulin injection)

Therapeutic: Antidiabetic (human insulin isophane suspension, human insulin injection)

Pregnancy category: B

Indications and Dosages

▶ *To control hyperglycemia in patients with diabetes mellitus*

S.C. INJECTION

Adults. Dosage highly individualized based on patient's metabolic needs, eating habits, and other lifestyle variables. Injected b.i.d. 30 to 60 minutes before a meal.

DOSAGE ADJUSTMENT Dosage reduced in patients with renal impairment and possibly those with hepatic impairment

---

Mechanism of Action

Human insulin isophane suspension and human insulin injection bind to insulin receptors in muscle and other tissues (except the brain), causing rapid intracellular transport of glucose and amino acids, promoting anabolism, and inhibiting protein catabolism. In the liver, insulin promotes uptake and storage of glucose as glycogen, inhibits gluconeogenesis, and promotes conversion of excess glucose into fat. All of these actions contribute to lowering blood glucose levels.

Contraindications

Episodes of hypoglycemia, diabetic ketoacidosis, hyperosmolar hyperglycemia, hypersensitivity to human insulin or its components

Interactions

DRUGS

human insulin isophane suspension and human insulin injection

anabolic steroids, baclofen, beta blockers, clonidine, corticosteroids, danazol, diuretics, estrogens, hormonal contraceptives, isoniazid, lithium salts, phenothiazines, some lipid-lowering drugs (such as niacin), somatropin, sympathomimetics, thyroid hormone: Possibly increased risk of hyperglycemia

ACE inhibitors, androgens, beta blockers, clonidine, disopyramide, fibrates, fluoxetine, inhibitors of pancreatic function (such as octreotide), lithium salts, MAO inhibitors, oral antidiabetics, propoxyphene, salicylates, sulfa antibiotics: Increased risk of hypoglycemia *beta blockers, clonidine, guanethidine, reserpine:* Possibly mask symptoms of hypoglycemia

pentamidine: Possibly hypoglycemia, sometimes followed by hyperglycemia

ACTIVITIES

alcohol use: Possibly increased or decreased blood glucose–lowering effect of insulin

Adverse Reactions

ENDO: Hypoglycemia, insulin resistance

SKIN: Injection site reaction, such as redness, swelling, or pruritus; lipodystrophy; whole-body pruritus or rash

Other: Anaphylaxis, hypokalemia, weight gain

Nursing Considerations

- Inject human insulin isophane suspension and human insulin injection subcutaneously, never intravenously. Rotate injection site within selected anatomical area.
- **WARNING** Monitor patient closely for hypoglycemia, the most common adverse effect of insulin therapy. Evidence may include sudden fatigue or weakness, irritability, shakiness, trouble concentrating, diaphoresis, headache, or change in mental status that may progress to coma, seizure, or neurologic impairment if treatment is delayed. Know that early warning symptoms may be different or less pronounced under certain conditions, such as long-term diabetes, presence of diabetic neuropathy, or use of beta blockers. More intensified diabetes control also increases risk of hypoglycemia.
- If hypoglycemia is suspected, obtain blood glucose level to confirm, and treat according to severity.
- For mild hypoglycemia, give 10 to 15 grams of a fast acting carbohydrate, such as 4 ounces of orange juice, 6 ounces of regular soda, 6 to 8 ounces of skim or 1% milk, 2 large lumps or teaspoons of sugar, 5 to 7 Lifesavers, or 2 to 5 glucose tablets. Wait 15 minutes; then retest patient's blood glucose level. If it's still low, treat again. If the patient's next meal or snack is more than 30 minutes away, also provide a follow-up snack. Determine the cause of hypoglycemia to prevent future episodes, if possible, and notify prescriber to determine next insulin dose.
- For severe hypoglycemia, expect to administer subcutaneous or intramuscular glucagon or concentrated intravenous glucose, as ordered. If glucagon is given, remember to keep patient's head turned to the side and elevated because vomiting may occur. If patient doesn't respond within 5 to 20 minutes, repeat glucagon

injection. Once patient is awake enough to swallow, provide clear liquids, such as regular non-cola soda, followed by a substantial snack, such as a roll with peanut butter or half of a cheese sandwich. Determine cause of hypoglycemia to prevent future episodes, if possible, and notify prescriber to determine next insulin dose.

- Monitor patient's blood glucose and glycosylated hemoglobin levels, as ordered to determine insulin dosage needs.
- Inspect patient's injection site regularly for signs of adverse reactions such as localized redness, swelling, pruritus, or lipodystrophy.
- Monitor patient's serum potassium level because hypokalemia may occur with insulin use, especially in patients with autonomic neuropathy, patients who are fasting (always check with prescriber before giving insulin to a patient who is fasting), or patients who are using potassium-lowering drugs or taking drugs known to alter serum potassium level.

PATIENT TEACHING
- Tell patient that human insulin isophane suspension and human insulin injection needs to be resuspended immediately before use. To resuspend, tell patient to roll the vial, cartridge or prefilled pen syringe between the palms of his hands 10 times. In addition, if the patient is using the prefilled cartridge or pen syringe form, tell him he must then turn the cartridge or syringe upside down so that the glass ball moves from one end of the delivery system to the other and keep turning it for at least 10 times to ensure solution becomes uniformly white and cloudy. If necessary, instruct patient to repeat rolling and turning procedure until the insulin solution is uniformly white and cloudy.
- Teach patient how to measure insulin dosage and use a standard insulin syringe, pen, or cartridge compatible delivery device prescribed. Inform patient that drug comes mixed as a 70% human insulin isophane suspension and 30% human insulin injection solution or as 50% human insulin isophane suspension and 50% human insulin injection solution and shouldn't be mixed with any other insulin.
- Instruct patient how to administer insulin subcutaneously. Review anatomical sites for insulin injection (abdomen [best site for absorption], thigh, upper arm) and stress the importance of rotating injection sites within the selected area. Alert patient that the rate of insulin absorption and consequently its onset of action can be affected by exercise and changing the injection

area; urge patient to follow guidelines provided by the prescriber.

- Caution patient to use human insulin isophane suspension and human insulin injection only if it appears uniformly cloudy after resuspension and not to use after its expiration date.
- Tell patient to keep spare insulin vials, cartridges, or pens in the refrigerator. Remind him that unrefrigerated vials must be used within 28 days of removing from the refrigerator or it must be discarded and unrefrigerated prefilled cartridges and pens must be used within 10 days or be discarded. Tell patient to keep the prefilled cartridge or pen currently in use at room temperature but as cool as possible.
- Caution patient to protect unrefrigerated insulin from direct heat and light.
- Instruct patient to measure insulin dosage carefully and inject it 30 to 60 minutes before a meal.
- Stress importance of following a regular meal plan and exercise program and of monitoring his blood glucose level regularly and glcosylated hemoglobin periodically.
- Explain signs and symptoms and proper management of hypoglycemia and hyperglycemia. Tell patient to notify prescriber if hypoglycemic episodes are frequent, severe, or difficult to bring under control.
- Stress importance of having follow-up appointments to determine effectiveness of prescribed insulin therapy and check for diabetes complications.
- Tell female patients to alert the prescriber if they become pregnant or intend to become pregnant because their insulin dosage will need to be adjusted.
- Advise patient to notify prescriber about changes in physical activity or usual meal plan because insulin dosage will need adjustment.
- Tell patient to notify prescriber if an illness, emotional disturbance, or other stress occurs because insulin dosage may need to be adjusted.
- Advise patient to obtain and wear medical alert identification showing that the patient takes insulin.
- Encourage family members to learn about the signs and symptoms of hypoglycemia and how to administer glucagon in an emergency.

75% insulin lispro protamine suspension and 25% insulin lispro injection
Humalog Mix 75/25

Class and Category
Chemical: Human insulin analogue (insulin lispro protamine suspension, insulin lispro injection)
Therapeutic: Antidiabetic (insulin lispro protamine suspension, insulin lispro injection)
Pregnancy category: B

Indications and Dosages
▶ *To control hyperglycemia in patients with diabetes mellitus*
S.C. INJECTION
Adults. Highly individualized dosage based on patient's metabolic needs, eating habits, and other lifestyle variables injected within 15 minutes before selected meals daily.
DOSAGE ADJUSTMENT Dosage reduced in patients with renal impairment and possibly those with hepatic impairment

---

Mechanism of Action
Insulin lispro protamine suspension and insulin lispro injection bind to insulin receptors located in muscle and other tissues (except brain), which causes rapid intracellular transport of glucose and amino acids, promotes anabolism, and inhibits protein catabolism. In the liver, insulin promotes the uptake and storage of glucose in the form of glycogen, inhibits gluconeogenesis, and promotes conversion of excess glucose into fat. All of these actions contribute to lowering blood glucose levels.

Contraindications
During episodes of hypoglycemia, diabetic coma, diabetic ketoacidosis, hyperosmolar hyperglycemic state, hypersensitivity to insulin lispro or any of its components

Interactions
DRUGS
insulin lispro protamine suspension and insulin lispro injection
anabolic steroids, baclofen, beta blockers, clonidine, corticosteroids, danazol, diuretics, estrogens, hormonal contraceptives, isoniazid, lithium salts, phenothiazines, certain lipid-lowering drugs (such as niacin), somatropin,

sympathomimetic agents, thyroid hormone: Increased hyperglycemic
activity
*ACE inhibitors, androgens, beta blockers, clonidine, disopyramide, fi-
brates, fluoxetine, inhibitors of pancreatic function (such as octreotide),
lithium salts, MAO inhibitors, oral antidiabetics, propoxyphene, salicylates, sulfa antibiotics:* Increased risk of hypoglycemia
beta blockers, clonidine, guanethidine, reserpine: Possibly masked
symptoms of hypoglycemia
pentamidine: Possibly hypoglycemia, sometimes followed by hyperglycemia
ACTIVITIES
**insulin lispro protamine suspension and insulin lispro
injection**
alcohol use: Possibly increased or decreased blood glucose–lowering
effects of insulin

Adverse Reactions
ENDO: Hypoglycemia, stimulation of insulin antibody production
SKIN: Injection site reaction, such as redness, swelling, or pruri-
tus; lipodystrophy; whole-body pruritus or rash
Other: Anaphylaxis, hypokalemia

Nursing Considerations
- Be aware that insulin lispro protamine suspension and insulin
  lispro injection has a more rapid onset of action and a shorter
  duration of action than regular human insulin, requiring that it
  be given within 15 minutes before a meal.
- Inject insulin lispro protamine suspension and insulin lispro injection subcutaneously, never intravenously. Rotate injection
  site within selected anatomical site.
- Be aware that 1 unit of insulin lispro protamine suspension and
  insulin lispro injection has the same glucose-lowering effect as
  1 unit of regular human insulin, but that its effect is more rapid
  and of shorter duration.
- **WARNING** Monitor patient closely for hypoglycemia, the
  most common adverse effect of insulin therapy. Evidence may
  include sudden fatigue or weakness, irritability, shakiness,
  trouble concentrating, diaphoresis, headache, or change in
  mental status that may progress to coma, seizure, or neurologic impairment if treatment is delayed. Know that early
  warning symptoms may be different or less pronounced under certain conditions, such as long-term diabetes, presence of
  diabetic neuropathy, or use of beta blockers. More intensified
  diabetes control also increases risk of hypoglycemia.

- If hypoglycemia is suspected, obtain blood glucose level to confirm, and treat according to severity.
- For mild hypoglycemia, give 10 to 15 grams of a fast-acting carbohydrate, such as 4 ounces of orange juice, 6 ounces of regular soda, 6 to 8 ounces of skim or 1% milk, 2 large lumps or teaspoons of sugar, 5 to 7 Lifesavers, or 2 to 5 glucose tablets. Wait 15 minutes; then retest patient's blood glucose. If blood glucose level is still low, treat again. If the patient's next meal or snack is more than 30 minutes away, also provide a follow-up snack. Determine cause of hypoglycemia to prevent future episodes, if possible, and notify prescriber to determine next insulin dose.
- For severe hypoglycemia, expect to give subcutaneous or intramuscular glucagon or concentrated intravenous glucose, as ordered. If glucagon is administered, remember to keep patient's head turned to the side and elevated because vomiting may occur. If patient doesn't respond within 5 to 20 minutes, repeat glucagon injection. Once the patient is awake enough to swallow, provide clear liquids, such as regular non-cola soda followed by a substantial snack, such as a roll with peanut butter or half of a cheese sandwich. Determine cause of hypoglycemia to prevent future episodes, if possible, and notify the prescriber to determine next insulin dose.
- Monitor patient's blood glucose and glycosylated hemoglobin levels, as ordered, to determine insulin dosage needs.
- Inspect the patient's injection site regularly for adverse reactions, such as localized redness, swelling or pruritus or lipodystrophy.
- Monitor patient's serum potassium level because hypokalemia may occur with insulin use, especially in patients with autonomic neuropathy, patients who are fasting (always check with prescriber before administering insulin in a patient who is fasting), or patients who are using potassium-lowering drugs or taking drugs known to alter the serum potassium level.

PATIENT TEACHING
- Tell patient how to measure insulin dosage using a standard insulin syringe or the Humalog Mix 75/25 pen. Inform patient that drug comes mixed as a 75% insulin lispro protamine suspension and 25% insulin lispro injection solution and shouldn't be mixed with any other insulin.
- Instruct patient how to administer insulin subcutaneously. Review anatomical sites for insulin injection (abdomen being the

best site for absorption) and stress importance of rotating injection sites within selected area. Alert patient that the rate of insulin absorption and consequently its onset of action can be affected by changes in injeciton site or exercise, and urge patient to adhere to guidelines provided by the prescriber.

- Caution patient to use insulin lispro protamine suspension and insulin lispro injection only if it appears uniformly cloudy after mixing and not to use after its expiration date.
- Tell patient to keep spare insulin vials or pens in the refrigerator. Remind him that unrefrigerated vials must be used within 28 days of removing from the refrigerator and unrefrigerated pens must be used within 10 days.
- Caution patient to protect unrefrigerated insulin from direct heat and light and to keep at a cool room temperature.
- Instruct patient to measure insulin dosage carefully and inject within 15 minutes before eating a meal.
- Stress importance of adhering to a regular meal plan and exercise program and of monitoring his blood glucose level regularly testing his glycosylated hemoglobin level periodically.
- Explain the signs and symptoms and proper management of hypoglycemia and hyperglycemia. Tell patient to notify prescriber if episodes freuquent, severe, or difficult to bring under control.
- Stress importance of adhering to follow-up appointments to determine effectiveness of prescribed insulin therapy and monitor for diabetes complications.
- Tell female patients to alert prescriber if they become pregnant or intend to become pregnant because their insulin dosage will need to be adjusted.
- Advise patient to notify prescriber about changes in their physical activity or usual meal plan because insulin dosage will need to be adjusted.
- Tell patient to notify prescriber if an illness, emotional disturbance, or other stress occurs because insulin dosage may need to be adjusted.
- Advise patient to obtain and wear medical alert identification showing that the patient takes insulin.
- Encourage family members to learn about the signs and symptoms of hypoglycemia and how to administer glucagon in an emergency.

levothyroxine sodium (T₄) and liothyronine sodium (T₃)
(liotrix)
Thyrolar ¼, Thyrolar ½, Thyrolar 1, Thyrolar 2, Thyrolar 3

Class and Category
Chemical: Thyroid hormones (levothyroxine, liothyronine)
Therapeutic: Thyroid hormone replacement (levothyroxine, liothyronine)
Pregnancy category: A

Indications and Dosages
▶ *To treat hypothyroidism without myxedema*
TABLETS
Adults. *Initial:* 25 mcg levothyroxine and 6.25 mcg liothyronine (one tablet of Thyrolar ½) daily, increased q 2 to 3 wks by 12.5 mcg levothyroxine and 3.1 mcg liothyronine until therapeutic effects occur. *Maintenance:* 50 mcg levothyroxine and 12.5 mcg liothyronine (one tablet of Thyrolar 1) to 100 mcg levothyroxine and 25 mcg liothyronine (one tablet of Thyrolar 2) daily.
▶ *To treat long-standing myxedema or hypothyroidism in patients with cardiovascular disease*
TABLETS
Adults. *Initial:* 12.5 mcg levothyroxine and 3.1 mcg liothyronine (one tablet of Thyrolar ¼) daily, increased q 2 to 3 wk by 12.5 mcg levothyroxine and 3.1 mcg liothyronine until therapeutic effects occur. *Maintenance:* 50 mcg levothyroxine and 12.5 mcg liothyronine (one tablet of Thyrolar 1) to 100 mcg levothyroxine and 25 mcg liothyronine (one tablet of Thyrolar 2) daily.
DOSAGE ADJUSTMENT For elderly patients, initial dose usually reduced to 25% to 50% of adult dose; dosage then doubled q 6 to 8 wk until therapeutic effects occur.
▶ *To treat congenital hypothyroidism in children*
TABLETS
Children age 12 and over. 75 mcg levothyroxine and 18.75 mcg liothyronine (one tablet of Thyrolar 1 and one tablet of Thyrolar ½) daily.
Children ages 6 to 12. 50 mcg levothyroxine and 12.5 mcg liothyronine (one tablet of Thyrolar 1) daily to 75 mcg levothyroxine and 18.75 mcg liothyronine (one tablet of Thyrolar 1 and one tablet of Thyrolar ½) daily.
Children ages 1 to 6. 37.5 mcg levothyroxine and 9.35 mcg liothyronine (one tablet of Thyrolar ½ and one tablet of Thyrolar ¼)

daily to 50 mcg levothyroxine and 12.5 mcg liothyronine (one tablet of Thyrolar 1) daily.

Children ages 6 months to 12 months. 25 mcg levothyroxine and 6.25 mcg liothyronine (one tablet of Thyrolar ½) daily to 37.5 mcg levothyroxine and 9.35 mcg liothyronine (one tablet of Thyrolar ½ and one tablet of Thyrolar ¼) daily.

Newborn infants to age 6 months. 12.5 mcg levothyroxine and 3.1 mcg liothyronine (one tablet of Thyrolar ¼) daily to 25 mcg levothyroxine and 6.25 mcg liothyronine (one tablet of Thyrolar ½) daily.

Mechanism of Action

Both levothyroxine and liothyronine are thyroid hormones and replace endogenous thyroid hormone, which may exert physiologic effects by controlling DNA transcription and protein synthesis. These hormones have all of the following actions of endogenous thyroid hormone. The combination drug:

* increases energy expenditure
* accelerates the rate of cellular oxidation, which stimulates growth, maturation, and metabolism of body tissues
* aids in myelination of nerves and development of synaptic processes in the nervous system
* enhances carbohydrate and protein metabolism, increasing gluconeogenesis and protein synthesis.

Contraindications

Hypersensitivity to levothyroxine, liothyronine, or their components; uncorrected adrenal insufficiency; untreated thyrotoxicosis

Interactions

DRUGS

levothyroxine and liothyronine

adrenocorticoids: Possibly need to adjust adrenocorticoid dosage as thyroid status changes

cholestyramine, colestipol: Decreased absorption of levothyroxine and liothyronine

digoxin: Possibly need to adjust digoxin dosage as thyroid status changes

estrogen: Reduced binding of levothyroxine and liothyronine to protein, possibly requiring increased thyroid hormone dosage

insulin, oral antidiabetics: Possibly need to adjust insulin or oral antidiabetic dosage as thyroid status changes

ketamine: Possibly hypertension and tachycardia

maprotiline: Increased risk of arrhythmias
oral anticoagulants: Altered anticoagulant activity, possibly need to adjust anticoagulant dosage
sympathomimetics: Increased effects of either drug; risk of coronary insufficiency in patients with coronary artery disease

Adverse Reactions

CNS: Anxiety, asthenia, depression, fatigue, headache, insomnia, sluggish feeling, tremor
CV: Arrhythmias, chest pain, hypertension, palpitations, tachycardia
EENT: Keratoconjunctivitis sicca
ENDO: Hyperthyroidism (with overdose), hypothyroidism, increase or decrease in TSH
GI: Nausea
MS: Arthralgia, myalgia
SKIN: Alopecia (transient), dry skin, hyperhidrosis, pruritus, rash, urticaria
Other: Allergic reactions, increased weight

Nursing Considerations

• Administer levothyroxine and liothyronine as a single daily dose before breakfast.
• Expect patient to undergo periodic thyroid function tests during levothyroxine and liothyronine therapy.
• Monitor PT of patient on anticoagulants; she may need a dosage adjustment.
• Monitor blood glucose level often in diabetic patient. Prescriber may adjust antidiabetic drug dosage as hormone replacement is achieved.

PATIENT TEACHING
• Inform patient that levothyroxine and liothyronine combination is usually taken for life. Caution her not to stop drug or change dosage unless instructed by prescriber.
• Instruct patient to take drug before breakfast because evening doses may cause insomnia.
• Advise patient to store tablets in refrigerator in a tightly sealed, light-resistant container.
• Instruct patient to report signs of hyperthyroidism, such as chest pain, excessive sweating, heat intolerance, insomnia, palpitations, and weight loss.
• Advise diabetic patient to monitor blood glucose level often because antidiabetic drug dosage may need to be adjusted.

- Inform patient that transient hair loss may occur during first few months of therapy.
- Inform patient of need for periodic thyroid hormone blood tests to monitor drug effectiveness.

norgestimate and ethinyl estradiol

Ortho-Cyclen, Ortho Tri-Cyclen

Class and Category

Chemical: Progesterone steroid hormone derivative (norgestimate), estrogenic steroid hormone derivative (ethinyl estradiol)
Therapeutic: Ovarian hormone replacement (norgestimate, ethinyl estradiol)
Pregnancy category: X

Indications and Dosages

▶ *To treat moderate acne vulgaris in patients who desire contraception having achieved menarche and who also are unresponsive to topical anti-acne medication*

TABLETS

Females age 15 and over. 0.180 mg, 0.215 mg, or 0.250 mg norgestimate and 0.035 mg ethinyl estradiol (1 active tablet) daily for 21 days starting first day of monthly menstruation followed by 0 mg norgestimate and 0 mg of ethinyl estradiol (1 inactive tablet) daily for 7 days; cycle repeated q 28 days. Alternatively, 0.180 mg, 0.215 mg, or 0.250 mg norgestimate and 0.035 mg ethinyl estradiol (1 active tablet) daily for 21 days starting the first Sunday after monthly menstruation begins, followed by 0 mg norgestimate and 0 mg of ethinyl estradiol (1 inactive tablet) daily for 7 days; cycle repeated q 28 days.

Contraindications

Active deep vein thrombosis, pulmonary embolism, or history of these conditions; cerebral vascular or coronary artery disease; hepatic disorders including cholestatic jaundice in previous pregnancy or prior oral contraceptive pill use; hypersensitivity to norgestimate, ethinyl estradiol, or their components; known or suspected breast cancer or history of breast cancer from estrogen use; known or suspected estrogen-dependent cancer; migraine with focal aura; new or recent (within past year) CVA or MI; pregnancy; undiagnosed abnormal genital bleeding

Mechanism of Action

Norgestimate as a progestin inhibits secretion of gonadotropins from the anterior pituitary to prevent ovulation and follicular maturation. It also thickens cervical secretions making it more difficult for sperm to enter the uterus and produces changes in the endometial lining of the uterus making it more unlikely for implantation to occur. These combined actions interfere with the normal mechanisms of reproduction to prevent pregnancy.

Ethinyl estradiol increases the rate of DNA and RNA synthesis in the cells of female reproductive organs, pituitary gland, hypothalamus, and other target organs. In the hypothalamus, estrogens reduce the release of gonadotropin-releasing hormone, which decreases pituitary release of follicle-stimulating hormone and luteinizing hormone, needed for ovulation and follicular maturation to occur. At the cellular level, estrogens also increase cervical secretions. These combined actions interfere with the normal mechanisms of reproduction to prevent pregnancy.

The combined effect of norgestimate and ethinyl estradiol may increase sex hormone binding globulin and decrease free testosterone, which in turn results in a decreased severity of facial acne.

Interactions

DRUGS

norgestimate and ethinyl estradiol

ampicillin, barbiturates, carbamazepine, griseofulvin, phenylbutazone, phenytoin, rifabutin, rifampin, St. John's Wort, tetracyclines, topiramate: Possibly reduced effectiveness of norgestimate and ethinyl estradiol; increased risk of breakthrough bleeding and menstrual irregularities

ethinyl estradiol component

corticosteroids: Increased therapeutic and toxic effects of corticosteroids

cyclosporine: Increased risk of hepatotoxicity and nephrotoxicity

hepatotoxic drugs (such as isoniazid): Increased risk of hepatitis and hepatotoxicity

oral antidiabetics: Decreased therapeutic effects of these drugs

warfarin: Decreased anticoagulant effect

FOODS

ethinyl estradiol component

grapefruit juice: Decreased metabolism and possibly increased adverse effects of ethinyl estradiol

ACTIVITIES
ethinyl estradiol component
smoking: Increased risk of CVA, pulmonary embolism, thrombophlebitis, and transient ischemic attack

Adverse Reactions

CNS: Chorea, CVA, dementia, depression, dizziness, exacerbation of epilepsy, headache, irritability, migraine headache, mood disturbances, nervousness, porphyria

CV: Hypertension, increased triglycerides, MI, peripheral edema, pulmonary embolism, thromboembolism, thrombophlebitis

EENT: Diplopia, intolerance of contact lenses, retinal vascular thrombosis, sinusitis, vision changes or loss

ENDO: Breast enlargement, pain, tenderness, or tumors; endometrial hyperplasia, galactorrhea; gynecomastia; hyperglycemia; nipple discharge

GI: Abdominal cramps or pain, aggravation of porphyria, anorexia, bloating, constipation, diarrhea, elevated liver function test results, enlargement of hepatic hemangiomas, flatulence, gallbladder obstruction, hepatitis, increased appetite, nausea, pancreatitis, vomiting

GU: Amenorrhea, breakthrough bleeding, cervical erosion, clear vaginal discharge, dysmenorrhea, endometiral or ovarian tumors, increased libido, increased size of uterine leiomyomata, leukorrhea, prolonged or heavy menstrual bleeding, urinary tract infection, vaginitis including vaginal candidiasis

MS: Arthralgias, back or extremity pain, leg cramps

RESP: Bronchitis, exacerbation of asthma, upper respiratory infection

SKIN: Alopecia, application site irritation, chloasma, erythema multiforme or nodosum, hirsutism, jaundice, melasma, pruritus, purpura, rash, urticaria

Other: Anaphylaxis, angioedema, flulike syndrome, folic acid deficiency, hypercalcemia (with bone metastases), hypocalcemia, hyperkalemia, hyponatremia, weight gain or loss

Nursing Considerations

- Use norgestimate and ethinyl estradiol cautiously in women with asthma, diabetes mellitus, epilepsy, migraines, porphyria, systemic lupus erythematosus, and hepatic hemangiomas because ethinyl estradiol can worsen these conditions.
- **WARNING** Assess patient for possible contact lens intolerance or changes in vision or visual acuity because estrogens can cause keratoconus. Be prepared to stop drug immediately,

as prescribed, if patient has sudden partial or complete loss of vision or sudden onset of diplopia or migraine.

- Monitor PT for loss of anticoagulant effect in patients taking warfarin because ethinyl estradiol increases production of clotting factors VII, VIII, IX, and X and promotes platelet aggregation.
- Watch for elevated liver function test results because progestins and estrogens may worsen such conditions as acute intermittent and variegate hepatic porphyria.
- Closely monitor patient's blood pressure. Some patients may have a substantial increase in blood pressure as an indiosyncratic reaction to ethinyl estradiol. Monitor patients who already have hypertension for increases in blood pressure because estrogens like ethinyl estradiol may cause fluid retention. Also monitor patients with asthma, heart disease, migraines, renal disease, or seizure disorder for worsening of these conditions.
- Monitor blood glucose level often in patients with diabetes mellitus because ethinyl estradiol may decrease insulin sensitivity and alter glucose tolerance.
- Expect to stop norgestimate and ethinyl estradiol therapy in any woman who develops dementia or signs or symptoms of cardiovascular disease, such as stroke, MI, pulmonary embolism, or venous thrombosis.
- Be aware that norgestimate and ethinyl estradiol may worsen mood disorders, including depression. Monitor patient for depression, mood changes, anxiety, fatigue, dizziness, or insomnia.
- **WARNING** Be aware that patients with breast cancer and bone metastasis may develop severe hypercalcemia because estrogens such as ethinyl estradiol influence calcium and phosphorus metabolism. Watch for toxic effects of increased calcium absorption in patients predisposed to hypercalcemia or nephrolithiasis.
- Assess skin for melasma (tan or brown patches), which may develop on forehead, cheeks, temples, and upper lip. These patches may persist after drug is stopped.
- Monitor thyroid function test results in patients with hypothyroidism because long-term use of the ethinyl estradiol may decrease effectiveness of thyroid therapy.
- Expect to stop norgestimate and ethinyl estradiol therapy several weeks before patient undergoes major surgery, as prescribed, because prolonged immobilization poses a risk of thromboembolism.

PATIENT TEACHING
- Before therapy starts, inform patient of risks involved in taking norgestimate and ethinyl estradiol, such as increased risk of cardiovascular disease, breast or endometrial cancer, dementia, gallbladder disease, and vision abnormalities.
- Alert patient to notify prescriber immediately if vaginal bleeding or any other abnormal signs and symptoms occur while using norgestimate and ethinyl estradiol.
- Advise patient to avoid smoking while using norgestimate and ethinyl estradiol.
- Stress importance of compliancy with follow up visits.
- Emphasize importance of good dental hygiene and regular dental checkups because an elevated progestin blood level increases the growth of normal oral flora, which may lead to gum tenderness, bleeding, or swelling.

pioglitazone hydrochloride and metformin hydrochloride

Actoplus Met

Class and Category

Chemical: Thiazolidinedione (pioglitazone), biguanide (metformin)
Therapeutic: Antidiabetic (pioglitazone, metformin)
Pregnancy category: C

Indications and Dosages

▶ *To reduce blood glucose level in patients with type 2 diabetes mellitus who have responded well to pioglitazone initially but need additional glycemic control*

TABLETS

Adults. *Initial:* 15 mg pioglitazone and 500 mg metformin (1 tablet) b.i.d. or 15 mg pioglitazone and 850 mg metformin (1 tablet) daily, gradually adjusted as needed.

▶ *To reduce blood glucose level in patients who haven't achieved adequate glycemic control with metformin alone*

TABLETS

Adults. *Initial:* 15 mg pioglitazone and 500 mg metformin (1 tablet) or 15 mg pioglitazone and 850 mg metformin (1 tablet) daily or b.i.d., gradually adjusted as needed.

▶ *To reduce blood glucose level in patients who already take pioglitazone and metformin separately*

TABLETS
Adults. *Initial:* 15 mg pioglitazone and 500 mg metformin
(1 tablet) or 15 mg pioglitazone and 850 mg metformin (1 tablet)
daily or b.i.d. depending on dose of pioglitazone and metformin
already being taken.

Mechanism of Action

Pioglitazone decreases insulin resistance by enhancing the sensitivity of
insulin-dependent tissues, such as adipose tissue, skeletal muscle, and the
liver, and reduces glucose output from the liver. Pioglitazone activates peroxisome proliferator-activated receptor-gamma (PRARy) receptors, which modu-
late transcription of insulin-responsive genes involved in glucose control and
lipid metabolism. In this way, pioglitazone reduces hyperglycemia, hyperinsu-
linemia, and hypertriglyceridemia in patients with type 2 diabetes mellitus
and insulin resistance. However to work effectively, pioglitazone depends on
the presence of endogenous insulin.

Metformin may promote storage of excess glucose as glycogen in the liver,
which reduces glucose production. Metformin also may improve glucose use
by skeletal muscle and adipose tissue by increasing glucose transport across
cell membranes. It also may increase the number of insulin receptors on cell
membranes and make them more sensitive to insulin. In addition, metformin
modestly decreases blood triglyceride and total cholesterol levels.

Contraindications

Hypersensitivity to pioglitazone, metformin, or their components;
impaired renal function; metabolic acidosis, including diabetic ketoacidosis; severe hepatic dysfunction; type 1 diabetes mellitus;
use of iodinated contrast media within preceding 48 hours

Interactions

DRUGS

pioglitazone component
hormonal contraceptives: Possibly decreased contraceptive effectiveness
insulin, oral antidiabetics: Increased risk of hypoglycemia
ketoconazole: Possibly decreased metabolism of pioglitazone
metformin component
*calcium channel blockers, corticosteroids, estrogens, hormonal contracep-
tives, isoniazid, nicotinic acid, phenothiazines, phenytoin, sympathomimetics, thiazide and other diuretics, thyroid drugs:* Possibly hyperglycemia
cationic drugs (such as amiloride, cimetidine, digoxin, morphine, pro-

cainamide, quinidine, quinine, ranitidine, triameterene, trimethoprim, vancomycin), nifedipine: Increased metformin level

clofibrate, MAO inhibitors, probenecid, propranolol, rifabutin, rifampin, salicylates, sulfonamides, sulfonylureas: Increased risk of hypoglycemia

furosemide: Possibly increased blood metformin level and decreased blood furosemide level

FOODS

metformin component

all foods: Possibly delayed metformin absorption

ACTIVITIES

metformin component

alcohol use: Increased risk of hypoglycemia and lactate formation

Adverse Reactions

CNS: Dizziness, headache

CV: Congestive heart failure, edema

EENT: Metallic taste, pharyngitis, sinusitis, tooth disorders

ENDO: Hyperglycemia, hypoglycemia

GI: Abdominal distention, anorexia, constipation, diarrhea, elevated liver transaminase levels, flatulence, indigestion, nausea, vomiting

GU: Urinary tract infection

HEME: Aplastic anemia, decreased hemoglobin and hematocrit, megaloblastic anemia, thrombocytopenia

MS: Myalgia

RESP: Upper respiratory tract infection

SKIN: Photosensitivity, rash

Other: Decreased vitamin B_{12} levels, lactic acidosis, weight gain or loss

Nursing Considerations

- Be aware that this therapy isn't recommended for patients with New York Heart Association Class III or IV status.
- Use drug cautiously in patients with edema because it may occur opr worsen as an adverse reaction to pioglitazone.
- Give pioglitazone and metformin tablets with meals to reduce the risk of adverse GI reactions.
- Expect prescriber to alter dosage if patient has a condition that decreases or delays gastric emptying, such as diarrhea, gastroparesis, GI obstruction, ileus, or vomiting.
- Withhold drug, as ordered, if patient becomes dehydrated because dehydration increases the risk of lactic acidosis.
- Be aware that iodinated contrast media used in radiographic studies increase the risk of renal failure and lactic acidosis dur-

ing pioglitazone and metformin therapy. Expect to withhold drug for 48 hours before and after testing.

- Be prepared to monitor liver function test results before therapy begins, every 2 months during the first year, and annually thereafter, as ordered, because drug is extensively metabolized in the liver. Be prepared to stop drug if patient develops jaundice or if ALT values are greater than 2½ times normal.

- Assess BUN and serum creatinine level, as appropriate, before and during long-term therapy in those at increased risk for lactic acidosis because of the metformin component of drug.

- **WARNING** Monitor patient for signs and symptoms of heart failure—such as shortness of breath, rapid weight gain, or edema—because pioglitazone can cause fluid retention that may lead to or worsen heart failure. Notify prescriber immediately about any deterioration in the patient's cardiac status, and expect to stop the drug, as ordered.

- Watch for signs and symptoms of hypoglycemia, especially if patient also takes another antidiabetic drug.

- Monitor fasting blood glucose level, as ordered, to evaluate effectiveness of therapy. Assess patient for hyperglycemia and the need for insulin during times of increased stress, such as infection or surgery.

- Monitor glycosylated hemoglobin level to assess long-term effectiveness of drug therapy.

- Be aware that patients with inadequate vitamin B_{12} or calcium intake or absorption may develop abnormal vitamin B_{12} levels. Vitamin B_{12} level should be measured every 2 to 3 years, as ordered.

- Expect to withhold drug temporarily, as ordered, before any surgical procedure except for minor procedures not associated with restricted intake of food and fluids. Don't resume drug until patient's oral intake has resumed and renal function is normal.

PATIENT TEACHING

- Stress the need for patient to continue exercise program, diet control, and weight management during pioglitazone and metformin therapy.

- Instruct patient to take drug with meals: at breakfast if taking drug once a day, or at breakfast and dinner if taking drug twice a day.

- Direct patient to take drug exactly as prescribed and not to change the dosage or frequency unless instructed.

- Advise patient to notify prescriber immediately if he has shortness of breath, fluid retention, or sudden weight gain because drug may need to be stopped.
- Teach patient how to measure his blood glucose level and recognize hyperglycemia and hypoglycemia. Urge him to notify prescriber about abnormal blood glucose level.
- Caution patient to avoid alcohol, which can increase the risk of hypoglycemia.
- Instruct patient to watch for early evidence of lactic acidosis, including drowsiness, hyperventilation, malaise, and muscle pain, and notify prescriber if such signs develop.
- Instruct patient to keep appointments for liver function tests, as ordered, typically every 2 months during first year of therapy and annually thereafter.
- Inform female patient who uses oral contraceptives that drug decreases their effectiveness; suggest that she use another method of contraception while taking pioglitazone and metformin.
- Warn women of childbearing age who are premenopausal and having periods of anovulation that pioglitazone and metformin may induce ovulation. Advise using adequate contraception while taking drug.

risedronate sodium and calcium carbonate
Actonel with Calcium

Class and Category
Chemical: Pyridinyl bisphosphonate (risedronate), elemental cation (calcium)
Therapeutic: Bone resorption inhibitor (risedronate, calcium)
Pregnancy category: C

Indications and Dosages
▶ *To prevent or treat osteoporosis in postmenopausal women*
TABLETS
Adult females. 35 mg risedronate (1 tablet) q wk on day 1 of 7-day treatment cycle followed by 1,250 mg calcium (1 tablet) daily on days 2 through 7 of 7-day treatment cycle.

Contraindications
Hypercalcemia; hypersensitivity to risedronate, calcium, or their components; hypocalcemia; inability to stand or sit uupright for

at least 30 minutes; renal calculi; severe renal impairment (creatinine clearance less than 30 ml/min)

Mechanism of Action

Risedronate inhibits osteoclasts at the cellular level. Normally, osteoclasts adhere to the bone surface; risedronate prevents them from doing so. This reduces the rate at which osteoclasts are resorbed by bone.

Calcium suppresses PTH secretion. Increased PTH levels contribute to age-related bone loss, especially at cortical sites, while increased bone turnover is an independent risk factor for fractures. With suppression of PTH secretion, bone turnover decreases.

Interactions

DRUGS

risedronate component

aspirin, NSAIDs: Increased risk of GI irritation

calcium-containing preparations, including antacids: Impaired absorption of risedronate

calcium component

bisphosphonates: Decreased absorption of the bisphosphonate

fluoroquinolones: Possibly decreased absorption of the fluoroquinolone

glucocorticoids (systemic): Decreased absorption of calcium

iron: Possibly decreased absorption of iron

levothyroxine: Decreased levothyroxine absorption and increased serum thyrotropin levels

tetracyclines: Possibly decreased absorption of tetracycline

thiazide diuretics: Reduced urinary excretion of calcium, possibly leading to adverse effects

vitamin D, vitamin D analgues (such as calcitriol, doxercalciferol, and paricalcitol): Possibly increased absorption of calcium

FOODS

risedronate component

all foods: Decreased risedronate bioavailability

calcium component

caffeine, high-fiber food: Possibly decreased calcium absorption

ACTIVITIES

calcium component

alcohol use (excessive), smoking: Possibly decreased calcium absorption

Adverse Reactions

CNS: Anxiety, asthenia, depression, dizziness, headache, hypertonia, insomnia, neuralgia, paresthesia, weakness, vertigo

CV: Angina, chest pain, hypertension, hypotension, peripheral edema

EENT: Amblyopia, cataract, onjunctivitis, dry eyes or mouth, otitis media, pharyngitis, rhinitis, sinusitis, tinnitus

ENDO: Hypercalcemia

GI: Abdominal pain, bloating, colitis, constipation, diarrhea, dysphagia, eructation, esophagitis, esophageal or gastric ulcer, flatulence, gastritis, heartburn, nausea

GU: UTI

HEME: Anemia

MS: Arthralgia; back, bone, or neck pain; bursitis; joint disorder; leg cramps; myasthenia; myalgia; osteonecrosis of the jaw; retrosternal pain

RESP: Bronchitis,dyspnea, pneumonia

SKIN: Bullous skin reactions, ecchymosis, pruritus, rash, skin carcinoma

Other: Angioedema, flulike symptoms

Nursing Considerations

- Use risedronate and calcium cautiously in patients with a history of kidney stones or hypercalciuria. Be prepared to monitor these patient's urinary calcium excretion regularly, as ordered.
- Check to determine if patient has had a dental examination before starting risedronate and calcium therapy, especially if patient has cancer; is receiving chemotherapy, head or neck radiation, or corticosteroids; or has poor oral hygiene. The risk of developing osteonecrosis is higher in these patients, and invasive dental procedures during risedronate and calcium therapy can exacerbate osteonecrosis.
- Be aware that bisphosphonates like risedronate may interfere with bone-imaging agents.
- Monitor patient's serum calcium levels and bone density scans regularly, as ordered to determine effectiveness of risedronate and calcium therapy.

PATIENT TEACHING

- Instruct patient to take risedronate with a full glass of water at least 30 minutes before she takes her first food or beverage (except water) of the day and not to lie down for 30 minutes. Instruct patient to take calcium tablets with food to improve absorption.

- Tell patient that if she misses taking her weekly risedronate tablet, to take it the morning after she remembers it and to return to taking 1 tablet of risedronate once a week, as originally scheduled on her chosen day. Stress that she should not take 2 risedronate tablets on the same day.
- Advise patient to avoid taking calcium within 2 hours of taking another oral drug because of risk of interaction.
- Caution patient to consult prescriber before taking OTC drugs because of risk of interactions.
- Tell patient to avoid excessive use of tobacco and excessive consumption of alcoholic beverages, caffeine-containing products and high-fiber foods because these substances may decrease calcium absorption.
- Instruct patient on proper oral hygiene and to notify prescriber before having any invasive dental procedure performed.
- Tell patient to notify prescriber if she develops difficulty or pain with swallowing, retrosternal pain, or severe persistent or worsening heartburn.

rosiglitazone maleate and metformin hydrochloride
Avandamet

Class and Category
Chemical: Thiazolidinedione (rosiglitazone), dimethylbiguanide (metformin)
Therapeutic: Antidiabetic
Pregnancy category: C

Indications and Dosages
▶ *To reduce blood glucose level as initial therapy in patients with type 2 diabetes mellitus who aren't adequately controlled with rosiglitazone alone*
TABLETS
Adults. *Initial:* 2 mg/500 mg b.i.d if patient was taking 4 mg daily of rosiglitazone monotherapy; 4 mg/500 mg b.i.d. if 8 mg daily of rosiglitazone monotherapy. Increased as needed after 1 to 2 wk if metformin dosage isn't sufficient or 8 to 12 wk if rosiglitazone dosage isn't sufficient. *Maximum:* 8 mg/2,000 mg/day.
▶ *To reduce blood glucose level as initial therapy in patients with type 2 diabetes mellitus who aren't adequately controlled with metformin alone*

TABLETS

Adults. *Initial:* 2 mg/500 mg b.i.d. if patient was taking 1,000 mg daily of metformin monotherapy; individualized if patient was taking 1,000 to 2,000 mg daily of metformin monotherapy; or 2 mg/1,000 mg (2 tablets, each 1 mg rosiglitazone and 500 mg metformin) b.i.d. if patient was taking 2,000 mg daily of metformin monotherapy. Dosage increased, as needed, after 1 to 2 wk if metformin dosage isn't sufficient or after 8 to 12 wk if rosiglitazone dosage isn't sufficient. *Maximum:* 8 mg rosiglitazone and 2,000 mg metformin daily.

DOSAGE ADJUSTMENT If patient has been taking rosiglitazone and metformin as separate tablets, usual starting dose of combination drug is that of rosiglitazone and metformin already being taken individually.

Mechanism of Action

Rosiglitazone and metformin each improve glucose control. Rosiglitazone increases tissue sensitivity to insulin. A peroxisome proliferator-activated receptor agonist, it regulates transcription of insulin-responsive genes in key target tissues, such as adipose tissue, skeletal muscle, and liver. Enhanced insulin sensitivity lowers blood glucose level.

Metformin may promote storage of excess glucose as glycogen in the liver, thus reducing glucose production. It also may improve glucose use by skeletal muscle and adipose tissue by facilitating glucose transport across cell membranes. Metformin also may increase the number of insulin receptors on cell membranes and make them more sensitive to insulin.

Contraindications

Diabetic coma; heart failure requiring drug treatment; hypersensitivity to metformin, rosiglitazone, or their components; ketoacidosis; metabolic acidosis (acute or chronic); renal disease or dysfunction (serum creatinine level of 1.5 mg/dl or more in men or 1.4 mg/dl or more in women); type 1 diabetes mellitus

Interactions

DRUGS

rosiglitazone component

CYP 2C8 inducers (such as rifampin): Possibly decreased effects of rosiglitazone

CYP 2C8 inhibitors (such as gemfibrozil): Possibly increased effects of rosiglitazone

metformin component

cimetidine: Increased blood metformin level; possibly increased risk of hypoglycemia
furosemide: Increased blood metformin level and decreased blood furosemide level
nifedipine: Enhanced metformin absorption
FOODS

metformin component
all foods: Delayed and reduced metformin absorption
ACTIVITIES

metformin component
alcohol use: Altered blood glucose control (usually hyperglycemia) and possibly potentiated metformin effect on lactate metabolism

Adverse Reactions
CNS: Fatigue, headache
CV: Edema, heart failure
EENT: Sinusitis
ENDO: Hyperglycemia, hypoglycemia
GI: Diarrhea, elevated liver function test results, hepatotoxicity
HEME: Anemia
MS: Arthralgia, back pain
RESP: Upper respiratory tract infection
SKIN: Urticaria
Other: Angioedema, lactic acidosis, viral infection, weight gain

Nursing Considerations
- **WARNING** Monitor renal function, as ordered, before starting rosiglitazone and metformin and at least annually thereafter because significant renal impairment can result in tissue hypoperfusion and hypoxemia, leading to lactic acidosis.
- Evaluate patient's liver function before starting drug and periodically throughout therapy, as ordered. Notify prescriber about abnormalities, such as nausea, vomiting, abdominal pain, fatigue, anorexia, and dark urine. Drug may need to be stopped.
- **WARNING** Expect to stop rosiglitazone and metformin for 48 hours before and after radiographic tests involving I.V. iodinated contrast media because of an increased risk of renal failure and lactic acidosis.
- **WARNING** Monitor malnourished or debilitated patients and those with renal, hepatic, pituitary, or adrenal insufficiency because they have an increased risk of hypoglycemia.
- Expect to monitor vitamin B_{12} blood levels at least every 2 to 3 years in patients with inadequate vitamin B_{12} or calcium in-

take or absorption because prolonged drug use may impair vitamin B_{12} absorption.

- Monitor fasting blood glucose level to determine patient's response to drug. Expect to monitor glycosylated hemoglobin (HbA_{1c}) level every 3 to 6 months, as ordered, to evaluate long-term blood glucose control.

- Monitor blood glucose level often to detect hyperglycemia and assess the need for supplemental insulin during circumstances of increased stress, such as infection, surgery, and trauma.

- Arrange for instruction about diabetes and consultation with a dietitian or certified diabetes educator, if possible.

- Monitor patient for evidence of heart failure, such as difficulty breathing, fatigue, abnormal heart sounds, and edema. Notify prescriber if such evidence occurs, and expect to stop drug.

PATIENT TEACHING

- Instruct patient to take rosiglitazone and metformin with morning and evening meals. Caution her not to skip the meal after taking the drug.

- Inform patient that drug is used with diet and exercise therapy and is not a substitute for these additional measures.

- Advise patient not to skip doses, stop drug, or take OTC drugs without first consulting prescriber because of the risk of hyperglycemia.

- Inform patient that the most common adverse effects are minor and typically occur during first few weeks of therapy.

- Teach patient how to monitor blood glucose level and when to report changes.

- Advise patient to expect laboratory monitoring of HbA_{1c} level every 3 months until blood glucose level is controlled.

- Instruct patient to report signs of hypoglycemia, such as anxiety, confusion, dizziness, excessive sweating, headache, and nausea.

- Advise patient to carry identification indicating that she has diabetes.

- Advise patient to avoid alcohol because it increases the risk of hypoglycemia.

- Instruct female patient of childbearing age to report suspected or confirmed pregnancy to prescriber because she may need to stop rosiglitazone and metformin therapy and switch to insulin therapy, as prescribed, during pregnancy.

testosterone cypionate and estradiol cypionate
Depo-Testadiol
testosterone enanthate and estradiol valerate
Valertest No. 1

Class and Category
Chemical: Androgen (testosterone), estrogen (estradiol)
Therapeutic: Hormone replacement (testosterone, estradiol)
Pregnancy category: X

Indications and Dosages
▶ *To treat moderate to severe vasomotor symptoms of menopause*
I.M. INJECTION (DEPO-TESTADIOL)
Adult females. 50 mg testosterone and 2 mg estradiol (1 ml) q 4 wk
I.M. INJECTION (VALERTEST NO. 1)
Adult females. 90 mg testosterone and 4 mg estradiol (1 ml) q 4 wk

---

Mechanism of Action
Testosterone esters such as cypionate and enanthate first undergo hydrolysis of the ester to the active form, free testosterone, in the liver. Free testosterone is further converted into two of the major active metabolites, DHT and estradiol. Thus, testosterone can produce estrogenic effects as a result of its conversion to estradiol to help maintain GU function and reduce vasomotor symptoms when estrogen production declines from menopause, surgical removal of the ovaries, or other estrogen deficiency.

Estradiol increases DNA and RNA synthesis in the cells of female reproductive organs, pituitary gland, hypothalamus, and other target organs. In the hypothalamus, estrogens decrease release of gonadotropin-releasing hormone, which reduces pituitary release of follicle-stimulating hormone and luteinizing hormone. In women, these hormones are required for normal GU and other essential body functions. At the cellular level, estrogens increase cervical secretions, cause endometrial cell proliferation, and improve uterine tone. Estrogen replacement helps maintain GU function and reduces vasomotor symptoms when estrogen production declines as a result of menopause, surgical removal of ovaries, or other estrogen deficiency.

Contraindications
Active thrombophlebitis or thromboembolic disorders; breastfeeding; hypersensitivity to testosterone, estradiol, or their compo-

nents; known or suspected breast cancer (except in select patients being treated for metastatic disease); known or suspected estrogen-dependent cancer; pregnancy; severe liver damage; undiagnosed abnormal genital bleeding

Interactions

DRUGS

testosterone and estradiol

corticosteroids: Increased therapeutic and toxic effects of corticosteroids

hepatotoxic drugs (such as isoniazid): Increased risk of hepatitis and hepatotoxicity

oral antidiabetics: Decreased or increased therapeutic effects of these drugs with risk of hyperglycemia or hypoglycemia

warfarin: Altered anticoagulant effect

testosterone component

cyclosporine: Possibly increased risk of nephrotoxicity

estradiol, estrogens: Enhanced estrogenic effects

propranolol: Increased clearance of propranolol

estradiol component

barbiturates, carbamazepine, hydantoins, rifabutin, rifampin: Possibly reduced activity of estradiol

FOODS

estradiol component

grapefruit juice: Decreased metabolism and possibly increased adverse effects of estradiol

ACTIVITIES

testosterone and estradiol

smoking: Increased risk of CVA, pulmonary embolism, thrombophlebitis, and transient ischemic attack

Adverse Reactions

CNS: Chorea, dementia, depression, dizziness, headache, migraine headache, stroke

CV: Elevated cholesterol and triglyceride levels, MI, peripheral edema, pulmonary embolism, thromboembolism, thrombophlebitis

EENT: Diplopia, intolerance of contact lenses, steepening of corneal curvature, vision changes or loss

ENDO: Breast enlargement, pain, tenderness or tumors; gynecomastia; hypercalcemia, hyperglycemia, hypoglycemia, virilization

GI: Abnormal cramps or pain, aggravation of hepatic porphyria , anorexia, constipation, diarrhea, elevated liver function test results, gallbladder obstruction, hepatitis, increased appetite, jaundice, nausea, pancreatitis, vomiting

GU: Alteration in amount of cervical secretions, amenorrhea, breakthrough bleeding, cervical erosion, clear vaginal discharge, dysmenorrhea, increased libido, increased size of uterine leiomyomata, prolonged or heavy menstrual bleeding, vaginal candidiasis

SKIN: Acne, alopecia, chloasma, erythema multiforme or nodosum, hemorrhagic eruption, hirsutism, jaundice, melasma, oily skin, purpura, rash, seborrhea, urticaria

Other: Anaphylaxis, folic acid deficiency, hypercalcemia (in metastatic bone disease), local injection site irritation, weight gain or loss

Nursing Considerations

- For I.M. injection of testosterone and estradiol, before withdrawing drug from vial, warm and shake vial to redissolve any crystals that may have formed during storage at temperatures lower than recommended.
- Give testosterone and estradiol only by I.M. injection.
- **WARNING** Be aware that patients with breast cancer and bone metastasis may develop severe hypercalcemia because estradiol influences calcium and phosphorus metabolism. Watch for toxic effects of increased calcium absorption in patients predisposed to hypercalcemia or nephrolithiasis.
- **WARNING** Assess patient for possible contact lens intolerance or changes in vision or visual acuity because estrogens such as estradiol can cause keratoconus. Be prepared to stop drug immediately, as prescribed, if patient has sudden partial or complete loss of vision or sudden diplopia or migraine.
- Monitor PT for change in anticoagulant effect in patients receiving warfarin because estradiol increases production of clotting factors VII, VIII, IX, and X and promotes platelet aggregation.
- Watch for elevated liver function test results because testosterone and estradiol may worsen such conditions as acute intermittent or variegate hepatic porphyria.
- Closely monitor patient's blood pressure. Some patients may have a substantial increase in blood pressure as an indiosyncratic reaction to estrogens. Monitor patients who already have hypertension for increased blood pressure because estrogens may cause fluid retention. Also monitor patients with asthma, heart disease, migraines, renal disease, or seizure disorder for worsening of these conditions.

- Watch for peripheral edema or mild weight gain because estradiol can cause sodium and fluid retention.
- Monitor blood glucose level often in patients who have diabetes mellitus because estradiol may decrease insulin sensitivity and alter glucose tolerance.
- **WARNING** Expect to stop testosterone and estradiol therapy in any woman who develops signs or symptoms of cardiovascular disease, such as stroke, MI, pulmonary embolism, or venous thrombosis.
- Be aware that estrogens such as estradiol may worsen mood disorders, including depression. Monitor patient for depression, mood changes, anxiety, fatigue, dizziness, or insomnia.
- Assess skin for melasma (tan or brown patches), which may develop on forehead, cheeks, temples, and upper lip. These patches may persist after drug is stopped.
- Monitor thyroid function test results in patients with hypothyroidism because long-term use of estradiol may decrease effectiveness of thyroid therapy.
- Expect to stop testosterone and estradiol therapy several weeks before patient undergoes major surgery, as prescribed, because prolonged immobilization poses a risk of thromboembolism.

PATIENT TEACHING
- Before therapy starts, inform patient of risks involved in testosterone and estradiol therapy, such as increased risk of cardiovascular disease, breast or endometrial cancer, dementia, gallbladder disease, and vision abnormalities.
- Inform patient receiving testosterone and estradiol that she should have an annual physical examination, including a pelvic examination, to screen for adverse effects such as cervical dysplasia.
- Inform patient that a cyclic combination regimen of testosterone and estradiol may cause monthly withdrawal bleeding; tell her to notify prescriber if this occurs.
- Instruct patient to notify prescriber about masculine changes, such as a deepening of the voice or facial hair growth.
- Also tell patient to notify prescriber of any unusual signs and symptoms because combination drug can cause serious adverse effects.
- Advise patient taking testosterone and estradiol not to smoke because smoking increases the risk of deep vein thrombosis, heart attack, and other thromboemolic disorders.

Eye and Ear Drugs

bacitracin zinc and polymyxin B sulfate
AK-Poly Bac Ophthalmic, Polysporin

Class and Category
Chemical: Bacillus subtilis derivative (bacitracin), bacillus polymyxa derivative (polymyxin B)
Therapeutic: Antibiotics (bacitracin, polymyxin B)
Pregnancy category: C

Indications and Dosages
▶ *To treat superficial ocular infections of the conjunctiva or cornea caused by gram-negative bacilli, including virtually all strains of* Pseudomonas aeruginosa *and* Haemophilus influenzae *and most gram-positive bacilli and cocci, including hemolytic streptococci*
OPHTHALMIC OINTMENT
Adults. Applied as a thin ribbon into conjunctival sac q 3 to 4 hr for 7 to 10 days, depending on severity of infection.

Mechanism of Action
Bacitracin interferes with bacterial cell wall synthesis by binding with iso-prenyl pyrophosphate (a lipid-carrying molecule that transports substances out of bacterial cells to help build new cell walls), forming an unusable complex in bacterial cells. This weakens the bacterial cell wall and causes lysis and death. Bacitracin is considered a bacteriostatic and bactericidal drug.

Polymyxin B binds to cell membrane phospholipids in gram-negative bacteria, increasing the permeability of the cell membrane. Polymyxin B also acts as a cationic detergent altering the osmotic barrier of the membrane and causing essential intracellular metabolites to leak out. Both actions lead to bacterial cell death.

Contraindications
Hypersensitivity to bacitracin, polymyxin B or their components

Adverse Reactions
EENT: Delayed corneal healing, secondary ocular infection

Nursing Considerations
• Monitor patient for evidence of secondary ocular infection, such as signs and symptoms not alleviated within 7 to 10 days. If infection continues after bacitracin and polymyxin B therapy, expect to obtain culture and sensitivity samples, as ordered, and administer additional antibiotic therapy as indicated.

PATIENT TEACHING

• Stress importance of using bacitracin and polymyxin B ophthalmic ointment exactly as prescribed, even if feeling better.
• Instruct patient or caregiver how to use ophthalmic ointment.
• Remind patients and caregivers to wash their hands before and after using drug.
• Caution patient or caregiver not to touch tube to eye or to share drug to avoid contaminatubg drug or spreading infection.
• Tell patient to notify prescriber if symptoms do not improve or become worse by the end of the prescribed therapy time.

chloroxylenol, pramoxine hydrochloride, and hydrocortisone
Cortane B Cortic, Cortic-ND, Otomar-HC, Oti-med, Tri-Otic

Class and Category
Chemical: Dimethylbenzene (chloroxylenol), morpholine derivative (pramoxine), glucocorticoid (hydrocortisone)
Therapeutic: Topical antiseptic, germicide and antifungal (chloroxylenol), local anesthetic (pramoxine), anti-inflammatory (hydrocortisone)
Pregnancy category: C

Indications and Dosages
▶ *To treat superficial infections of external auditory canal caused by sensitive gram-positive and gram-negative bacteria, such as* Streptococcus pneumoniae *and* Haemophilus influenzae
EARDROPS

Adults. Wick saturated with drug and inserted into ear canal followed by instillation of several drops as often as needed to keep wick moistened for 24 hr. Wick removed at end of 24 hr, followed by instillation of 5 drops, t.i.d. or q.i.d. Or, drops instilled without use of wick t.i.d. or q.i.d.

Children. Wick saturated with drug and inserted into ear canal followed by instillation of several drops as often as needed to keep wick moistened for 24 hr. Wick removed at end of 24 hr, followed by instillation of 3 drops, t.i.d. or q.i.d. Or, drops instilled without use of wick t.i.d. or q.i.d.

▶ *To prevent superficial infection of the external auditory canal in an unaffected ear when infection is present in the other ear*
EARDROPS
Adults. 5 drops instilled t.i.d.

Mechanism of Action

Chloroxylenol destroys bacterial microorganisms by breaking down the bacterial cell wall. This results in cell death.

Hydrocortisone binds to intracellular glucocorticoid receptors in the ear and suppresses the inflammatory and immune responses by:

• inhibiting neutrophil and monocyte accumulation at the inflammation site and suppressing their phagocytic and bactericidal activity
• stabilizing lysosomal membranes
• suppressing the antigen response of macrophages and helper T cells
• inhibiting the synthesis of cellular mediators of the inflammatory response, such as cytokines, interleukins, and prostaglandins.

Pramoxine provides temporary relief from auricular itching and pain by stabilizing the neuronal membrane of nerve endings with which it comes into contact.

Contraindications
Hypersensitivity to chloroxylenol, hydrocortisone, other steroids, pramoxine, or their components; ophthalmic use; perforated eardrums; presence of varicella or vaccinia infections

Adverse Reactions
EENT: Ear canal burning, dryness, irritation or pruritus
ENDO: Systemic hypercorticoidism (with prolonged use)
SKIN: Acneform eruptions, folliculitis, hypertrichosis, hypopigmentation

Nursing Considerations
• Before inserting wick into ear canal, carefully remove all cerumen and debris.
• Monitor patient closely for signs and symptoms of systemic hypercorticoidism if drug is given over prolonged period of time because hydrocortisone may be absorbed enough to increase glucocorticoid blood levels.

- Inspect ear canal for evidence of irritation or allergic response. If present, stop drug and notify prescriber.

PATIENT TEACHING
- Instruct patient or caregiver to use chloroxylenol, pramoxine, and hydrocortisone eardrops exactly as prescribed.
- Show the patient or caregiver how to use eardrops, if necessary.
- Tell patient to stop using drug and notify prescriber if allergic response or local irritation occurs.

ciprofloxacin hydrochloride 0.3% and dexamethasone 0.1%

Ciprodex

Class and Category

Chemical: Fluoroquinolone derivative (ciprofloxacin), glucocoritcoid (dexamethasone)
Therapeutic: Antibiotic (ciprofloxacin), anti-inflammatory (dexamethasone)
Pregnancy category: C

Indications and Dosages

▶ *To treat acute otitis media caused by* Staphylococcus aureus, Streptococcus pneumoniae, Haemophilus influenzae, Moraxella catarrhalis, *or* Pseudomonas aeruginosa

SUSPENSION

Children age 6 months and over with tympanostomy tube or tubes. 4 drops in affected ear or ears b.i.d. for 7 days.

▶ *To treat acute otitis externa caused by* S. aureus *or* P. aeruginosa

SUSPENSION

Adults and children age 6 months and over. 4 drops instilled into affected ear or ears b.i.d. for 7 days.

Contraindications

Hypersensitivity to ciprofloxacin, other quinolone antibiotics, dexamethasone, other corticosteroids, or their components; viral infection of external ear canal such as herpes simplex or varicella

Adverse Reactions

CNS: Irritability
EENT: Decreased hearing; ear congestion, discomfort, erythema, pain, precipitate, or pruritus; taste perversion; secondary ear infection
SKIN: Rash

Mechanism of Action

Ciprofloxacin inhibits the enzyme DNA gyrase, which is responsible for the unwinding and supercoiling of bacterial DNA before it replicates. By inhibiting this enzyme, ciprofloxacin causes bacterial cells to die.

Dexamethasone binds to intracellular glucocorticoid receptors in external and media ear tissue and suppresses the inflammatory and immune responses by:

• inhibiting neutrophil and monocyte accumulation at the inflammation site and suppressing their phagocytic and bactericidal activity
• stabilizing lysosomal membranes
• suppressing the antigen response of macrophages and helper T cells
• inhibiting the synthesis of cellular mediators of the inflammatory response, such as cytokines, interleukins, and prostaglandins.

Nursing Considerations

• Don't instill ciprofloxacin and dexamethasone otic suspension into eye or inject parenterally.
• If patient develops a rash, stop drug and notify prescriber.
• If there's no improvement in 1 week, obtain culture and sensitivity samples, as ordered, to rule out possibility of secondary infection, particularly fungal infection.

PATIENT TEACHING

• Instruct patient or caregiver to use ciprofloxacin and dexamethasone eardrops exactly as prescribed, for length of time prescribed, even if feeling better.
• Show patient or caregiver how to use eardrops, if necessary, telling him to lie down with the affected ear upward before instilling the drops. Following instillation, tell him to maintain this position for 30 to 60 seconds so that the drops can penetrate into the ear.
• Tell patient to shake suspension well before using and to warm bottle by holding it in his hands for 1 or 2 minutes to avoid dizziness that may occur with the instillation of a cold solution into the ear canal.
• Tell patient to protect bottle from light.
• Tell patient to stop using drug and notify prescriber if a rash occurs.
• Advise patient to contact prescriber if signs and symptoms worsen or do not improve in 7 days.

ciprofloxacin hydrochloride and hydrocortisone

Cipro HC Otic

Class and Category

Chemical: Fluoroquinolone derivative (ciprofloxacin), glucocoritcoid (hydrocortisone)

Therapeutic: Antibiotic (ciprofloxacin), anti-inflammatory (hydrocortisone)

Pregnancy category: C

Indications and Dosages

▶ *To treat otitis externa caused by* Pseudomonas aeruginosa, Staphylococcus aureus, *or* Proteus mirabilis

SUSPENSION

Adults and children age 1 and over. 3 drops instilled into affected ear b.i.d. for 7 days.

Mechanism of Action

Ciprofloxacin inhibits the enzyme DNA gyrase, which is responsible for the unwinding and supercoiling of bacterial DNA before it replicates. By inhibiting this enzyme, ciprofloxacin causes bacterial cells to die.

Hydrocortisone binds to intracellular glucocorticoid receptors in external ear tissue and suppresses the inflammatory and immune responses by:

- inhibiting neutrophil and monocyte accumulation at the inflammation site and suppressing their phagocytic and bactericidal activity
- stabilizing lysosomal membranes
- suppressing the antigen response of macrophages and helper T cells
- inhibiting the synthesis of cellular mediators of the inflammatory response, such as cytokines, interleukins, and prostaglandins.

Contraindications

Hypersensitivity to ciprofloxacin, other quinolone antibiotics, hydrocortisone, other corticosteroids or their components; perforated tympanic; viral infections of the external ear canal such as herpes simplex or varicella

Adverse Reactions

CNS: Headache including migraine, hyperesthesia, paresthesia

EENT: Secondary fungal ear infection

RESP: Cough

SKIN: Alopecia, fungal dermatitis, pruritus, rash, urticaria

Nursing Considerations
- Don't instill ciprofloxacin and hydrocortisone otic suspension into eye or inject it parenterally.
- Stop drug and notify prescriber about rash or other symptoms of hypersensitivity, such as pruritus or urticaria, because systemic quinolones could cause an anaphylactic reaction; ensure immediate emergency treatment.
- If there's no improvement in 1 week, obtain culture and sensitivity samples, as ordered, to rule out possibility of secondary infection, particularly fungal infection.

PATIENT TEACHING
- Instruct patient or caregiver to administer ciprofloxacin and hydrocortisone eardrops exactly as prescribed for length of time prescribed, even if feeling better.
- Show patient or caregiver how to administer eardrops, if necessary, telling him to lie down with the affected ear upward before instilling the drops. Following instillation, tell him to maintain this position for 30 to 60 seconds so that the drops can penetrate into the ear.
- Tell patient to shake suspension well before using and to warm bottle by holding it in his hands for 1 or 2 minutes to avoid dizziness that may occur with the instillation of a cold solution into the ear canal.
- Tell patient to protect bottle from light.
- Tell patient to stop using drug and notify prescriber if allergic response or local irritation occurs.
- Advise patient to contact prescriber if signs and symptoms worsen or do not improve in 7 days.

colistin sulfate, neomycin sulfate, thonzonium bromide, hydrocortisone acetate
Coly-Mycin S, Cortisporin-TC

Class and Category
Chemical: Polypeptide (colistin), aminoglucoside (neomycin), unclassified (thonzonium), glucocorticoid (hydrocortisone)
Therapeutic: Antibiotics (colistin, neomycin), surface activator (thonzonium), anti-inflammatory (hydrocortisone)
Pregnancy category: C

Indications and Dosages

▶ *To treat superficial bacterial infections of the external auditory canal or mastoidectomy and fenestration cavities caused by* Enterobacter aerogenes, Escherichia coli, Klebsiella pneumoniae, Pseudomonas aeruginosa, *or* Staphylococcus aureus

OTIC SUSPENSION

Adults. 5 drops instilled into the affected ear or ears t.i.d. or q.i.d. for 10 days. Or, cotton wick inserted into ear canal and then saturated with solution followed by repeat saturation q 4 hr with cotton wick replaced q 24 hr for 10 days.

Children. 4 drops instilled into the affected ear or ears t.i.d. or q.i.d. for 10 days. Or, cotton wick inserted into ear canal and then saturated with solution followed by repeat saturation q 4 hr with cotton wick replaced q 24 hr for 10 days.

Mechanism of Action

Colistin penetrates and disrupts bacterial cell membranes, killing the cells.

Neomycin competes with messenger RNA to bind with a receptor protein on the 30S ribosomal subunit of DNA in bacterial cells. This action causes abnormal, nonfunctioning proteins to form, which kills the cells.

Thonzonium is a surface-active agent that promotes tissue contact among other drugs in the mix. It does this by dispersing and penetrating cellular debris and exudate.

Hydrocortisone binds to intracellular glucocorticoid receptors in the ear and suppresses inflammatory and immune responses by:

• inhibiting neutrophil and monocyte accumulation at the inflammation site and suppressing their phagocytic and bactericidal activity
• stabilizing lysosomal membranes
• suppressing the antigen response of macrophages and helper T cells
• inhibiting the synthesis of cellular mediators of the inflammatory response, such as cytokines, interleukins, and prostaglandins.

These actions inhibit the edema, fibrin deposition, capillary dilation, leukocyte migration, capillary proliferation, fibroblast proliferation, deposition of collagen, and scar formation associated with inflammation.

Contraindications

Hypersensitivity to colistin, neomycin, thonzonium, hydrocortisone, or their components; presence of or suspected external auditory canal viral infection caused by herpes simplex virus or varicella zoster virus

Adverse Reactions

EENT: Ear canal edema, erythema, irritation or pruritis; hearing loss, ototoxicity
GU: Nephrotoxicity
SKIN: Rash

Nursing Considerations

- Use cautiously in patients with perforated tympanic membrane.
- Don't administer otic suspension into eye or inject parenterally.
- Stop drug and notify prescriber about rash or localized reactions, such as ear canal edema, erythema, irritation, or pruritus.
- Monitor patient's hearing. If hearing loss develops, stop drug immediately and notify prescriber.
- If there's no improvement in 1 week, obtain culture and sensitivity samples, as ordered, to rule out possibility of secondary infection, particularly fungal infection.

PATIENT TEACHING

- Instruct patient or caregiver to administer eardrops exactly as prescribed for length of time prescribed even if feeling better.
- Tell patient or caregiver to clean external auditory canal and dry with sterile cotton applicator before instilling drops.
- Tell patient to shake suspension well before using and to warm bottle by holding it in his hands for 1 or 2 minutes to avoid dizziness that may occur with the instillation of a cold solution.
- Show patient or caregiver how to administer eardrops, if necessary. Tell patient to lie down with the affected ear upward before instilling the drops. After instillation, tell him to keep this position for 5 minutes so the drops can penetrate into the ear.
- Caution patient not to touch tip of dropper to ear, fingers, or other surfaces to avoid contamination.
- Tell patient to stop using drug and notify prescriber if allergic response or local irritation occurs.
- Advise patient to contact prescriber if signs and symptoms worsen or do not improve in 7 days.

cyclopentolate hydrochloride 0.2% and phenylephrine 1%

Cyclomydril

Class and Category

Chemical: Tertiary amine (cyclopentolate), sympathomimetic amine (phenylephrine)

Therapeutic: Mydriatic and cycloplegic (cyclopentolate), vasoconstrictor (phenylephrine)
Pregnancy category: C

Indications and Dosages

▶ *To produce mydriasis and cycloplegia before diagnostic ophthalmic procedures are performed*

SOLUTION

Adults and children age 1 and over. 1 drop instilled in each eye, repeated q 5 to 10 minutes, as needed. *Maximum:* 3 drops per eye.

Mechanism of Action

Cyclopentolate blocks the action of acetylcholine, which causes relaxation of the cholinergically innervated sphincter muscle of the iris. The drug also blocks cholinergic stimulation of the accommodative ciliary muscle of the lens, resulting in dilation of the pupil and paralysis of accommodation.

Phenylephrine stimulates alpha-adrenergic receptors and inhibits activity of the intracellular enzyme adenyl cyclase, which then inhibits production of cAMP. The inhibition of cAMP causes constriction of the arterioles. Phenylephrine also acts directly on the adrenergic receptors in the eye producing contraction of the dilator muscles.

Contraindications

Angle-closure glaucoma; hypersensitivity to cyclopentolate, phenylephrine or their components; severe coronary artery disease or hypertension; use within 14 days of MAO inhibitor therapy; ventricular tachycardia

Interactions

DRUGS

phenylephrine component

MAO inhibitors: Increased and prolonged cardiac stimulation, increased vasopressor effect, increased risk of severe cardiovascular and cerebrovascular effects, hyperpyrexia, vomiting

Adverse Reactions

CNS: Confusion, dizziness, excitation, headache, insomnia, nervousness, paresthesia, psychotic reactions (children), restlessness, tremor, weakness

CV: Angina, bradycardia, hypertension, hypotension, palpitations, peripheral vasoconstriction that may lead to necrosis or gangrene, tachycardia, ventricular arrhythmias

EENT: Blocked lacrimal drainage system, blurred vision, dry mouth, increased intraocular pressure, superficial punctate epithelial ocular lesions, transient ocular burning, ocular erythema or irritation
GI: Constipation, nausea, vomiting
GU: Urinary hesitancy or retention
RESP: Dyspnea
SKIN: Photophobia
Other: Allergic reaction

Nursing Considerations
- Use cautiously in elderly patients and those predisposed to increased intraocular pressure. Prepare these patients to have a tonometric examination, as ordered, and an estimation of the depth of the angle of the posterior chamber before instillation of cyclopentolate and phenylephrine drops.
- After administering eyedrops, compress lacrimal sac for several minutes to minimize systemic absorption.
- Be aware that patients with heavily pigmented irises may need a higher dosage to obtain same effect.
- Monitor patient closely for adverse reactions. Systematic reactions may occur because of absorption. Notify prescriber if present and be prepared to provide supportive treatment, as ordered until effects of drug has worn off (typically 24 hours but may persist for several days).
- Monitor children, patients with Down syndrome, and the elderly who are more susceptible to adverse reactions, especially psychotic reactions and excitation that often occur within 30 to 45 minutes following administration of drug.
- Observe patient for signs and symptoms of an allergic response such as persistent irritation and diffuse redness of eyes that occurs within minutes of administering drug.

PATIENT TEACHING
- Warn patient that cyclopentolate and phenylephrine may cause a transient burning sensation when instilled.
- Caution patient to avoid potentially hazardous activities until the effects of the drug has worn off.

dorzolamide hydrochloride and timolol maleate
Cosopt

Class and Category
Chemical: Carbonic anhydrase inhibitor (dorzolamide), beta blocker (timolol)
Therapeutic: Ocular Antihypertensives (dorzolamide, timolol)
Pregnancy category: C

Indications and Dosages
▶ *To reduce elevated intraocular pressure in patients with open-angle glaucoma or ocular hypertension who have not responded well to beta blocker alone*
OPHTHALMIC SOLUTION
Adults and children age 2 and over. 1 drop instilled into affected eye or eyes b.i.d.

Mechanism of Action
Dorzolamide inhibits human carbonic anhydrase II. When carbonic anhydrase II is inhibited in the ciliary processes of the eye, aqueous humor secretion is decreased because the formation of bicarbonate ions is slowed reducing sodium and fluid transport. This results in lowered intraocular pressure.

Timolol reduces acqueous humor secretion by blocking $beta_1$ and $beta_2$ receptors in the ciliary processes of the eye. It also slightly increases the outflow of aqueous humor. These combined actions lowers intraocular pressure.

Contraindications
Bronchial asthma including history; cardiogenic shock; hypersensitivity to dorzolamide, timolol, or their components; overt cardiac failure; second or third degree atrioventricular block; severe chronic obstructive pulmonary disease; sinus bradycardia

Interactions
DRUGS
dorzolamide component
carbonic anhydrase inhibitors: Possibly additive effects
salicylate (high-dose): Increased risk of salicylate toxicity
timolol component
beta blockers (oral): Possibly additive beta blocker effect
calcium antagonists: Possibly increased risk of atrioventricular conduction disturbances, left ventricular failure, and hypotension
catecholamine-depleting agents, such as reserpine: Possibly additive effects and development of hypotension or marked bradycardia
clonidine: Increased risk of rebound hypertension when clonidine is discontinued

digitalis and calcium antagonists: Possibly additive effects in prolonging atrioventricular conduction time

epinephrine (injectable): Possibly unresponsive therapeutic effect to epinephrine use in treatment of anaphylaxis

quinidine: Possibly decreased heart rate

Adverse Reactions

CNS: Dizziness, headache

CV: Hypertension

EENT: Blepharitis; blurred or cloudy vision; bitter, sour, or unusual taste; conjunctiva discharge, edema, hyperemia, infection, or pain; corneal erosion or staining; cortical lens opacity; dry eyes; eyelid edema, erythema, exudates, pain or scales; foreign body sensation; glaucomatous cupping; lens nucleus coloration, or opacity; ocular burning, discharge, pain, pruritus, stinging, or tearing; pharyngitis; post-subcapsular cataract; sinusitis; superficial punctate keratitis; visual field defect; vitreous detachment

GI: Abdominal pain, dyspepsia, nausea

GU: UTI

MS: Back pain

RESP: Bronchitis, cough, upper respiratory infection

Nursing Considerations

- Be aware that dorzolamide and timolol shouldn't be given to patients with severe renal impairment because drug is excreted mainly by the kidneys and its effects on such patients are unknown.
- Administer dorzolamide and timolol cautiously in patients with diabetes mellitus or hyperthyroidism because timolol, a beta blocker, may mask signs and symptoms of acute hypoglycemia and thyrotoxicosis. Also administer cautiously in patients with hepatic dysfunction because adverse effects of this drug aren't known in this patient population.
- Monitor patient closely for systemic adverse reactions because even though drug is administered topically, it's absorbed systemically and can cause severe reactions. If patient develops a systemic adverse reaction, withhold drug and notify prescriber
- Monitor patient closely for adverse reactions associated with sulfonamide use because dorzolamide is a sulfonamide. Although these reactions haven't occurred with dorzolamide and timolol, the possibility exists for serious reactions, such as Stevens-Johnson syndrome, toxic epidermal necrolysis, fulminant hepatic necrosis, agranulocytosis, aplastic anemia, and other blood dyscrasias. If these types of adverse reactions occur

during therapy with dorzolamide and timolol, withhold drug and notify prescriber.
- Also monitor the patient closely for adverse reactions associated with beta blocker use because timolol is a beta blocker. Although these reactions haven't occurred with dorzolamide and timolol, the possibility exists. For example, beta-adrenergic blockade may precipitate heart failure or increase muscle weakness in patients with myasthenia gravis. If these types of adverse reactions occur during therpy with dorzolamide and timolol, withhold drug and notify prescriber.
- Inspect patient for ocular adverse reactions. If reactions such as conjunctivitis and lid reactions occur suggesting the presence of an allergic response, notify prescriber and expect dorzolamide and timolol to be discontinued.

PATIENT TEACHING
- Instruct patient to use dorzolamide and timolol solution exactly as prescribed.
- Show patient how to open the bottle for the first time by unscrewing the cap as indicated by the arrows on the top of the cap. Warn him that if cap is pulled directly up and away from the bottle, the dispenser will not work properly.
- Teach patient how to use eyedrops, if necessary.
- Instruct patient not to touch the bottle tip to his eyelids or any other surface and not to share the drug with anyone else to avoid contaminating drug and spreading eye infection.
- If patient wears soft contact lenses, tell him to remove them before using drug and to wait 15 minutes before reinserting them.
- Tell patient that if other topical eye drugs are used, he should space them at least 10 minutes apart.
- Advise patient to withhold dorzolamide and timolol and notify prescriber if serious or unusual reactions occur or if indications of a localized allergic response such as conjunctivitis or eyelid abnormalities appear while using the drug.
- Caution patient that if trauma or infection occurs in a treated eye, he should contact prescriber for advice on continuing therapy with dorzolamide and timolol.

fluorescein sodium 0.25% and benoxinate hydrochloride 0.4%
Fluress, Flurate

Class and Category

Chemical: Water-soluble dibasic acid xanthine dye (fluorescein), diethylamino ethyl amino butoxybenzoate (benoxinate)
Therapeutic: Disclosing agent (fluorescein), local anesthetic (benoxinate)
Pregnancy category: NR

Indications and Dosages

▶ *To prevent eye pain and identify corneal scratches or tears during ophthalmic procedures such as tonometry, gonioscopy, removal of corneal foreign bodies, and other short corneal or conjunctival procedures*
OPHTHALMIC SOLUTION
Adults. 1 or 2 drops instilled into affected eye or eyes as a one-time instillation before surgery.
▶ *To provide deep ophthalmic anesthesia*
OPTHTHALMIC SOLUTION
Adults. 2 drops instilled into affected eye or eyes at 90-second intervals for three instillations.

Mechanism of Action

Fluorescein reveals defects in the corneal epithelium because any break in the normally intact epithelium will allow the dye to penetrate, causing a green color at the site. Intact corneal epithelium resists fluorescein penetration and doesn't change color. Precorneal tear film will appear yellow or orange. If epithelial loss is extensive, topical fluorescein penetrates into the aqueous humor and can be seen biomicroscopically as a green flare.

Benoxinate stabilizes the neuronal membrane so the neuron is less permeable to ions. This prevents the initiation and transmission of nerve impulses, thereby preventing the perception of eye pain.

Contraindications

Hypersensitivity to fluorescein, benoxinate, or any of their components

Adverse Reactions

EENT: Acute, diffuse epithelial keratitis; corneal filaments; gray, ground, glass corneal appearance; iritis with descemetitis; sloughing of necrotic epithelium; temporary burning, conjunctival redness, or stinging
SKIN: Contact allergic dermatitis with drying and fissuring of fingertips

Nursing Considerations

- Use cautiously in patients with allergies, cardiac disease, or hyperthyroidism because they're at increased risk for adverse reactions to fluorescein and benoxinate.
- Monitor patient closely after instillation of fluorescein and benoxinate drops for adverse systemic effects because, although rare, toxicity causing central nervous system stimulation followed by depression may occur.
- Protect treated eyes from irritating chemicals and foreign bodies until effects of anesthesia have worn off.

PATIENT TEACHING

- Warn patient that instillation of fluorescein and benoxinate eyedrops may cause a transient burning or stinging.
- Caution patient not to touch or rub affected eye or eyes until the effects of anesthesia is gone.

fluorescein sodium 0.25% and proparacaine hydrochloride 0.5%

Fluoracaine

Class and Category

Chemical: Water-soluble dibasic acid xanthine dye (fluorescein), diethylamino ethyl ester (proparacaine)
Therapeutic: Disclosing agent (fluorescein), local anesthetic (proparacaine)
Pregnancy category: NR

Indications and Dosages

▶ *To prevent or relieve eye pain and identify corneal scratches or tears during ophthalmic procedures such as tonometry, gonioscopy, removal of corneal foreign bodies, and other short corneal or conjunctival procedures*
OPHTHALMIC SOLUTION
Adults. 1 or 2 drops instilled in affected eye or eyes as a one-time instillation before surgery.
▶ *To provide deep ophthalmic anesthesia*
OPTHTHALMIC SOLUTION
Adults. 1 drop instilled in affected eye or eyes q 5 to 10 minutes for 5 to 7 doses.

Contraindications

Hypersensitivity to fluorescein, proparacaine, or their components

Mechanism of Action

Fluorescein reveals defects in the corneal epithelium because any break in the normally intact corneal epithelium will allow the dye to penetrate, causing a green color at the site. Intact corneal epithelium resists fluorescein penetration and doesn't change color. Precorneal tear film will appear yellow or orange. If epithelial loss is extensive, topical fluorescein penetrates into the aqueous humor and can be seen biomicroscopically as a green flare.

Proparacaine stabilizes the neuronal membrane so the neuron is less permeable to ions. This prevents the initiation and transmission of nerve impulses, thereby preventing the perception of eye pain.

Adverse Reactions

EENT: Acute, diffuse epithelial keratitis; corneal filaments; gray, ground, glass corneal appearance; iritis with descemetitis; sloughing of necrotic epithelium; temporary burning, conjunctival redness, or stinging

SKIN: Contact allergic dermatitis with drying and fissuring of fingertips

Nursing Considerations

- Use cautiously in patients with allergies, cardiac disease, or hyperthyroidism because they're at increased risk for adverse reactions to fluorescein and proparacaine.
- Monitor patient closely for adverse systemic effects after instillation of fluorescein and proparacaine drops because, although rare, toxicity causing CNS stimulation followed by depression may occur.
- Apply an eye patch, as ordered, following instillation of fluoresceine and proparacaine eyedrops, and protect treated eye from irritating chemicals and foreign bodies until effects of anesthesia have worn off.

PATIENT TEACHING

- Warn patient that fluorescein and proparacaine eyedrops may cause burning or stinging several hours after instillation.
- Caution patient not to touch or rub his eye and to leave the eye patch on, if present, until the effects of anesthesia is gone.

fluorometholone 0.1% and sulfacetamide sodium 10%

FML-S

Class and Category

Chemical: Fluorinated glucocorticoid (fluorometholone), sulfona-mide (sulfacetamide sodium)

Therapeutic: Anti-inflammatory (fluorometholone), antibiotic (sul-facetamide sodium)

Pregnancy category: C

Indications and Dosages

▶ *To treat inflammatory ocular conditions of the palpebral and bulbar conjunctiva, cornea, and anterior segment of the globe; chronic anterior uveitis and corneal injury from chemical, radiation, or thermal burns or penetration of foreign bodies when superficial ocular infection is present (or risk is high) caused by* Enterobacter *species,* Escherichia coli, Klebsiella species, Staphylococcus aureus, Streptococcus pneumoniae, *and* Streptococcus viridans *group*

OPHTHALMIC SUSPENSION

Adults. 1 drop instilled into conjunctival sac q.i.d.

Mechanism of Action

Fluorometholone binds to intracellular glucocorticoid receptors in the eye and suppresses inflammatory and immune responses by:

• inhibiting neutrophil and monocyte accumulation at the inflammation site and suppressing their phagocytic and bactericidal activity

• stabilizing lysosomal membranes

• suppressing the antigen response of macrophages and helper T cells

• inhibiting the synthesis of cellular mediators of the inflammatory response, such as cytokines, interleukins, and prostaglandins.

These actions inhibit the edema, fibrin deposition, capillary dilation, leukocyte migration, capillary proliferation, fibroblast proliferation, deposition of colla-gen and scar formation associated with inflammation.

Sulfacetamide sodium interferes with utilization of para-aminobenzoic acid (PABA) thus inhibiting biosynthesis of folic acid, which is essential for growth of susceptible organisms.

Incompatibilities

Silver preparations are incompatible with sulfonamide prepara-tions such as sulfacetamide

Contraindications

Fungal diseases affecting ocular structures; hypersensitivity to flu-orometholone, other corticosteroids, sulfacetamide sodium, other sulfonamides, or their components; mycobacterial infection of the eye; viral diseases of the cornea and conjunctiva, including epithelial herpes simplex keratitis, vaccinia, and varicella

Interactions
DRUGS

fluorometholone component
corticosteroids: Increased risk of cross-sensitivity
sulfacetamide sodium component
local anesthetics: Possibly antagonized effects of sulfacetamide
sulfonamides: Increased risk of cross-sensitivity

Adverse Reactions
EENT: Acute anterior uveitis; conjunctivitis; conjunctival hyperemia, corneal ulcers or secondary fungal infections; elevated intraocular pressure; eye irritation; glaucoma; keratitis; loss of accommodation; mydriasis; optic nerve damage; perforation of the globe; posterior subcapsular cataract formation; ptosis; secondary ocular bacterial infections
ENDO: Systemic hypercorticoidism (with prolonged use)
GI: Fulminant hepatic necrosis
HEME: Agranulocytosis, aplastic anemia, blood dyscrasias
SKIN: Stevens-Johnson syndrome, toxic epidermal necrolysis
Other: Allergic reactions, delayed wound healing

Nursing Considerations
- Use fluorometholone and sulfacetamide sodium with great caution in the patient with a history of herpes simplex because use of an ocular steroid preparation such as fluorometholone may exacerbate the severity of many ocular viral infections.
- Use cautiously in patients with glaucoma because the fluorometholone component of drug may cause elevated intraocular pressure. Be prepared to monitor patient's intraocular pressure frequently in patients with glaucoma or routinely if drug is used for 10 days or longer in patients without glaucoma.
- Obtain eyelid culture and sensitivity tests as ordered before giving first dose, if infection is already present. Expect to begin drug therapy before test results are known.
- Be aware that the use of topical corticosteroids like fluorometholone in the presence of thin corneal or scleral tissue may lead to perforation.
- Assess patient's vision, and inspect eyes for abnormalities because prolonged use of ophthalmic corticosteroids may cause glaucoma, damage to the optic nerve, defects in visual acuity and fields of vision, and posterior subcapsular cataract forma-

tion. Prolonged use also increases risk of secondary ocular infections.

- Question patient about eye discomfort because fluorometholone may mask signs and symptoms of acute purulent eye infections.
- **WARNING** Don't inject fluorometholone and sulfacetamide sodium suspension into the eye.
- Monitor patient for serious adverse reactions including allergic response. If suspected, notify prescriber, withhold fluorometholone and sulfacetamide sodium, and be prepared to administer appropriate supportive treatment.
- If patient has persistent corneal ulceration and has used fluorometholone and sulfacetamide sodium suspension long-term, obtain fungal cultures because fungal corneal infections are particularly likely with long-term local corticosteroid use.

PATIENT TEACHING
- Instruct patient to use fluorometholone and sulfacetamide sodium suspension exactly as prescribed.
- Teach patient how to use eyedrops, if necessary.
- Tell patient to shake the bottle well before using.
- Caution patient to discard the suspension if it appears dark brown and obtain a new suspension.
- Advise patient to discontinue using fluorometholone and sulfacetamide sodium and notify prescriber if signs and symptoms such as ocular pain or inflammation do not improve after two days or becomes worse.
- Instruct patient to take care not to touch the bottle tip to eyelids or any other surface to avoid contamination.
- Inform patient that no one else should use the drug because infection may be spread in this manner.

neomycin sulfate, polymyxin B sulfate, and bacitracin zinc

AK-Spore, Neocidin, Neosporin Ointment, Neotal, Ocu-Spor-B, Ocusporin, Ocutricin, Spectro-Sporin, Triple Antibiotic

Class and Category

Chemical: Aminoglucoside (neomycin), bacillus polymyxa derivative (polymyxin B), bacillus subtilis derivative (bacitracin)
Therapeutic: Antibiotics (neomycin, polymyxin B, bacitracin
Pregnancy category: C

Indications and Dosages

▶ *To treat superficial bacterial infections of the external eye and surrounding area, such as conjunctivitis, keratitis, keratoconjunctivitis, blepharitis, or blepharoconjunctivitis caused by* Enterobacter *species,* Escherichia coli, Haemophilus influenzae, Klebsiella species, Neisseria *species,* Pseudomonas aeruginosa, Staphylococcus aureus, *and streptococci, including* Streptococcus pneumoniae

OPHTHALMIC OINTMENT

Adults. Thin ribbon (about ½ inch) applied into conjunctival sac of affected eye or eyes q 3 or 4 hr for 7 to 10 days

---

Mechanism of Action

Neomycin competes with messenger RNA to bind with a receptor protein on the 30S ribosomal subunit of DNA in bacterial cells. This action causes abnormal, nonfunctioning proteins to form, which kills the cells.

Polymyxin B binds to cell membrane phospholipids in gram-negative bacteria, increasing cell membrane permeability. Polymyxin B also acts as a cationic detergent, altering the osmotic barrier of the membrane and causing essential intracellular metabolites to leak. Both actions lead to cell death.

Bacitracin interferes with bacterial cell wall synthesis by binding with isoprenyl pyrophosphate (a lipid-carrying molecule that transports substances out of bacterial cells to help build new cell walls), forming an unusable complex in bacterial cells. This weakens cell walls and causes cell lysis and death. Bacitracin is bacteriostatic and bactericidal.

Contraindications

Hypersensitivity to neomycin, polymyxin B, bacitracin, or their components

Adverse Reactions

EENT: Conjunctival or eyelid edema, erythema, or pruritis; delayed eye wound healing; elevation of intraocular pressure; glaucoma; local eye irritation, optic nerve damage; posterior subcapsular cataract formation; secondary eye infection
GU: Nephrotoxicity
SKIN: Pruritis, rash, urticaria
Other: Allergic reactions, anaphylaxis

Nursing Considerations

• Obtain eyelid culture and sensitivity tests as ordered before giving first dose, if infection is already present. Expect to begin drug therapy before test results are known.

- Monitor patient for signs of hypersensitivity such as conjunctiva and eyelid edema, erythema, or pruritis and notify prescriber, if present, and expect to discontinue drug. Be aware that failure to heal may also be a sensitization reaction.
- Monitor patient for secondary ocular infections because overgrowth of nonsusceptible organisms including fungi may occur.
- Notify prescriber if patient's eye discomfort or inflammation does not improve or purulent discharge becomes worse.

PATIENT TEACHING
- Instruct patient to use neomycin, polymyxin B, and bacitracin ointment exactly as prescribed, even when feeling better.
- Teach patient how to administer eye ointment, if appropriate.
- Advise patient to stop using neomycin, polymyxin B, and bacitracin and notify prescriber if ocular pain or inflammation don't improve, becomes worse or an allergic reaction occurs.
- Instruct patient to take care not to touch the tube tip to eyelids or any other surface to avoid contamination.
- Inform patient that no one else should use the drug because infection may be spread in this manner.

neomycin sulfate, polymyxin B sulfate, bacitracin zinc, and hydrocortisone

AK-Spore HC, Cortisporin

Class and Category

Chemical: Aminoglucoside (neomycin), bacillus polymyxa derivative (polymyxin B), bacillus subtilis derivative (bacitracin), synthetic glucocorticoid (hydrocortisone)
Therapeutic: Antibiotics (neomycin, polymyxin B, bacitracin), antiinflammatory (hydrocortisone)
Pregnancy category: C

Indications and Dosages

▶ *To treat inflammatory ocular conditions of the palpebral and bulbar conjunctiva, cornea, and anterior segment of the globe; chronic anterior uveitis and corneal injury from chemical, radiation, or thermal burns or penetration of foreign bodies when superficial ocular infection is present (or risk is high) caused by* Enterobacter *species,* Escherichia coli, Haemophilus influenzae, Klebsiella *species,* Neisseria *species,* Pseudomonas aeruginosa, Staphylococcus aureus, *and streptococci, including* Streptococcus pneumoniae

OPHTHALMIC OINTMENT
Adults. Thin ribbon (about ½ inch) applied into conjunctival sac of affected eye or eyes q 3 or 4 hr.

Mechanism of Action

Neomycin competes with messenger RNA to bind with a receptor protein on the 30S ribosomal subunit of DNA in bacterial cells. This action causes abnormal, nonfunctioning proteins to form, which kills the cells.

Polymyxin B binds to cell membrane phospholipids in gram-negative bacteria, increasing cell membrane permeability. Polymyxin B also acts as a cationic detergent, altering the osmotic barrier of the membrane and causing essential intracellular metabolites to leak. Both actions lead to cell death.

Bacitracin interferes with bacterial cell wall synthesis by binding with isoprenyl pyrophosphate (a lipid-carrying molecule that transports substances out of bacterial cells to help build new cell walls), forming an unusable complex in bacterial cells. This weakens cell walls and causes lysis and death. Bacitracin is bacteriostatic and bactericidal.

Hydrocortisone binds to intracellular glucocorticoid receptors in the eye and suppresses inflammatory and immune responses by:
• inhibiting neutrophil and monocyte accumulation at the inflammation site and suppressing their phagocytic and bactericidal activity
• stabilizing lysosomal membranes
• suppressing the antigen response of macrophages and helper T cells
• inhibiting the synthesis of cellular mediators of the inflammatory response, such as cytokines, interleukins, and prostaglandins.
These actions inhibit the edema, fibrin deposition, capillary dilation, leukocyte migration, capillary proliferation, fibroblast proliferation, deposition of collagen and scar formation associated with inflammation.

Contraindications

Fungal diseases affecting ocular structures; hypersensitivity to neomycin, polymyxin B, bacitracin, hydrocortisone, other corticosteroids, or their components; mycobacterial infection of the eye; viral diseases of the cornea and conjunctiva, including epithelial herpes simplex keratitis, vaccinia, and varicella

Adverse Reactions

EENT: Conjunctival or eyelid edema, erythema, or pruritis; delayed eye wound healing; elevation of intraocular pressure; glaucoma; local eye irritation; optic nerve damage; posterior subcapsular cataract formation; secondary eye infection
GU: Nephrotoxicity

SKIN: Pruritis, rash, urticaria
Other: Allergic reactions, anaphylaxis

Nursing Considerations

- Use neomycin, polymyxin B, bacitracin, and hydrocortisone with great caution if patient has a history of herpes simplex because ocular steroids such as hydrocortisone may worsen the severity of many ocular viral infections.
- Use cautiously in patients with glaucoma because the hydrocortisone component of drug may cause elevated intraocular pressure. Be prepared to monitor patient's intraocular pressure frequently in patients with glaucoma or routinely if drug is used for 10 days or longer in patients without glaucoma.
- Obtain eyelid culture and sensitivity tests as ordered before giving first dose, if infection is already present. Expect to begin drug therapy before test results are known.
- Be aware that the use of topical corticosteroids like hydrocortisone in the presence of thin corneal or scleral tissue may lead to perforation.
- Assess patient's vision and inspect eyes for abnormalities because prolonged use of ophthalmic corticosteroids may cause glaucoma, with damage to the optic nerve, defects in visual acuity and fields of vision, and forkation of posterior subcapsular cataracts. Prolonged use also increases risk of secondary ocular infections.
- Notify prescriber if patient's eye discomfort or inflammation does not improve within 48 hours or worsens.
- Question patient regarding the presence of eye discomfort because hydrocortisone may mask signs and symptoms of acute purulent infections.
- **WARNING** Do not inject neomycin, polymyxin B, bacitracin, and hydrocortisone solution into the eye or introduce it directly into the anterior chamber of the eye.
- If patient has persistent corneal ulceration and has used neomycin, polymyxin B, bacitracin, and hydrocortisone suspension long-term, obtain fungal cultures because fungal corneal infections are particularly likely with long-term local corticosteroid use.

PATIENT TEACHING

- Instruct patient to administer neomycin, polymyxin B, bacitracin, and hydrocortisone ointment exactly as prescribed, even when feeling better.
- Teach patient how to use eye ointment, if appropriate.

- Advise patient to stop using neomycin, polymyxin B, bacitracin, and hydrocortisone and notify prescriber if ocular pain or inflammation don't improve within 48 hours, become worse, or patient has an allergic reaction.
- Instruct patient to take care not to touch the tube tip to eyelids or any other surface to avoid contamination.
- Inform patient that no one else should use the drug because infection may be spread in this manner.

neomycin sulfate, polymyxin B sulfate, and dexamethasone sodium phosphate

AK-Trol, Dexacine, Maxitrol

Class and Category

Chemical: Aminoglucoside (neomycin), bacillus polymyxa derivative (polymyxin B), synthetic glucocorticoid (dexamethasone)
Therapeutic: Antibiotics (neomycin, polymyxin B), anti-inflammatory (dexamethasone)
Pregnancy category: C

Indications and Dosages

▶ *To treat inflammatory ocular conditions of the palpebral and bulbar conjunctiva, cornea, and anterior segment of the globe; chronic anterior uveitis and corneal injury from chemical, radiation, or thermal burns or penetration of foreign bodies when superficial ocular infection is present (or risk is high) caused by* Enterobacter *species,* Escherichia coli, Haemophilus influenzae, Klebsiella *species,* Neisseria *species,* Pseudomonas aeruginosa, *and* Staphylococcus aureus

OPHTHALMIC SUSPENSION

Adults. If severe, 1 or 2 drops instilled into conjuctival sac of affected eyes hourly and then tapered to discontinuation as infection and inflammation subsides. If mild, 1 or 2 drops instilled into conjunctival sac of affected eyes 4 to 6 times daily and then tapered to discontinuation as infection and inflammation subsides.

OPTHALMIC OINTMENT

Adults. Applied as a thin ribbon (about ½ inch) into conjunctival sac t.i.d. or q.i.d.

Contraindications

Fungal diseases affecting ocular structures; hypersensitivity to neomycin, polymyxin B, dexamethasone, other corticosteroids, or their components; mycobacterial infection of the eye; viral diseases of the cornea and conjunctiva, including epithelial herpes simplex keratitis, vaccinia, and varicella

---

Mechanism of Action

Neomycin competes with messenger RNA to bind with a receptor protein on the 30S ribosomal subunit of DNA in bacterial cells. This action causes abnormal, nonfunctioning proteins to form, which kills the cells.

Polymyxin B binds to cell membrane phospholipids in gram-negative bacteria, increasing the permeability of the cell membranes. Polymyxin B also acts as a cationic detergent, altering the osmotic barrier of the membrane and causing essential intracellular metabolites to leak. Both actions lead to cell death.

Dexamethasone binds to intracellular glucocorticoid receptors in the eye and suppresses inflammatory and immune responses by:
* inhibiting neutrophil and monocyte accumulation at the inflammation site and suppressing their phagocytic and bactericidal activity
* stabilizing lysosomal membranes
* suppressing the antigen response of macrophages and helper T cells
* inhibiting the synthesis of cellular mediators of the inflammatory response, such as cytokines, interleukins, and prostaglandins.

These actions inhibit the edema, fibrin deposition, capillary dilation, leukocyte migration, capillary proliferation, fibroblast proliferation, deposition of collagen and scar formation associated with inflammation.

Adverse Reactions

EENT: Delayed eye wound healing, elevation of intraocular pressure, glaucoma, optic nerve damage, posterior subcapsular cataract formation, secondary eye infection
SKIN: Pruritis, rash, urticaria
Other: Allergic reactions

Nursing Considerations

* Use neomycin, polymyxin B, and dexamethasone with great caution in the patient with a history of herpes simplex because use of an ocular steroid preparation such as dexamethasone may exacerbate the severity of many ocular viral infections.
* Use cautiously in patients with glaucoma because the dexamethasone component of drug may cause elevated intraocular pressure. Be prepared to monitor patient's intraocular pressure frequently in patients with glaucoma or routinely if drug is used for 10 days or longer in patients without glaucoma.

- Obtain eyelid culture and sensitivity tests as ordered before giving first dose, if infection is already present. Expect to begin drug therapy before test results are known.
- Be aware that topical corticosteroids such as dexamethasone may lead to perforation if the patient has thin corneal or scleral tissue.
- Assess patient's vision and inspect eyes for abnormalities as prolonged use of ophthalmic corticosteroids may cause glaucoma, damage to the optic nerve, defects in visual acuity and fields of vision, and posterior subcapsular cataract formation. Prolonged use also increases risk of secondary ocular infections.
- Notify prescriber if patient's eye discomfort or inflammation worsens.
- Question patient about eye discomfort because dexamethasone may mask signs and symptoms of acute purulent eye infections.
- **WARNING** Don't inject neomycin, polymyxin B, and dexamethasone solution into the eye.
- If patient has persistent corneal ulceration and has used neomycin, polymyxin B, and dexamethasone suspension longterm, obtain fungal cultures because fungal corneal infections are particularly likely with long-term local corticosteroid use.

PATIENT TEACHING
- Instruct patient to use neomycin, polymyxin B and dexamethasone solution exactly as prescribed.
- If needed, teach patient how to use eyedrops or ointment.
- If patient will use suspension form, tell him to shake the container first.
- Advise patient to discontinue using neomycin, polymyxin B, and dexamethasone and notify prescriber if signs and symptoms such as ocular pain or inflammation do not improve after 2 days or becomes worse or if an allergic reaction occurs.
- Instruct patient to take care not to touch the bottle tip or tube tip to eyelids or any other surface to avoid contamination.
- Inform patient that no one else should use the drug because infection may be spread in this manner.

neomycin, polymyxin B sulfate, and gramicidin
Neosporin Solution

Class and Category
Chemical: Aminoglucoside (neomycin), bacillus polymyxa derivative (polymyxin B), and bacillus brevis derivative (gramicidin)

Therapeutic: Antibiotics (neomycin, polymyxin B, gramicidin)
Pregnancy category: C

Indications and Dosages

▶ *To treat superficial infections of the external eye and surrounding area, such as conjunctivitis, keratitis, keratoconjunctivitis, blepharitis, and blepharoconjunctivitis caused by susceptible bacteria*

OPHTHALMIC SOLUTION

Adults. For severe infections, 2 drops instilled into affected eye or eyes q 1 hr initially. With positive response, taper to q 2 to 4 hr for total of 7 to 10 days. For mild to moderate infections, 1 or 2 drops instilled into affected eye or eyes q 2 to 4 hr for 7 to 10 days.

Mechanism of Action

Neomycin competes with messenger RNA to bind with a receptor protein on the 30S ribosomal subunit of DNA in bacterial cells. This action causes abnormal, nonfunctioning proteins to form, which kills the cells.

Polymyxin B binds to cell membrane phospholipids in gram-negative bacteria, increasing cell membrane permeability. Polymyxin B also acts as a cationic detergent, altering the osmotic barrier of the membrane and causing essential intracellular metabolites to leak. Both actions lead to cell death.

Gramicidin increases bacterial cell membrane permeability to inorganic cations by forming a network of channels through the normal lipid bilayer of the membrane. This results in the death of susceptible gram-positive bacteria.

Contraindications

Hypersensitivity to neomycin, polymyxin B, gramicidin, or their components

Adverse Reactions

EENT: Conjunctival or eyelid edema, erythema, or pruritus; delayed healing; local eye irritation; secondary eye infection
SKIN: Rash
Other: Anaphylaxis

Nursing Considerations

- **WARNING** Be aware that neomycin, polymyxin B, and gramicidin should never be introduced into the anterior chamber of the eye or injected subconjunctivally.
- Monitor patient for evidence of allergic reaction, such as rash, localized conjunctival or eyelid edema, erythema, or pruritus. If present, withhold drug and notify prescriber.

- Know that if an allergic reaction occurs, patient may also be allergic to gentamicin, kanamycin, paromomycin, and streptomycin because of cross-sensitivity.
- Monitor patient for evidence of secondary ocular infection such as signs and symptoms not alleviated within 7 to 10 days. If infection is not eradicated at completion of neomycin, polymyxin B, and gramicidin therapy, expect to obtain culture and sensitivity samples, as ordered, and administer additional antibiotic therapy as indicated.

PATIENT TEACHING

- Stress importance of administering neomycin, polymyxin B, and gramicidin ophthalmic solution exactly as prescribed, even when feeling better.
- Instruct patient or caregiver how to use eyedrops, if necessary.
- Remind patients and caregivers to wash their hands before and after administering drug.
- Caution patient or caregiver not to touch eye with tip of dropper or to share the drug with anyone else because of risk of contamination or spread of infection.
- Tell patient to notify prescriber if symptoms do not improve or become worse by the end of the prescribed therapy time.

neomycin sulfate, polymyxin B sulfate, and hydrocortisone

Antibiotic Ear Suspension, Cortisporin Ophthalmic Solution, Cortisporin Otic, Octicair, Pediotic

Class and Category

Chemical: Aminoglucoside (neomycin), bacillus polymyxa derivative (polymyxin B),synthetic glucocorticoid (hydrocortisone)
Therapeutic: Antibiotics (neomycin, polymyxin B), anti-inflammatory (hydrocortisone)
Pregnancy category: C

Indications and Dosages

▶ *To treat inflammatory ocular conditions of the palpebral and bulbar conjunctiva, cornea, and anterior segment of the globe; chronic anterior uveitis and corneal injury from chemical, radiation, or thermal burns or penetration of foreign bodies when superficial ocular infection is present (or risk is high) from bacteria caused by* Enterobacter *species,* Escherichia coli, Haemophilus influenzae, Klebsiella species, Neisseria *species,* Pseudomonas aeruginosa, *and* Staphylococcus

aureus
OPHTHALMIC SUSPENSION

Adults. 1 or 2 drops instilled into the affected eye or eyes q 3 or 4 hr.

▶ *To treat superficial bacterial infections of the external auditory canal or mastoidectomy and fenestration cavities caused by* Enterobacter *species,* Escherichia coli, Haemophilus influenzae, Klebsiella *species,* Neisseria *species,* Pseudomonas aeruginosa, *and* Staphylococcus aureus

OTIC SOLUTION

Adults. 4 drops instilled into the affected ear or ears t.i.d. or q.i.d. for 10 days. Or, cotton wick inserted into ear canal and then saturated with solution followed by repeat saturation q 4 hr, with cotton wick replaced q 24 hr for 10 days.

Children age 2 and over. 3 drops instilled into the affected ear or ears t.i.d. or q.i.d. for 10 days. Or, cotton wick inserted into ear canal and then saturated with solution followed by repeat saturation q 4 hr, with cotton wick replaced q 24 hr for 10 days.

Mechanism of Action

Neomycin competes with messenger RNA to bind with a receptor protein on the 30S ribosomal subunit of DNA in bacterial cells. This action causes abnormal, nonfunctioning proteins to form, which kills the cells.

Polymyxin B binds to cell membrane phospholipids in gram-negative bacteria, increasing cell membrane permeability. Polymyxin B also acts as a cationic detergent, altering the osmotic barrier of the membrane and causing essential intracellular metabolites to leak. Both actions lead to cell death.

Hydrocortisone binds to intracellular glucocorticoid receptors in the eye and ear and suppresses inflammatory and immune responses by:
• inhibiting neutrophil and monocyte accumulation at the inflammation site and suppressing their phagocytic and bactericidal activity
• stabilizing lysosomal membranes
• suppressing the antigen response of macrophages and helper T cells
• inhibiting the synthesis of cellular mediators of the inflammatory response, such as cytokines, interleukins, and prostaglandins.

These actions inhibit the edema, fibrin deposition, capillary dilation, leukocyte migration, capillary proliferation, fibroblast proliferation, deposition of collagen and scar formation associated with inflammation.

Contraindications

Fungal diseases affecting ocular or auricular structures; hypersensitivity to neomycin, polymyxin B, hydrocortisone, other corticosteroids, or their components; mycobacterial infection of the eye or ear; viral diseases of the cornea, conjunctiva and ear, including epithelial herpes simplex keratitis, vaccinia, and varicella

Adverse Reactions

EENT: Burning or stinging in ear (if drug has gained access to middle ear); conjunctival, eyelid or ear canal edema, erythema, or pruritis; delayed eye or ear wound healing; elevation of intraocular pressure; glaucoma; hearing loss; optic nerve damage; ototoxicity; posterior subcapsular cataract formation; secondary eye infection
GU: Nephrotoxicity
SKIN: Pruritis, rash, urticaria
Other: Allergic reactions

Nursing Considerations

- Use neomycin, polymyxin B, and hydrocortisone with great caution in patients with a history of herpes simplex because ocular or otic steroids such as hydrocortisone may worsen the severity of many ocular or otic viral infections.
- Use cautiously in patients with glaucoma because hydrocortisone may increase intraocular pressure. Monitor intraocular pressure often in patients with glaucoma and routinely if drug is used for 10 days or longer in patients without glaucoma.
- If infection is already present, obtain eyelid or ear culture and sensitivity tests as ordered before giving first dose. Expect to begin drug therapy before test results are known.
- Be aware that topical corticosteroids like hydrocortisone may lead to perforation if patient has thin corneal or scleral tissue.
- Assess patient's vision and inspect eyes for abnormalities because prolonged use of ophthalmic corticosteroids may cause glaucoma, damage to the optic nerve, defects in visual acuity and fields of vision, and posterior subcapsular cataract formation. Prolonged use also increases the risk of secondary ocular or otic infections.
- Notify prescriber if patient's discomfort or inflammation worsens.
- Question patient about eye or ear discomfort because hydrocortisone may mask evidence of acute purulent infections.
- **WARNING** Don't inject neomycin, polymyxin B, and hydrocortisone solution into the eye.
- If patient has persistent corneal ulceration and has used neomycin, polymyxin B, and hydrocortisone suspension long-term, obtain fungal cultures because fungal corneal infections are particularly likely with long-term local corticosteroid use.

PATIENT TEACHING
- Instruct patient to use neomycin, polymyxin B, and hydrocortisone solution exactly as prescribed, even when feeling better.
- Teach patient how to use eyedrops or eardrops, if appropriate.
- Instruct patient prescribed suspension form of drug to shake container well before administering.
- Advise patient to discontinue using neomycin, polymyxin B, and hydrocortisone and notify prescriber if signs and symptoms such as ocular or ear pain or inflammation do not improve or becomes worse or if an allergic reaction occurs.
- Instruct patient to take care not to touch the bottle tip to eyelids or ear or any other surface to avoid contamination.
- Inform patient that no one else should use the drug because infection may be spread in this manner.

neomycin sulfate, polymyxin B sulfate, and prednisolone
Poly-Pred Liquifilm

Class and Category
Chemical: Aminoglucoside (neomycin), bacillus polymyxa derivative (polymyxin B), glucocorticoid (prednisolone)
Therapeutic: Antibiotics (neomycin, polymyxin B), anti-inflammatory (prednisolone)
Pregnancy category: C

Indications and Dosages
▶ *To treat inflammatory ocular conditions of the palpebral and bulbar conjunctiva, cornea, and anterior segment of the globe; chronic anterior uveitis and corneal injury from chemical, radiation, or thermal burns or penetration of foreign bodies when superficial ocular infection is present (or risk is high) caused by* Enterobacter *species,* Escherichia coli, Haemophilus influenzae, Klebsiella *species,* Neisseria *species,* Pseudomonas aeruginosa, *and* Staphylococcus aureus
OPHTHALMIC SUSPENSION
Adults. For severe eye infection, 1 or 2 drops instilled into affected eye or eyes q 30 minutes, decreasing in frequency as infection is controlled. For mild to moderate eye infection, 1 or 2 drops instilled into affected eye or eyes q 3 to 4 hr. For eyelid infection, 1 or 2 drops instilled in the eye; then have patient close the eye, and rub excess on lid and lid margins q 3 to 4 hr.

Mechanism of Action

Neomycin competes with messenger RNA to bind with a receptor protein on the 30S ribosomal subunit of DNA in bacterial cells. This action causes abnormal, nonfunctioning proteins to form, which kills the cells.

Polymyxin B binds to cell membrane phospholipids in gram-negative bacteria, increasing cell membrane permeability. Polymyxin B also acts as a cationic detergent, altering the osmotic barrier of the membrane and causing essential intracellular metabolites to leak. Both actions lead to cell death.

Prednisolone binds to intracellular glucocorticoid receptors in the eye and suppresses inflammatory and immune responses by:

- inhibiting neutrophil and monocyte accumulation at the inflammation site and suppressing their phagocytic and bactericidal activity
- stabilizing lysosomal membranes
- suppressing the antigen response of macrophages and helper T cells
- inhibiting the synthesis of cellular mediators of the inflammatory response, such as cytokines, interleukins, and prostaglandins.

These actions inhibit the edema, fibrin deposition, capillary dilation, leukocyte migration, capillary proliferation, fibroblast proliferation, deposition of collagen and scar formation associated with inflammation.

Contraindications

Fungal diseases affecting ocular structures; hypersensitivity to neomycin, polymyxin B, prednisolone, other corticosteroids, or their components; mycobacterial infection of the eye; uncomplicated removal of a corneal foreign body; viral diseases of the cornea and conjunctiva, including epithelial herpes simplex keratitis, vaccinia, and varicella

Adverse Reactions

EENT: Conjunctival or eyelid edema, erythema, or pruritis; delayed eye wound healing; elevation of intraocular pressure; glaucoma; optic nerve damage; posterior subcapsular cataract formation; secondary eye infection

SKIN: Pruritis, rash, urticaria

Other: Allergic reactions

Nursing Considerations

- Use neomycin, polymyxin B, and prednisolone with great caution if patient has a history of herpes simplex because ocular steroids such as prednisolone may worsen the severity of many ocular viral infections.

- Use cautiously in patients with glaucoma because prednisolone may increase intraocular pressure. Be prepared to check intraocular pressure often in patients with glaucoma and routinely when therapy lasts 10 days in patients without glaucoma.
- Obtain eyelid culture and sensitivity tests as ordered before giving first dose, if infection is already present. Expect to begin drug therapy before test results are known.
- Be aware that topical corticosteroids such as prednisolone may lead to perforation if patient has thin corneal or scleral tissue.
- Assess patient's vision and inspect eyes for abnormalities as prolonged use of ophthalmic corticosteroids may cause glaucoma, damage to the optic nerve, defects in visual acuity and fields of vision, and posterior subcapsular cataract formation. Prolonged use also increases risk of secondary ocular infections.
- Notify prescriber if patient's eye discomfort or inflammation does not improve within 48 hours or worsens.
- Question patient regarding the presence of eye discomfort as the prednisolone component of drug may mask signs and symptoms of acute purulent infections.
- **WARNING** Do not inject neomycin, polymyxin B, and prednisolone subconjunctivally nor should the drug be introduced directly into the anterior chamber of the eye.
- If patient has persistent corneal ulceration and has used neomycin, polymyxin B, and prednisolone suspension longterm, obtain fungal cultures because fungal corneal infections are particularly likely with long-term local corticosteroid use.

PATIENT TEACHING
- Instruct patient to use neomycin, polymyxin B, and prednisolone suspension exactly as prescribed, even when feeling better.
- Teach patient how to use eyedrops, if appropriate.
- Tell patient to shake suspension well before using drops.
- Advise patient to discontinue using neomycin, polymyxin B, and prednisolone and notify prescriber if signs and symptoms such as ocular pain or inflammation do not improve within 48 hours, becomes worse or an allergic reaction occurs.
- Instruct patient to take care not to touch the eyedropper to eyelids or any other surface to avoid contamination.
- Inform patient that no one else should use the drug because infection may be spread in this manner.

oxytetracycline hydrochloride and polymyxin B sulfate

Terramycin with Polymyxin B Sulfate Ophthalmic Ointment

Class and Category

Chemical: Tetracycline derived from *Streptomyces rimosus* (oxytetracycline), *Bacillus polymyxa* derivative (polymyxin B)

Therapeutic: Antibiotics (oxytetracycline, polymyxin B)

Pregnancy category: C

Indications and Dosages

▶ *To treat superficial ocular infection involving the conjunctiva or cornea caused by susceptible strains of staphylococci, streptococci, pneumococci,* Hemophilus influenzae, Pseudomonas aeruginosa, *Koch-Weeks bacillus, or* Proteus

OPHTHALMIC OINTMENT

Adults. Applied as a thin ribbon (about ½ inch) into conjunctival sac b.i.d. to q.i.d.

Mechanism of Action

Oxytetracycline binds with ribosomal subunits of susceptible bacteria and alters the cytoplasmic membrane, inhibiting bacterial protein synthesis and rendering the organism ineffective.

Polymyxin B binds to cell membrane phospholipids in gram-negative bacteria, increasing cell membrane permeability. Polymyxin B also acts as a cationic detergent, altering the osmotic barrier of the membrane and causing essential intracellular metabolites to leak. Both actions lead to cell death.

Contraindications

Hypersensitivity to oxytetracycline, polymyxin B, or their components

Adverse Reactions

EENT: Erythema, pruritus, rash, or swelling of eye and surrounding area; secondary eye infection

Nursing Considerations

• Assess patient for adverse reactions. If signs and symptoms of an allergic response such as local rash or pruritus occur, withhold drug and notify prescriber.

• Monitor patient for evidence of secondary ocular infection. If infection remains when oxytetracycline and polymyxin B therapy ends, expect to obtain culture and sensitivity samples, as ordered, and give additional antibiotic therapy as indicated.

PATIENT TEACHING
- Stress importance of instilling oxytetracycline and polymyxin B ophthalmic ointment exactly as prescribed, even when eye(s) is feeling better.
- Instruct patient or caregiver how to use ophthalmic ointment.
- Remind patients and caregivers to wash their hands before and after administering drug.
- Caution patient or caregiver not to touch eye with tip of tube or to share the drug with anyone else because of risk of contamination or spread of infection.
- Tell patient to notify prescriber if symptoms do not improve or become worse by the end of the prescribed therapy time.

phenylephrine hydrochloride 0.25%, antipyrine 5%, and benzocaine 5%

Tympagesic

Class and Category

Chemical: Sympathomimetic amine (phenylephrine), pyrazolone derivative (antipyrine), ethyl aminobenzoate (benzocaine)
Therapeutic: Vasoconstrictor and decongestant (phenylephrine), analgesic (antipyrine) and local anesethetic (benzocaine)
Pregnancy category: C

Indications and Dosages

▶ *To relieve ear pain in treatment of painful ear conditions, such as acute otitis media*
OTIC SOLUTION
Adults. External ear canal filled with solution followed by insertion of cotton pledget moistened with otic solution. Pledget moistened q 2 to 4 hr, as needed, until pain is relieved

Contraindications

Hypersensitivity to phenylephrine, antipyrine, benzocaine or their components; perforated tympanic membrane; presence of ear discharge

Interactions

DRUGS
phenylephrine component
beta blockers, MAO inhibitors: Enhanced sympathomimetic effects
benzocaine component
sulfonamides: Reduced sulfonamide effectiveness

Mechanism of Action

Phenylephrine stimulates alpha-adrenergic receptors and inhibits the activity of the intracellular enzyme adenyl cyclase, which then inhibits production of cAMP. Inhibition of cAMP causes arteriole constriction, which decreases blood flow and mucosal edema. Phenylephrine also enhances the effects of anesthetics such as benzocaine by decreasing their rate of absorption and prolonging their duration of action.

Antipyrine blocks conduction of nerve impulses to the brain, thereby disrupting impulse transmission and preventing the perception of ear pain.

Benzocaine blocking nerve conduction, first in autonomic and then in sensory and finally in motor nerve fibers. Its effect appears to stem from decreased permeability of nerve cell membranes to sodium ions or competition with calcium ions for membrane binding sites.

Adverse Reactions

CNS: Anxiety, chills, dizziness, headache, nervousness, restlessness, weakness
EENT: Ear canal irritation, redness, or swelling; tinnitus
GI: Nausea, vomiting
HEME: Agranulocytosis
SKIN: Contact dermatitis, erythema, pallor, pruritus, rash, urticaria, vesiculation with oozing

Nursing Considerations

• Use cautiously in elderly patients and those with hypertension, increased intraocular pressure, diabetes mellitus, ischemic heart disease, hyperthyroidism, or prostatic hypertrophy because of the vasoconstrictive properties of phenylephrine.
• Monitor patient closely for systematic adverse reactions, although they're rare because absorption from the eardrum or external ear canal is minimal. If irritation or an allergic response occurs, such as rash, pruritus, or urticaria, withhold drug and notify prescriber.
• Be aware that drug contains a sulfite that can cause serious to life-threatening allergic-type reactions, including anaphylaxis, in susceptible patients such as those with asthma.
• Withhold drug and notify prescriber if patient has nausea, vomiting, and CNS stimulation because these rare symptoms may signal high levels antipyrine and benzocaine.
PATIENT TEACHING
• Instruct patient or caregiver to use phenylephrine, antipyrine, and benzocaine eardrops exactly as prescribed.

- Show patient or caregiver how to administer eardrops, if necessary, telling him to use the dropped to fill the ear canal with the drug and then insert a cotton pledget saturated with the drug into the ear canal until the next application. Remind him to replace the dropper into the bottle without rinsing it.
- Tell patient to stop using drug and notify prescriber if allergic response or local irritation occurs.
- Inform patient that drug may be stopped when ear pain has stopped. If pain persists, tell patient to notify prescriber because drug is intended only for short-term use.

prednisolone acetate and gentamicin sulfate

Pred-G, Pred G Liquilfilm, Pred-G S.O.P.

Class and Category

Chemical: Glucocorticoid (prednisolone), aminoglycoside derived from *Micromonospora purpurea* (gentamicin)
Therapeutic: Anti-inflammatory (prednisolone), antibiotic (gentamicin)
Pregnancy category: C

Indications and Dosages

▶ *To treat inflammatory ocular conditions of the palpebral and bulbar conjunctiva, cornea, and anterior segment of the globe; chronic anterior uveitis and corneal injury from chemical, radiation, or thermal burns or penetration of foreign bodies when superficial ocular infection is present (or risk is high) caused by* Enterobacter aerogenes, Escherichia coli, Hemophilus influenzae, Klebsiella pneumoniae, Neisseria gonorrhoeae, Pseudomonas aeruginosa, Serratia marcescens, Staphylococcus aureus, Streptococcus pneumoniae, *or* Streptococcus pyogenes

OINTMENT

Adults. A small ribbon (about ½ inch) applied into the conjunctival sac once daily to t.i.d.

SUSPENSION

Adults. If severe infection, 1 drop instilled into conjunctival sac of affected eye or eyes q 1 hr and then tapered to b.i.d. to q.i.d. with positive response. If mild to moderate infection, 1 drop instilled into conjunctival sac b.i.d. to q.i.d.

Contraindications

Fungal diseases affecting ocular structures; hypersensitivity to gentamicin, prednisolone, other corticosteroids, or their components; mycobacterial infection of the eye; viral diseases of the cornea and conjunctiva, including epithelial herpes simplex keratitis, vaccinia, and varicella

---

Mechanism of Action

Prednisolone binds to intracellular glucocorticoid receptors in the eye and suppresses inflammatory and immune responses by:

- inhibiting neutrophil and monocyte accumulation at the inflammation site and suppressing their phagocytic and bactericidal activity
- stabilizing lysosomal membranes
- suppressing the antigen response of macrophages and helper T cells
- inhibiting the synthesis of cellular mediators of the inflammatory response, such as cytokines, interleukins, and prostaglandins.

These actions inhibit the edema, fibrin deposition, capillary dilation, leukocyte migration, capillary proliferation, fibroblast proliferation, deposition of collagen, and scar formation associated with inflammation.

Gentamicin binds to negatively charged sites on the outer cell membrane of bacteria, thereby disrupting the membrane's integrity. Gentamicin also binds to bacterial ribosomal subunits and inhibits protein synthesis. Both actions lead to cell death.

Adverse Reactions

EENT: Conjunctival or eyelid edema, erythema, or pruritis; delayed eye wound healing; elevation of intraocular pressure; glaucoma; local eye burning, irritation, or stinging; optic nerve damage; posterior subcapsular cataract formation; secondary eye infection; superficial punctate keratitis

Nursing Considerations

- Use prednisolone and gentamicin with great caution in patients with a history of herpes simplex because ocular steroids such as prednisolone may worsen the severity of ocular viral infections.
- Use cautiously in patients with glaucoma because prednisolone may increase intraocular pressure. Be prepared to monitor intraocular pressure often in patients with glaucoma or routinely if therapy lasts 10 days or more in patients without glaucoma.
- If infection is already present, obtain eyelid culture and sensitivity tests, as ordered, before giving first dose. Expect to start drug therapy before test results are known.
- Be aware that topical corticosteroids such as prednisolone may lead to perforation if patient has thin corneal or scleral tissue.

- Assess patient's vision and inspect eyes for abnormalities as prolonged use of ophthalmic corticosteroids may cause glaucoma, damage to the optic nerve, defects in visual acuity and fields of vision, and posterior subcapsular cataract formation. Prolonged use also increases risk of secondary ocular infections.
- Notify prescriber if patient's eye discomfort or inflammation doesn't improve within 48 hours or it worsens.
- Question patient about eye discomfort because prednisolone may mask signs and symptoms of acute purulent infections.
- **WARNING** Do not inject prednisolone and gentamicin suspension subconjunctivally nor should the drug be introduced directly into the anterior chamber of the eye.
- If patient has persistent corneal ulceration and has used prednisolone and gentamicin solution long-term, obtain fungal cultures because fungal corneal infections are particularly likely with long-term local corticosteroid use.

PATIENT TEACHING
- Instruct patient to use prednisolone and gentamicin suspension or ointment exactly as prescribed, even when feeling better.
- Teach patient how to use eyedrops or ointment, if appropriate.
- Tell patient to shake suspension well before using eyedrops.
- Advise patient to stop using prednisolone and gentamicin and to notify prescriber if ocular pain or inflammation don't improve within 48 hours, they become worse, or patient has an allergic reaction.
- Instruct patient to take care not to touch the eyedropper or tube tip to eyelids or any other surface to avoid contamination.
- Inform patient that no one else should use the drug because infection may be spread in this manner.

prednisolone acetate and sulfacetamide sodium

Blephamide, Cetapred, Isopto, Metimyd, Sulster, Vasocidin

Class and Category

Chemical: Glucocorticoid (prednisolone), sulfonamide (sulfacetamide sodium)
Therapeutic: Anti-inflammatory (prednisolone), antibiotic (sulfacetamide sodium)
Pregnancy category: C

Indications and Dosages

▶ *To treat inflammatory ocular conditions of the palpebral and bulbar conjunctiva, cornea, and anterior segment of the globe; chronic anterior uveitis and corneal injury from chemical, radiation, or thermal burns or penetration of foreign bodies when superficial ocular infection is present (or risk is high) caused by* Enterobacter *species,* Escherichia coli, Haemophilus influenzae, Klebsiella *species,* Staphylococcus aureus, Streptococcus pneumoniae, *and* Streptococcus viridans *group*
OPHTHALMIC SUSPENSION
Adults. 2 drops instilled into conjunctival sac q 4 hr while awake and h.s.

Mechanism of Action

Prednisolone binds to intracellular glucocorticoid receptors in the eye and suppresses inflammatory and immune responses by:
• inhibiting neutrophil and monocyte accumulation at the inflammation site and suppressing their phagocytic and bactericidal activity
• stabilizing lysosomal membranes
• suppressing the antigen response of macrophages and helper T cells
• inhibiting the synthesis of cellular mediators of the inflammatory response, such as cytokines, interleukins, and prostaglandins.
These actions inhibit the edema, fibrin deposition, capillary dilation, leukocyte migration, capillary proliferation, fibroblast proliferation, deposition of collagen, and scar formation associated with inflammation.
Sulfacetamide sodium hinders bacterial cell growth by restricting the synthesis of folic acid required for growth through competition with para-aminobenzoic acid (PABA).

Incompatibilities

Silver preparations are incompatible with sulfacetamide preparations

Contraindications

Fungal diseases affecting ocular structures; hypersensitivity to prednisolone, other corticosteroids, sulfacetamide sodium, other sulfonamides, or their components; mycobacterial infection of the eye; viral diseases of the cornea and conjunctiva, including epithelial herpes simplex keratitis, vaccinia, and varicella

Interactions
DRUGS

prednisolone component
corticosteroids: Increased risk of cross-sensitivity

sulfacetamide sodium component

local anesthetics: Possibly antagonized effects of sulfacetamide sodium

sulfonamides: Increased risk of cross-sensitivity

Adverse Reactions

EENT: Acute anterior uvetitis, conjunctivitis, conjunctival hyperemia, corneal ulcers or secondary fungal infections, elevated intraocular pressure, eye irritation, glaucoma, keratitis, loss of accommodation, mydriasis, optic nerve damage, perforation of the globe of the eye, posterior subcapsular cataract formation, ptosis, secondary ocular bacterial infections

ENDO: Systemic hypercorticoidism

GI: Fulminant hepatic necrosis

HEME: Agranulocytosis, aplastic anemia, blood dyscrasias

SKIN: Stevens-Johnson syndrome, toxic epidermal necrolysis

Other: Allergic reactions, delayed wound healing

Nursing Considerations

- Use prednisolone and sulfacetamide sodium with great caution in patients with a history of herpes simplex because ocular steroids such as prednisolone may worsen the severity of many ocular viral infections.
- Use cautiously in patients with glaucoma because prednisolone may increase intraocular pressure. Be prepared to monitor intraocular pressure often in patients with glaucoma or routinely if therapy lasts 10 days or longer in patients without glaucoma.
- Also use cautiously in African-Americans, who have a greater risk of acute anterior uveitis than other populations do when using this drug.
- If infection is already present, obtain eyelid culture and sensitivity tests as ordered before giving first dose. Expect to start drug therapy before test results are known.
- Be aware that topical corticosteroids such as prednisolone may lead to perforation if patient has thin corneal or scleral tissue.
- Assess patient's vision and inspect eyes for abnormalities as prolonged use of ophthalmic corticosteroids may cause glaucoma, with damage to the optic nerve, defects in visual acuity, and fields of vision and in posterior subcapsular cataract formation. Prolonged use also increases risk of secondary ocular infections.
- Notify prescriber if patient's eye discomfort or inflammation worsens.
- Question patient about eye discomfort because prednisolone may mask signs and symptoms of acute purulent eye infections.

- **WARNING** Don't inject prednisolone and sulfacetamide sodium suspension into the eye.
- Monitor patient for serious adverse reactions, including allergic response. If suspected, notify prescriber, withhold prednisolone and sulfacetamide sodium, and be prepared to administer appropriate supportive treatment.
- If patient has persistent corneal ulceration and has used prednisolone and sulfacetamide suspension long-term, obtain fungal cultures because fungal corneal infections are particularly likely with long-term local corticosteroid use.

PATIENT TEACHING
- Instruct patient to use prednisolone and sulfacetamide sodium suspension exactly as prescribed even when feeling better.
- Teach patient how to administer eyedrops, if necessary.
- Tell patient to shake the bottle well before using.
- Caution patient to discard the suspension if it appears dark brown and obtain a new suspension.
- Advise patient to stop using prednisolone and sulfacetamide sodium and notify prescriber if ocular pain or inflammation don't improve or they worsen after 2 days.
- Instruct patient to take care not to touch the bottle tip to eyelids or any other surface to avoid contamination.
- Inform patient that no one else should use the drug because infection may be spread in this manner.

scopolamine hydrobromide 0.3% and phenylephrine 10%

Murocoll-2

Class and Category

Chemical: Naturally occurring tertiary amine (scopolamine), sympathomimetic amine (phenylephrine)
Therapeutic: Mydriatic and cycloplegic (scopolamine), mydriatic (phenylephrine)
Pregnancy category: NR

Indications and Dosages

▶ *To produce mydriasis for diagnostic eye exam*
SOLUTION
Adults. 1 or 2 drops instilled into each eye, repeated in 5 minutes if needed.
▶ *To break posterior synechiae in iritis*

SOLUTION
Adults. 1 or 2 drops instilled into affected eye or eyes t.i.d. to q.i.d. postoperatively.

Mechanism of Action

Scopolamine blocks the action of acetylcholine, which relaxes the cholinergically innervated sphincter muscle of the iris. The drug also blocks cholinergic stimulation of the accommodative ciliary muscle of the lens, resulting in dilation of the pupil and paralysis of accommodation.

Phenylephrine acts on adrenergic receptors in the eye, contracting the dilator muscle of the pupil and constricting the arterioles of the conjunctiva.

Contraindications

Angle-closure glaucoma; hypersensitivity to scopolamine, phenylephrine, sulfites or their components; severe coronary artery disease or hypertension; use within 14 days of MAO inhibitor therapy; ventricular tachycardia

Interactions
DRUGS

phenylephrine component
MAO inhibitors: Increased and prolonged cardiac stimulation, increased vasopressor effect, increased risk of severe cardiovascular and cerebrovascular effects, hyperpyrexia, and vomiting

Adverse Reactions

CNS: Amnesia, confusion, dizziness, excitation, hallucinations, headache, insomnia, nervousness, paresthesia, psychotic reactions, restlessness, somnolence, tremor, weakness
CV: Angina, bradycardia, hypertension, hypotension, palpitations, peripheral vasoconstriction that may lead to necrosis or gangrene, tachycardia, ventricular arrhythmias
EENT: Blocked lacrimal drainage system; blurred vision; dry mouth; follicular conjunctivitis; increased intraocular pressure; ocular vascular congestion, edema, erythema, irritation or exudates
GI: Constipation, nausea, vomiting
GU: Urinary hesitancy, incontinence or retention
MS: Spastic extremities
RESP: Dyspnea
SKIN: Photophobia
Other: Allergic reaction, anaphylaxis

Nursing Considerations

- Use cautiously in elderly patients and those predisposed to increased intraocular pressure. Prepare these patients to have an estimation of the depth of the angle of their anterior chamber before instillation of scopolamine and phenylephrine drops.
- Monitor patient closely for adverse reactions. Systematic reactions may occur because of absorption. If they occur, notify prescriber and be prepared to give supportive treatment until effects of drug have worn off—which may take several days.
- Monitor elderly patients and those with Down syndrome, who are more susceptible to adverse reactions, especially psychotic reactions and excitation that often occur within 30 to 45 minutes after administration.
- **WARNING** Be aware that scopolamine and phenylephrine contains a bisulfite that may cause severe allergic-type reactions, especially in patients with asthma. Monitor these patients closely for anaphylaxis, and withhold drug and be prepared to provide supportive care, if indicated.
- Observe patient for signs and symptoms of an allergic response such as persistent irritation and diffuse redness of eyes that occurs within minutes of administering drug.

PATIENT TEACHING

- Instruct patient or caregiver how to administer eyedrops.
- Advise patient or caregiver to press a finger on the lacrimal sac for 1 to 2 minutes after administration.
- Stress importance of using eyedrops exactly as prescribed.
- Caution patient to avoid potentially hazardous activities until the CNS effects of the drug are known.
- Tell patient to withhold drug and notify prescriber if allergic reaction occurs.
- Instruct patient to take care not to touch the eyedropper to eyelids or any other surface to avoid contamination.

tobramycin and dexamethasone

TobraDex

Class and Category

Chemical: Aminoglycoside (tobramycin), synthetic glucocorticoid (dexamethasone)
Therapeutic: Antibiotic (tobramycin), anti-inflammatory (dexamethasone)
Pregnancy category: C

Indications and Dosages

▶ *To treat inflammatory ocular conditions of the palpebral and bulbar conjunctiva, cornea, and anterior segment of the globe; chronic anterior uveitis and corneal injury from chemical, radiation, or thermal burns or penetration of foreign bodies when superficial ocular infection is present (or risk is high) caused by* Acinetobacter calcoaceticus, Enterobacter aerogenes, Escherichia coli, Haemophilus influenzae, Haemophilus aegyptius, Klebsiella pneumoniae, Moraxella lacunata, Morganella morganii, *most* Proteus vulgaris *strains,* Proteus mirabilis, Pseudomonas aeruginosa, Staphylococcus aureus, Staphylococcus epidermidis, Streptococcus pneumoniae, *some* Streptococcus *group A beta-hemolytic and nonhemolytic species, or some* Neisseria *species*

OPHTHALMIC SUSPENSION

Adults and children age 2 and over. *Initial:* 1 or 2 drops instilled into conjunctival sac q 2 hr for 24 to 48 hr, followed by 1 or 2 drops instilled into conjunctival sac q 4 to 6 hr. Or, 1 or 2 drops instilled into conjunctival sac q 4 to 6 hr.

OPHTHALMIC OINTMENT

Adults and children age 2 and over. Applied as a thin ribbon (about ½ inch) into conjunctival sac t.i.d. or q.i.d.

Mechanism of Action

Tobramycin inhibits bacterial protein synthesis by binding irreversibly to one of two aminoglycoside-binding sites on the 30S ribosomal subunit, resulting in bacteriostatic effects. Bactericidal effects may stem from accumulation of tobramycin in cells, so intracellular drug level exceeds the extracellular level.

Dexamethasone binds to intracellular glucocorticoid receptors in the eye and suppresses inflammatory and immune responses by:

• inhibiting neutrophil and monocyte accumulation at the inflammation site and suppressing their phagocytic and bactericidal activity

• stabilizing lysosomal membranes

• suppressing the antigen response of macrophages and helper T cells

• inhibiting the synthesis of cellular mediators of the inflammatory response, such as cytokines, interleukins, and prostaglandins.

These actions inhibit the edema, fibrin deposition, capillary dilation, leukocyte migration, capillary proliferation, fibroblast proliferation, deposition of collagen and scar formation associated with inflammation.

Contraindications

Fungal diseases affecting ocular structures; hypersensitivity to tobramycin, other aminoglycosides, dexamethasone, other corticosteroids, or their components; mycobacterial infection of the eye; viral diseases of the cornea and conjunctiva, including epithelial herpes simplex keratitis, vaccinia, and varicella

Interactions
DRUGS
tobramycin component
aminoglycosides: Increased risk of cross-sensitivity
dexamethasone component
corticosteroids: Increased risk of cross-sensitivity

Adverse Reactions
EENT: Conjunctival erythema, delayed eye wound healing, elevation of intraocular pressure, eyelid itching and swelling, glaucoma, optic nerve damage, posterior subcapsular cataract formation, secondary eye infection
SKIN: Pruritis, rash, urticaria
Other: Allergic reactions

Nursing Considerations
- Use tobramycin and dexamethasone with great caution in the patient with a history of herpes simplex because use of an ocular steroid preparation such as dexamethasone may exacerbate the severity of many ocular viral infections.
- Use cautiously in patients with glaucoma because the dexamethasone component of drug may cause elevated intraocular pressure. Be prepared to monitor patient's intraocular pressure frequently in patients with glaucoma or routinely if drug is used for 10 days or longer in patients without glaucoma.
- Obtain eyelid culture and sensitivity tests as ordered before giving first dose, if infection is already present. Expect to begin drug therapy before test results are known.
- Be aware that topical corticosteroids such as dexamethasone may lead to perforation if patient has thin corneal or scleral tissue.
- Assess patient's vision and inspect eyes for abnormalities as prolonged use of ophthalmic corticosteroids may cause glaucoma, damage to the optic nerve, defects in visual acuity and fields of vision and posterior subcapsular cataract formation. Prolonged use also increases risk of secondary ocular infections.
- Tell prescriber if patient's discomfort or inflammation worsens.
- Question patient about eye discomfort because dexamethasone may mask signs and symptoms of acute purulent eye infections.
- **WARNING** Don't inject tobramycin and dexamethasone suspension into the eye.

- Monitor patient for serious eye adverse reactions including allergic response. If suspected, notify prescriber, withhold tobramycin and dexamethasone, and be prepared to administer appropriate supportive treatment.
- If patient has persistent corneal ulceration and has used tobramycin and dexamethasone suspension long-term, obtain fungal cultures because fungal corneal infections are particularly likely with long-term local corticosteroid use.

PATIENT TEACHING

- Instruct patient to use tobramycin and dexamethasone exactly as prescribed.
- Teach patient how to use eyedrops or ointment, if necessary.
- Tell patient to shake suspension well before using.
- Advise patient to discontinue using tobramycin and dexamethasone and notify prescriber if signs and symptoms such as ocular pain or inflammation do not improve after 2 days or becomes worse or if an allergic reaction occurs.
- Instruct patient to take care not to touch the bottle or tube tip to eyelids or any other surface to avoid contamination.
- Inform patient that no one else should use the drug because infection may be spread in this manner.

trimethoprim sulfate and polymyxin B sulfate

Polytrim

Class and Category

Chemical: Dihydrofolic acid analogue (trimethorprim), bacillus polymyxa derivative (polymyxin B)
Therapeutic: Antibiotics (trimethorprim, polymyxin B)
Pregnancy category: C

Indications and Dosages

▶ *To treat mild to moderate superficial ocular bacterial infections including acute bacterial conjunctivitis and blepharoconjunctivitis caused by susceptible strains of* Staphylococcus aureus, Staphylococcus epidermidis, Streptococcus pneumoniae, Streptococcus viridans, Haemophilus influenzae, *and* Pseudomonas aeruginosa

OPHTHALMIC SOLUTION

Adults and children age 2 months and over. 1 drop instilled into affected eye or eyes q 3 hr while awake for 7 to 10 days. *Maximum:* 6 drops per eye daily.

Mechanism of Action

Trimethorprim inhibits formation of tetrahydrofolic acid, the metabolically active form of folic acid, in susceptible bacteria. This action depletes folate, an essential component of bacterial development, thereby disrupting production of bacterial nucleic acid and protein.

Polymyxin B binds to cell membrane phospholipids in gram-negative bacteria, increasing cell membrane permeability. Polymyxin B also acts as a cationic detergent, altering the osmotic barrier of the membrane and causing essential intracellular metabolites to leak. Both actions lead to cell death.

Contraindications

Hypersensitivity to trimethorprim, polymyxin B, or their components

Adverse Reactions

EENT: Circumocular rash surrounding eye; eyelid or local burning, edema, itching, increased redness and stinging; secondary eye infection; tearing

Nursing Considerations

- Be aware that trimethorprim and polymyxin B shouldn't be used to prevent or treat ophthalmic neonatorium.
- **WARNING** Don't inject drug solution into the eye.
- Monitor patient for sensitivity reaction, such as rash. If present, notify prescriber and expect drug to be stopped.
- Monitor patient for evidence of secondary eye infection, such as discharge or the failure of signs and symptoms to improve. Notify prescriber, and expect to obtain culture and sensitivity samples and to implement appropriate measures, as indicated and ordered.

PATIENT TEACHING

- Instruct patient to use trimethorprim and polymyxin B solution exactly as prescribed even when feeling better.
- Teach patient how to administer eyedrops, if necessary.
- Advise patient to stop using trimethorprim and polymyxin B and to notify prescriber if redness, irritation, swelling, or pain persists or increases.
- Instruct patient to take care not to touch the bottle tip to eyelids or any other surface to avoid contamination.
- Inform patient that no one else should use the drug because infection may be spread in this manner.

Gastrointestinal Drugs

bismuth subsalicylate, metronidazole, and tetracycline hydrochloride

Helidac Therapy

Class and Category

Chemical: 2-hydroxybenzoic acid bismuth salt and salicylic acid (bismuth subsalicylate), synthetic nitroimidazole derivative (metronidazole), chlortetracycline derivative (tetracycline)

Therapeutic: Antibiotic (bismuth, metronidazole, tetracycline)

Pregnancy category: D

Indications and Dosages

▶ *To eradicate* Helicobacter pylori *infection in patients with duodenal ulcer, given with an H₂ antagonist approved to treat acute duodenal ulcer*

CHEWABLE TABLETS (BISMUTH SUBSALICYLATE), TABLETS (METRONIDAZOLE), CAPSULES (TETRACYCLINE)

Adults. 525 mg bismuth subsalicyate (2 chewable tablets), 250 mg metronidazole (1 tablet), and 500 mg tetracycline (1 capsule) q.i.d. for 14 days.

Mechanism of Action

Bismuth subsalicylate is almost completely hydrolyzed in the GI tract to bismuth and salicylic acid. It disrupts the integrity of *Helicobacter pylori* cells and prevents their adhesion to the gastric epithelium. It also kills *H. pylori* by inhibiting its urease, phospholipase, and proteolytic activity.

Metronidazole is un-ionized at physiologic pH and is readily taken up by *H. pylori* cells. Once inside the cells, metronidazole is reduced to unidentified polar products that lack the nitro group; they disrupt bacterial DNA and inhibit nucleic acid synthesis to cause cell death.

Tetracycline exerts a bacteriostatic effect against *H. pylori* by passing through the bacterial lipid bilayer, where it binds reversibly to 30S ribosomal subunits. Bound tetracycline blocks the binding of aminoacyl transfer RNA to messenger RNA, thus inhibiting bacterial protein synthesis.

Contraindications

Breastfeeding; children; hepatic or renal impairment; hypersensitivity to bismuth subsalicylate, aspirin, other salicylates, metronidazole, other nitromidazole derivatives, tetracycline, other tetracyclines, or their components; pregnancy

Interactions

DRUGS

bismuth subsalicylate, metronidazole, and tetracycline
anticogulants: Increased risk for bleeding

bismuth subsalicylate component

aspirin, insulin, oral antidiabetics, probenecid, sulfinpyrazone: Increased risk of hypoglycemia

metronidazole component

cimetidine: Possibly prolonged metronidazole half-life and decreased plasma clearance
disulfiram: Increased risk of psychotic reactions
lithium: Increased serum lithium level and toxicity
phenobarbital, phenytoin: Reduced metronidazole plasma level and possibly impaired phenytoin clearance

tetracycline component

aluminum-, calcium-, or magnesium-containing antacids; iron supplements (oral); magnesium-containing laxatives; magnesium salicylate; multivitamins (containing manganese or zinc salts); sodium bicarbonate: Possibly impaired absorption of tetracycline and formation of nonabsorbable complexes
cholestyramine, colestipol: Possibly impaired tetracycline absorption
digoxin: Possibly increased blood digoxin level
methoxyflurane: Possibly nephrotoxicity
oral contraceptives (containing estrogen): Possibly reduced contraceptive reliability
penicillins: Possibly decreased bactericidal effect of penicillins

FOODS

tetracycline component

dairy products, other foods: Possibly impaired tetracycline absorption

ACTIVITIES

metronidazole component

alcohol use: Possibly increased incidence of abdominal cramps, nausea, vomiting, headache, and flushing

Adverse Reactions

CNS: Asthenia, cerebral ischemia, depression, dizziness, headache, insomnia, malaise, nervousness, paresthesia, peripheral neuropathy, seizures, somnolence, syncope, weakness

CV: Chest pain, hypertension, MI

EENT: Conjunctivitis, discolored tongue, dry mouth, enamel hypoplasia, glossitis, metallic taste, oral candidiasis, rhinitis, sinusitis, stomatitis, taste perversion

GI: Abdominal pain, anal discomfort, anorexia, constipation, diarrhea, duodenal ulcer, dyspepsia, dysphagia, elevated liver enzymes, flatulence, GI hemorrhage, hepatotoxicity, intestinal obstruction, melena, nausea, rectal candidiasis or hemorrhage, vomiting

GU: Incontinence, UTI, vaginal candidiasis

HEME: Mild leukopenia

MS: Arthritis, musculoskeletal pain, rheumatoid arthritis, tendonitis

RESP: Upper respiratory infection

SKIN: Acne, ecchymosis, photosensitivity, pruritus, rash

Other: Flulike syndrome, neoplasms

Nursing Considerations

- Use cautiously in patients with CNS disease; those with blood dyscrasia or a history of it; and elderly patients who may have asymptomatic renal and hepatic dysfunction.
- Be aware that drug is packaged in 14 blister cards, each containing the following daily dose: eight chewable 262.4-mg bismuth subsalicylate tablets, four 250-mg metronidazole tablets, and four 500-mg tetracycline capsules.
- Know that bismuth subsalicylate is used in this combination for its antimicrobial effects and not for relief of upset stomach.
- Monitor anticoagulant therapy closely because triple therapy may interact with anticoagulants.
- Monitor diabetic patients receiving insulin or oral antidiabetic agents for hypoglycemia.
- Monitor patient for signs of central nervous system effects such as seizures and peripheral neuropathy. If present, contact prescriber and expect to discontinue triple therapy.
- Be aware that if candidiasis infection occurs, it will require treatment with a candicidal agent.

PATIENT TEACHING

- Instruct patient to take bismuth subsalicylate, metronidazole, and tetracycline triple therapy exactly as prescribed for length of time prescribed.

- Tell patient to chew and then swallow bismuth subsalicylate pink tablets and then swallow the metronidazole white tablet and tetracycline white capsule whole with a full glass of water.
- Instruct patient to avoid antacids; preparations containing iron, zinc, or sodium bicarbonate; and milk or dairy products while taking triple therapy.
- If patient misses a dose, caution against doubling the next dose. Instead, tell him to make up the missed dose by continuing the normal dose schedule until the drug is gone. If he misses more than four doses, instruct patient to notify prescriber.
- Caution patient to avoid alcohol during drug therapy and for at least 1 day after taking all doses.
- Tell patient that bismuth subsalicylate may cause a transient and harmless darkening of his tongue and black stool.
- Instruct patient to report blood in his stool or any other troublesome or serious adverse effect, such as a yeast infection.
- Warn patient to avoid sun exposure as much as possible and to use sunscreen when out of doors.
- Tell women using oral contraceptives to use an additional or different form of contraception throughout bismuth subsalicylate, metronidazole, and tetracycline triple therapy.

chlordiazepoxide hydrochloride and clidinium bromide

Clindex, Clinoxide, Clipoxide, Librax, Lidox, Lidoxide, Zebrax

Class, Category, and Schedule

Chemical: Benzodiazepine (chlordiazepoxide), synthetic quaternary ammonium derivative (clidinium)
Therapeutic: Sedative (chlordiazepoxide), anticholinergic (clidinium)
Pregnancy category: NR
Controlled substance: Schedule IV

Indications and Dosages

▶ *As adjunct therapy in the treatment of peptic ulcer; to treat irritable bowel syndrome and acute enterocolitis*
CAPSULE
Adults. 5 to 10 mg clordiazepoxide and 2.5 to 5 mg clidinium (1 to 2 capsules) daily up to q.i.d. 30 to 60 minutes before meals or food intake

Mechanism of Action

Chlordiazepoxide may potentiate the effects of gamma-aminobutyric acid (GABA) and other inhibitory neurotransmitters by binding to specific benzodiazepine receptors in limbic and cortical areas of the CNS. By binding to these receptors, chlordiazepoxide increases GABA's inhibitory effects and blocks cortical and limbic arousal, which helps relax and slow the digestive system.

Clidinium inhibits acetylcholine's muscarinic actions at postganglionic parasympathetic receptor sites, including smooth muscles, secretory glands, and the CNS. These actions relax smooth muscles, including those in the GI tract, and diminish GI and biliary tract secretions to reduce gastric acid formation.

Contraindications

Angle-closure glaucoma; benign bladder neck obstruction; hypersensitivity to chlordiazepoxide, clidinium, or their components; ileus, intestinal atony (elderly or debilitated patients), intestinal obstruction, myasthenia gravis; myocardial ischemia; ocular adhesions between lens and iris; prostatic hypertrophy; renal disease; severe ulcerative colitis; tachycardia; toxic megacolon; unstable cardiovascular status in acute hemorrhage

Interactions

DRUGS

chlordiazepoxide and clidinium

antidiarrheal drugs containing attapulgitel or kaolin: Decreased blood levels of chlordiazepoxide and clidinium
CNS depressants: Increased clidinium and CNS effects
ketoconazole: Decreased blood level of ketoconazole
oral potassium chloride: Increased risk of causing or worsening gastric or intestinal ulceration

chlordiazepoxide component

antacids: Altered rate of chlordiazepoxide absorption
cimetidine, disulfiram, fluoxetine, hormonal contraceptives, isoniazid, ketoconazole, metoprolol, propoxyphene, propranolol, valproic acid: Increased blood chlordiazepoxide level
digoxin: Increased blood digoxin level and risk of digitalis toxicity
levodopa: Decreased efficacy of levodopa's antiparkinsonian effects
neuromuscular blockers: Potentiated, counteracted, or diminished effects of neuromuscular blockers
phenytoin: Possibly increased phenytoin toxicity

probenecid: Shortened onset of action or prolonged effect of chlordiazepoxide
rifampin: Decreased chlordiazepoxide effect
theophyllines: Antagonized sedative effects of chlordiazepoxide
clidinium component
amantadine: Increased risk of clidinium adverse effects
atenolol: Increased atenolol effects
other anticholinergics: Possibly increased adverse effects
phenothiazines: Decreased antipsychotic effectiveness
tricyclic antidepressants: Increased clidinium adverse effects
ACTIVITIES
chlordiazepoxide and clindinium
alcohol use: Increased CNS effects

Adverse Reactions

CNS: Ataxia, confusion, depression, dizziness, drowsiness, excitement, fever, headache, insomnia, irritability, memory loss, nervousness, weakness
CV: Bradycardia, hypotension, palpitations, tachycardia
EENT: Blurred vision, cycloplegia, dry mouth, increased intraocular pressure, loss of taste, mydriasis, nasal congestion, pharyngitis, photophobia
GI: Bloating, constipation, dysphagia, heartburn, hepatic dysfunction, jaundice, ileus, nausea, vomiting
GU: Impotence, urinary hesitancy, urine retention
HEME: Agranulocytosis
RESP: Dyspnea, shortness of breath
SKIN: Decreased sweating, flushing, rash, urticaria

Nursing Considerations

- Use chlordiazepoxide and clidinium cautiously in patients with heart failure, arrhythmias, hypertension, autonomic neuropathy, hyperthyroidism, allergies, asthma, debilitating chronic lung disease, renal or hepatic impairment, or porphyria.
- **WARNING** Be aware that prolonged use of therapeutic doses can lead to dependence.
- Monitor liver function test results during therapy.
- If patient has a history of psychiatric disorders, monitor for paradoxical reactions, such as excitement, stimulation, and acute rage, during first 2 weeks of therapy.
- **WARNING** Monitor for excitement, agitation, drowsiness, and confusion in elderly patients because they're more sensitive to the clidinium component's effects. If these reactions occur, notify prescriber and expect to decrease dosage.

- Take safety precautions to protect patient from falling.

PATIENT TEACHING
- Instruct patient to take drug 30 to 60 minutes before meals.
- Tell patient to take chlordiazepoxide and clidinium exactly as prescribed and not to alter dosage or dosing frequency without consulting prescriber first.
- Alert patient that chlordiazepoxide and clidinium may become habit forming, causing mental or physical dependence. Stress importance of not abruptly stopping chlordiazepoxide and clidinium therapy because withdrawal symptoms, such as vomiting, diaphoresis, and dizziness may occur.
- Caution patient to avoid potentially hazardous activities until drug's CNS effects are known.
- Instruct patient to avoid alcohol and other CNS depressants during chlordiazepoxide and clidinium therapy.
- Advise patient to avoid using antacids during chlordiazepoxide and clidinium therapy.
- Instruct patient to report adverse effects, such as constipation, vision changes, sore throat, trouble urinating, and palpitations.
- Tell patient to avoid taking chlordiazepoxide and clidinium within an hour of antidiarrheal drugs because chlordiazepoxide and clidinium will be less effective.
- Alert patient that drug will make him sweat less, which may cause his body temperature to increase, especially during exercise, hot weather, or hot baths or saunas. Advise using extra care not to become overheated as heat stroke could occur.
- Advise patient to use sugarless candy or gum, melt bits of ice in his mouth, or use a saliva substitute if his mouth, nose, or throat feels dry. If mouth dryness continues for more than 2 weeks, tell patient to contact prescriber because continued dryness may increase his risk for dental disease, which can include tooth decay, gum disease, and fungus infections.

diphenoxylate hydrochloride and atropine sulfate
Lofene, Logen, Lomocot, Lomotil, Lonox, Vi-Atro

Class, Category, and Schedule
Chemical: Belladonna alkaloid, tertiary amine (atropine), phenylpiperidine derivative opioid (diphenoxylate)
Therapeutic: Antidiarrheal

Pregnancy category: C
Controlled substance: Schedule V

Indications and Dosages

▶ *To treat acute and chronic diarrhea*
ORAL SOLUTION, TABLETS
Adults and adolescents. *Initial:* 5 mg of diphenoxylate and
0.05 mg of atropine t.i.d. or q.i.d. *Maintenance:* 5 mg of diphenoxylate and 0.05 mg of atropine daily, p.r.n. *Maximum:* 20 mg of
diphenoxylate daily.
DOSAGE ADJUSTMENT Dosage reduced as soon as symptoms are controlled. Expect prescriber to consider alternative
treatment if no improvement occurs after 10 days at maximum
dosage. Dosage also reduced in elderly or very ill patients and
in those with respiratory problems.

Mechanism of Action

Diphenoxylate directly affects circular smooth muscles of the GI tract, reducing intestinal motility.
 Subtherapeutic doses of atropine are added to diphenoxylate to reduce its
potential for abuse.

Contraindications

Diarrhea caused by pseudomembranous enterocolitis or entero-
toxin-producing bacteria; hypersensitivity to atropine, diphenoxylate, or their components; obstructive jaundice; ulcerative colitis

Interactions

DRUGS
anticholinergics: Possibly enhanced effects of atropine
barbiturates, tranquilizers, and other habit-forming CNS depressants: Potentiated CNS depression; possibly increased risk of drug dependence
MAO inhibitors: Possibly hypertensive crisis
naltrexone: Withdrawal symptoms if patient is physically dependent on diphenoxylate
opioid analgesics: Increased risk of severe constipation; additive
CNS depression
ACTIVITIES
alcohol use: Possibly potentiated CNS depression

Adverse Reactions

CNS: Confusion, depression, dizziness, drowsiness, euphoria,

fever, headache, hyperthermia, lethargy, malaise, paresthesia, restlessness, sedation
CV: Tachycardia
EENT: Gingival hyperplasia
GI: Abdominal cramps or pain, anorexia, ileus, nausea, pancreatitis, toxic megacolon, vomiting
GU: Urine retention
RESP: Respiratory depression
SKIN: Dry skin and mucous membranes, flushing, pruritus, urticaria
Other: Anaphylaxis, physical and psychological dependence

Nursing Considerations

- **Warning** Use diphenoxylate-atropine combination with extreme caution in patients with abnormal hepatic or renal function because drug can cause hepatic coma. Monitor liver function test results as appropriate during long-term therapy.
- **Warning** Monitor for respiratory depression, especially in elderly or very ill patients and in those with respiratory problems; expect to give lower doses as prescribed.
- If severe fluid or electrolyte imbalance develops, expect to withhold drug as ordered until imbalance is corrected. Drug-induced ileus or toxic megacolon may cause fluid retention in the intestine, aggravating dehydration and electrolyte imbalance.
- Closely monitor patient with ulcerative colitis because drug has caused toxic megacolon. Notify prescriber immediately about unexpected adverse reactions, especially abdominal distention and hypoactive or absent bowel sounds.
- During long-term therapy, assess for tolerance to drug's antidiarrheal effects.

PATIENT TEACHING
- Caution patient not to exceed the prescribed dosage because of the risk of adverse reactions, including drug dependence.
- Stress the importance of keeping drug away from children because overdose can cause permanent brain damage in them.
- Instruct patient to take drug with food if GI distress occurs.
- Advise patient to avoid potentially hazardous activities until drug's CNS effects are known.
- Urge patient to avoid alcohol and CNS depressants because of additive effects.
- Instruct patient to notify prescriber if diarrhea isn't improved or controlled within 48 hours or if a fever develops.

lansoprazole, amoxicillin, and clarithromycin
Prevpac

Class and Category
Chemical: Substituted benzimidazole (lansoprazole), aminopeni-cillin (amoxicillin), macrolide derivative (clarithromycin)
Therapeutic: Antisecretory, antiulcer (lansoprazole), antiobiotics (amoxicillin, clarithromycin)
Pregnancy category: C

Indications and Dosages
▶ *To reduce the risk of duodenal ulcer recurrence by eradicating the presence of* Helicobacter pylori *in the stomach*
E.R. CAPSULES (LANSOPRAZOLE), CAPSULES (AMOXICILLIN), TABLETS (CLARITHROMYCIN)
Adults. 30 mg lansoprazole, 1 gram amoxicillin, and 500 mg clarithromycin (one 30-mg capsule lansoprazole, two 500-mg capsules amoxicillin, and one 500-mg tablet clarithromycin) b.i.d. morning and evening for 10 to 14 days.
DOSAGE ADJUSTMENT For patients with renal impairment (creatinine clearance less than normal but greater than 30 ml/min), hepatic impairment, or both, clarithromycin dosage may need to be reduced or dosing interval increased.

Mechanism of Action
Lansoprazole binds to and inactivates the hydrogen-potassium-adenosine triphosphate enzyme system (also called the proton pump) in gastric parietal cells. This action blocks the final step of gastric acid production.

Amoxicillin kills bacteria by binding to and inactivating penicillin-binding proteins on the inner membrane of bacterial cell walls. Penicillin-binding proteins play a role in bacterial cell wall synthesis and cell division. By binding to these proteins, the drug weakens bacterial cell walls and causes lysis.

Clarithromycin inhibits RNA-dependent protein synthesis in many types of aerobic, anaerobic, gram-positive, and gram-negative bacteria. By binding with the 50S ribosomal subunit of the bacterial 70S ribosome, clarithromycin causes bacterial cells to die.

Contraindications
Concurrent therapy with astemizole, cisapride, pimozide, or terfe-nadine; hypersensitivity to lansoprazole, amoxicillin, other peni-

cillins, clarithromycin, erythromycin, other macrolides, or their components

Interactions

DRUGS

lansoprazole component

ampicillin, digoxin, iron salts, ketoconazole, other drugs that depend on low gastric pH for bioavailability: Inhibited absorption of these drugs
fluvoxamine: Elevated plasma lansoprozole level
sucralfate: Delayed lansoprazole absorption
theophylline: Slightly decreased blood theophylline level
warfarin: Possibly increased risk of bleeding

amoxicillin component

allopurinol: Possibly increased incidence of rash
chloramphenicol, macrolides, sulfonamides, tetracyclines: Reduced bactericidal effect of amoxicillin
methotrexate: Increased risk of methotrexate toxicity
oral contraceptives with estrogen: Possibly reduced contraceptive effectiveness
probenecid: Increased amoxicillin effects

clarithromycin component

astemizole, disopyramide, quinidine: Possibly prolonged QT interval or torsades de pointes
carbamazepine, other drugs metabolized by cytochrome P450 enzyme system: Increased blood levels of these drugs
cisapride, disopyramide, pimozide, quinidine, terfenadine: Increased risk of arrhythmias
digoxin: Increased serum digoxin level
dihydroergotamine, ergotamine: Risk of acute ergot toxicity
lovastatin, simvastatin: Risk of rhabdomyolysis
oral anticoagulants: Potentiated anticoagulant effects
rifabutin, rifampin: Decreased blood clarithromycin level by more than 50%
sildenafil: Possibly prolonged blood sildenafil level
theophylline: Increased blood theophylline level
triazolam: Possibly increased CNS effects
zidovudine: Decreased blood zidovudine level

FOODS

lansoprazole component

all food: Possibly reduced absorption of lansoprazole

Adverse Reactions

CNS: Agitation, anxiety, behavior changes, confusion, dizziness, fatigue, headache, insomnia, reversible hyperactivity, seizures, somnolence, vertigo

CV: QT-interval prolongation, torsades de pointes, ventricular arrhythmias

EENT: Altered taste, glossitis, hearing loss, oral moniliasis, stomatitis, tongue discoloration

ENDO: Hypoglycemia

GI: Abdominal pain, anorexia, constipation, diarrhea, elevated liver enzymes, hepatitis, jaundice, increased appetite, indigestion, nausea, pancreatitis, pseudomembranous colitis, vomiting

GU: Elevated BUN level

HEME: Anemia, eosinophilia, granulocytosis, leukopenia, neutropenia, thrombocytopenia, thrombocytopenic purpura

MS: Arthralgia

SKIN: Acute generalized exanthematous pustulosis, erythema multiforme, erythematous maculopapular rash, exfoliative dermatitis, Stevens-Johnson syndrome, toxic epidermal necrolysis, pruritus, rash, urticaria

Other: Allerigc reaction, anaphylaxis, serum sickness–like reactions, superinfection

Nursing Considerations

• Use lansoprazole, amoxicillin, and clarithromycin cautiously in patients with renal impairment because of the clarithromycin component and in patients with infectious mononucleosis or who are breastfeeding because of the amooxicillin component.

• Administer lansoprazole, amoxicillin, and clarithromycin 30 minutes before breakfast and dinner.

• **WARNING** If allergic reaction occurs, stop lansoprazole, amoxicillin, and clarithromycin immediately and start emergency care as indicated and ordered. It may include epinephrine, oxygen, intravenous steroids, and airway management.

• Monitor patient closely for diarrhea, which may be caused by antibiotic-induced pseudomembranous colitis. If diarrhea occurs, notify prescriber and expect to withhold drug therapy and administer treatment for diarrhea, as ordered.

PATIENT TEACHING

• Instruct patient to take lansoprazole, amoxicillin, and clarithromycin exactly as prescribed even when feeling better.

• Tell patient to swallow each capsule and tablet whole.

• Let patient know he may take antacids with lansoprazole, amoxicillin, and clarithromycin therapy.

- Advise patient to report diarrhea, severe headache, severe nausea, rash, itching, or worsening of symptoms immediately to prescriber.

phenobarbital, hyoscyamine sulfate (or hydrobromide), atropine sulfate, and scopolamine hydrobromide

Barophen, Donnamor, Daonnapine, Donnatal, Donnatal Extentabs, Hyosophen, Kinesed, Spasmophen, Spasquid, Susano

Class and Category

Chemical: Barbiturate (phenobarbital), tertiary amine (hyoscyamine, atropine, scopolamine)

Therapeutic: Sedative-hypnotic (phenobarbital), anticholinergic (hyoscyamine, atropine, scopolamine)

Pregnancy category: C

Indications and Dosages

▶ *As adjunct to treat irritable bowel syndrome, acute enterocolitis, and duodenal ulcer*

CAPSULE, TABLET

Adults and adolescents. 16 to 32 mg phenobarbital, 0.104 to 0.208 mg hyoscyamine, 0.0194 to 0.0388 mg atropine, and 0.0065 to 0.0125 mg scopolamine (1 or 2 capsules or tablets) b.i.d. to q.i.d.

CHEWABLE TABLETS

Adults and adolescents. 16 to 32 mg phenobarbital, 0.12 to 0.24 mg hyoscyamine, 0.12 to 0.24 mg atropine, and 0.007 to 0.014 mg scopolamine (1 or 2 tablets) b.i.d. to q.i.d.

E.R. TABLETS

Adults and adolescents. 48.6 mg phenobarbital, 0.3111 mg hyoscyamine, 0.0582 mg atropine, and 0.0195 mg scopolamine (1 tablet) q 8 to 12 hr.

ELIXIR

Adults and adolescents. 16 to 32 mg phenobarbital, 0.104 to 0.208 mg hyoscyamine, 0.0194 to 0.0388 mg atropine, and 0.0065 to 0.0125 mg scopolamine (5 or 10 ml) b.i.d. to q.i.d.

Contraindications

Acute intermittent porphyria; glaucoma; hiatal hernia associated with reflux esophagitis; hypersensitivity to phenobarbital, other barbiturates, hyoscyamine, atropine, scopolamine or their components; idiosyncratic reaction of phenobarbital-induced excitement or restlessness; intestinal atony in elderly or debilitated patients; myasthenia gravis; paralytic ileus; obstructive uropathy or GI disorders; severe ulcerative colitis; toxic megacolon; unstable cardiovascular status in acute hemorrhage

---

Mechanism of Action

Phenobarbital inhibits ascending conduction in the reticular formation, which produces drowsiness, hypnosis, and sedation. Phenobarbital also decreases the spread of seizure activity in the cortex, thalamus, and limbic system.

Belladonna alkaloids (hyoscyamine, atropine, scopolamine) inhibit acetylcholine's muscarinic actions at postganglionic parasympathetic receptor sites, including smooth muscles, secretory glands, and CNS. These actions relax smooth muscles and diminish GI, GU, and biliary tract secretions.

Interactions

DRUGS

phenobarbital component

acetaminophen: Decreased acetaminophen effectiveness with long-term phenobarbital therapy

amphetamines: Delayed intestinal absorption of phenobarbital

anesthetics (halogenated hydrocarbon): Possibly hepatotoxicity

anticonvulsants (hydantoin): Unpredictable effects anticonvulsant metabolism

anticonvulsants (succinimide), including carbamazepine: Decreased blood levels and elimination half-lives of these drugs

calcium channel blockers: Possibly excessive hypotension

carbonic anhydrase inhibitors: Enhanced osteopenia induced by phenobarbital

chloramphenicol, corticosteroids, cyclosporine, dacarbazine, digoxin, metronidazole, quinidine: Decreased effectiveness of these drugs from enhanced metabolism

CNS depressants: Additive CNS depression

cyclophosphamide: Possibly reduced half-life and increased leukopenic activity of cyclophosphamide

disopyramide: Possibly ineffectiveness of disopyramide

doxycycline, fenoprofen: Shortened half-life of these drugs

griseofulvin: Possibly decreased absorption and effectiveness of griseofulvin

guanadrel, guanethidine: Possibly increased orthostatic hypotension

haloperidol: Decreased seizure threshold, decreased blood haloperidol level *ketamine (high doses):* Increased risk of hypotension and respiratory depression

leucovorin: Interference with phenobarbital's anticonsulsant effect

levothyroxine, oral contraceptives, phenylbutazone, tricyclic antidepressants: Decreased effectiveness of these drugs

loxapine, phenothiazines, thioxanthenes: Decreased seizure threshold

MAO inhibitors: Prolonged phenobarbital effects and possibly altered pattern of seizure activity

maprotiline: Increased CNS depression, decreased seizure threshold at high doses, and decreased phenobarbital effectiveness

methoxyflurane: Possibly hepatotoxicity and nephrotoxicity

methylphenidate: Increased risk of phenobarbital toxicity

mexiletine: Decreased blood mexiletine level

oral anticoagulants: Decreased anticoagulant activity and increased risk of bleeding when phenobarbital is discontinued

pituitary hormones (posterior): Increased risk of arrhythmias and coronary insufficiency

primidone: Altered pattern of seizures and increased CNS effects of both drugs

valproate, valproic acid: Decreased phenobarbital metabolism and increased risk of barbiturate toxicity

vitamin D: Decreased phenobarbital effectiveness

xanthines: Increased xanthine metabolism and antagonized hypnotic effect of phenobarbital

belladonna alkaloids component

amantadine: Increased adverse anticholinergic effects

atenolol, digoxin: Possibly increased therapeutic and adverse effects of these drugs

phenothiazines: Possibly decreased phenothiazine effectiveness and increased adverse effects of belladonna alkaloids

tricyclic antidepressants: Possibly increased adverse anticholinergic effects

ACTIVITIES

phenobarbital component

alcohol use: Additive CNS depression

Adverse Reactions

CNS: Anxiety, CNS stimulation (with high doses), confusion, depression, dizziness, drowsiness, headache, insomnia, irritability, lethargy, mood changes, nervousness, paradoxical stimulation, sedation, vertigo, weakness

CV: Bradycardia, hypotension, palpitations, tachycardia

EENT: Altered taste, blurred vision, cycloplegia, dry mouth, in-

creased intraocular pressure, miosis, mydriasis, nasal congestion, photophobia, ptosis
ENDO: Suppression of lactation
GI: Bloating, constipation, diarrhea, dysphagia, heartburn, ileus, nausea, vomiting
GU: Decreased libido, impotence, urinary hesitancy, urine retention
MS: Arthralgia, bone tenderness, musculoskeletal pain
RESP: Bronchospasm, respiratory depression
SKIN: Decreased sweating, dermatitis, flushing, photosensitivity, rash, urticaria, xerostomia
Other: Anaphylaxis, physical and psychological dependence

Nursing Considerations

- Be aware that drug shouldn't be given during third trimester of pregnancy because repeated use of phenobarbital can cause dependence in neonate. Drug also shouldn't be given to breastfeeding women because it may cause CNS depression in infants.
- Use drug cautiously in patients with allergies, arrhythmias, asthma, autonomic neuropathy, coronary artery disease, debilitating chronic lung disease, heart failure, hepatic or renal dysfunction, hypertension, hyperthyroidism, tachycardia, and prostatic hypertrophy because of adverse effects of drug.
- Monitor patient's respiratory status before each dose because drug can cause respiratory depression, especially in patient with bronchopneumonia, pulmonary disease, respiratory tract infection, or status asthmaticus.
- Monitor patient for diarrhea, which may be an early sign of incomplete intestinal obstruction, especially in patients with ileostomy or colostomy. If present, withhold drug and notify prescriber.
- **WARNING** Monitor elderly patients for excitement, agitation, drowsiness, and confusion, even with small doses. Elderly patients are more sensitive to the effects of the combination drug and are more likely to develop these adverse reactions. If they develop, notify prescriber because dosage may need to be decreased.
- Anticipate that phenobarbital may worsen major depression, suicidal tendencies, or other mental disorders.
- Monitor patient receiving anticoagulant therapy because phenobarbital may necessitate larger doses of the anticoagulant for optimal effect. When drug is stopped, the anticoagulant dose may have to be decreased.

- Take safety precautions to protect patient from injury from falling.
- If patient has received drug for a prolonged period, expect to taper dosage slowly to prevent withdrawal symptoms when drug is discontinued because of phenobarbital component.

PATIENT TEACHING
- Tell patient to take drug exactly as prescribed and not to increased dosage or dosing frequency without consulting prescriber because drug may become habit forming.
- Instruct patient to take elixir form undiluted or to mix it with water, milk, or fruit juice and to use a calibrated device to ensure accurate dosage.
- Tell patient to notify prescriber if she has persistent or severe diarrhea, constipation, or difficulty urinating.
- Caution patient to avoid driving and similar activities until the effects of the drug is known.
- **WARNING** Urge patient to avoid extremely hot or humid conditions because heatstroke may occur.
- Urge patient to avoid alcohol during therapy.
- Caution patient on prolonged therapy to abruptly stopping drug as withdrawal symptoms may occur because of the phenobarbital component of drug.
- Alert female patient to notify prescriber about suspected, known, or intended pregnancy. Advise against breastfeeding during therapy.

Genitourinary Drugs

belladonna and opium

B & O Suppositories, B & O Supprettes No. 15A,
B & O Supprettes No. 16A

Class, Category, and Schedule

Chemical: Naturally occurring belladonna leaf herb (belladonna), naturally occurring dried milky exudate of the Papaver somniferum Linne or its variety album De Candolle plant (opium)
Therapeutic: Geniturinary analgesic
Pregnancy category: C
Controlled substance: Schedule II

Indications and Dosages

▶ *To relieve moderate to severe pain from ureteral spasm following GU surgery that is unresponsive to nonopioid analgesics*
SUPPOSITORY
Adults. 16.2 mg belladonna and 30 mg opium (1 suppository) or 16.2 mg belladonna and 60 mg opium (1 suppository) daily or b.i.d.

Mechanism of Action

Belladonna leaf contains several alkaloids, mainly L-hyoscyamine (which probably racemizes to atropine during extraction) and scopolamine. Atropine dominates belladonna's effect, inhibiting acetylcholine's muscarinic action at the neuroeffector junctions of smooth muscles of the urinary bladder. It decreases urinary tract motility and smooth muscle contractions, thereby relieving ureteral spasms and pain.

Opium contains several opioid alkaloids, including morphine. Morphine dominates the effect of opium binding with and activating opioid receptors (primarily mu receptors) in the brain and spinal cord to produce analgesia and euphoria.

Contraindications

Acute alcoholism, angle-closure glaucoma; asthma; GI obstructive disease (alchalasia, pyloric obstruction, pyloroduodenal stenosis); hepatic disease; hypersensitivity to belladonna, atropine, opium, morphine, or their components; ileus; intestinal atony; labor (with premature delivery); myasthenia gravis; myocardial ischemia; obstructive uropathy; renal disease; respiratory depression, severe ulcerative colitis; tachycardia; toxic megacolon; unstable cardiovascular status in acute hemorrhage; upper airway obstruction

Interactions

DRUGS

belladonna and opium

anticholinergics: Increased risk of severe constipation leading to ileus, urine retention

antihistamines: Possibly excessive anticholinergic activity

belladonna component

amantadine, antidyskinetics, meperidine, muscle relaxants, phenothiazines, tricyclic antidepressants and other drugs with anticholinergic properties including antiarrhythmics (disopyramide, procainamide, quinidine), buclizine, meclizine: Increased anticholinergic effect

antimyasthenics: Reduced intestinal motility

cyclopropane: Increased risk of ventricular arrhythmias

metoclopramide: Decreased effect on GI motility

opioid analgesics: Increased risk of ileus, severe constipation, and urine retention

potassium chloride, especially wax-matrix forms: Possibly GI ulcers

opium component

amitriptyline, clomipramine, nortriptyline: Increased CNS and respiratory depression

anticholinergics: Possibly severe constipation leading to ileus, urine retention

antidiarrheals such as loperamide and paregoric: CNS depression, possibly severe constipation

antihistamines, chloral hydrate, glutethimide, MAO inhibitors, methocarbamol: Increased CNS and respiratory depressant effects of opium

antihypertensives, hypotension-producing drugs: Increased hypotension, risk of orthostatic hypotension

buprenorphine: Decreased therapeutic effects of morphine, increased respiratory depression, possibly withdrawal symptoms

cimetidine: Increased analgesic and CNS and respiratory depressant effects of opium

CNS depressants: Possibly coma, hypotension, respiratory depression, severe sedation
diuretics: Decreased diuretic efficacy
metoclopramide: Possibly antagonized metoclopramide effect on GI motility
mixed agonist-antagonist analgesics: Possibly withdrawal symptoms
naloxone: Antagonized analgesic and CNS and respiratory depressant effects of opium (morphine), possibly withdrawal symptoms
naltrexone: Possibly induction or worsening of withdrawal symptoms if opium given within 7 to 10 days before naltrexone
neuromuscular blockers: Increased or prolonged respiratory depression
opioid analgesics: Increased CNS and respiratory depression, increased hypotension
ACTIVITIES
opium component
alcohol use: Increased CNS and respiratory depression, increased hypotension

Adverse Reactions

CNS: Agitation, amnesia, anxiety, ataxia, Babinski's or Chaddock's reflex, behavioral changes, coma, confusion, decreased concentration, decreased tendon reflexes, delirium, delusions, depression, dizziness, drowsiness, euphoria, fever, hallucinations, headache, hyperreflexia, insomnia, lethargy, light-headedness, malaise, mania, nervousness, paranoia, psychosis, restlessness, sedation, seizures, somnolence, stupor, syncope, tremor, vertigo, weakness
CV: Arrhythmias, bradycardia, cardiac arrest, cardiac dilation, chest pain, hypertension, hypotension, orthostatic hypotension, left ventricular failure, MI, palpitations, shock, tachycardia, weak or impalpable peripheral pulses
EENT: Acute angle-closure glaucoma, altered taste, blepharitis, blindness, blurred vision, conjunctivitis, cyclophoria, cycloplegia, decreased visual acuity or accommodation, diplopia, dry mouth, eye irritation, eyelid crusting, heterophoria, increased intraocular pressure, keratoconjunctivitis, lacrimation, laryngitis, laryngeal edema or laryngospasm (allergic), miosis, mydriasis, nasal congestion, nystagmus, oral lesions, photophobia, pupils poorly reactive to light, rhinitis, strabismus, tongue chewing
GI: Abdominal cramps or distention, abdominal pain, anorexia, biliary tract spasm, bloating, constipation, decreased bowel sounds, delayed gastric emptying, diarrhea, dysphagia, elevated

liver function test results, gastroesophageal reflux, heartburn, hiccups, ileus and toxic megacolon in patients with inflammatory bowel disease, intestinal obstruction, indigestion, nausea, vomiting

GU: Bladder distention, decreased ejaculate potency, decreased libido, difficult ejaculation, enuresis, impotence, prolonged labor, urinary hesitancy, urinary urgency, urine retention

HEME: Anemia, leukopenia, thrombocytopenia

MS: Arthralgia, dysarthria, hypertonia, muscle twitching

RESP: Apnea, asthma exacerbation, atelectasis, bradypnea, bronchospasm, depressed cough reflex, dyspnea, hypoventilation, inspiratory stridor, pulmonary edema, respiratory depression or arrest, shallow breathing, subcostal recession, tachypnea, wheezing

SKIN: Cold skin, cyanosis, decreased sweating, dermatitis, diaphoresis, flushing, pallor, pruritus, rash, urticaria

Other: Allergic reaction, anaphylaxis, dehydration, facial edema, physical and psychological dependence, polydipsia, sensations of warmth, withdrawal symptoms

Nursing Considerations

- Before therapy begins, assess patient's current drug use, including all prescription and OTC drugs.
- If rectal suppository is too soft to insert, chill it in refrigerator for 30 minutes or run wrapped suppository under cold water.
- **WARNING** Monitor respiratory and cardiovascular status carefully and frequently during belladonna and opium therapy. Be alert for changes in vital signs that could signal presence of arrhythmias, respiratory depression, and hypotension.
- Evaluate patient for therapeutic response, including report of decreased pain and body movements that suggest pain relief.
- Watch for excessive or persistent sedation; if patient is on higher dosage of opium, it may need to be lowered.
- Be aware that belladonna and opium may cause physical and psychological dependence; watch carefully for drug tolerance and withdrawal symptoms, such as body aches, diaphoresis, diarrhea, fever, piloerection, rhinorrhea, sneezing, and yawning.
- Be aware that opium may have a prolonged duration and cumulative effect in patients with impaired hepatic or renal function. Monitor patient carefully.
- Assess bowel and bladder elimination. Notify prescriber if diarrhea, constipation, urinary hesitancy, or urine retention develop.

PATIENT TEACHING
- Instruct patient to take belladonna and opium exactly as prescribed and not to change dosage without consulting prescriber.
- Tell patient to moisten rectal suppository before inserting it.
- Urge patient to avoid alcohol and other CNS depressants during belladonna and opium therapy.
- Advise patient to avoid potentially hazardous activities while taking belladonna and opium until the CNS effects are known.
- Teach patient to change position slowly to minimize effects of orthostatic hypotension.
- Instruct patient to notify prescriber about worsening or breakthrough pain.
- Inform patient that belladonna and opium may be habit-forming. Urge him to notify prescriber if he experiences anxiety, decreased appetite, excessive tearing, irritability, muscle aches or twitching, rapid heart rate, or yawning.
- Advise patient to notify prescriber if he has persistent or severe diarrhea, constipation, or difficulty urinating.

citric acid monohydrate, potassium citrate monohydrate, and sodium citrate dihydrate

Tricitrates

Class and Category

Chemical: Base (citric acid), potassium derivative of base (potassium citrate), sodium derivative of base (sodium citrate)
Therapeutic: Urinary alkalinizers (citric acid, potassium citrate, sodium citrate)
Pregnancy category: NR

Indications and Dosages

▶ *To provide long-term maintenance of alkaline urine when managing chronic metabolic acidosis caused by such conditions as chronic renal insufficiency or renal tubular acidosis*
SOLUTION
Adults. 1,002 to 2,004 mg citric acid, 1,650 to 3,300 mg potassium citrate, and 1,500 to 3,000 mg sodium citrate (15 to 30 ml) q.i.d. after meals and h.s.
Children. 334 to 1,002 mg citric acid, 550 to 1,650 mg potassium citrate, and 500 to 1,500 mg sodium citrate (5 to 15 ml) q.i.d. after meals and h.s.

> ## Mechanism of Action
> Citrate acid, potassium citrate, and sodium citrate are oxidized in the body to form bicarbonate, a buffer, which increases urinary pH as it is readily excreted in urine.

Contraindications
Azotemia, hyperkalemia, hypernatremia, oliguria, severe myocardial damage or renal impairment, untreated Addison's disease, use with sodium restricted diets

Adverse Reactions
GI: Laxative effect, nausea, vomiting
Other: Hyperkalemia, hypernatremia, metabolic alkalosis

Nursing Considerations
• Use with extreme caution in patients who need to limit intake of sodium and potassium and in patients with heart failure, hypertension, renal dysfunction, peripheral or pulmonary edema, or toxemia of pregnancy.
• Use cautiously in patients with low urine output.
• Monitor patient's serum electrolyte and acid-base status, as ordered, because electrolyte imbalance or metabolic alkalosis may occur, especially in patients with renal impairment.

PATIENT TEACHING
• Instruct patient to take citric acid, potassium citrate, and sodium citrate exactly as prescribed because excessive amounts can cause tetany or depress heart function.
• Instruct patient to store drug solution in a tight container and protect from extreme heat or cold.
• Tell patient to take drug after meals and at bedtime to minimize the laxative effect of the drug.
• Reassure patient that the drug is pleasant tasting.

neomycin sulfate and polymyxin B sulfate irrigant
Neosporin G.U. Irrigant

Class and Category
Chemical: Aminoglycoside (neomycin), polypeptide (polymyxin B sulfate)

Therapeutic: Antibiotic
Pregnancy category: D

Indications and Dosages

▶ *To prevent bacteriuria and gram-negative rod septicemia associated with the use of indwelling catheters*
IRRIGANT
Adults. 1-ml ampule diluted in 1,000 ml of isotonic saline solution, continuously irrigating the urinary bladder over 24 hr via a three-way catheter every day for up to 10 days.

Mechanism of Action

Both neomycin and polymyxin B are bactericidal. Neomycin competes with messenger RNA in bacterial cells to bind with a specific receptor protein on the 30S ribosomal subunit of DNA. This action causes abnormal, nonfunctioning proteins to form. A lack of functional proteins causes bacterial cell death.

Polymyxin B binds to cell membrane phospholipids in gram-negative bacteria, increasing the permeability of the cell membrane. It also acts as a cationic detergent, altering the osmotic barrier of the membrane and causing essential intracellular metabolites to leak. These actions results in cell death.

Contraindications

Bladder mucosa or wall tears, bladder surgery involving bladder wall, hypersensitivity to neomycin, other aminoglycosides, polymyxin B or other polymyxins or their components, or history of a serious reaction to neomycin or other aminoglycosides

Interactions

DRUGS
neomycin and polymyxin B
general anesthetics, neuromuscular blockers, skeletal muscle relaxants: Increased or prolonged skeletal muscle relaxation, possibly respiratory paralysis
neomycin component
dimenhydrinate: Possibly masked symptoms of neomycin-induced ototoxicity
oral anticoagulants: Possibly potentiated anticoagulant effects
polymyxin B component
nephrotoxic and neurotoxic drugs (such as aminoglycosides, amphotericin B, colistin, sodium citrate, streptomycin, tobramycin, and vancomycin): Increased risk of nephrotoxicity and neurotoxicity

Adverse Reactions

EENT: Hearing impairment (only if absorption inadvertently occurs), tinnitis (only if absorption inadvertently occurs)

GU: Irritation of urinary bladder mucosa, renal dysfunction (only if absorption inadvertently occurs)

Nursing Considerations

- Add 1 ampule of neomycin and polymyxin B to a 1,000-ml container of isotonic saline solution using aseptic technique. Use within 48 hours. When ready to use, connect the 1,000-ml container to the inflow lumen of the three-way urinary catheter and begin flow.
- Monitor flow rate of the irrigation solution to deliver 1,000 ml continuously over 24 hours. If the patient's urine output exceeds 2 liters in 24 hours, notify prescriber to determine if rate should be adjusted to deliver 2,000 ml of neomycin and polymyxin B solution over 24 hours.
- Don't interrupt the flow of irrigation solution into the bladder for longer than a few minutes, and only if absolutely necessary because effectiveness to prevent a bladder infection will be compromised with less than continuous irrigation.
- Obtain urine specimens for urinalysis and culture and sensitivity testing routinely throughout neomycin and polymyxin B therapy, as ordered. Notify prescriber of any abnormal findings.
- Be aware that neomycin and polymyxin B usually isn't absorbed systemically as long as the irrigation does not go beyond 10 days.
- Watch closely for neuromuscular blockade, nephrotoxicity, or ototoxicity if patient is receiving high doses or prolonged treatment or patient is elderly, dehydrated, or has impaired renal function.

PATIENT TEACHING

- Advise patient to notify prescriber about hearing loss or ringing in the ears.
- Tell patient to alert prescriber if she suspects or knows she is pregnant because the neomycin portion of the drug can cross the placenta if it is inadvertently absorbed.

potassium acid phosphate and sodium acid phosphate

K-Phos M.F., K Phos No. 2

Class and Category
Chemical: Electrolyte minerals (potassium acid phosphate, sodium acid phosphate)
Therapeutic: Urinary acidifiers (potassium acid phosphate, sodium acid phosphate)
Pregnancy category: C

Indications and Dosages
▶ *To acidify urine and lower urinary calcium concentration*
TABLETS
Adults. 155 mg to 610 mg potassium acid phosphate and 350 mg to 1,400 mg sodium acid phosphate (1 to 2 tablets depending on product used) q.i.d. *Maximum:* 8 tablets daily.

Mechanism of Action
Potassium acid phosphate and sodium acid phosphate increases serum phosphate levels. At the renal distal tubule, hydrogen secretion by the tubular cell in exchange for sodium in the tubular urine converts dibasic phosphate salts to monobasic phosphate salts. This causes large amounts of acid to be excreted without lowering urine pH to a degree that would block hydrogen transport by a high concentration gradient between the tubular cell and luminal fluid. Phosphate salts lower urinary calcium level because an increase in serum phosphorus level causes a decrease in calcium level. This effect may involve increased bone formation, movement of calcium into cells, decreased bone resorption, or decreased calcium absorption.

Contraindications
Hyperkalemia, hyperphosphatemia, infected magnesium ammonium phosphate stones, renal insufficiency less than 30% normal

Interactions
DRUGS
potassium acid phosphate and sodium acid phosphate
potassium supplements: Increased risk of hyperkalemia
salicylates: Reduced excretion of salicylates which may lead to salicylate toxicity
FOODS
potassium acid phosphate and sodium acid phosphate
sodium-rich foods, salt: Increased risk of hypernatremia

Adverse Reactions
CNS: Confusion, dizziness, headache, numbness, seizures, thirst, tingling, tiredness, weakness

CV: Irregular heartbeat, peripheral edema, tachycardia
EENT: Numbness or tingling around lips
GI: Abdominal discomfort, diarrhea, nausea, vomiting
GU: Low urine output
MS: Bone and joint pain, heaviness of legs, muscle cramps, pain or weakness in hands and feet
RESP: Shortness of breath
Other: Weight gain

Nursing Considerations
- Use cautiously in patients with cardiac disease (including heart failure), Addison's disease, acute dehydration, hepatic or renal impairment, extensive tissue breakdown (as with burns), congenital myotonia, hypernatremia, hypertension, toxemia of pregnancy, hypoparathyroidism, acute panceatitis, and rickets.
- Monitor renal function and serum electrolyte test results, as ordered because electrolyte imbalances can result in serious adverse effects.
- Be aware that high serum phosphate levels increase the risk of extra skeletal calcification.

PATIENT TEACHING
- Instruct patient to take potassium acid phosphate and sodium acid phosphate exactly as prescribed.
- Tell patient to take drug with a full glass of water.
- Caution patient to avoid eating excessive amounts of potassium- or sodium-rich foods and to limit salt intake.
- Advise patient to notify prescriber if abdominal pain, nausea, or vomiting occurs.
- Warn patient with kidney stones of the possibility of passing old stones when phosphate therapy is started.
- Instruct patient to avoid antacids that contain aluminum, calcium, or magnesium while taking phosphate drug because they may hinder phosphate absorption.

potassium citrate monohydrate and citric acid monohydrate
Cytra-K Crystals, Polycitra-L Crystals, Cytra-K, Polycitra-K

Class and Category
Chemical: Potassium derivative of base (potassium citrate), base (citric acid)
Therapeutic: Urinary alkalinizes (potassium citrate, citric acid)

Pregnancy category: NR

Indications and Dosages

▶ *To provide long-term maintenance of alkaline urine in the management of chronic metabolic acidosis caused by such conditions as chronic renal insufficiency or renal tubular acidosis*

POWDER FOR MIX (CYTRA-L CRYSTALS, POLYCITRA-K CRYSTALS)

Adults. 3,300 mg potassium citrate monohydrate and 1,002 mg citric acid monohydrate (number of packets varies depending on manufacturer) q.i.d. after meals and h.s.

SOLUTION, SYRUP (CYTRA-K, POLYCITRA-K)

Adults. 3,300 to 6,600 mg potassium citrate monohydrate and 1,002 to 2,004 mg citric acid monohydrate (15 to 30 ml) q.i.d. after meals and h.s.

Children. 1,100 to 3,300 mg potassium citrate monohydrate and 334 to 1,002 mg citric acid monohydrate (5 to 15 ml) q.i.d. after meals and h.s.

Mechanism of Action

Potassium citrate and citrate acid are oxidized in the body to form bicarbonate, a buffer, which increases urinary pH as it is readily excreted in urine.

Contraindications

Acute dehydration, adynamia episodica hereditaria, anuria, azotemia, heat cramps, hyperkalemia, oliguria, severe myocardial damage or renal impairment, untreated Addison's disease

Adverse Reactions

GI: Laxative effect, nausea, vomiting
Other: Hyperkalemia, metabolic alkalosis

Nursing Considerations

• Use with extreme caution in patients who need to limit intake of potassium.
• Monitor patient's serum electrolytes and acid-base status, as ordered, because hyperkalemia or metabolic alkalosis may occur, especially in patients with renal impairment.

PATIENT TEACHING

• Instruct patient to take potassium citrate and citric acid exactly as prescribed because excessive amounts can cause tetany or depress heart function.
• Instruct patient to mix drug exactly as described on packets and to protect packets from extreme heat or cold.

- Instruct patient prescribed solution form to store in a tight container and protect from extreme heat or cold.
- Tell patient to take drug after meals and at bedtime to minimize the GI effects of the drug.
- Reassure patient that the drug is pleasant tasting.

probenecid and colchicine
ColBenemid, Col-Probenecid, Proben-C

Class and Category
Chemical: Sulfonamide derivative (probenecid), colchicium alkaloid derivative (colchicine)
Therapeutic: Antigout
Pregnancy category: Not rated

Indications and Dosages
▶ *To treat chronic gouty arthritis in patients who experience frequent attacks*
TABLETS
Adults. *Initial:* 500 mg of probenecid and 0.5 mg of colchicine (1 tablet) daily for 1 wk; then increased to maintenance dosage. *Maintenance:* 1 tablet b.i.d.; if not effective or if 24-hr uric acid excretion isn't greater than 700 mg, dosage increased by 1 tablet daily q 4 wk, as needed and prescribed, up to a maximum of 4 tablets daily. If no acute gout attacks occur over next 6 mo and serum uric acid level is within normal limits, dosage decreased, as prescribed, by 1 tablet q 6 mo until lowest effective maintenance dose is reached.
DOSAGE ADJUSTMENT Dosage possibly increased for patients with mild renal dysfunction.

Mechanism of Action
Reduces the frequency of gout attacks through several mechanisms. Probenecid increases urinary excretion of uric acid and reduces serum uric acid level, which may prevent or resolve urate deposits, tophus formation, and joint changes. Eventually, the incidence of acute gout attacks may decrease.

Colchicine helps to stop inflammation, probably by disrupting microtubules in leukocytes. Microtubules contribute to cell structure and movement. When colchicine binds to tubulin (the protein from which microtubules are made), it causes microtubules to fall apart. This, in turn, disrupts cell function and prevents leukocytes from continuing to invade joints and produce inflammation.

Contraindications

Age less than 2 years; blood dyscrasias; hypersensitivity to colchicine, probenecid, or their components; renal calculi (urate)

Interactions

DRUGS

acyclovir: Decreased renal tubular secretion of acyclovir

allopurinol: Additive antihyperuricemic effects

aminosalicylate sodium, cephalosporins, ciprofloxacin, clofibrate, dapsone, ganciclovir, imipenem, methotrexate, nitrofurantoin, norfloxacin, penicillins: Increased and possibly prolonged blood levels of these drugs and increased risk of toxicity

antineoplastics (rapidly cytolytic): Possibly uric acid nephropathy

cyclosporine: Possibly impaired renal function and risk of nephrotoxicity

diazoxide, mecamylamine, pyrazinamide: Increased risk of hyperuricemia; decreased probenecid effectiveness

dyphylline: Increased half-life of dyphylline

erythromycin: Impaired metabolism of colchicine

furosemide: Increased blood furosemide level

heparin: Increased and prolonged anticoagulant effect

indomethacin, ketoprofen, other NSAIDs: Possibly increased adverse effects

lorazepam, oxazepam, temazepam: Increased effects of these drugs and, possibly, excessive sedation

riboflavin: Decreased GI absorption of riboflavin

rifampin, sulfonamides: Increased blood levels of these drugs and, possibly, toxicity

salicylates: Decreased uricosuric effects of probenecid and colchicine

sodium benzoate and sodium phenylacetate: Decreased renal elimination of these drugs

sulfonylureas: Increased sulfonylurea half-life

thiopental: Prolonged thiopental effect

vitamin B_{12} (cyanocobalamin): Reversible decrease in blood vitamin B_{12} level

zidovudine: Increased risk of zidovudine toxicity

ACTIVITIES

alcohol use: Increased risk of hyperuricemia, decreased antigout effects

Adverse Reactions

CNS: Dizziness, fever, headache, peripheral neuritis

EENT: Sore gums

GI: Abdominal pain, anorexia, diarrhea, hepatic necrosis, nausea, vomiting

GU: Hematuria, nephropathy (urate), nephrotic syndrome, renal calculi (urate), renal colic, urinary frequency

HEME: Agranulocytosis, anemia, aplastic anemia, hemolytic anemia, leukopenia

MS: Back or rib pain, gout attacks, muscle weakness

SKIN: Alopecia, dermatitis, flushing, purpura

Other: Anaphylaxis

Nursing Considerations

- Be aware that probenecid and colchicine therapy shouldn't be started until acute gout attack has subsided. If acute gout attack begins during therapy, however, expect to continue therapy.
- Use drug cautiously in patients with peptic ulcer disease.
- Expect to give sodium bicarbonate (3 to 7.5 g daily) or potassium citrate (7.5 g daily), as prescribed, to keep urine alkaline and prevent renal calculus formation.
- Monitor CBC, serum uric acid level, and liver and renal function test results during therapy.
- Closely monitor patients receiving intermittent therapy because they're more prone to allergic reactions.
- Monitor blood glucose level often in diabetic patient who takes a sulfonylurea because of the risk of drug interactions.

PATIENT TEACHING

- Advise patient to take probenecid and colchicine with meals to minimize stomach upset.
- Encourage increased fluid intake (up to 3 liters daily, if not contraindicated) to help prevent renal calculus formation.
- Instruct patient to notify prescriber immediately if she has a gouty arthritis flare-up (joint pain, swelling, and redness) or signs of kidney stones, such as flank pain and blood in urine.
- Caution patient against taking salicylates during therapy. Instead, urge her to use acetaminophen for mild pain or fever.

sodium citrate dihydrate and citric acid monohydrate

Bicitra, Cytra-2, Oracit, Shohl's Solution

Class and Category

Chemical: Salt derivative of base (sodium citrate), base (citric acid)

Therapeutic: Urinary alkalinizes (sodium citrate, citric acid)
Pregnancy category: NR

Indications and Dosages

▶ *To provide long-term maintenance of alkaline urine in the management of chronic metabolic acidosis associated with conditions such as chronic renal insufficiency or renal tubular acidosis*

SOLUTION (ORACIT)

Adults. 980 to 2,940 mg sodium citrate dihydrate and 1,280 to 3,840 mg citric acid monohydrate (10 to 30 ml) q.i.d. after meals and h.s.

Children. 490 to 1,470 mg sodium citrate dihydrate and 640 to 1,920 mg citric acid monohydrate (5 to 15 ml) q.i.d. after meals and h.s.

SOLUTION (BICITRA, CYTRA-2, SHOHL'S SOLUTION)

Adults. 1,000 to 3,000 mg sodium citrate dihydrate and 668 to 2,004 mg citric acid monohydrate (10 to 30 ml) q.i.d. after meals and h.s.

Children. 500 to 1,500 mg sodium citrate dihydrate and 334 to 1,002 mg citric acid monohydrate (5 to 15 ml) q.i.d. after meals and h.s.

Mechanism of Action

Sodium citrate dihydrate and citrate acid monohydrate are oxidized in the body to form bicarbonate, a buffer, which increases urinary pH as it is readily excreted in urine.

Contraindications

Severe renal impairment, sodium-restricted diet

Adverse Reactions

GI: Laxative effect, nausea, vomiting
Other: Hypernatremia, metabolic alkalosis

Nursing Considerations

- Use with extreme caution in patients with heart failure, hypertension, renal dysfunction, peripheral or pulmonary edema, or toxemia of pregnancy.
- Use with caution in patients with low urine output.
- Monitor patient's serum electrolytes and acid-base status, as ordered, because hypernatremia or metabolic alkalosis may occur, especially in patients with renal impairment.

PATIENT TEACHING
- Instruct patient to take drug exactly as prescribed because excessive amounts can cause tetany or depress heart function.
- Tell patient to take drug after meals and at bedtime to minimize the GI effects of the drug.
- Reassure patient that the drug is pleasant tasting.
- Instruct patient to store drug solution in a tight container and protect from extreme heat or cold.

trimethoprim, sulfamethoxazole, and phenazopyridine hydrochoride
Zotrim

Class and Category
Chemical: Dihydrofolic acid analogue (trimethoprim), sulfonamide derivative (sulfamethoxazole, azo dye (phenazopyridine)
Therapeutic: Antibiotics (trimethoprim, sulfamethoxazole), urinary analgesic (phenazopyridine)
Pregnancy category: C

Indications and Dosages
▶ *To treat urinary tract infections caused by susceptible strains of* Escherichia coli, Enterobacer *or* Klebsiella *species,* Morganella morganii, Proteus mirabilis, *and* Proteus vulgaris
DOUBLE-STRENGTH TABLET (TRIMETHOPRIM AND SULFAMETHOXAZOLE)
Adults. 160 mg trimethoprim and 800 mg sulfamethoxazole (1 tablet) q 12 hr for 10 days.
DOSAGE ADJUSTMENT For patients with creatinine clearance between 15 ml/min and 30 ml/min, dosage decreased by half.
▶ *To relieve pain, burning, urgency, frequency, and other discomforts caused by infection-related irritation of the lower urinary tract mucosa*
TABLET (PHENAZOPYRIDINE)
Adults. 200 mg phenazopyridine (1 tablet) t.i.d. after meals for no longer than 2 days.

Contraindications
Age less than 2 months; breastfeeding; hypersensitivity to trimethoprim, sulfamethoxazole, other sulfonamides, phenazopyridine, or their components; megaloblastic anemia caused by folate deficiency; renal insufficiency (creatinine clearance less than 15 ml/min); term pregnancy

Mechanism of Action

Trimethoprim and sulfamethoxazole block two consecutive steps in the formation of essential nucleic acids and proteins in susceptible organisms. Sulfamethoxazole inhibits synthesis of dihydrofolic acid (a nucleic acid) by completing with para-aminobenzoic acid. Trimethoprim inhibits the action of the enzyme dihydro-folate reductase, thus blocking production of tetrahydrofolic acid. These actions result in bacterial cell death.

Phenazopyridine exerts a topical or local anesthetic effect on the mucosa of the urinary tract as drug is excreted in urine to relieve discomfort associated with urinary tract infection.

Interactions

DRUGS

trimethoprim and sulfamethoxazole components

ACE inhibitors: Possibly increased risk of hyperkalemia in elderly patients

cyclosporine: Decreased blood level and therapeutic effectiveness of cyclosporine, increased risk of nephrotoxicity

digoxin: Possibly increased blood digoxin level resulting in increased risk of digoxin toxicity

diuretics: Increased risk of thrombocytopenic purpura in elderly patients

indomethacin: Possibly increased blood trimethoprim and sulfamethoxazole levels

methotrexate: Increased blood methotrexate level and risk of methotrexate toxicity

phenytoin: Possibly decreased hepatic clearance and prolonged half-life of phenytoin

pyrimethamine (dosage greater than 25 mg/wk): Increased risk of megaloblastic anemia

sulfonylureas: Possibly increased hypoglycemic effects of sulfonylureas

tricyclic antidepressants: Decreased effectiveness of tricyclic antidepressant

warfarin: Increased anticoagulant effects

Adverse Reactions

CNS: Anxiety, aseptic meningitis ataxia, chills, depression, fatigue, hallucinations, headache, insomnia, seizures, vertigo

EENT: Glossitis, stomatitis

GI: Abdominal pain, anorexia, diarrhea, hepatitis, indigestion, nausea, pancreatitis, pseudomembranous enterocolitis, vomiting

GU: Crystalluria, reddish orange urine, renal failure, toxic nephrosis
HEME: Agranulocytosis, eosinophilia, hemolytic anemia, leukopenia, methemoglobinemia, neutropenia, thrombocytopenia
RESP: Cough, dyspnea
SKIN: Dermatitis, erythema, photosensitivity, pruritus, rash, Stevens-Johnson syndrome, toxic epidermal necrolysis, urticaria
Other: Anaphylaxis, discoloration of body fluids

Nursing Considerations
• Be aware that blister card contains 20 double-strength tri-methoprim and sulfamethoxazole tablets and 6 phenazopyridine tablets.
• Expect to obtain culture and sensitivity test results before starting antibiotic therapy with trimethroprin and sulfamethoxazole.
• Assess patient for evidence of blood dyscrasia, including bleeding, ecchymosis, and joint pain. This is especially important in elderly patients who also take a thiazide diuretic during the 10 days of trimethroprin and sulfamethoxazole therapy.
• Notify prescriber if yellowish skin or sclera develop in patient during 2-day therapy with phenazopyridine because this may indicate drug accumulation from impaired renal excretion. Expect prescriber to discontinue drug.

PATIENT TEACHING
• If GI distress develops, advise patient to take drug with meals.
• Instruct patient not to take phenazopyridine in package for longer than 2 days and to notify prescriber if symptoms persist beyond that time.
• Warn patient that during use of phenazopyridine, his urine will turn orange to red and other body fluids such as tears may become discolored. Explain that this effect is harmless and will resolve when drug is stopped.
• Advise patient not to wear contact lenses while using phenazopyridine because they may become stained from discoloration of tears.
• Instruct patient to notify prescriber immediately if rash, severe diarrhea, or other serious adverse reactions occur.
• To minimize photosensitivity, advise patient to avoid direct sunlight and to use sunscreen.

Respiratory Drugs

acrivastine and pseudoephedrine sulfate

Semprex-D

Class and Category

Chemical: Alkylamine antihistamine (acrivastine), sympatho-mimetic amine (pseudoephedrine)

Therapeutic: Antihistaminic (acrivastine), decongestant (pseudoephedrine)

Pregnancy category: B

Indications and Dosages

▶ *To relieve symptoms of seasonal allergic rhinitis*

CAPSULES

Adults and children age 12 and over. 8 mg acrivastine and 60 mg pseudoephedrine (1 capsule) q 4 to 6 hr. *Maximum:* 8 mg acrivastine and 60 mg pseudoephedrine (1 capsule) q 4 to 6 hr daily.

Mechanism of Action

Acrivastine competes with histamine for histamine H_1 receptor sites on effector cells and antagonizes the vasodilator effect of endogenously released histamine. This prevents vascular engorgement, mucosal edema, sneezing, and profuse watery secretion and irritation that normally result from histamine action on peripheral afferent nerve terminals.

Pseudoephedrine acts on alpha$_1$-adrenergic receptors in the mucosa of the respiratory tract to produce vasoconstriction. This process shrinks swollen nasal mucous membranes; reduces tissue hyperemia, edema, and nasal congestion; and increases nasal airway patency. It also may increase drainage of sinus secretions and open obstructed eustachian ostia.

Contraindications

Hypersensitivity or idiosyncractic reactions to acrivastine, other alkylamine antihistamines, pseudoephedrine, other sympathomimetic amines, or their components; severe coronary artery disease or hypertension; use within 14 days of MAO inhibitor therapy

Interactions

DRUGS

acrivastine component

barbiturates, CNS depressants, tricyclic antidepressants: Additive effects

pseudoephedrine component

antacids: Increased absorption of pseudoephedrine

antihypertensives, diuretics: Possibly decreased antihypertensive effects

beta blockers: Decreased therapeutic effects of both drugs

citrates: Possibly inhibited urinary excretion and prolonged duration of action of pseudoephedrine

CNS stimulants, sympathomimetics: Possibly increased additive CNS stimulation to excessive levels

cocaine (mucosal-local): Possibly increased cardiovascular effects of either drug and CNS stimulation

digoxin, levodopa: Increased risk of cardiac arrhythmias

hydrocarbon inhalation anesthetics: Increased risk of serious arrhythmias

kaolin: Decreased pseudoephedrine absorption

MAO inhibitors: Increased and prolonged cardiac stimulation, increased vasopressor effect, increased risk of severe cardiovascular and cerebrovascular effects, hyperpyrexia, and vomiting

nitrates: Reduced antianginal effects of nitrates

rauwolfia alkaloids: Possibly inhibited pseudoephedrine action

thyroid hormones: Increased cardiovascular effects of both drugs

ACTIVITIES

acrivastine component

alcohol use: Additive effects

Adverse Reactions

CNS: Asthenia, dizziness, headache, insomnia, light-headedness, nervousness, restlessness, somnolence, trembling, weakness

CV: Palpitations, tachycardia

EENT: Dry mouth, pharyngitis

ENDO: Dysmenorrhea

GI: Dyspepsia, nausea, vomiting

GU: Dysuria
RESP: Bronchospasm, increased cough
SKIN: Diaphoresis, erythema multiforme, pallor
Other: Anaphylaxis, angioedema

Nursing Considerations

- Use cautiously in patients with diabetes, hypertension, increased intraocular pressure, ischemic heart disease, prostatic hypertrophy, stenosing peptic ulcer, or pyloroduodenal obstruction because of the vasoconstrictive action of pseudoephedrine.
- Monitor elderly patients closely for dizziness, sedation, confusion, hallucinations, convulsions, CNS depression, and hypotension because these patients are more likely to develop such adverse effects.
- Monitor renal function, as ordered, because pseudoephedrine is substantially excreted by the kidneys. Be aware that drug isn't recommended for patients with impaired renal function.
- Evaluate effectiveness of acrivastine and pseudoephedrine in relieving symptoms of seasonal allergic rhinitis, such as sneezing, rhinorrhea, pruritus, lacrimation, and nasal congestion.
- Be aware that patient shouldn't undergo intradermal allergen tests within 4 days of receiving drug because the results may be altered.

PATIENT TEACHING

- Urge patient to avoid alcohol, other antidepressants, and OTC medications containing other antihistamines or sympathomimetics while taking acrivastine and pseudoephedrine.
- Instruct patient to avoid potentially hazardous activities until drug's CNS effects are known.
- Suggest that patient relieve dry mouth with frequent rinsing and use of sugarless gum or hard candy.

azatadine maleate and pseudoephedrine sulfate

Trinalin Repetabs

Class and Category

Chemical: Piperidine derivative (azatadine), sympathomimetic amine (pseudoephedrine)
Therapeutic: Antihistamine (azatadine), decongestant (pseudoephedrine)
Pregnancy category: NR

Indications and Dosages

▶ *To relieve symptoms of upper respiratory mucosal congestion in perennial and allergic rhinitis; to relieve nasal congestion and eustachian tube congestion*

E.R. TABLETS

Adults. 1 mg azatadine and 120 mg pseudoephedrine (1 tablet) b.i.d.

Mechanism of Action

Azatadine competes with histamine for histamine H_1 receptor sites on effector cells and antagonizes the vasodilator effect of endogenously released histamine. This prevents vascular engorgement, mucosal edema and profuse watery secretion, irritation, and sneezing that normally result from histamine action on peripheral afferent nerve terminals in nasal passages.

Pseudoephedrine acts on alpha$_1$-adrenergic receptors in the mucosa of the respiratory tract to produce vasoconstriction. This process shrinks swollen nasal mucous membranes; reduces tissue hyperemia, edema, and nasal congestion; and increases nasal airway patency. It also may increase drainage of sinus secretions and open obstructed eustachian ostia.

Contraindications

Hypersensitivity or idiosyncractic reactions to azatadine, pseudoephedrine or their components; hyperthyroidism; narrow-angle glaucoma; severe coronary artery disease or hypertension; urine retention; use within 14 days of MAO inhibitor therapy

Interactions

DRUGS

azatadine component

barbiturates, CNS depressants, tricyclic antidepressants: Additive effects

pseudoephedrine component

antacids: Increased pseudoephedrine absoprtion

antihypertensives, diuretics: Possibly decreased antihypertensive effects

beta blockers: Decreased therapeutic effects of both drugs

citrates: Possibly inhibited urinary excretion and prolonged duration of pseudoephedrine action

CNS stimulants, sympathomimetics: Possibly increased additive CNS stimulation to excessive levels

cocaine (mucosal-local): Possibly increased cardiovascular effects of either drug and CNS stimulation

digoxin, levodopa: Increased risk of cardiac arrhythmias

hydrocarbon inhalation anesthetics: Increased risk of serious arrhythmias

kaolin: Decreased pseudoephedrine absorption

MAO inhibitors: Increased and prolonged cardiac stimulation, increased vasopressor effect, increased risk of severe cardiovascular and cerebrovascular effects, hyperpyrexia, and vomiting

nitrates: Reduced antianginal effects of nitrates

rauwolfia alkaloids: Possibly inhibited action of pseudoephedrine

thyroid hormones: Increased cardiovascular effects of both drugs

ACTIVITIES

azatadine component

alcohol use: Additive effects

Adverse Reactions

CNS: Anxiety, CNS stimulation or depression, confusion, disturbed coordination, dizziness, drowsiness, fear, hallucinations, headache, insomnia, light-headedness, mood shifts, nervousness, restlessness, sedation, seizures, sleepiness, tenseness, trembling, weakness

CV: Arrhythmias, hypertension, hypotension, palpitations, tachycardia

EENT: Dry mouth, nose, or throat

GI: Abdominal pain, epigastric distress, nausea, vomiting

GU: Dysuria, urine retention

HEME: Hemolytic anemia, pancytopenia, thrombocytopenia

RESP: Dyspnea, thickened bronchial secretions

SKIN: Diaphoresis, pallor, rash

Nursing Considerations

- Use cautiously in patients with bladder neck obstruction, cardiovascular disease, diabetes, increased intraocular pressure, pyloroduodenal obstruction, prostatic hypertrophy, or stenosing peptic ulcer because of the vasoconstrictive action of pseudoephedrine. Also use cautiously in patients with a history of bronchial asthma because of the atropine-like action of azatadine.
- Monitor elderly patients for dizziness, sedation, confusion, hallucinations, CNS depression, hypotension, and seizures because these patients are more likely to develop such adverse effects.
- Monitor renal function, as ordered, because pseudoephedrine is substantially excreted by the kidneys.
- Regularly evaluate effectiveness of azatadine and pseudoephedrine in relieving upper respiratory congestion.

- Be aware that patient shouldn't undergo intradermal allergen tests within 4 days of receiving drug because the results may be altered.

PATIENT TEACHING

- Urge patient to avoid alcohol, other antidepressants and OTC medications containing other antihistamines or sympathomimetics while taking azatadine and pseudoepherine.
- Instruct patient to avoid potentially hazardous activities until drug's CNS effects are known.
- Suggest that patient relieve dry mouth with frequent rinsing and use of sugarless gum or hard candy.

brompheniramine maleate and pseudoephedrine hydrochloride
AccuHist Pediatric Drops, Andehist, Brofed, Bromadrine TR, Bromfed, Bromfed-PD, Bromfenex, Bromfenex PD, Dimetapp Cold & Allergy, Histex SR, Iofed, Iofed PD, Lodrane, Lodrane 12 D, Lodrane LD, Respahist, Rondec, Rondec Chewables, Touro, UTRAbrom, UTRAbrom PD

dexbrompheniramine maleate and pseudoephedrine sulfate
Dexaphen SA, Disobrom

Class and Category
Chemical: Propylamine derivative (brompheniramine, dexbrompheniramine), sympathomimetic amine (pseudoephedrine)
Therapeutic: Antihistamines (brompheniramine, dexbrompheniramine), decongestant (pseudoephedrine)
Pregnancy category: B

Indications and Dosages
▶ *To relieve persistent runny nose, sneezing, and nasal congestion caused by upper respiratory infections, sinus inflammation, or hay fever*
E.R. CAPSULES
Adults and children age 12 and over. 6 or 12 mg brompheniramine and 60 or 120 mg pseudoephedrine (1 to 2 capsules depending on product used) q 12 hr.
Children ages 6 to 12. 6 mg brompheniramine and 60 mg pseudoephedrine (1 capsule) q 12 hr.

TABLETS, CHEWABLE TABLETS
Adults and children age 12 and over. 4 mg brompheniramine and 60 mg pseudoephedrine (1 tablet) q 4 hr.
Children ages 6 to 12. 2 mg brompheniramine and 30 mg pseudoephedrine (½ tablet) q 4 hr.
E.R. TABLETS
Adults. 6 to 12 mg brompheniramine or dexbrompheniramine and 45 to 120 mg pseudoephedrine (1 or 2 tablets depending on product used) q 12 hr.
ORAL SOLUTION
Adults and children age 12 and over. 8 mg brompheniramine and 60 mg pseudoephedrine (10 ml) q 8 hr. Or, 4 mg brompheniramine and 60 mg pseudoephedrine (5 ml) q 4 to 6 hr.
Children ages 6 to 12. 4 mg brompheniramine and 30 mg pseudoephedrine (5 ml) q 8 hr.
Children ages 2 to 6. 2 mg bromopheniramine and 15 mg pseudoephedrine (2.5 ml) q 8 hr.
SYRUP
Adults and children age 12 and over. 4 mg brompheniramine and 60 mg pseudoephedrine (10 ml) q 4 to 6 hr.
Children ages 6 to 12. 2 mg brompheniramine and 30 mg pseudoephedrine (5 ml) q 4 to 6 hr.
DROPS
Children ages 12 months to 24 months. 1 mg brompheniramine and 15 mg pseudoephedrine (1 ml) q.i.d.
Children ages 6 to 12 months. 0.75 mg brompheniramine and 11.25 mg pseudoephedrine (0.75 ml) q.i.d.
Infants ages 3 months to 6 months. 0.5 mg brompheniramine and 7.5 mg pseudoephedrine (0.5 ml) q.i.d.
Infants ages 1 month to 3 months. 0.25 mg brompheniramine and 3.75 mg pseudoephedrine (0.25 ml) q.i.d.

Mechanism of Action
Brompheniramine and dexbrompheniramine compete with histamine for H_1 receptor sites, thereby antagonizing many histamine effects and reducing allergy signs and symptoms.

Pseudoephedrine acts on alpha$_1$-adrenergic receptors in the mucosa of the respiratory tract to produce vasoconstriction. This process shrinks swollen nasal mucous membranes; reduces tissue hyperemia, edema, and nasal congestion; and increases nasal airway patency. It also may increase drainage of sinus secretions and open obstructed eustachian ostia.

Contraindications

Breastfeeding; hypersensitivity or idiosyncractic reactions to bromseniramine, dexbrompheniramine, pseudoephedrine, or their components; hyperthyroidism; narrow-angle glaucoma; severe coronary artery disease or hypertension; urine retention; use within 14 days of MAO inhibitor therapy

Interactions

DRUGS

bromopheniramine, dexbrompheniramine, and pseudo-ephedrine

MAO inhibitors: Increased and prolonged cardiac stimulation, increased vasopressor effect, increased risk of severe cardiovascular and cerebrovascular effects, hyperpyrexia, and vomiting

bromopheniramine and dexbrompheniramine components

anticholinergics: Additive anticholinergic effects
CNS depressants: Additive CNS effects

pseudoephedrine component

antacids: Increased pseudoephedrine absorption
antihypertensives, diuretics: Possibly decreased antihypertensive effects
beta blockers: Decreased therapeutic effects of both drugs
citrates: Possibly inhibited urinary excretion and prolonged duration of pseudoephedrine action
CNS stimulants, sympathomimetics: Possibly increased additive CNS stimulation to excessive levels
cocaine (mucosal-local): Possibly increased cardiovascular effects of either drug and CNS stimulation
digoxin, levodopa: Increased risk of cardiac arrhythmias
hydrocarbon inhalation anesthetics: Increased risk of serious arrhythmias
kaolin: Decreased pseudoephedrine absorption
nitrates: Reduced antianginal effects of nitrates
rauwolfia alkaloids: Possibly inhibited pseudoephedrine action
thyroid hormones: Increased cardiovascular effects of both drugs

ACTIVITIES

bromopheniramine and dexbrompheniramine components

alcohol use: Additive CNS effects

Adverse Reactions

CNS: Anxiety, chills, confusion, coordination disturbance, dizziness, drowsiness, excitation (children), fatigue, fear, hallucinations, headache, hysteria, insomnia, irritability, light-headedness, nervousness, numbness, restlessness, sedation, seizures, tenseness, trembling, vertigo, weakness

CV: Arrhythmias, chest tightness, hypotension, palpitations, tachycardia

EENT: Blurred or double vision; dry mouth, nose, and throat; nasal congestion; tinnitus

ENDO: Early menstruation

GI: Anorexia, constipation, diarrhea, nausea, stomach upset or pain, vomiting

GU: Dysuria, frequent urination, urinary hesitancy, urine retention

HEME: Anemia, unusual bleeding or bruising

RESP: Dyspnea, increased chest congestion, wheezing

SKIN: Diaphoresis, pallor, photosensitivity, rash, urticaria

Other: Anaphylaxis

Nursing Considerations

- Use cautiously in patients with asthma, cardiovascular disease, diabetes, emphysema or other chronic lung disease, hypertension, peptic ulcer, hyperthyroidism, narrow-angle glaucoma, or prostatic hypertrophy.
- Monitor children for excitation and elderly patients for dizziness, sedation, and hypotension; such patients may have an increased risk for these effects.
- Monitor renal function, as ordered, because pseudoephedrine is substantially excreted by the kidneys.
- Regularly evaluate effectiveness of brompheniramine or dexbrompheniramine and pseudoephedrine in reducing upper respiratory symptoms.
- Be aware that patient shouldn't undergo intradermal allergen tests within 72 hours of receiving drug because results may be altered.

PATIENT TEACHING

- Instruct patient to use a calibrated measuring device for syrup or oral solution form of brompheniramine and pseudoephedrine to ensure accurate dose.
- Urge patient to avoid alcohol and other antidepressants while taking brompheniramine or dexbrompheniramine and pseudoephedrine.
- Instruct patient to avoid potentially hazardous activities until drug's CNS effects are known.
- Suggest that patient relieve dry mouth with frequent rinsing and use of sugarless gum or hard candy.

• Tell patient to take last dose of the day a few hours before bedtime if brompheniramine or dexbrompheniramine and pseudoephedrine makes him nervous or restless.

carbetapentane tannate and chlorpheniramine tannate

Tannic-12, Trionate, Tussi-12, Tussi-12 S, Tussizone-12 RF

Class and Category

Chemical: Cyclopentane carbolic ester (carbetapentane), propylamine derivative (chlorpheniramine)

Therapeutic: Antitussive (carbetapentane) and antihistaminic (chlorpheniramine)

Pregnancy category: C

Indications and Dosages

▶ *To relieve cough in such respiratory tract conditions as the common cold, bronchial asthma, and acute and chronic bronchitis*

TABLETS

Adults. 60 or 120 mg carbetapentane and 5 or 10 mg chlorpheniramine (1 or 2 tablets) q 12 hr.

SUSPENSION

Adults and children age 6 and over. 30 or 60 mg carbetapentante and 4 or 8 mg chlorpheniramine (5 or 10 ml) q 12 hr.

Children ages 2 to 6. 15 or 30 mg carbetapentante and 2 or 4 mg chlorpheniramine (2.5 or 5 ml) q 12 hr.

Mechanism of Action

Carbetapentane has atropine-like and local anesthetic actions that suppresses the cough reflex through selective depression of the medullary cough center in the brain.

Chlorpheniramine competes with histamine for H_1 receptor sites, thereby antagonizing many histamine effects and reducing allergy effects.

Contraindications

Breastfeeding; hypersensitivity to carbetapentane, chlorpheniramine, or their components; use of MAO inhibitors within 14 days

Interactions

DRUGS

carbetapentane and chlorpheniramine (suspension form)

tartrazine (FD & C Yellow No. 5): Possibly induced allergic-type reactions in susceptible people
chlorpheniramine component
CNS depressants: Additive CNS effects
MAO inhibitors: Possibly prolonged and intensified anticholinergic effects of chlorpheniramine
phenytoin: Possibly increased serum phenytoin levels and toxicity
ACTIVITIES
chlorpheniramine component
alcohol use: Additive CNS effects

Adverse Reactions

CNS: Confusion, dizziness, drowsiness, excitation (children), hallucinations, headache, insomnia, restlessness, sedation
CV: Bradycardia, hypotension, palpitations, tachycardia
EENT: Blurred vision, dry mouth or eyes
GI: Abdominal pain, constipation, nausea, vomiting
GU: Urinary hesitancy, urine retention
HEME: Agranulocytosis, aplastic anemia, thrombocytopenia

Nursing Considerations

- Use cautiously in patients with cardiovascular disease, hypertension, hyperthyroidism, narrow-angle glaucoma, or prostatic hypertrophy.
- Monitor children for excitation and elderly patients for dizziness, sedation, and hypotension; such patients may have an increased risk for these effects.
- Monitor patient's CBC and platelet count, as ordered. Rarely, drug may cause serious adverse reactions, such as agranulocytosis, aplastic anemia, and thrombocytopenia.
- Regularly evaluate effectiveness of carbetapentane and chlorpheniramine in reducing cough and allergy symptoms.
- Be aware that patient shouldn't have intradermal allergen tests within 72 hours of receiving drug because results may be altered.

PATIENT TEACHING

- Instruct patient to use a calibrated measuring device for suspension form of carbetapentane and chlorpheniramine to ensure accurate dose.
- Urge patient to avoid alcohol and other antidepressants while taking carbetapentane and chlorpheniramine.
- Instruct patient to avoid potentially hazardous activities until drug's CNS effects are known.
- Suggest that patient relieve dry mouth with frequent rinsing and use of sugarless gum or hard candy.

carbetapentane tannate, chlorpheniramine tannate, ephedrine tannate, and phenylephrine tannate

Quad Tann, Renatamine Pediatric Suspension, Rynatuss, Rynatuss Pediatric Suspension

Class and Category

Chemical: Cyclopentane carbolic ester (carbetapentane), propylamine derivative (chlorpheniramine), sympathomimetic amines (ephedrine, phenylephrine)

Therapeutic: Antitussive (carbetapentane), antihistaminic (chlorpeniramine), bronchodilator (ephedrine), decongestant (phenylephrine)

Pregnancy category: C

Indications and Dosages

▶ *To relieve cough in such respiratory tract conditions as the common cold, bronchial asthma, and acute and chronic bronchitis*

TABLETS

Adults. 60 or 120 mg carbetapentane, 5 or 10 mg chlorpheniramine, 10 or 20 mg ephedrine, and 10 or 20 mg phenylephrine (1 or 2 tablets) q 12 hr.

SUSPENSION

Adults and children age 6 and over. 30 or 60 mg carbetapentante, 4 or 8 mg chlorpheniramine, 5 or 10 mg ephedrine, and 5 or 10 mg phenylephrine (5 or 10 ml) q 12 hr.

Children ages 2 to 6. 15 or 30 mg carbetapentante, 2 or 4 mg chlorpheniramine, 2.5 or 5 mg ephedrine and 2.5 or 5 mg phenylephrine (2.5 or 5 ml) q 12 hr.

Mechanism of Action

Carbetapentane has atropine-like and local anesthetic actions that suppress the cough reflex in the medullary cough center in the brain.

Chlorpheniramine competes with histamine for H_1 receptor sites, thereby antagonizing many histamine effects and reducing allergy effects.

Ephedrine stimulates beta-adrenergic receptors in the lungs, relaxing bronchial smooth muscle and relieving bronchospasm. It also stimulates alpha-adrenergic receptors in nasal passages to produce vasoconstriction and a drying effect on nasal mucous membranes.

Phenylephrine stimulates alpha-adrenergic receptors and inhibits the intracellular enzyme adenyl cyclase, which then inhibits production of cAMP. Inhibition of cAMP causes arterial and venous constriction in nasal passages, which decreases blood flow and mucosal edema caused by allergic response.

Contraindications

Breastfeeding; hypersensitivity to carbetapentane, chlorpheniramine, ephedrine, or phenylephrine or their components; use of MAO inhibitors within 14 days

Interactions

DRUGS

carbetapentane, chlorpheniramine, ephedrine, and phenylephrine (suspension form)
tartrazine (FD & C Yellow No. 5): Possibly induced allergic-type reactions in susceptible persons
chlorpheniramine, ephedrine, and phenylephrine components
MAO inhibitors: Possibly prolonged and intensified anticholinergic effects
phenytoin: Possibly increased serum phenytoin levels and toxicity
chlorpheniramine and phenylephrine components
CNS depressants: Additive CNS effects
ephedrine and phenylephrine components
alpha blockers, haloperidol, loxapine, phenothiazines, thioxanthenes: Possibly decreased vasoconstrictor effect of phenylephrine
beta blockers: Decreased therapeutic effects of each drug
ergot alkaloids: Possibly rupture of cerebral blood vessel, increased vasopressor effect, peripheral vascular ischemia, and gangrene (with ergotamine)
hydrocarbon inhalation anesthetics: Increased risk of serious arrhythmias
thyroid hormones: Increased cardiovascular effects of each drug
ephedrine component
guanadrel, guanethidine: Possibly decreased hypotensive effects of these agents
guanethidine, methyldopa, reserpine: Reduced pressor response of ephedrine
theophylline: Possibly enhanced toxicity, especially increased nausea, nervousness, and insomnia
tricyclic antidepressants: Possibly increased pressor response
urinary acidifers: May decrease half-life of ephedrine, which may lead to decreased effects
urinary alkalizers: May increase ephadrine half-life and effects
phenylephrine component
antihypertenisves, diuretics: Possibly decreased antihypertensive effects
atropine: Possibly enhanced vasopressor effect of phenylephrine

bretylium: Possibly potentiated vaopressor effect and arrhythmias
doxapram: Increased vasopressor effect of both drugs
guanadrel, guanethidine: Increased vasopressor effect of phenylephrine; increased risk of severe hypertension and arrhythmias
mecamylamine, methyldopa: Decreased hypotensive effects of these drugs; increased vasopressor effect of phenylephrine
nitrates: Possibly decreased vasopressor effect of phenylephrine and decreased antianginal effect of nitrates
oxytocin: Possibly severe, persistent hypertension
phenoxybenzamine: Decreased vasoconstrictor effect of phenylephrine; possibly hypotension and tachycardia
theophylline: Possibly enhanced toxicity (including cardiac toxicity)
ACTIVITIES
chlorpheniramine and phenylephrine components
alcohol use: Additive CNS effects

Adverse Reactions

CNS: Confusion, dizziness, drowsiness, excitation (children), headache, impaired cognition, insomnia, nervousness, paresthesia, restlessness, sedation, tremor, weakness
CV: Angina, bradycardia, hypertension, hypotension, palpitations, peripheral vasoconstriction that may lead to necrosis or gangrene, tachycardia, ventricular arrhythmias
EENT: Blurred vision, dry eyes or mouth
GI: Abdominal pain, constipation, nausea, vomiting
GU: Urinary hesitancy, urine retention
HEME: Agranulocytosis, aplastic anemia, thrombocytopenia
RESP: Dyspnea

Nursing Considerations

• Use cautiously in patients with cardiovascular disease, diabetes, hypertension, hyperthyroidism, narrow-angle glaucoma, or prostatic hypertrophy.
• Monitor children for excitation and elderly patients for dizziness, sedation, and hypotension; such patients may have an increased risk for these effects.
• Monitor patient's CBC and platelet counts, as ordered, because, although rare, drug may cause serious hematologic adverse reactions such as agranulocytosis, aplastic anemia, and thrombocytopenia.
• Regularly evaluate effectiveness of carbetapentane, chlorpheniramine, ephedrine, and phenylephrine in reducing cough and allergy symptoms.

- Be aware that patient shouldn't have intradermal allergen tests within 72 hours of receiving drug because results may be altered.

PATIENT TEACHING
- Instruct patient to use a calibrated measuring device for suspension form of carbetapentane, chlorpheniramine, ephedrine, and phenylephrine to ensure accurate dose.
- Urge patient to avoid alcohol and other antidepressants while taking drug.
- Instruct patient to avoid potentially hazardous activities until drug's CNS effects are known.
- Suggest that patient relieve dry mouth with frequent rinsing and use of sugarless gum or hard candy.

carbetapentane citrate, phenylephrine hydrochloride, and guaifenesin
Levall

Class and Category
Chemical: Cyclopentane carbolic ester (carbetapentane), sympathomimetic amine (phenylephrine), glyceryl guaiacolate (guaifenesin)
Therapeutic: Antitussive (carbetapentane), decongestant (phenylephrine), expectorant (guaifenesin)
Pregnancy category: C

Indications and Dosages
▶ *To provide temporary relief of nonproductive cough and nasal congestion from the common cold, bronchitis, or sinusitis*
ORAL SOLUTION
Adults. 20 mg carbetapentane, 15 mg phenylephrine, and 100 mg guaifenesin (5 ml) q 4 to 6 hr. *Maximum:* 20 ml daily.

Mechanism of Action
Carbetapentane has atropine-like and local anesthetic actions, which suppress the cough reflex in the medullary, cough center in the brain.

Phenylephrine stimulates alpha-adrenergic receptors and inhibits the intracellular enzyme adenyl cyclase, which then inhibits production of cAMP. Inhibition of cAMP causes arterial and venous constriction in nasal passages, which decreases blood flow and mucosal edema caused by allergic response.

Guaifenesin increases fluid and mucus removal from the upper respiratory tract by increasing the volume of secretions and reducing their adhesiveness and surface tension.

Contraindications

Hypersensitivity to bisulfites, carbetapentane, phenylephrine, guaifenesin, or their components; severe coronary artery disease or hypertension; use within 14 days of MAO inhibitor therapy; ventricular tachycardia

Interactions

DRUGS

phenylephrine component

alpha blockers, haloperidol, loxapine, phenothiazines, thioxanthenes: Possibly decreased vasoconstrictor effect of phenylephrine

antihypertenisves, diuretics: Possibly decreased antihypertensive effects

atropine: Possibly enhanced vasopressor effect of phenylephrine

beta blockers: Decreased therapeutic effects of both drugs

bretylium: Possibly potentiated vaopressor effect and arrhythmias

doxapram: Increased vasopressor effect of both drugs

ergot alkaloids: Possibly cerebral blood vessel rupture, increased vasopressor effect, peripheral vascular ischemia, and gangrene (with ergotamine)

guanadrel, guanethidine: Increased vasopressor effect of phenylephrine; increased risk of severe hypertension and arrhythmias

hydrocarbon inhalation anesthetics: Increased risk of serious arrhythmias

MAO inhibitors: Increased and prolonged cardiac stimulation, increased vasopressor effect, increased risk of severe cardiovascular and cerebrovascular effects, hyperpyrexia, and vomiting

maprotiline, tricyclic antidepressants: Increased risk of severe cardiovascular effects (including arrhythmias, hyperpyrexia, severe hypertension)

mecamylamine, methyldopa: Decreased hypotensive effects of these drugs and increased vasopressor effect of phenylephrine

nitrates: Possibly decreased vasopressor effect of phenylephrine and decreased antianginal effect of nitrates

oxytocin: Possibly severe, persistent hypertension

phenoxybenzamine: Decreased vasoconstrictor effect of phenylephrine and possible hypotension and tachycardia

theophylline: Possibly enhanced toxicity (including cardiac toxicity)

thyroid hormones: Increased cardiovascular effects of each drug

Adverse Reactions

CNS: Anxiety, confusion, dizziness, hallucinations, headache, insomnia, nervousness, paresthesia, restlessness, tremor, weakness

CV: Angina, bradycardia, hypertension, hypotension, palpitations, peripheral vasoconstriction that may lead to necrosis or gangrene, tachycardia, ventricular arrhythmia

GI: Nausea, vomiting
GU: Dysuria, urine retention
RESP: Dyspnea
SKIN: Pallor, rash, urticaria
Other: Allergic reaction

Nursing Considerations

- Assess patient for signs and symptoms of angina, arrhythmias, and hypertension because phenylephrine may increase myocardial oxygen demand and the risk of proarrhythmias and blood pressure changes.
- **WARNING** Monitor patient with thyroid disease for increased sensitivity to catecholamines and for possible thyrotoxicity or cardiotoxicity.
- Regularly evaluate effectiveness of carbetapentane, phenylephrine, and guaifenesin in relieving cough and other upper respiratory symptoms. Notify prescriber if symptoms don't improve or if they worsen.

PATIENT TEACHING

- Caution patient to take drug exactly as prescribed and not to increase dosage or frequency without first consulting prescriber.
- Instruct patient to increase fluid intake (unless contraindicated) to help thin secretions.
- Advise patient to avoid potentially hazardous activities until drug's CNS effects are known.

carbetapentane tannate, phenylephrine tannate, and pyrilamine tannate

Tussi-12D, Tussi-12D S

Class and Category

Chemical: Cyclopentane carbolic ester (carbetapentane), sympathomimetic amine (phenylephrine), ethylenediamine antihistamine (pyrilamine)

Therapeutic: Antitussive (carbetapentane), decongestant (phenylephrine), antihistaminic (pyrilamine)

Pregnancy category: C

Indications and Dosages

▶ *To relieve cough and nasal congestion from the common cold, sinusitis, allergic rhinitis, and other upper respiratory tract conditions*

SUSPENSION
Adults. 30 to 60 mg carbetapentane, 5 to 10 mg phenylephrine, and 30 to 60 mg pyrilamine (5 to 10 ml) q 12 hr.
TABLETS
Adults. 60 to 120 mg carbetapentane, 10 to 20 mg phenylephrine, and 40 to 80 mg pyrilamine (1 to 2 tablets) q 12 hr.

Mechanism of Action

Carbetapentane has atropine-like and local anesthetic actions that suppress the cough reflex in the medullary cough center in the brain.

Phenylephrine stimulates alpha-adrenergic receptors and inhibits the intracellular enzyme adenyl cyclase, which then inhibits production of cAMP. Inhibition of cAMP causes arterial and venous constriction in nasal passages, which decreases blood flow and mucosal edema caused by allergic response.

Pyrilamine competes with histamine for H_1 receptor sites, thereby antagonizing many histamine effects to reduce allergy signs and symptoms.

Contraindications

Acute MI; angina; breastfeeding; cardiac arrhythmias; coronary artery disease; hypersensitivity to carbetapentane, phenylephrine, pyrilamine or their components; use of MAO inhibitors within 14 days; ventricular tachycardia

Interactions

DRUGS
phenylephrine and pyrilamine
MAO inhibitors: Possibly prolonged and intensified anticholinergic effects of pyrilamine and overall effects of phenylephrine
carbetapentane component
tartrazine (FD & C Yellow No. 5 contained in certain products): Possibly induced allergic-type reactions in susceptible persons
phenylephrine component
alpha blockers, haloperidol, loxapine, phenothiazines, thioxanthenes: Possibly decreased vasoconstrictor effect of phenylephrine
antihypertenisves, diuretics: Possibly decreased antihypertensive effects
atropine: Possibly enhanced vasopressor effect of phenylephrine
beta blockers: Decreased therapeutic effects of both drugs
bretylium: Possibly potentiated vaopressor effect and arrhythmias
doxapram: Increased vasopressor effect of both drugs
ergot alkaloids: Possibly cerebral blood vessel rupture, increased vasopressor effect, peripheral vascular ischemia, and gangrene (with ergotamine)

guanadrel, guanethidine: Increased vasopressor effect of phenylephrine, increased risk of severe hypertension and arrhythmias
hydrocarbon inhalation anesthetics: Increased risk of serious arrhythmias
maprotiline, tricyclic antidepressants: Increased risk of severe cardiovascular effects (including arrhythmias, hyperpyrexia, severe hypertension)
mecamylamine, methyldopa: Decreased hypotensive effects of these drugs, increased vasopressor effect of phenylephrine
nitrates: Possibly decreased vasopressor effect of phenylephrine and decreased antianginal effect of nitrates
oxytocin: Possibly severe, persistent hypertension
phenoxybenzamine: Decreased vasoconstrictor effect of phenylephrine, possibly hypotension and tachycardia
theophylline: Possibly enhanced toxicity (including cardiac toxicity)
thyroid hormones: Increased cardiovascular effects of each drug
chlorpheniramine component
CNS depressants: Additive CNS effects
ACTIVITIES
chlorpheniramine component
alcohol use: Additive CNS effects

Adverse Reactions
CNS: Confusion, dizziness, drowsiness, hallucinations, headache, insomnia, nervousness, paresthesia, restlessness, sedation, seizures, tremor, weakness
CV: Angina, bradycardia, hypertension, hypotension, palpitations, peripheral vasoconstriction that may lead to necrosis or gangrene, tachycardia, ventricular arrhythmias
EENT: Blurred vision; dry eyes, mouth, and nose
GI: Constipation, nausea, vomiting
GU: Urinary hesitancy, urine retention
RESP: Dyspnea

Nursing Considerations
• Use cautiously in patients with cardiovascular disease, diabetes, hypertension, hyperthyroidism, narrow-angle glaucoma, or prostatic hypertrophy.
• Monitor patients who may be more susceptible to dizziness, sedation, and hypotension, such as the elderly.
• Regularly evaluate effectiveness of carbetapentane, phenylephrine, and pyrilamine in reducing cough and nasal congestion.
• Be aware that patient shouldn't have intradermal allergen tests within 72 hours of receiving drug because results may be altered.

PATIENT TEACHING
• Instruct patient to use a calibrated measuring device when using suspension form of carbetapentane, phenylephrine, and pyrilamine to ensure accurate dose.
• Instruct patient to take drug exactly as prescribed and not to increase dosage or frequency without consulting prescriber.
• Urge patient to avoid alcohol and other antidepressants while taking carbetapentane, phenylephrine, and pyrilamine.
• Instruct patient to avoid potentially hazardous activities until drug's CNS effects are known.
• Suggest that patient relieve dry mouth with frequent rinsing and use of sugarless gum or hard candy.

carbinoxamine maleate and pseudoephedrine hydrochloride

Andehist Drops, Cardec-S, Coldec D, CP Oral, Mooredec, Palgic-D, Rinade B.I.D. Tablets, Rondec, Rondec Drops, Rondec-TR

Class and Category

Chemical: Ethanolamine derivative (carbinoxamine), sympathomimetic amine (pseudoephedrine)
Therapeutic: Antihistaminic (carbinoxamine), decongestant (pseudoephedrine)
Pregnancy category: C

Indications and Dosages

▶ *To relieve persistent runny nose, sneezing, and nasal congestion caused by upper respiratory infections, sinus inflammation, hay fever, or the common cold*

E.R. TABLETS
Adults. 6 to 8 mg carbinoxamine and 60 to 120 mg pseudoephedrine (1 tablet) q 12 hr.

TABLETS
Adults. 4 mg carbinoxamine and 120 mg pseudoephedrine (1 tablet) q 12 hr. Or, 4 mg carbinoxamine and 60 mg pseudoephedrine (1 tablet) q 6 hr. Or, 8 mg carbinoxamine and 90 mg pseudoephedrine (1 tablet) q 12 hr.
Children age 6 and over. 4 mg carbinoxamine and 60 mg pseudoephedrine (1 tablet) q 6 hr.

CHEWABLE TABLETS
Adults and children age 12 and over. 4 mg carbinoxamine and 60 mg pseudoephedrine (1 tablet) q 4 hr.

Children ages 6 to 12. 2 mg carbinoxamine and 30 mg pseudo-ephedrine (½ tablet) q 4 hr.

SYRUP

Adults and children age 6 and over. 4 mg carbinoxamine and 60 mg pseudoephedrine (5 ml) q 6 hr.

Children age 18 months to 6 years. 2 mg carbinoxamine and 30 mg pseudoephedrine (2.5 ml) q 6 hr.

ORAL SOLUTION

Children ages 9 months to 18 months. 2 mg carbinoxamine and 25 mg pseudoephedrine (1 ml) q 6 hr.

Children ages 6 months to 9 months. 1.5 mg carbinoxamine and 18.75 mg pseudoephedrine (0.75 ml) q 6 hr.

Infants ages 3 months to 6 months. 1 mg carbinoxamine and 12.5 mg pseudoephedrine (0.5 ml) q 6 hr.

Infants ages 1 month to 3 months. 0.5 mg carbinoxamine and 6.25 mg pseudoephedrine (0.25 ml) q 6 hr.

DROPS

Children ages 12 months to 24 months. 1 or 2 mg carbinox-amine and 15 mg pseudoephedrine (1 ml) q.i.d.

Children ages 6 months to 12 months. 0.75 or 1.5 mg carbinoxamine and 11.25 mg psuedoephedrine (0.75 ml) q.i.d.

Infants ages 3 months to 6 months. 0.5 or 1 mg carbinoxa-mine and 7.5 mg pseudoephedrine (0.5 ml) q.i.d.

Infants ages 1 month to 3 months. 0.25 or 0.5 mg carbinox-amine and 3.75 mg pseudoephedrine (0.25 ml) q.i.d.

Mechanism of Action

Carbinoxamine competes with histamine for H_1 receptor sites, thereby antag-onizing many histamine effects and reducing allergy signs and symptoms.

Pseudoephedrine acts on $alpha_1$-adrenergic receptors in the mucosa of the respiratory tract to produce vasoconstriction. This process shrinks swollen nasal mucous membranes; reduces tissue hyperemia, edema, and nasal con-gestion; and increases nasal airway patency. It also may increase drainage of sinus secretions and open obstructed eustachian ostia.

Contraindications

Angina; breastfeeding; cardiac arrhythmias; hypersensitivity or idiosyncratic reactions to carbinoxamine, pseudoephedrine, or their components; hyperthyroidism; MI; narrow-angle glaucoma; severe coronary artery disease or hypertension; urine retention; use within 14 days of MAO inhibitor therapy

Interactions

DRUGS

carbinoxamine and pseudoephedrine

MAO inhibitors: Increased and prolonged cardiac stimulation, increased vasopressor effect, increased risk of severe cardiovascular and cerebrovascular effects, hyperpyrexia, and vomiting

carbinoxamine component

anticholinergics: Additive anticholinergic effects

CNS depressants: Additive CNS effects

pseudoephedrine component

antacids: Increased absorption of pseudoephedrine

antihypertensives, diuretics: Possibly decreased antihypertensive effects

beta blockers: Decreased therapeutic effects of both drugs

citrates: Possibly inhibited urinary pseudoephedrine excretion and prolonged duration of action

CNS stimulants, sympathomimetics: Possibly increased additive CNS stimulation to excessive levels

cocaine (mucosal-local): Possibly increased cardiovascular effects of either drug and CNS stimulation

digoxin, levodopa: Increased risk of cardiac arrhythmias

hydrocarbon inhalation anesthetics: Increased risk of serious arrhythmias

kaolin: Decreased pseudoephedrine absorption

MAO inhibitors: Increased and prolonged cardiac stimulation, increased vasopressor effect, increased risk of severe cardiovascular and cerebrovascular effects, hyperpyrexia, and vomiting

nitrates: Reduced antianginal effects of nitrates

rauwolfia alkaloids: Possibly inhibited pseudoephedrine action

thyroid hormones: Increased cardiovascular effects of both drugs

ACTIVITIES

carbinoxamine component

alcohol use: Additive CNS effects

Adverse Reactions

CNS: Anxiety, chills, confusion, coordination disturbance, dizziness, drowsiness, excitation (children), fatigue, fear, hallucinations, headache, hysteria, insomnia, irritability, light-headedness, nervousness, numbness, restlessness, sedation, seizures, tenseness, trembling, vertigo, weakness

CV: Angina, arrhythmias, chest tightness, hypertension, palpitations, tachycardia

EENT: Blurred or double vision; dry eyes, mouth, nose, and throat; nasal congestion; tinnitus
ENDO: Early menstruation
GI: Anorexia, constipation, diarrhea, nausea, stomach upset or pain, vomiting
GU: Dysuria, frequent urination, urinary hesitancy, urine retention
HEME: Anemia, unusual bleeding or bruising
RESP: Dyspnea, increased chest congestion, wheezing
SKIN: Diaphoresis, pallor, photosensitivity, rash, urticaria
Other: Anaphylaxis

Nursing Considerations

- Use cautiously in patients with asthma, cardiovascular disease, diabetes, emphysema or other chronic lung disease, hypertension, peptic ulcer, hyperthyroidism, narrow-angle glaucoma, or prostatic hypertrophy.
- Monitor children for excitation and elderly patients for dizziness, sedation, and hypotension; such patients may have an increased risk for these effects.
- Monitor renal function, as ordered, because pseudoephedrine is substantially excreted by the kidneys.
- Regularly evaluate effectiveness of carbinoxamine and pseudoephedrine in reducing upper respiratory symptoms.
- Be aware that patient shouldn't have intradermal allergen tests within 72 hours of receiving drug because results may be altered.

PATIENT TEACHING

- Instruct patient to use a calibrated measuring device for syrup or oral solution form of carbinoxamine and pseudoephedrine to ensure accurate dose.
- Urge patient to avoid alcohol and other antidepressants while taking carbinoxamine and pseudoephedrine.
- Instruct patient to avoid potentially hazardous activities until drug's CNS effects are known.
- Suggest that patient relieve dry mouth with frequent rinsing and use of sugarless gum or hard candy.
- Tell patient to take last dose of the day a few hours before bedtime if carbinoxamine and pseudoephedrine makes her nervous or restless.

cetirizine hydrochloride and pseudoephedrine hydrochloride
Zyrtec-D 12 Hour

Class and Category
Chemical: H$_1$ receptor antagonist (cetirizine), sympathomimetic amine (pseudoephedrine)
Therapeutic: Antihistamine (cetirizine), decongestant (pseudoephedrine)
Pregnancy category: C

Indications and Dosages
▶ *To relieve nasal and non-nasal symptoms of seasonal or perennial allergic rhinitis*
E.R. TABLETS
Adults and children age 12 and over. 5 mg cetirizine and 120 mg pseudoephedrine (1 tablet) q 12 hr.
DOSAGE ADJUSTMENT For patients with decreased renal function (creatinine clearance of 11 to 31 ml/min/1.73 m^2), patients on hemodialysis (creatinine clearance less than 7 ml/min/1.73 m^2), or patients with decreased hepatic function, dosage decreased to 5 mg cetirizine and 120 mg pseudoephedrine (1 tablet) q 24 hr.

Mechanism of Action
Cetirizine competes with histamine for histamine H$_1$ receptor sites on effector cells and antagonizes the vasodilator effect of endogenously released histamine. This prevents the peripheral vascular engorgement, mucosal edema, sneezing, and profuse watery nasal secretion and irritation that normally result from histamine action on peripheral afferent nerve terminals.

Pseudoephedrine acts on alpha$_1$-adrenergic receptors in the mucosa of the respiratory tract to produce vasoconstriction. This process shrinks swollen nasal mucous membranes; reduces tissue hyperemia, edema, and nasal congestion; and increases nasal airway patency. It also may increase drainage of sinus secretions and open obstructed eustachian ostia.

Contraindications
Angina; cardiac arrhythmias; hypersensitivity or idiosyncratic reactions to cetirizine, pseudoephedrine, or their components; hyperthyroidism; narrow-angle glaucoma; severe coronary artery disease or hypertension; urine retention; use within 14 days of MAO inhibitor therapy

Interactions
DRUGS
cetirizine component
barbiturates, CNS depressants, tricyclic antidepressants: Additive effects

theophylline: Possibly decreased cetirizine clearance
pseudoephedrine component
antacids: Increased pseudoephedrine absorption
antihypertensives, diuretics: Possibly decreased antihypertensive effects
beta blockers: Decreased therapeutic effects of both drugs
citrates: Possibly inhibited urinary pseudoephedrine excretion and prolonged duration of action
CNS stimulant, other sympathomimetics: Possibly increased additive CNS stimulation to excessive levels
cocaine (mucosal-local): Possibly increased cardiovascular effects of either drug and CNS stimulation
digoxin, levodopa: Increased risk of cardiac arrhythmias
hydrocarbon inhalation anesthetics: Increased risk of serious arrhythmias
kaolin: Decreased pseudoephedrine absorption
MAO inhibitors: Increased and prolonged cardiac stimulation, increased vasopressor effect, increased risk of severe cardiovascular and cerebrovascular effects, hyperpyrexia, vomiting
nitrates: Reduced antianginal effects of nitrates
rauwolfia alkaloids: Possibly inhibited pseudoephedrine action
thyroid hormones: Increased cardiovascular effects of both drugs
ACTIVITIES
cetirizine component
alcohol use: Additive effects

Adverse Reactions
CNS: Anxiety, dizziness, drowsiness, excitability, fatigue, fear, hallucinations, headache, insomnia, light-headedness, nervousness, restlessness, seizures, somnolence, trembling, weakness
CV: Angina, arrhythmias, hypertension, palpitations, tachycardia
EENT: Dry mouth, epistaxis, ocular hypertension, pharyngitis, sinusitis
GI: Nausea, vomiting
GU: Dysuria
RESP: Dyspnea
SKIN: Diaphoresis, pallor

Nursing Considerations
• Use cautiously in patients with hypertension, diabetes mellitus, ischemic heart disease, increased intraocular pressure, hyperthyroidism, renal impairment, or prostatic hypertrophy because of pseudoephedrine component of the drug.

- Monitor children for excitation and elderly patients for dizziness, sedation, and hypotension; such patients may have an increased risk for these effects.
- Monitor renal function, as ordered, because pseudoephedrine is substantially excreted by the kidneys.
- Evaluate effectiveness of cetirizine and pseudoephedrine in relieving seasonal or perennial allergic rhinitis.
- Be aware that patient shouldn't have intradermal allergen tests within 4 days of receiving drug because results may be altered.

PATIENT TEACHING
- Urge patient to avoid alcohol, other antidepressants, and OTC medication containing other antihistamines or sympathomimetics while taking cetirizine and pseudoephedrine.
- Instruct patient to avoid potentially hazardous activities until drug's CNS effects are known.
- Suggest that patient relieve dry mouth with frequent rinsing and use of sugarless gum or hard candy.

chlorpheniramine maleate and hydrocodone bitartrate
S-T Forte 2
chlorpheniramine polistirex and hydrocodone polistirex
Tussionex Pennkinetic Suspension

Class, Category, and Schedule
Chemical: Alkylamine (chlorpheniramine), opioid and phenanthrene derivative (hydrocodone)
Therapeutic: Antihistamine (chlorpheniramine), antitussive (hydrocodone),
Pregnancy category: C
Controlled substance: Schedule III

Indications and Dosages
▶ *To relieve cough and respiratory symptoms from colds and allergies*
SUSPENSION
Adults. 8 mg chlorpheniramine and 10 mg hydrocodone (5 ml) q 12 hr. *Maximum:* 16 mg chlorpheniramine and 20 mg hydrocodone q 24 hr.
Children age 6 and over. 4 mg chlorpheniramine and 5 mg hydrocodone (2.5 ml) q 12 hr. *Maximum:* 8 mg chlorpheniramine and 10 mg hydrocodone q 24 hr.

ORAL SOLUTION
Adults and children age 12 and over. 2 mg chlorpheniramine
and 2.5 mg hydrocodone (5 ml) q 6 to 8 hr.
Children ages 3 to 12. 1 mg chlorpheniramine and 1.25 mg hydrocodone (2.5 ml) q 6 to 8 hr.

Mechanism of Action

Chlorpheniramine competes with histamine for H$_1$ receptor sites, thereby antagonizing many histamine effects and reducing allergy signs and symptoms.
 Hydrocodone suppresses cough by acting directly on opiate receptors in
the medulla's cough center.

Contraindications

Hypersensitivity to chlorpheniramine, hydrocodone, other opioids, or their components; respiratory depression; severe asthma;
upper airway obstruction; use of MAO inhibitors within 14 days

Interactions

DRUGS
chlorpheniramine and hydrocodone
anticholinergics, paregoric: Possibly intensified anticholinergic adverse effects, such as paralytic ileus
CNS depressants: Additive CNS effects
MAO inhibitors: Increased and prolonged cardiac stimulation, increased vasopressor effect, increased risk of severe cardiovascular
and cerebrovascular effects, hyperpyrexia, and vomiting
chlorpheniramine component
phenytoin: Possibly increased serum phenytoin levels and toxicity
hydrocodone component
antihypertensives, diuretics: Potentiated hypotensive effects
buprenorphine: Decreased hydrocodone effectiveness
hydroxyzine: Increased hydrocodone analgesic effect; increased
CNS depressant and hypotensive effects
metoclopramide: Antagonized effect of metoclopramide on GI
motility
naloxone: Antagonized hydrocodone analgesic effect
naltrexone: Precipitated withdrawal symptoms in hydrocodone-
dependent patients
neuromuscular blockers: Additive respiratory depressant effects
opioids: Additive CNS and respiratory depressants effects and hypotensive effects

ACTIVITIES
chlorpheniramine and hydrocodone
alcohol use: Additive CNS effects

Adverse Reactions
CNS: Anxiety, confusion, decreased mental and physical performance, depression, dizziness, drowsiness, euphoria, faintness, fear, headache, light-headedness, mood changes, nervousness, restlessness, sedation, seizures, tiredness, weakness
CV: Bradycardia, chest tightness, hypotension, palpitations, tachycardia
EENT: Blurred or double vision, dry mouth, laryngeal edema, laryngospasm
GI: Anorexia, constipation, nausea, paralytic ileus, toxic megacolon, vomiting
GU: Dysuria, frequent urination
RESP: Dyspnea, shortness of breath, slow or irregular breathing, wheezing
Skin: Diaphoresis, facial flushing, pruritis, rash, uriticaria
Other: Angioedema, atelectasis, mental or physical dependence

Nursing Considerations
• Use cautiously in patients with a recent head injury and those with Addison's disease, asthma or other chronic respiratory disease, increased intraocular pressure, hypothyroidism, liver or renal impairment, or prostatic hypertrophy.
• Monitor children for excitation and elderly patients for dizziness, sedation, and hypotension; they have an increased risk.
• Regularly evaluate effectiveness of chlorpheniramine and hyrdocodone in reducing symptoms.
• Be aware that patient shouldn't have intradermal allergen tests within 72 hours of receiving drug because results may be altered.
PATIENT TEACHING
• Instruct patient to shake suspension well before measuring dose and to use a calibrated device to ensure accurate dose.
• Urge patient to avoid alcohol and other antidepressants while taking chlorpheniramine and hydrocodone.
• Instruct patient to avoid potentially hazardous activities until drug's CNS effects are known.
• Suggest that patient relieve dry mouth with frequent rinsing and use of sugarless gum or hard candy.
• Tell patient to take last dose of the day a few hours before bedtime if chlorpheniramine and hydrocodone makes her nervous or restless.

chlorpheniramine maleate, hydrocodone bitartrate, and phenylephrine hydrochloride

Atuss MS, Chlorgest-HD, Comtussin HC, Cytuss HC, ED-TLC, ED Tuss HC, Endagen-HD, Endal HD, Endal HD Plus, Histinex HC, Histussin HC, Hydrocodone CP, Hydrocodone HD, Hydron CP, Hydro-PC, Hydro-PC II, Iodal HD, Iotussin HC, Maxi-Tuss HC, Poly-Tussin, Unituss HC, Vanex-HD, Z-Cof HC

Class, Category, and Schedule

Chemical: Alkylamine (chlorpheniramine), opioid and phenanthrene derivative (hydrocodone), and sympathomimetic amine (phenylephrine)

Therapeutic: Antihistamine (chlorpheniramine), antitussive (hydrocodone), and decongestant (phenylephrine)

Pregnancy category: C

Controlled substance: Schedule III

Indications and Dosages

▶ *To relieve cough and upper respiratory symptoms of colds and allergies*

SYRUP, ORAL SOLUTION

Adults and children age 12 and over. 2 to 4 mg chlorpheniramine, 1.67 mg to 5 mg hydrocodone, and 5 to 10 mg phenylephrine (5 to 10 ml depending on product used) q 4 hr or t.i.d. to q.i.d. Or, 8 mg chlorpheniramine, 3.34 mg hydrocodone, and 10 mg phenylephrine (10 ml) q 6 to 8 hr. *Maximum:* 4 doses daily.

Children age 6 to 12. 2 to 4 mg chlorpheniramine, 1.25 to 2.5 mg hydrocodone, and 5 to 10 mg phenylephrine (2.5 or 5 ml depending on product) q 4 to 8 hr. *Maximum:* 4 doses daily.

Children age 2 to 6. 1 mg chlorpheniramine, 0.625 mg hydrocodone, and 2.5 mg phenylephrine (1.25 ml) q 4 to 6 hr.

DOSAGE ADJUSTMENT For patients with renal impairment, dosage may need to be reduced.

Contraindications

Breastfeeding; closed-angle glaucoma; hypersensitivity to chlorpheniramine, hydrocodone, other opioids, phenylephrine, or their components; prostate disease; respiratory depression; severe asthma; thyroid disease; upper airway obstruction, use of MAO inhibitors within 14 days

---

Mechanism of Action

Chlorpheniramine competes with histamine for H_1 receptor sites, thereby antagonizing many histamine effects and reducing allergy signs and symptoms.

Hydrocodone suppresses cough by directly acting on opiate receptors in the medulla's cough center.

Phenylephrine stimulates alpha-adrenergic receptors and inhibits the intracellular enzyme adenyl cyclase, which then inhibits production of cAMP. Inhibition of cAMP causes arterial and venous constriction in nasal passages, which decreases blood flow and mucosal edema caused by allergic response.

Interactions

DRUGS

chlorpheniramine, hydrocodone and phenylephrine

MAO inhibitors: Increased and prolonged cardiac stimulation, increased vasopressor effect, increased risk of severe cardiovascular and cerebrovascular effects, hyperpyrexia, vomiting

chlorpheniramine and hydrocodone

anticholinergics: Possibly intensified anticholinergic adverse effects

CNS depressants: Additive CNS effects

chlorpheniramine component

phenytoin: Possibly increased serum phenytoin levels and toxicity

hydrocodone component

antihypertensives, diuretics: Potentiated hypotensive effects

buprenorphine: Decreased effectiveness of hydrocodone

hydroxyzine: Increased hydrocodone analgesic effect; increased CNS depressant and hypotensive effects

metoclopramide: Antagonized effect of metoclopramide on GI motility

naloxone: Antagonized hydrocodone analgesic effect

naltrexone: Precipitated withdrawal symptoms in hydrocodone-dependent patients

neuromuscular blockers: Additive respiratory depressant effects

opioids: Additive CNS and respiratory depressants effects and hypotensive effects

phenylephrine component

alpha blockers, haloperidol, loxapine, phenothiazines, thioxanthenes: Possibly decreased vasoconstrictor effect of phenylephrine

antihypertenisves, diuretics: Possibly decreased antihypertensive effects

atropine: Possibly enhanced vasopressor effect of phenylephrine

beta blockers: Decreased therapeutic effects of both drugs

bretylium: Possibly potentiated vaopressor effect and arrhythmias
doxapram: Increased vasopressor effect of both drugs
ergot alkaloids: Possibly cerebral blood vessel rupture, increased vasopressor effect, peripheral vascular ischemia, and gangrene (with ergotamine)
guanadrel, guanethidine: Increased vasopressor effect of phenylephrine, increased risk of severe hypertension and arrhythmias
hydrocarbon inhalation anesthetics: Increased risk of serious arrhythmias
maprotiline, tricyclic antidepressants: Increased risk of severe cardiovascular effects (including arrhythmias, hyperpyrexia, severe hypertension)
mecamylamine, methyldopa: Decreased hypotensive effects of these drugs, increased vasopressor effect of phenylephrine
nitrates: Possibly decreased vasopressor effect of phenylephrine and decreased antianginal effect of nitrates
oxytocin: Possibly severe, persistent hypertension
phenoxybenzamine: Decreased vasoconstrictor effect of phenylephrine, possibly hypotension and tachycardia
theophylline: Possibly enhanced toxicity (including cardiac toxicity)
thyroid hormones: Increased cardiovascular effects of each drug
ACTIVITIES
chlorpheniramine and hydrocodone
alcohol use: Additive CNS effects

Adverse Reactions

CNS: Anxiety, confusion, decreased mental and physical performance, depression, dizziness, drowsiness, excitation (children), euphoria, faintness, fear, hallucinations, headache, insomnia, irritability, lethargy, light-headedness, mood changes, nervousness, paresthesia, psychosis, restlessness, sedation, seizures, tiredness, tremor, weakness
CV: Angina, bradycardia, chest tightness, hypertension, hypotension, palpitations, peripheral vasoconstriction, tachycardia, ventricular arrhythmias
EENT: Blurred or double vision, dry mouth, laryngeal edema, laryngospasm, mydriasis, ocular hypertension, photophobia
GI: Abdominal pain, anorexia, constipation, nausea, paralytic ileus, toxic megacolon, vomiting
GU: Dysuria, frequent urination, urinary hesitancy or retention
RESP: Dyspnea, shortness of breath, slow or irregular breathing, wheezing
Skin: Diaphoresis, facial flushing, pruritis, rash, uriticaria

Other: Angioedema, anaphylaxis, physical or psychological dependence

Nursing Considerations
- Use cautiously in patients with a recent head injury and those with Addison's disease, asthma or other chronic respiratory disease, increased intraocular pressure, hypothyroidism, or liver or renal impairment.
- Monitor children for excitation and elderly patients for dizziness, sedation, and hypotension; such patients may have an increased risk for these effects.
- Regularly evaluate effectiveness of chlorpheniramine, hydrocodone, and phenylephrine in reducing cough and upper respiratory symptoms.
- Be aware that patient shouldn't have intradermal allergen tests within 72 hours of receiving drug because results may be altered.

PATIENT TEACHING
- Instruct patient to use a calibrated measuring device to ensure accurate dose of chlorpheniramine, hydrocodone, and phenylephrine.
- Urge patient to avoid alcohol and other antidepressants while taking chlorpheniramine, hydrocodone, and phenylephrine.
- Instruct patient to avoid potentially hazardous activities until drug's CNS effects are known.
- Suggest that patient relieve dry mouth with frequent rinsing and use of sugarless gum or hard candy.
- Tell patient to take last dose of the day a few hours before bedtime if chlorpheniramine, hydrocodone, and phenylephrine makes him nervous or restless.

chlorpheniramine maleate, hydrocodone bitartrate, and pseudoephedrine hydrochloride

Histinex PV, Hydro-Tussin HC, Hydron PSC, Hyphed, P-V Tussin, Pancof-HC, Tussend

Class, Category, and Schedule
Chemical: Alkylamine (chlorpheniramine), opioid and phenanthrene derivative (hydrocodone), sympathomimetic amine (pseudoephedrine)
Therapeutic: Antihistamine (chlorpheniramine), antitussive (hydrocodone), decongestant (pseudoephedrine)

Pregnancy category: C
Controlled substance: Schedule III

Indications and Dosages

▶ *To relieve cough and upper respiratory symptoms of colds and allergies*

ORAL SOLUTION, SYRUP

Adults and children age 12 and over. 2 to 4 mg chlorpheniramine, 3 to 6 mg hydrocodone, and 15 to 60 mg pseudoephedrine (5 to 10 ml depending on product) q 4 to 6 hr. Or, doses may be given t.i.d or q.i.d. *Maximum:* 4 doses daily.

Children ages 6 to 12. 2 mg chlorpheniramine, 2.5 mg hydrocodone, and 30 mg pseudoephedrine (5 ml) q 4 to 6 hr. *Maximum:* 4 doses daily.

Children ages 2 to 6. 1 mg chlorpheniramine, 1.25 mg hydrocodone, and 15 mg pseudoephedrine (2.5 ml) q 4 to 6 hr. *Maximum:* 4 doses daily.

TABLETS

Adults. 4 mg chlorpheniramine, 5 mg hydrocodone, and 60 mg pseudoephedrine (1 tablet) q 6 hr.

Mechanism of Action

Chlorpheniramine competes with histamine for H_1 receptor sites, thereby antagonizing many histamine effects and reducing allergy signs and symptoms.

Hydrocodone suppresses cough by directly acting on opiate receptors in the medulla's cough center.

Pseudoephedrine acts on $alpha_1$-adrenergic receptors in the mucosa of the respiratory tract to produce vasoconstriction. This process shrinks swollen nasal mucous membranes; reduces tissue hyperemia, edema, and nasal congestion; and increases nasal airway patency. It also may increase drainage of sinus secretions and open obstructed eustachian ostia.

Contraindications

Hypersensitivity or idiosyncractic reactions to chlorpheniramine, hydrocodone, other opioids, pseudodephedrine, or their components; hyperthyroidism; narrow-angle glaucoma; prostatic hypertrophy; respiratory depression; severe asthma, coronary artery disease or hypertension; upper airway obstruction, urine retention, use of MAO inhibitors within 14 days

Interactions

DRUGS

chlorpheniramine, hydrocodone, and pseudoephedrine

MAO inhibitors: Increased and prolonged cardiac stimulation, increased vasopressor effect, increased risk of severe cardiovascular and cerebrovascular effects, hyperpyrexia, and vomiting

chlorpheniramine and hydrocodone

anticholinergics, paregoric: Possibly intensified anticholinergic adverse effects

CNS depressants: Additive CNS effects

chlorpheniramine component

phenytoin: Possibly increased serum phenytoin level and toxicity

hydrocodone component

antihypertensives, diuretics: Potentiated hypotensive effects

buprenorphine: Decreased hydrocodone effectiveness

hydroxyzine: Increased hydrocodone analgesic effect; increased CNS depressant and hypotensive effects

metoclopramide: Antagonized effect of metoclopramide on GI motility

naloxone: Anatagonized hydrocodone analgesic effect

naltrexone: Precipitated withdrawal symptoms in hydrocodone-dependent patients

neuromuscular blockers: Additive respiratory depressant effects

opioids: Additive CNS and respiratory depressants effects and hypotensive effects

pseudoephedrine component

antacids: Increased pseudoephedrine absorption

antihypertensives, diuretics: Possibly decreased antihypertensive effects

beta blockers: Decreased therapeutic effects of both drugs

citrates: Possibly inhibited urinary pseudoephedrine excretion and prolonged duration of action

CNS stimulant, other sympathomimetics: Possibly increased additive CNS stimulation to excessive levels

cocaine (mucosal-local): Possibly increased cardiovascular effects of either drug and CNS stimulation

digoxin, levodopa: Increased risk of cardiac arrhythmias

hydrocarbon inhalation anesthetics: Increased risk of serious arrhythmias

kaolin: Decreased pseudoephedrine absorption

nitrates: Reduced antianginal effects of nitrates

rauwolfia alkaloids: Possibly inhibited pseudoephedrine action

thyroid hormones: Increased cardiovascular effects of both drugs

ACTIVITIES

chlorpheniramine and hydrocodone

alcohol use: Additive CNS effects

Adverse Reactions

CNS: Angina, anxiety, arrhythmia exacerbation, confusion, decreased mental and physical performance, depression, dizziness, drowsiness, excitation (children), euphoria, faintness, fear, headache, insomnia, light-headedness, mood changes, nervousness, restlessness, sedation, seizures, tiredness, trembling, weakness
CV: Bradycardia, chest tightness, hypotension, palpitations, tachycardia
EENT: Blurred or double vision, dry mouth, laryngeal edema, laryngospasm, photophobia
GI: Anorexia, constipation, nausea, paralytic ileus, toxic megacolon, vomiting
GU: Dysuria, frequent urination, urine retention
RESP: Dyspnea, shortness of breath, slow or irregular breathing, wheezing
Skin: Diaphoresis, facial flushing, pallor, pruritis, rash, uriticaria
Other: Angioedema, atelectasis, mental or physical dependence

Nursing Considerations

- Use cautiously in patients with a recent head injury and those with Addison's disease, asthma or other chronic respiratory disease, increased intraocular pressure, or liver or renal impairment.
- Monitor children for excitation and elderly patients for dizziness, sedation, and hypotension; such patients may have an increased risk for these effects.
- Monitor renal function, as ordered, because pseudoephedrine is substantially excreted by the kidneys.
- Regularly evaluate effectiveness of chlorpheniramine, hydrocodone, and pseudoephedrine in reducing symptoms.
- Be aware that patient shouldn't have intradermal allergen tests within 72 hours of receiving drug because it may alter results.

PATIENT TEACHING
- Instruct patient to use a calibrated measuring device to ensure accurate dose.
- Urge patient to avoid alcohol and other antidepressants while taking chlorpheniramine, hydrocodone, and pseudoephedrine.
- Instruct patient to avoid potentially hazardous activities until drug's CNS effects are known.
- Suggest that patient relieve dry mouth with frequent rinsing and use of sugarless gum or hard candy.
- Tell patient to take last dose of the day a few hours before bedtime if chlorpheniramine, hydrocodone, and pseudoephedrine makes her nervous or restless.

chlorpheniramine maleate, hydrocodone bitartrate, pseudoephedrine hydrochloride, and guaifenesin

Ztuss Expectorant

Class, Category, and Schedule

Chemical: Alkylamine (chlorpheniramine), opioid and phenanthrene derivative (hydrocodone), sympathomimetic amine (pseudoephedrine), glyceryl guaiacolate (guaifenesin)
Therapeutic: Antihistamine (chlorpheniramine), antitussive (hydrocodone), decongestant (pseudoephedrine), expectorant (guaifenesin)
Pregnancy category: C
Controlled substance: Schedule III

Indications and Dosages

▶ *To relieve cough and upper respiratory symptoms of colds and allergies*

ORAL SOLUTION

Adults. 4 mg chlorpheniramine, 5 mg hydrocodone, 30 mg pseudoephedrine, and 200 mg guaifenesin (10 ml) q 4 to 6 hr.

Mechanism of Action

Chlorpheniramine competes with histamine for H_1 receptor sites, thereby antagonizing many histamine effects and reducing allergy signs and symptoms.

Hydrocodone suppresses cough by directly acting on opiate receptors in the medulla's cough center.

Pseudoephedrine acts on alpha$_1$-adrenergic receptors in the mucosa of the respiratory tract to produce vasoconstriction. This process shrinks swollen nasal mucous membranes; reduces tissue hyperemia, edema, and nasal congestion; and increases nasal airway patency. It also may increase drainage of sinus secretions and open obstructed eustachian ostia.

Guaifenesin increases fluid and mucus removal from the upper respiratory tract by increasing the volume of secretions and reducing their adhesiveness and surface tension.

Contraindications

Hypersensitivity or idiosyncratic reactions to chlorpheniramine, hydrocodone, other opioids, pseuodephedrine, guaifenesin, or their components; hyperthyroidism; narrow-angle glaucoma; prostatic hypertrophy; respiratory depression; severe asthma, coronary artery disease or hypertension; upper airway obstruction, urine retention, use of MAO inhibitors within 14 days

Interactions

DRUGS

chlorpheniramine, hydrocodone, and pseudoephedrine

MAO inhibitors: Increased and prolonged cardiac stimulation, increased vasopressor effect, increased risk of severe cardiovascular and cerebrovascular effects, hyperpyrexia, and vomiting

chlorpheniramine and hydrocodone

anticholinergics, paregoric: Possibly intensified adverse anticholinergic effects

CNS depressants: Additive CNS effects

chlorpheniramine component

phenytoin: Possibly increased serum phenytoin level and toxicity

hydrocodone component

antihypertensives, diuretics: Potentiated hypotensive effects

buprenorphine: Decreased hydrocodone effectiveness

hydroxyzine: Increased hydrocodone analgesic effect; increased CNS depressant and hypotensive effects

metoclopramide: Antagonized effect of metoclopramide on GI motility

naloxone: Anatagonized hydrocodone analgesic effect

naltrexone: Precipitated withdrawal symptoms in hydrocodone-dependent patients

neuromuscular blockers: Additive respiratory depressant effects

opioids: Additive CNS and respiratory depressants effects and hypotensive effects

pseudoephedrine component

antacids: Increased pseudoephedrine absorption

antihypertensives, diuretics: Possibly decreased antihypertensive effects

beta blockers: Decreased therapeutic effects of both drugs

citrates: Possibly inhibited urinary excretion and prolonged duration of pseudoephedrine action

CNS stimulant, other sympathomimetics: Possibly increased additive CNS stimulation to excessive levels

cocaine (mucosal-local): Possibly increased cardiovascular effects of either drug and CNS stimulation

digoxin, levodopa: Increased risk of cardiac arrhythmias

hydrocarbon inhalation anesthetics: Increased risk of serious arrhythmias

kaolin: Decreased pseudoephedrine absorption

nitrates: Reduced antianginal effects of nitrates
rauwolfia alkaloids: Possibly inhibited pseudoephedrine action
thyroid hormones: Increased cardiovascular effects of both drugs
ACTIVITIES
chlorpheniramine and hydrocodone
alcohol use: Additive CNS effects

Adverse Reactions

CNS: Anxiety, confusion, decreased mental and physical performance, depression, dizziness, drowsiness, euphoria, faintness, fear, headache, insomnia, light-headedness, mood changes, nervousness, restlessness, sedation, seizures, tiredness, trembling, weakness
CV: Angina, arrhythmia exacerbation, bradycardia, chest tightness, hypotension, palpitations, tachycardia
EENT: Blurred or double vision, dry mouth, laryngeal edema, laryngospasm, photophobia
GI: Anorexia, constipation, nausea, paralytic ileus, toxic megacolon, vomiting
GU: Dysuria, frequent urination, urine retention
RESP: Dyspnea, shortness of breath, slow or irregular breathing, wheezing
Skin: Diaphoresis, facial flushing, pallor, pruritis, rash, uriticaria
Other: Angioedema, atelectasis, mental or physical dependence

Nursing Considerations

• Use cautiously in patients with a recent head injury and in those with Addison's disease, asthma or other chronic respiratory disease, increased intraocular pressure, or liver or renal impairment.
• Monitor patients who may be more susceptible to dizziness, sedation, and hypotension, such as the elderly.
• Monitor renal function, as ordered, because pseudoephedrine is substantially excreted by the kidneys.
• Regularly evaluate effectiveness of chlorpheniramine, hydrocodone, pseudoephedrine, and guaifenesin in reducing symptoms.
• Be aware that patient shouldn't have intradermal allergen tests within 72 hours of receiving drug because results may be altered.
PATIENT TEACHING
• Instruct patient to use a calibrated measuring device to ensure accurate dose.

- Urge patient to avoid alcohol and other antidepressants while taking chlorpheniramine, hydrocodone, pseudoephedrine, and guaifenesin.
- Instruct patient to avoid potentially hazardous activities until drug's CNS effects are known.
- Suggest that patient relieve dry mouth with frequent rinsing and use of sugarless gum or hard candy.
- Tell patient to take last dose of the day a few hours before bedtime if chlorpheniramine, hydrocodone, pseudoephedrine, and guaifenesin makes him nervous or restless.

chlorpheniramine maleate and pseudoephedrine hydrochloride
Amerifed, Anaplex, Atrohist Pediatric, Biohist-LA, Chlordrine S.R., Chlorfed-A, Chlor-Trimeton Allergy Decongestant, Codimal LA, Colfed-A, Deconamine, Deconamine SR, Deconomed SR, Dura-Tap PD, Histade, Histex, Kronofed-A, Kronofed-A Jr., ND Clear, ND Clear T.D., Novafed A, Pseudo-Chlor, Rescon, Rescon-ED, Rescon-JR, Rinade B.I.D. Capsules, Ryna, Sudafed Cold & Allergy, Time-Hist

chlorpheniramine tannate and pseudoephedrine tannate
C-PHED, CP-TANNIC, Tanafed

Class and Category
Chemical: Alkylamine (chlorpheniramine), sympathomimetic amine (pseudoephedrine)
Therapeutic: Antihistamine (chlorpheniramine), decongestant (pseudoephedrine)
Pregnancy category: C

Indications and Dosages
▶ *To relieve persistent runny nose, sneezing, and nasal congestion caused by upper respiratory infections, sinus inflammation, or hay fever; to relieve sinus pressure and drain sinuses*
SYRUP
Adults and children age 12 and over. 2 to 4 mg chlorpheniramine and 30 to 60 mg pseudoephedrine (5 to 10 ml) q 6 to 8 hr.
Children ages 6 to 12. 1 to 2 mg chlorpheniramine and 15 to 30 mg pseudoephedrine (2.5 to 5 ml) q 6 to 8 hr.

Children ages 2 to 6. 1 mg chlorpheniramine and 15 mg pseudoephedrine (2.5 ml) q 6 to 8 hr.

ORAL SOLUTION

Adults. 4 mg chlorpheniramine and 60 mg pseudoephedrine (10 ml) q 4 to 6 hr. Alternatively, 4 mg chlorpheniramine and 80 mg pseudoephedrine (5 ml) q 8 hr.

SUSPENSION (TANNATE)

Adults and children age 12 and over. 9 to 18 mg chlorpheniramine and 150 to 300 mg pseudoephedrine (10 to 20 ml) q 12 hr.

Children ages 6 to 12. 4.5 to 9 mg chlorpheniramine and 75 to 150 mg pseudoephedrine (5 to 10 ml) q 12 hr.

Children ages 2 to 6. 2.25 to 4.5 mg chlorpheniramine and 37.5 to 75 mg pseudoephedrine (2.5 to 5 ml) q 12 hr.

TABLETS

Adults. 4 mg chlorpheniramine and 60 mg pseudoephedrine (1 tablet) q 4 to 8 hr. *Maximum:* 4 doses daily.

E.R. TABLETS

Adults. 6 to 12 mg chlorpheniramine and 60 to 120 mg pseudoephedrine (½ to 1 tablet depending on product) q 12 hr.

E.R. CAPSULES

Adults and children age 12 and over. 4 to 8 mg chlorpheniramine and 60 to 120 mg pseudoephedrine (1 or 2 capsules depending on product) q 12 hr.

Children ages 6 to 12. 4 mg chlorpheniramine and 60 mg pseudoephedrine (1 capsule) q 12 hr.

Mechanism of Action

Chlorpheniramine competes with histamine for H_1 receptor sites, thereby antagonizing many histamine effects and reducing allergy signs and symptoms.

Pseudoephedrine acts on $alpha_1$-adrenergic receptors in the mucosa of the respiratory tract to produce vasoconstriction. This process shrinks swollen nasal mucous membranes; reduces tissue hyperemia, edema, and nasal congestion; and increases nasal airway patency. It also may increase drainage of sinus secretions and open obstructed eustachian ostia.

Contraindications

Breastfeeding; hypersensitivity or idiosyncractic reactions to chlorpheniramine, pseudoephedrine, or their components; hyperthyroidism; narrow-angle glaucoma; severe coronary artery disease or hypertension; urine retention; use within 14 days of MAO inhibitor therapy

Interactions
DRUGS
chlorpheniramine and pseudoephedrine
MAO inhibitors: Increased and prolonged cardiac stimulation, increased vasopressor effect, increased risk of severe cardiovascular and cerebrovascular effects, hyperpyrexia, and vomiting
chlorpheniramine component
anticholinergics: Additive anticholinergic effects
CNS depressants: Additive CNS effects
phenytoin: Possibly increased serum phenytoin levels and toxicity
pseudoephedrine component
antacids: Increased pseudoephedrine absorption
antihypertensives, diuretics: Possibly decreased antihypertensive effects
beta blockers: Decreased therapeutic effects of both drugs
citrates: Possibly inhibited urinary excretion and prolonged duration of pseudoephedrine action
CNS stimulant, other sympathomimetics: Possibly increased additive CNS stimulation to excessive levels
cocaine (mucosal-local): Possibly increased cardiovascular effects of either drug and CNS stimulation
digoxin, levodopa: Increased risk of cardiac arrhythmias
hydrocarbon inhalation anesthetics: Increased risk of serious arrhythmias
kaolin: Decreased pseudoephedrine absorption
nitrates: Reduced antianginal effects of nitrates
rauwolfia alkaloids: Possibly inhibited pseudoephedrine action
thyroid hormones: Increased cardiovascular effects of both drugs
ACTIVITIES
chlorpheniramine component
alcohol use: Additive CNS effects

Adverse Reactions
CNS: Anxiety, chills, confusion, coordination disturbance, dizziness, drowsiness, excitation (children), fatigue, fear, hallucinations, headache, hysteria, insomnia, irritability, light-headedness, nervousness, numbness, restlessness, sedation, seizures, tenseness, trembling, vertigo, weakness
CV: Arrhythmias, chest tightness, hypotension, palpitations, tachycardia
EENT: Blurred or double vision; dry mouth, nose, and throat; nasal congestion, tinnitus
ENDO: Early menstruation

GI: Anorexia, constipation, diarrhea, nausea, stomach upset or pain, vomiting
GU: Dysuria, frequent urination, urinary hesitancy or retention
HEME: Anemia, unusual bleeding or bruising
RESP: Dyspnea, increased chest congestion, wheezing
SKIN: Diaphoresis, pallor, photosensitivity, rash, urticaria
Other: Anaphylaxis

Nursing Considerations

• Use cautiously in patients with asthma, cardiovascular disease, diabetes, emphysema or other chronic lung disease, hypertension, peptic ulcer, narrow-angle glaucoma, or prostatic hypertrophy.
• Monitor children for excitation and elderly patients for dizziness, sedation, and hypotension; such patients may have an increased risk for these effects.
• Monitor renal function, as ordered, because pseudoephedrine is substantially excreted by the kidneys.
• Regularly evaluate effectiveness of chlorpheniramine and pseudoephedrine in reducing upper respiratory symptoms regularly.
• Be aware that patient shouldn't have intradermal allergen tests within 72 hours of receiving drug because results may be altered.

PATIENT TEACHING
• Instruct patient to use a calibrated measuring device when using syrup form of chlorpheniramine and pseudoephedrine to ensure accurate dose.
• Urge patient to avoid alcohol and other antidepressants while taking chlorpheniramine and pseudoephedrine.
• Instruct patient to avoid potentially hazardous activities until drug's CNS effects are known.
• Suggest that patient relieve dry mouth with frequent rinsing and use of sugarless gum or hard candy.
• Tell patient to take last dose of the day a few hours before bedtime if chlorpheniramine and pseudoephedrine makes her nervous or restless.

chlorpheniramine maleate, pseudoephedrine hydrochloride, and methscopolamine nitrate

CPM 8/PSE 90/MSC 2.5, Durahist, Mescolor, Pannaz, Rescon-MX, Xiral

Class and Category

Chemical: Alkylamine (chlorpheniramine), sympathomimetic amine (pseudoephedrine), hyoscine methobromide (methscopolamine)

Therapeutic: Antihistamine (chlorpheniramine), decongestant (pseudoephedrine), anticholingeric (methscopolamine)

Pregnancy category: C

Indications and Dosages

▶ *To relieve persistent runny nose, sneezing, and nasal congestion caused by upper respiratory infections, sinus inflammation, or hay fever; to relieve sinus pressure and drain sinuses*

E.R. TABLETS

Adults. 8 mg chlorpheniramine, 120 mg pseudoephedrine, and 2.5 mg methscopolamine (1 tablet) q 12 hr. *Maximum:* 16 mg chlorpheniramine, 240 mg pseudoephedrine, and 5 mg methscopolamine in 24 hr.

Children ages 6 to 12. 4 mg chlorpheniramine, 60 mg pseudoephedrine, and 1.25 mg methscopolamine (½ tablet) q 12 hr. *Maximum:* 8 mg chlorpheniramine, 120 mg pseudoephedrine, and 2.5 mg methscopolamine in 24 hr.

Mechanism of Action

Chlorpheniramine competes with histamine for H_1 receptor sites, thereby antagonizing many histamine effects and reducing allergy signs and symptoms.

Pseudoephedrine acts on $alpha_1$-adrenergic receptors in the mucosa of the respiratory tract to produce vasoconstriction. This process shrinks swollen nasal mucous membranes; reduces tissue hyperemia, edema, and nasal congestion; and increases nasal airway patency. It also may increase drainage of sinus secretions and open obstructed eustachian ostia.

Methscopolamine competitively inhibits acetylcholine at autonomic postganglionic cholinergic receptors. Because the most sensitive receptors are in salivary, bronchial, and sweat glands, this action reduces secretions from these glands. It also reduces nasal, oropharyngeal, and bronchial secretions and decreases airway resistance by relaxing smooth muscles in the bronchi and bronchioles.

Contraindications

Breastfeeding; cardiac disease such as arrhythmias, congestive heart failure, coronary artery disease, severe hypertension, and mitral stenosis; hemorrhage with hemodynamic instability; hepatic dysfunction; hypersensitivity or idiosyncractic reactions to chlorpheniramine, pseudoephedrine, methscopolamine, or their components; hyperthyroidism; ileus; intestinal atony; myasthenia gravis; narrow-angle glaucoma; obstructive GI or uropathic disease; prostatic hypertrophy; renal impairment; toxic megacolon; ulcerative colitis; urine retention; use within 14 days of MAO inhibitor therapy

Interactions

DRUGS

chlorpheniramine and pseudoephedrine

MAO inhibitors: Increased and prolonged cardiac stimulation, increased vasopressor effect, increased risk of severe cardiovascular and cerebrovascular effects, hyperpyrexia, and vomiting

chlorpheniramine and methscopolamine

anticholinergics: Additive anticholinergic effects
CNS depressants: Additive CNS effects

chlorpheniramine component

phenytoin: Possibly increased serum phenytoin level and toxicity

pseudoephedrine component

antacids: Increased pseudoephedrine absorption
antihypertensives, diuretics: Possibly decreased antihypertensive effects
beta blockers: Decreased therapeutic effects of both drugs
citrates: Possibly inhibited urinary excretion and prolonged duration of pseudoephedrine action
CNS stimulant, other sympathomimetics: Possibly increased additive CNS stimulation to excessive levels
cocaine (mucosal-local): Possibly increased cardiovascular effects of either drug and CNS stimulation
digoxin, levodopa: Increased risk of cardiac arrhythmias
hydrocarbon inhalation anesthetics: Increased risk of serious arrhythmias
kaolin: Decreased pseudoephedrine absorption
nitrates: Reduced antianginal effects of nitrates
rauwolfia alkaloids: Possibly inhibited action of pseudoephedrine
thyroid hormones: Increased cardiovascular effects of both drugs

methscopolamine component

adsorbent antidiarrheals, antacids: Decreased absorption and therapeutic effects of methoscopolamine
antimyasthenics: Possibly reduced intestinal motility
CNS depressants: Possibly potentiated effects of either drug, resulting in additive sedation
haloperidol: Decreased antipsychotic effect of haloperidol

ketoconazole: Decreased ketoconazole absorption
lorazepam (parenteral): Possibly hallucinations, irrational behavior, and sedation
metoclopramide: Possibly antagonized effect of metoclopramide on GI motility
opioid analgesics: Increased risk of severe constipation and ileus
potassium chloride: Possibly increased severity of potassium chloride-induced GI lesions
sildenafil, tadalafil, vardenafil: Possibly increased risk of hypotension
urinary alkalizers (antacids, carbonic anhydrase inhibitors, citrates, sodium bicarbonate): Delayed excretion of methscopolamine, possibly leading to increased therapeutic and adverse effects

ACTIVITIES

chlorpheniramine and methscopolamine
alcohol use: Additive CNS effects

Adverse Reactions

CNS: Anxiety, chills, confusion, coordination disturbance, dizziness, drowsiness, euphoria, fatigue, fear, hallucinations, headache, hysteria, insomnia, irritability, light-headedness, memory loss, nervousness, numbness, paradoxical stimulation, restlessness, sedation, seizures, tenseness, trembling, vertigo, weakness
CV: Arrhythmias, chest tightness, hypotension, palpitations, tachycardia
EENT: Blurred or double vision; dry eyes, mouth, nose, and throat; mydriasis; nasal congestion; tinnitus
ENDO: Early menstruation
GI: Anorexia, constipation, diarrhea, dysphagia, nausea, stomach upset or pain, vomiting
GU: Dysuria, frequent urination, urinary hesitancy or retention
HEME: Anemia, unusual bleeding or bruising
RESP: Dyspnea, increased chest congestion, wheezing
SKIN: Decreased sweating, diaphoresis, dry skin, flushing, pallor, photosensitivity, rash, urticaria
Other: Anaphylaxis

Nursing Considerations

- Use cautiously in patients with asthma, diabetes, emphysema or other chronic lung disease, hypertension, or peptic ulcer.
- Monitor patients who may be more susceptible to dizziness, sedation, and hypotension, such as the elderly.
- Monitor renal function, as ordered, because pseudoephedrine is substantially excreted by the kidneys.

- Regularly evaluate effectiveness of chlorpheniramine, pseudoephedrine, and methscopolamine in reducing upper respiratory symptoms.
- Be aware that patient shouldn't have intradermal allergen tests within 72 hours of receiving drug because results may be altered.

PATIENT TEACHING

- Urge patient to avoid alcohol and other antidepressants while taking chlorpheniramine, pseudoephedrine, and methscopolamine.
- Instruct patient to avoid potentially hazardous activities until drug's CNS effects are known.
- Suggest that patient relieve dry mouth with frequent rinsing and use of sugarless gum or hard candy. Suggest lubricating drops for dry eyes.
- Tell patient to take last dose of the day a few hours before bedtime if chlorpheniramine, pseudoephedrine, and methscopolamine makes him nervous or restless.

chlorpheniramine maleate, pyrilamine maleate, hydrocodone bitartrate, phenylephrine hydrochloride, and pseudoephedrine hydrochloride

Statuss Green

Class, Category, and Schedule

Chemical: Alkylamine (chlorpheniramine), ethylenediamine antihistamine (pyrilamine), opioid and phenanthrene derivative (hydrocodone), sympathomimetic amines (phenylephrine, pseudoephedrine)

Therapeutic: Antihistamines (chlorpheniramine, pyrilamine), antitussive (hydrocodone), decongestants (phenylephrine, pseudoephedrine)

Pregnancy category: C

Controlled substance: Schedule III

Indications and Dosages

▶ *To relieve cough and upper respiratory symptoms of colds and allergies*

ORAL SOLUTION

Adults. 4 mg chlorpheniramine, 6.6 mg pyrilamine, 5 mg hydrocodone, 10 mg phenylephrine, and 6.6 mg pseudoephedrine (10 ml) q 4 to 6 hr. *Maximum:* 40 ml daily.

Mechanism of Action

Chlorpheniramine and pyrilamine competes with histamine for H_1 receptor sites, thereby antagonizing many histamine effects and reducing allergy signs and symptoms.

Hydrocodone suppresses cough by acting directly on opiate receptors in the medulla's cough center.

Phenylephrine stimulates alpha-adrenergic receptors and inhibits the intracellular enzyme adenyl cyclase, which then inhibits production of cAMP. Inhibition of cAMP causes arterial and venous constriction in nasal passages, which decreases blood flow and mucosal edema caused by allergic response.

Pseudoephedrine acts on $alpha_1$-adrenergic receptors in the mucosa of the respiratory tract to produce vasoconstriction. This process shrinks swollen nasal mucous membranes; reduces tissue hyperemia, edema, and nasal congestion; and increases nasal airway patency. It also may increase drainage of sinus secretions and open obstructed eustachian ostia.

Contraindications

Breastfeeding; hypersensitivity or idiosyncractic reactions to chlorpheniramine, pyrilamine, hydrocodone, other opioids, phenylephrine, pseuodephedrine, or their components; hyperthyroidism; narrow-angle glaucoma; prostatic hypertrophy; respiratory depression; severe asthma, coronary artery disease or hypertension; upper airway obstruction; urine retention; use of MAO inhibitors within 14 days

Interactions

DRUGS

chlorpheniramine, pyrilamine, and hydrocodone components

CNS depressants: Additive CNS effects

chlorpheniramine, hydrocodone, and pseudoephedrine components

MAO inhibitors: Increased and prolonged cardiac stimulation, increased vasopressor effect, increased risk of severe cardiovascular and cerebrovascular effects, hyperpyrexia, and vomiting

chlorpheniramine and hydrocodone components

anticholinergics, paregoric: Possibly intensified anticholinergic adverse effects

chlorpheniramine component

phenytoin: Possibly increased serum phenytoin level and toxicity

hydrocodone component

antihypertensives, diuretics: Potentiated hypotensive effects

buprenorphine: Decreased hydrocodone effectiveness
hydroxyzine: Increased hydrocodone analgesic effect; increased CNS depressant and hypotensive effects
metoclopramide: Antagonized effect of metoclopramide on GI motility
naloxone: Anatagonized hydrocodone analgesic effect
naltrexone: Precipitated withdrawal symptoms in hydrocodone-dependent patients
neuromuscular blockers: Additive respiratory depressant effects
opioids: Additive CNS and respiratory depressants effects and hypotensive effects

phenylephrine component
alpha blockers, haloperidol, loxapine, phenothiazines, thioxanthenes: Possibly decreased vasoconstrictor effect of phenylephrine
antihypertenisves, diuretics: Possibly decreased antihypertensive effects
atropine: Possibly enhanced vasopressor effect of phenylephrine
beta blockers: Decreased therapeutic effects of both drugs
bretylium: Possibly potentiated vaopressor effect and arrhythmias
doxapram: Increased vasopressor effect of both drugs
ergot alkaloids: Possibly cerebral blood vessel rupture, increased vasopressor effect, peripheral vascular ischemia, and gangrene (with ergotamine)
guanadrel, guanethidine: Increased vasopressor effect of phenylephrine; increased risk of severe hypertension and arrhythmias
hydrocarbon inhalation anesthetics: Increased risk of serious arrhythmias
maprotiline, tricyclic antidepressants: Increased risk of severe cardiovascular effects (including arrhythmias, hyperpyrexia, severe hypertension)
mecamylamine, methyldopa: Decreased hypotensive effects of these drugs, increased vasopressor effect of phenylephrine
nitrates: Possibly decreased vasopressor effect of phenylephrine and decreased antianginal effect of nitrates
oxytocin: Possibly severe, persistent hypertension
phenoxybenzamine: Decreased vasoconstrictor effect of phenylephrine, possibly hypotension and tachycardia
theophylliine: Possibly enhanced toxicity (including cardiac toxicity)
thyroid hormones: Increased cardiovascular effects of each drug

pseudoephedrine component
antacids: Increased pseudoephedrine absorption
antihypertensives, diuretics: Possibly decreased antihypertensive effects

beta blockers: Decreased therapeutic effects of both drugs
citrates: Possibly inhibited urinary excretion and prolonged duration of action of pseudoephedrine
CNS stimulant, other sympathomimetics: Possibly increased additive CNS stimulation to excessive levels
cocaine (mucosal-local): Possibly increased cardiovascular effects of either drug and CNS stimulation
digoxin, levodopa: Increased risk of cardiac arrhythmias
hydrocarbon inhalation anesthetics: Increased risk of serious arrhythmias
kaolin: Decreased pseudoephedrine absorption
nitrates: Reduced antianginal effects of nitrates
rauwolfia alkaloids: Possibly inhibited pseudoephedrine action
thyroid hormones: Increased cardiovascular effects of both drugs
ACTIVITIES
chlorpheniramine, pyrilamine, and hydrocodone components
alcohol use: Additive CNS effects

Adverse Reactions

CNS: Anxiety, confusion, decreased mental and physical performance, depression, dizziness, drowsiness, euphoria, faintness, fear, headache, insomnia, light-headedness, mood changes, nervousness, paresthesia, restlessness, sedation, seizures, tiredness, trembling, weakness
CV: Angina, bradycardia, chest tightness, hypertension, hypotension, palpitations, tachycardia, ventricular arrhythmias
EENT: Blurred or double vision, dry mouth, laryngeal edema, laryngospasm, photophobia
GI: Anorexia, constipation, nausea, paralytic ileus, toxic megacolon, vomiting
GU: Dysuria, frequent urination, urinary hesitancy or retention
RESP: Dyspnea, shortness of breath, slow or irregular breathing, wheezing
Skin: Diaphoresis, facial flushing, pallor, pruritis, rash, uriticaria
Other: Angioedema, atelectasis, mental or physical dependence

Nursing Considerations

• Use cautiously in patients with a recent head injury and those with Addison's disease, asthma or other chronic respiratory disease, increased intraocular pressure, or liver or renal impairment.
• Monitor patients who may be more susceptible to dizziness, sedation, and hypotension, such as the elderly.

- Monitor renal function, as ordered, because pseudoephedrine is substantially excreted by the kidneys.
- Regularly evaluate effectiveness of chlorpheniramine, pyrilamine, hydrocodone, phenylephrine, and pseudoephedrine in reducing symptoms.
- Be aware that patient shouldn't have intradermal allergen tests within 72 hours of receiving drug because results may be altered.

PATIENT TEACHING
- Instruct patient to use a calibrated measuring device to ensure accurate dose.
- Urge patient to avoid alcohol and other antidepressants while taking drug.
- Instruct patient to avoid potentially hazardous activities until drug's CNS effects are known.
- Suggest that patient relieve dry mouth with frequent rinsing and use of sugarless gum or hard candy.
- Tell patient to take last dose of the day a few hours before bedtime if drug makes her nervous or restless.

codeine polistirex and chlorpheniramine polistirex

Codeprex Pennkinetic

Class, Category, and Schedule

Chemical: Opioid and phenanthrene derivative (codeine), alkylamine (chlorpheniramine)
Therapeutic: Antitussive (codeine), antihistamine (chlorpheniramine),
Pregnancy category: C
Controlled substance: Schedule III

Indications and Dosages

▶ *To relieve cough and upper respiratory symptoms due to hay fever, other upper respiratory allergies, or allergic rhinitis*

E.R. SUSPENSION
Adults and children age 12 and over. 40 mg codeine and 8 mg chlorpheniramine (10 ml) q 12 hr.
Children ages 6 to 12. 20 mg codeine and 4 mg chlorpheniramine (5 ml) q 12 hr.

Contraindications

Breastfeeding; constipation; hypersensitivity to codeine, chlorpheniramine, other opioids or their components; inflammatory bowel disease; prostatic hypertrophy; respiratory depression; severe asthma; upper airway obstruction, use of MAO inhibitors within 14 days

---

Mechanism of Action
Codeine suppresses cough by directly acting on opiate receptors in the medulla's cough center.

Chlorpheniramine competes with histamine for H_1 receptor sites, thereby antagonizing many histamine effects and reducing allergy signs and symptoms.

Interactions
DRUGS
codeine and chlorpheniramine
anticholinergics, paregoric: Possibly intensified adverse anticholinergic effects
CNS depressants: Additive CNS effects
MAO inhibitors: Increased and prolonged cardiac stimulation, increased vasopressor effect, increased risk of severe cardiovascular and cerebrovascular effects, hyperpyrexia, and vomiting
codeine component
antihypertensives, diuretics: Potentiated hypotensive effects
buprenorphine: Decreased codeine effectiveness
hydroxyzine: Increased codeine analgesic effect; increased CNS depressant and hypotensive effects
metoclopramide: Antagonized effect of metoclopramide on GI motility
naloxone: Antagonized codeine analgesic effect
naltrexone: Precipitated withdrawal symptoms in codeine-dependent patients
neuromuscular blockers: Additive respiratory depressant effects
opioids: Additive CNS and respiratory depressants effects and hypotensive effects
tricyclic antidepressants: Possibly increased effect of either the antidepressant or codeine
chlorpheniramine component
phenytoin: Possibly increased serum phenytoin level and toxicity
ACTIVITIES
codeine and chlorpheniramine
alcohol use: Additive CNS effects

Adverse Reactions

CNS: Asthenia, anxiety, confusion, dizziness, depression, drowsiness, dyskinesia, euphoria, excitability (especially in children) faintness, hallucinations, headache, impaired cognition, insomnia, irritability, light-headedness, nervousness, restlessness, sedation, syncope, tiredness, tremor, vertigo, weakness
CV: Bradycardia, hypertension, hypotension, orthostatic hypotension, palpitation, tachycardia
ENDO: Decreased lactation, early menses, gynecomastia, hyperglycemia, hypoglycemia
EENT: Blurred vision; diplopia; dry mouth, pharynx, and respiratory passages; hypermetropia; increased lacrimation; labyrinthitis; laryngismus; mydriasis; nasal stuffiness; photophobia; tinnitus
GI: Abdominal distention or pain, acute pancreatitis, anorexia, constipation, diarrhea, dyspepsia, epigastric distress, esophageal reflux, increased appetite, nausea, vomiting
GU: Decreased or increased libido, dysuria, urinary frequency or hesitancy, urine retention, ureteral spasm
RESP: Dyspnea, respiratory depression, wheezing
SKIN: Dermatitis, diaphoresis, erythema, flushing, pruritus, rash, urticaria
Other: Drug fever, emotional or physical dependence

Nursing Considerations

- Use cautiously in patients with a recent head injury and in those with Addison's disease, asthma or other chronic respiratory disease, increased intraocular pressure, hypothyroidism, or liver or renal impairment.
- **WARNING** Monitor respiratory function because codeine and chlorpheniramine may suppress the cough reflex and cause thickening of bronchial secretions, aggravating such conditions as asthma and COPD and, in rare cases, may depress respirations and induce apnea. Notify prescriber immediately if respiratory rate drops below 10 breaths/minute.
- Monitor children for excitation and elderly patients for dizziness, sedation, and hypotension; such patients may have an increased risk for these effects.
- Regularly evaluate effectiveness of codeine and chlorpheniramine in reducing symptoms.
- Be aware that patient shouldn't have intradermal allergen tests within 72 hours of receiving drug because results may be altered.

PATIENT TEACHING
- Instruct patient to shake suspension well before measuring dose and to use a calibrated device to ensure accurate dose.
- Tell patient that codeine and chlorpheniramine must not be diluted with fluids or mixed with other drugs.
- Urge patient to avoid alcohol and other antidepressants while taking codeine and chlorpheniramine.
- Instruct patient to avoid potentially hazardous activities until drug's CNS effects are known.
- Suggest that patient relieve dry mouth with frequent rinsing and use of sugarless gum or hard candy.
- Tell patient to take last dose of the day a few hours before bedtime if codeine and chlorpheniramine makes him nervous or restless.

codeine phosphate, chlorpheniramine maleate, and pseudoephedrine sulfate

Decohistine DH, Dihistine DH, Novahistine DH, Ryna-C

Class, Category, and Schedule

Chemical: Opioid and phenanthrene derivative (codeine), alkylamine (chlorpheniramine), sympathomimetic amine (pseudoephedrine)

Therapeutic: Antitussive (codeine), antihistamine (chlorpheniramine), decongestant (pseudoephedrine)

Pregnancy category: C

Controlled substance: Schedule V

Indications and Dosages

▶ *To relieve cough and upper respiratory symptoms of hay fever, other upper respiratory allergies, and allergic rhinitis*

ELIXIR, ORAL SOLUTION

Adults and children age 12 and over. 10 to 20 mg codeine, 2 to 4 mg chlorpheniramine, and 30 to 60 mg pseudoephedrine (5 to 10 ml depending on product) q 4 to 6 hr. *Maximum:* 40 ml daily.

Children ages 6 to 12. 10 mg codeine, 2 mg chlorpheniramine, and 30 mg peudoephedrine (5 ml) q 6 hr.

Contraindications

Constipation; hypersensitivity or idiosyncractic reactions to codeine, chlorpheniramine, other opioids, pseudoephedrine, or their components; hyperthyroidism; inflammatory bowel disease;

narrow-angle glaucoma; prostatic hypertrophy; respiratory depression; severe asthma, coronary artery disease or hypertension; upper airway obstruction, urine retention; use of MAO inhibitors within 14 days

---

Mechanism of Action

Codeine suppresses cough by directly acting on opiate receptors in the medulla's cough center.

Chlorpheniramine competes with histamine for H_1 receptor sites, thereby antagonizing many histamine effects and reducing allergy signs and symptoms.

Pseudoephedrine acts on alpha$_1$-adrenergic receptors in the mucosa of the respiratory tract to produce vasoconstriction. This process shrinks swollen nasal mucous membranes; reduces tissue hyperemia, edema, and nasal congestion; and increases nasal airway patency. It also may increase drainage of sinus secretions and open obstructed eustachian ostia.

Interactions

DRUGS

codeine, chlorpheniramine, and pseudoephedrine

MAO inhibitors: Increased and prolonged cardiac stimulation, increased vasopressor effect, increased risk of severe cardiovascular and cerebrovascular effects, hyperpyrexia, vomiting

codeine and chlorpheniramine

anticholinergics, paregoric: Possibly intensified anticholinergic adverse effects

CNS depressants: Additive CNS effects

ACTIVITIES

alcohol use: Additive CNS effects

codeine component

antihypertensives, diuretics: Potentiated hypotensive effects

buprenorphine: Decreased codeine effectiveness

hydroxyzine: Increased codeine analgesic effect; increased CNS depressant and hypotensive effects

metoclopramide: Antagonized effect of metoclopramide on GI motility

naloxone: Antagonized codeine analgesic effect

naltrexone: Precipitated withdrawal symptoms in codeine-dependent patients

neuromuscular blockers: Additive respiratory depressant effects

opioids: Additive CNS and respiratory depressants effects and hypotensive effects

tricyclic antidepressants: Possibly increased effect of either the antidepressant or codeine

chlorpheniramine component

phenytoin: Possibly increased serum phenytoin levels and toxicity

pseudoephedrine component

antacids: Increased absorption of pseudoephedrine

antihypertensives, diuretics: Possibly decreased antihypertensive effects

beta blockers: Decreased therapeutic effects of both drugs

citrates: Possibly inhibited urinary excretion and prolonged duration of pseudoephedrine action

CNS stimulant, other sympathomimetics: Possibly increased additive CNS stimulation to excessive levels

cocaine (mucosal-local): Possibly increased cardiovascular effects of either drug and CNS stimulation

digoxin, levodopa: Increased risk of cardiac arrhythmias

hydrocarbon inhalation anesthetics: Increased risk of serious arrhythmias

kaolin: Decreased pseudoephedrine absorption

nitrates: Reduced antianginal effects of nitrates

rauwolfia alkaloids: Possibly inhibited action of pseudoephedrine

thyroid hormones: Increased cardiovascular effects of both drugs

Adverse Reactions

CNS: Asthenia, anxiety, confusion, dizziness, depression, drowsiness, dyskinesia, euphoria, excitability, faintness, hallucinations, headache, impaired cognition, insomnia, irritability, light-headedness, nervousness, restlessness, sedation, syncope, tiredness, tremor, vertigo, weakness

CV: Bradycardia, hypertension, hypotension, orthostatic hypotension, palpitation, tachycardia

ENDO: Decreased lactation, early menses, gynecomastia, hyperglycemia, hypoglycemia

EENT: Blurred vision; diplopia; dry mouth, pharynx, and respiratory passages; hypermetropia; increased lacrimation; labyrinthitis; laryngismus; mydriasis; nasal stuffiness; photophobia; tinnitus

GI: Abdominal distention or pain, acute pancreatitis, anorexia, constipation, diarrhea, dyspepsia, epigastric distress, esophageal reflux, increased appetite, nausea, vomiting

GU: Decreased or increased libido, dysuria, urinary frequency or hesitancy, urine retention, ureteral spasm

RESP: Dyspnea, respiratory depression, wheezing

SKIN: Dermatitis, diaphoresis, erythema, flushing, pallor, pruritus, rash, urticaria
Other: Drug fever, emotional or physical dependence

Nursing Considerations

- Use cautiously in patients with a recent head injury and those with Addison's disease, asthma or other chronic respiratory disease, increased intraocular pressure, or liver or renal impairment.
- **WARNING** Monitor respiratory function because codeine, chlorpheniramine, and pseudoephedrine may suppress the cough reflex and cause thickening of bronchial secretions, aggravating such conditions as asthma and COPD. In rare cases, it may depress respirations and induce apnea. Notify prescriber immediately if respiratory rate drops below 10 breaths/minute.
- Monitor patients who may be more susceptible to dizziness, sedation, and hypotension, such as the elderly.
- Monitor renal function, as ordered, because pseudoephedrine is substantially excreted by the kidneys.
- Regularly evaluate effectiveness of codeine, chlorpheniramine, and pseudoephedrine in reducing symptoms.
- Be aware that patient shouldn't have intradermal allergen tests within 72 hours of receiving drug because results may be altered.

PATIENT TEACHING

- Explain that codeine, chlorpheniramine, and pseudoephedrine must not be diluted with fluids or mixed with other drugs.
- Urge patient to avoid alcohol and other antidepressants while taking codeine, chlorpheniramine, and pseudoephedrine.
- Instruct patient to avoid potentially hazardous activities until drug's CNS effects are known.
- Suggest that patient relieve dry mouth with frequent rinsing and use of sugarless gum or hard candy.
- Tell patient to take last dose of the day a few hours before bedtime if codeine, chlorpheniramine, and pseudoephedrine makes her nervous or restless.

codeine phosphate, phenylephrine hydrochloride, and pyrilamine maleate
Codimal PH

Class, Category, and Schedule
Chemical: Opioid and phenanthrene derivative (codeine), sympa-

thomimetic amine (phenylephrine), ethylenediamine antihistamine (pyrilamine)

Therapeutic: Antitussive (codeine), decongestant (phenylephrine), antihistaminic (pyrilamine)

Pregnancy category: C

Schedule Category: V

Indications and Dosages

▶ *To relieve cough and upper respiratory symptoms of hay fever, other upper respiratory allergies, allergic rhinitis, and the common cold*

SYRUP

Adults. 10 to 20 mg codeine, 5 to 10 mg phenylephrine and 8.33 to 16.66 mg pyrilamine (5 to 10 ml) q 4 to 6 hr.

Children ages 6 to 12. 10 mg codeine, 5 mg phenylephrine, and 8.33 mg pyrilamine (5 ml) q 4 to 6 hr.

Mechanism of Action

Codeine suppresses cough by directly acting on opiate receptors in the medulla's cough center.

Phenylephrine stimulates alpha-adrenergic receptors and inhibits the intracellular enzyme adenyl cyclase, which then inhibits production of cAMP. Inhibition of cAMP causes arterial and venous constriction in nasal passages, which decreases blood flow and mucosal edema caused by allergic response.

Pyrilamine competes with histamine for H_1 receptor sites, thereby antagonizing many histamine effects to reduce allergy signs and symptoms.

Contraindications

Acute MI; angina; arrhythmias; breastfeeding, coronary artery disease; hypersensitivity to codeine, other opioids, phenylephrine, pyrilamine, or their components; irritable bowel syndrome; paralytic ileus; prostatic hypertrophy; respiratory depression; severe asthma; upper airway obstruction; use of MAO inhibitors within 14 days

Interactions

DRUGS

codeine and phenylephrine

MAO inhibitors: Increased and prolonged cardiac stimulation, increased vasopressor effect, increased risk of severe cardiovascular and cerebrovascular effects, hyperpyrexia, and vomiting

codeine and pyrilamine

anticholinergics, paregoric: Possibly intensified anticholinergic adverse effects

CNS depressants: Additive CNS effects
codeine component
antihypertensives, diuretics: Potentiated hypotensive effects
antidiarrheals: Increased risk of severe constipation
buprenorphine: Decreased codeine effectiveness
hydroxyzine: Increased codeine analgesic effect; increased CNS depressant and hypotensive effects
metoclopramide: Antagonized effect of metoclopramide on GI motility
naloxone: Antagonized codeine analgesic effect
naltrexone: Precipitated withdrawal symptoms in codeine-dependent patients
neuromuscular blockers: Additive respiratory depressant effects
opioids: Additive CNS and respiratory depressants effects and hypotensive effects
tricyclic antidepressants: Possibly increased effect of either the antidepressant or codeine
phenylephrine component
alpha blockers, haloperidol, loxapine, phenothiazines, thioxanthenes: Possibly decreased vasoconstrictor effect of phenylephrine
antihypertenisves, diuretics: Possibly decreased antihypertensive effects
atropine: Possibly enhanced vasopressor effect of phenylephrine
beta blockers: Decreased therapeutic effects of both drugs
bretylium: Possibly potentiated vaopressor effect and arrhythmias
doxapram: Increased vasopressor effect of both drugs
ergot alkaloids: Possibly cerebral blood vessel rupture, increased vasopressor effect, peripheral vascular ischemia, and gangrene (with ergotamine)
guanadrel, guanethidine: Increased vasopressor effect of phenylephrine; increased risk of severe hypertension and arrhythmias
hydrocarbon inhalation anesthetics: Increased risk of serious arrhythmias
maprotiline, tricyclic antidepressants: Increased risk of severe cardiovascular effects (including arrhythmias, hyperpyrexia, severe hypertension)
mecamylamine, methyldopa: Decreased hypotensive effects of these drugs; increased vasopressor effect of phenylephrine
nitrates: Possibly decreased vasopressor effect of phenylephrine and decreased antianginal effect of nitrates
oxytocin: Possibly severe, persistent hypertension
phenoxybenzamine: Decreased vasoconstrictor effect of phenylephrine; possibly hypotension and tachycardia

theophylline: Possibly enhanced toxicity (including cardiac toxicity)
thyroid hormones: Increased cardiovascular effects of each drug
ACTIVITIES
codeine and pyrilamine
alcohol use: Additive CNS effects

Adverse Reactions

CNS: Asthenia, anxiety, confusion, dizziness, depression, drowsiness, dyskinesia, euphoria, faintness, headache, insomnia, irritability, light-headedness, nervousness, paresthesia, restlessness, sedation, syncope, tiredness, tremor, vertigo, weakness
CV: Angina, bradycardia, hypertension, hypotension, orthostatic hypotension, palpitations, peripheral vasoconstriction that may lead to necrosis or gangrene, tachycardia, ventricular arrhythmias
ENDO: Decreased lactation, early menses, gynecomastia, hyperglycemia, hypoglycemia
EENT: Blurred vision; diplopia; dry mouth, pharynx, and respiratory passages; hypermetropia; increased lacrimation; labyrinthitis; laryngismus; mydriasis; nasal stuffiness; photophobia; tinnitus
GI: Abdominal distention or pain, acute pancreatitis, anorexia, constipation, diarrhea, dyspepsia, epigastric distress, esophageal reflux, increased appetite, nausea, vomiting
GU: Dysuria, increased libido, urinary frequency or hesitancy, urine retention, ureteral spasm
RESP: Dyspnea, respiratory depression, wheezing
SKIN: Dermatitis, diaphoresis, erythema, flushing, pruritus, rash, urticaria
Other: Drug fever, emotional or physical dependence

Nursing Considerations

- Use cautiously in patients with recent head injury and in those with Addison's disease, asthma or other chronic respiratory disease, cardiovascular disease, diabetes, hypertension, liver or renal impairment, narrow-angle glaucoma, or thyroid imbalance.
- **WARNING** Monitor respiratory function because codeine, phenylephrine, and pyrilamine may suppress the cough reflex and cause thickening of bronchial secretions, aggravating such conditions as asthma and COPD. In rare cases, it may depress respirations and induce apnea. Notify prescriber immediately if respiratory rate drops below 10 breaths/minute.
- Monitor patients who may be more susceptible to dizziness, sedation, and hypotension, such as the elderly.
- Regularly evaluate effectiveness of codeine, phenylephrine, and pyrilamine in reducing cough and upper respiratory symptoms.

- Be aware that patient shouldn't undergo have allergen tests within 72 hours of receiving drug because results may be altered.

PATIENT TEACHING

- Instruct patient to use a calibrated measuring device to ensure accurate dose.
- Urge patient to avoid alcohol and other antidepressants while taking codeine, phenylephrine, and pyrilamine.
- Instruct patient to avoid potentially hazardous activities until drug's CNS effects are known.
- Suggest that patient relieve dry mouth with frequent rinsing and use of sugarless gum or hard candy.
- Tell patient to take last dose of the day a few hours before bedtime if codeine, phenylephrine, and pyrilamine makes him nervous or restless.

codeine phosphate and pseudoephedrine hydrochloride

Cycofed, Nucofed

Class, Category, and Schedule

Chemical: Opioid and phenanthrene derivative (codeine), sympathomimetic amine (pseudoephedrine)

Therapeutic: Antitussive (codeine), decongestant (pseudoephedrine)

Pregnancy category: C

Controlled substance: Schedule III

Indications and Dosages

▶ *To relieve cough and other symptoms of allergies and the common cold*

CAPSULES

Adults. 20 mg codeine and 60 mg pseudoephedrine (1 capsule) q 6 hr.

SYRUP

Adults and children age 12 and over. 20 mg codeine and 60 mg pseudoephedrine (5 ml) q 6 hr.

Children ages 6 to 12. 10 mg codeine and 30 mg pseudoephedrine (2.5 ml) q 6 hr.

Children ages 2 to 6. 5 mg codeine and 15 mg pseudoephedrine (1.25 ml) q 6 hr.

Contraindications

Hypersensitivity or idiosyncractic reactions to codeine, other opioids, pseudoephedrine, or their components; hyperthyroidism; irritable bowel syndrome; narrow-angle glaucoma; paralytic ileus; prostatic hypertrophy; respiratory depression; severe asthma, coronary artery disease, or hypertension; upper airway obstruction; urine retention; use of MAO inhibitors within 14 days

Mechanism of Action

Codeine suppresses cough by directly acting on opiate receptors in the medulla's cough center.

Pseudoephedrine acts on $alpha_1$-adrenergic receptors in the mucosa of the respiratory tract to produce vasoconstriction. This process shrinks swollen nasal mucous membranes; reduces tissue hyperemia, edema, and nasal congestion; and increases nasal airway patency. It also may increase drainage of sinus secretions and open obstructed eustachian ostia.

Interactions

DRUGS

codeine and pseudoephedrine

MAO inhibitors: Increased and prolonged cardiac stimulation, increased vasopressor effect, increased risk of severe cardiovascular and cerebrovascular effects, hyperpyrexia, and vomiting

codeine component

anticholinergics, paregoric: Possibly intensified anticholinergic adverse effects

antidiarrheals: Increased risk for severe constipation

antihypertensives, diuretics: Potentiated hypotensive effects

buprenorphine: Decreased codeine effectiveness

CNS depressants: Additive CNS effects

hydroxyzine: Increased codeine analgesic effect; increased CNS depressant and hypotensive effects

metoclopramide: Antagonized effect of metoclopramide on GI motility

naloxone: Antagonized codeine analgesic effect

naltrexone: Precipitated withdrawal symptoms in codeine-dependent patients

neuromuscular blockers: Additive respiratory depressant effects

opioids: Additive CNS and respiratory depressants effects and hypotensive effects

tricyclic antidepressants: Possibly increased effect of either the antidepressant or codeine

pseudoephedrine component

antacids: Increased pseudoephedrine absorption

antihypertensives, diuretics: Possibly decreased antihypertensive effects

beta blockers: Decreased therapeutic effects of both drugs

citrates: Possibly inhibited urinary pseudoephedrine excretion and prolonged duration of action

CNS stimulant, other sympathomimetics: Possibly increased additive CNS stimulation to excessive levels

cocaine (mucosal-local): Possibly increased cardiovascular effects of either drug and CNS stimulation

digoxin, levodopa: Increased risk of cardiac arrhythmias

hydrocarbon inhalation anesthetics: Increased risk of serious arrhythmias

kaolin: Decreased pseudoephedrine absorption

nitrates: Reduced antianginal effects of nitrates

rauwolfia alkaloids: Possibly inhibited action of pseudoephedrine

thyroid hormones: Increased cardiovascular effects of both drugs

ACTIVITIES

codeine component

alcohol use: Additive CNS effects

Adverse Reactions

CNS: Confusion, dizziness, drowsiness, euphoria, faintness, hallucinations, headache, insomnia, lack of coordination, lethargy, light-headedness, nervousness, restlessness, seizures, tiredness, trembling, weakness

CV: Angina, bradycardia, hypertension, hypotension, palpitations, tachycardia

EENT: Blurred or double vision, dry mouth, laryngeal edema, laryngospasm

GI: Abdominal cramps or pain, anorexia, constipation, nausea, paralytic ileus, toxic megacolon, vomiting

GU: Decreased libido, dysuria, frequent urination, impotence

RESP: Dyspnea, respiratory depression, shortness of breath, slow or irregular breathing, wheezing

Skin: Diaphoresis, facial flushing, pallor, pruritis, rash, uriticaria

Other: Angioedema, atelectasis

Nursing Considerations

- Use cautiously in patients with hypertension, diabetes mellitus, ischemic heart disease, increased intraocular pressure, or renal impairment because of pseudoephedrine component.
- **WARNING** Monitor respiratory function because codeine may suppress the cough reflex and cause thickening of bronchial secretions, aggravating such conditions as asthma

and COPD. In rare cases, it may depress respirations and induce apnea. Notify prescriber immediately if respiratory rate drops below 10 breaths/minute.

- Monitor renal function, as ordered, because pseudoephedrine is substantially excreted by the kidneys.
- Regularly evaluate effectiveness of codeine and pseudoephedrine in reducing cough and allergy symptoms.

PATIENT TEACHING

- Instruct patient to use a calibrated measuring device to ensure accurate dose of codeine and pseudoephedrine.
- Urge patient to avoid alcohol and other antidepressants while taking codeine and pseudoephedrine.
- Instruct patient to avoid potentially hazardous activities until drug's CNS effects are known.
- Suggest that patient relieve dry mouth with frequent rinsing and use of sugarless gum or hard candy.
- Tell patient to take last dose of the day a few hours before bedtime if codeine and pseudoephedrine makes her nervous or restless.

codeine phosphate, triprolidine hydrochloride, and pseudoephedrine hydrochloride

Triacin-C, Triafed w/Codeine

Class, Category, and Schedule

Chemical: Opioid and phenanthrene derivative (codeine), alkylamine antihistamine (triprolidine), sympathomimetic amine (pseudoephedrine)
Therapeutic: Antitussive (codeine), antihistamine (triprolidine), decongestant (pseudoephedrine)
Pregnancy category: C
Controlled substance: Schedule V

Indications and Dosages

▶ *To relieve cough and upper respiratory symptoms of hay fever, other upper respiratory allergies, and allergic rhinitis*

SYRUP

Adults and children age 12 and over. 20 mg codeine, 2.5 mg triprolidine, and 60 mg pseudoephedrine (10 ml) q 4 to 6 hr.
Children ages 6 to 12. 10 mg codeine, 1.25 mg triprolidine, and 30 mg pseudoephedrine (5 ml) q 4 to 6 hr.

Children age 2 to 6. 5 mg codeine, 0.625 mg triprolidine, and 15 mg pseudoephedrine (2.5 ml) q 4 to 6 hr.

Mechanism of Action

Codeine suppresses cough by directly acting on opiate receptors in the medulla's cough center.

Triprolidine competes with histamine for H_1 receptor sites, thereby antagonizing many histamine effects and reducing allergy signs and symptoms.

Pseudoephedrine acts on $alpha_1$-adrenergic receptors in the mucosa of the respiratory tract to produce vasoconstriction. This process shrinks swollen nasal mucous membranes; reduces tissue hyperemia, edema, and nasal congestion; and increases nasal airway patency. It also may increase drainage of sinus secretions and open obstructed eustachian ostia.

Contraindications

Acute MI; angina; hypersensitivity or idiosyncractic reactions to codeine, other opioids, triprolidine, pseudoephedrine, or their components; hyperthyroidism; narrow-angle glaucoma; paralytic ileus; prostatic hypertrophy; respiratory depression; severe asthma, corornary artery disease or hypertension; upper airway obstruction, urine retention; use of MAO inhibitors within 14 days

Interactions

DRUGS

codeine and pseudoephedrine

MAO inhibitors: Increased and prolonged cardiac stimulation, increased vasopressor effect, increased risk of severe cardiovascular and cerebrovascular effects, hyperpyrexia, and vomiting

codeine and triprolidine

anticholinergics, paregoric: Possibly intensified anticholinergic adverse effects

CNS depressants: Additive CNS effects

codeine component

antihypertensives, diuretics: Potentiated hypotensive effects

antidiarrheals: Increased risk of severe constipation

buprenorphine: Decreased codeine effectiveness

hydroxyzine: Increased codeine analgesic effect; increased CNS depressant and hypotensive effects

metoclopramide: Antagonized effect of metoclopramide on GI motility

naloxone: Anatagonized codeine analgesic effect

naltrexone: Precipitated withdrawal symptoms in codeine-dependent patients

neuromuscular blockers: Additive respiratory depressant effects

opioids: Additive CNS and respiratory depressants effects and hypotensive effects

tricyclic antidepressants: Possibly increased effect of either the antidepressant or codeine

triprolidine component

MAO inhibitors: Prolonged and intensified anticholinergic (drying) effects of triprolidine

pseudoephedrine component

antacids: Increased pseudoephedrine absorption

antihypertensives, diuretics: Possibly decreased antihypertensive effects

beta blockers: Decreased therapeutic effects of both drugs

citrates: Possibly inhibited urinary pseudoephedrine excretion and prolonged duration of action

CNS stimulant, other sympathomimetics: Possibly increased additive CNS stimulation to excessive levels

cocaine (mucosal-local): Possibly increased cardiovascular effects of either drug and CNS stimulation

digoxin, levodopa: Increased risk of cardiac arrhythmias

hydrocarbon inhalation anesthetics: Increased risk of serious arrhythmias

kaolin: Decreased pseudoephedrine absorption

nitrates: Reduced antianginal effects of nitrates

rauwolfia alkaloids: Possibly inhibited pseudoephedrine action

thyroid hormones: Increased cardiovascular effects of both drugs

ACTIVITIES

codeine and triprolidine

alcohol use: Additive CNS effects

Adverse Reactions

CNS: Asthenia, anxiety, confusion, dizziness, depression, drowsiness, dyskinesia, euphoria, excitability, faintness, headache, insomnia, irritability, light-headedness, nervousness, restlessness, sedation, syncope, tiredness, tremor, vertigo, weakness

CV: Bradycardia, hypertension, hypotension, orthostatic hypotension, palpitation, tachycardia

ENDO: Decreased lactation, early menses, gynecomastia, hyperglycemia, hypoglycemia

EENT: Blurred vision; diplopia; dry mouth, pharynx, and respira-

tory passages; hypermetropia; increased lacrimation; labyrinthitis; laryngismus; mydriasis; nasal stuffiness; photophobia; tinnitus
GI: Abdominal distention or pain, acute pancreatitis, anorexia, constipation, diarrhea, dyspepsia, epigastric distress, esophageal reflux, increased appetite, nausea, vomiting
GU: Decreased libido, dysuria, urinary frequency or hesitancy, urine retention, ureteral spasm
RESP: Dyspnea, respiratory depression, wheezing
SKIN: Dermatitis, diaphoresis, erythema, flushing, pallor, pruritus, rash, urticaria
Other: Drug fever, emotional or physical dependence

Nursing Considerations

- Use cautiously in patients with recent head injury and those with Addison's disease, asthma or other chronic respiratory disease, increased intraocular pressure, or liver or renal impairment.
- **WARNING** Monitor respiratory function because codeine, triprolidine, and pseudoephedrine may suppress cough reflex and cause thickening of bronchial secretions, aggravating such conditions as asthma and COPD. In rare cases, it may depress respirations and induce apnea. Notify prescriber immediately if respiratory rate drops below 10 breaths/minute.
- Monitor patients who may be more susceptible to dizziness, sedation, and hypotension, such as the elderly.
- Monitor renal function, as ordered, because pseudoephedrine is substantially excreted by the kidneys.
- Regularly evaluate effectiveness of codeine, triprolidine, and pseudoephedrine in reducing symptoms.
- Be aware that patient shouldn't have intradermal allergen tests within 72 hours of receiving drug because results may be altered.

PATIENT TEACHING
- Instruct patient to use a calibrated measuring device.
- Tell patient that codeine, triprolidine, and pseudoephedrine must not be diluted with fluids or mixed with other drugs.
- Urge patient to avoid alcohol and other antidepressants while taking codeine, triprolidine, and pseudoephedrine.
- Instruct patient to avoid potentially hazardous activities until drug's CNS effects are known.
- Suggest that patient relieve dry mouth with frequent rinsing and use of sugarless gum or hard candy.
- Tell patient to take last dose of the day a few hours before bedtime if codeine, triprolidine, and pseudoephedrine makes him nervous or restless.

desloratadine and pseudoephedrine sulfate

Clarinex-D 24 Hour

Class and Category

Chemical: Active metabolite of loratadine a long-acting tricyclic histamine antagonist (desloratadine), sympathomimetic amine (pseudoephedrine)

Therapeutic: Antihistamine (desloratadine), decongestant (pseudo-ephedrine)

Pregnancy category: C

Indications and Dosages

▶ *To relieve nasal and non-nasal symptoms of seasonal allergic rhinitis, including nasal congestion*

E.R. TABLETS

Adults. 5 mg desloratadine and 240 mg pseudoephedrine (1 tablet) daily.

DOSAGE ADJUSTMENT For patients with renal impairment, 5 mg desloratadine and 240 mg pseudoephedrine (1 tablet) q 48 hr.

Mechanism of Action

Desloratadine is an active metabolite of loratadine that competes with free histamine for histamine H_1 receptor sites. Without histamine, vascular engorgement, mucosal edema, profuse watery secretion, local irritation, and sneezing that normally result from histamine action on afferent nerve terminals in nasal passages cannot occur.

Pseudoephedrine acts on $alpha_1$-adrenergic receptors in the mucosa of the respiratory tract to produce vasoconstriction. This process shrinks swollen nasal mucous membranes; reduces tissue hyperemia, edema, and nasal congestion; and increases nasal airway patency. It also may increase drainage of sinus secretions and open obstructed eustachian ostia.

Contraindications

Angina; hepatic insufficiency; hypersensitivity or idiosyncractic reactions to desloratadine, loratadine, pseudoephedrine, or their components; hyperthyroidism; narrow-angle glaucoma; prostatic hypertrophy; severe coronary artery disease or hypertension; urine retention; use within 14 days of MAO inhibitor therapy

Interactions

DRUGS

desloratadine component

barbiturates, CNS depressants, tricyclic antidepressants: Additive effects

pseudoephedrine component

antacids: Increased pseudoephedrine absorption

beta blockers, diuretics, methyldopa, mecamylamine, reserpine, veratum alkaloids: Decreased antihypertensive effects of these drugs

citrates: Possibly inhibited urinary pseudoephedrine excretion and prolonged duration of action

CNS stimulant, other sympathomimetics: Possibly increased additive CNS stimulation to excessive levels

cocaine (mucosal-local): Possibly increased cardiovascular effects of either drug and CNS stimulation

digoxin, levodopa: Increased risk of cardiac arrhythmias

hydrocarbon inhalation anesthetics: Increased risk of serious arrhythmias

kaolin: Decreased pseudoephedrine absorption

MAO inhibitors: Increased and prolonged cardiac stimulation, increased vasopressor effect, increased risk of severe cardiovascular and cerebrovascular effects, hyperpyrexia, and vomiting

nitrates: Reduced antianginal effects of nitrates

rauwolfia alkaloids: Possibly inhibited pseudoephedrine action

ACTIVITIES

desloratadine component

alcohol use: Additive effects

Adverse Reactions

CNS: Agitation, anxiety, dizziness, fatigue, headache, hyperactivity, insomnia, light-headedness, nervousness, restlessness, seizures, somnolence, trembling, weakness

CV: Angina, arrhythmia exacerbation, hypertension, palpitations, tachycardia

EENT: Dry mouth, pharyngitis, photophobia, ocular hypertension

ENDO: Dysmenorrhea

GI: Anorexia, nausea, vomiting

GU: Dysuria, urine retention

RESP: Bronchospasm, coughing, dyspnea

SKIN: Diaphoresis, pallor, pruritus, rash

Nursing Considerations

• Be aware that desloratadine and pseudodoephedrine therapy isn't recommended for patients with renal impairment.

- Use cautiously in patients with diabetes, hypertension, increased intraocular pressure, ischemic heart disease, or renal disease because of the pseudoephedrine component.
- Monitor elderly patients closely because they're more prone to developing adverse effects.
- Monitor renal function, as ordered, because pseudoephedrine is substantially excreted by the kidneys.
- Regularly evaluate effectiveness of desloratadine and pseudoephedrine in relieving seasonal and nonseasonal allergic rhinitis.
- Be aware that patient shouldn't have intradermal allergen tests within 4 days of receiving drug because results may be altered.

PATIENT TEACHING
- Instruct patients to take desloratadine and pseudoephedrine with a full glass of water and not to break or chew the tablet but to swallow it whole.
- Urge patient to avoid alcohol, other antidepressants, and OTC medication containing other antihistamines or sympathomimetics while taking desloratadine and pseudoephedrine.
- Instruct patient to avoid potentially hazardous activities until drug's CNS effects are known.
- Suggest that patient relieve dry mouth with frequent rinsing and use of sugarless gum or hard candy.

dexchlorpheniramine tannate and pseudoephedrine tannate
Tanafed DP

Class and Category
Chemical: Alkylamine (dexchlorpheniramine), sympathomimetic amine (pseudoephedrine)
Therapeutic: Antihistamine (dexchlorpheniramine), decongestant (pseudoephedrine)
Pregnancy category: C

Indications and Dosages
▶ *To relieve persistent runny nose, sneezing and nasal congestion caused by upper respiratory infection, sinus inflammation, or hay fever; to relieve sinus pressure and drain sinuses*
SUSPENSION
Adults. 5 to 10 mg dexchlorpheniramine and 150 to 300 mg pseudoephedrine (10 to 20 ml) q 12 hr.

Mechanism of Action

Dexchlorpheniramine competes with histamine for H_1 receptor sites, antagonizing many histamine effects and reducing allergy signs and symptoms.

Pseudoephedrine acts on $alpha_1$-adrenergic receptors in the mucosa of the respiratory tract to produce vasoconstriction. This process shrinks swollen nasal mucous membranes; reduces tissue hyperemia, edema, and nasal congestion; and increases nasal airway patency. It also may increase drainage of sinus secretions and open obstructed eustachian ostia.

Contraindications

Angina; breastfeeding; hypersensitivity or idiosyncractic reactions to dexchlorpheniramine, pseudoephedrine, or their components; hyperthyroidism; narrow-angle glaucoma; prostatic hypertrophy; severe coronary artery disease or hypertension; urine retention; use within 14 days of MAO inhibitor therapy

Interactions

DRUGS

dexchlorpheniramine component

anticholinergics: Additive anticholinergic effects

CNS depressants: Additive CNS effects

MAO inhibitors: Prolonged and intensified anticholinergic (drying) effect of dexchlorpheniramine

phenytoin: Possibly increased serum phenytoin levels and toxicity

pseudoephedrine component

antacids: Increased pseudoephedrine absorption

antihypertensives, diuretics: Possibly decreased antihypertensive effects

beta blockers: Decreased therapeutic effects of both drugs

citrates: Possibly inhibited urinary pseudoephedrine excretion and prolonged duration of action

CNS stimulant, other sympathomimetics: Possibly increased additive CNS stimulation to excessive levels

cocaine (mucosal-local): Possibly increased cardiovascular effects of either drug and CNS stimulation

digoxin, levodopa: Increased risk of cardiac arrhythmias

hydrocarbon inhalation anesthetics: Increased risk of serious arrhythmias

kaolin: Decreased pseudoephedrine absorption

MAO inhibitors: Increased and prolonged cardiac stimulation, increased vasopressor effect, increased risk of severe cardiovascular and cerebrovascular effects, hyperpyrexia, vomiting

nitrates: Reduced antianginal effects of nitrates
rauwolfia alkaloids: Possibly inhibited pseudoephedrine action
thyroid hormones: Increased cardiovascular effects of both drugs
ACTIVITIES
dexchlorpheniramine component
alcohol use: Additive CNS effects

Adverse Reactions

CNS: Anxiety, chills, confusion, coordination disturbance, dizziness, drowsiness, excitation (children), fatigue, fear, hallucinations, headache, hysteria, insomnia, irritability, light-headedness, nervousness, numbness, restlessness, sedation, seizures, tenseness, trembling, vertigo, weakness
CV: Arrhythmias, chest tightness, hypertension, palpitations, tachycardia
EENT: Blurred or double vision; dry mouth, nose, and throat; nasal congestion, tinnitus
ENDO: Early menstruation
GI: Anorexia, constipation, diarrhea, nausea, stomach upset or pain, vomiting
GU: Dysuria, frequent urination, urinary hesitancy, urine retention
HEME: Anemia, unusual bleeding or bruising
RESP: Dyspnea, increased chest congestion, wheezing
SKIN: Diaphoresis, pallor, photosensitivity, rash, urticaria
Other: Anaphylaxis

Nursing Considerations

• Use cautiously in patients with asthma, cardiovascular disease, diabetes, emphysema or other chronic lung disease, hypertension, peptic ulcer, or narrow-angle glaucoma.
• Monitor patients who may be more susceptible to dizziness, sedation and hypotension, such as the elderly.
• Monitor renal function, as ordered, because pseudoephedrine is substantially excreted by the kidneys.
• Regularly evaluate effectiveness of dexchlorpheniramine and pseudoephedrine in reducing upper respiratory symptoms.
• Be aware that patient shouldn't undergo allergen tests within 72 hours of receiving drug because results may be altered.
PATIENT TEACHING
• Instruct patient to use a calibrated measuring device to ensure accurate dose.
• Urge patient to avoid alcohol and other antidepressants while taking dexchlorpheniramine and pseudoephedrine.

- Instruct patient to avoid potentially hazardous activities until drug's CNS effects are known.
- Suggest that patient relieve dry mouth with frequent rinsing and use of sugarless gum or hard candy.
- Tell patient to take last dose of the day a few hours before bedtime if dexchlorpheniramine and pseudoephedrine makes him nervous or restless.

dextromethorphan hydrobromide, brompheniramine maleate, and phenylephrine hydrochloride
Alacol DM

Class and Category
Chemical: D-isomer codeine analog of levorphanol (dextromethorphan), alkylamine derivative (brompheniramine), sympathomimetic amine (phenylephrine)
Therapeutic: Antitussive (dextromethorphan), antihistaminic (brompheniramine), decongestant (phenylephrine)
Pregnancy category: C

Indications and Dosages
▶ *To relieve cough and nasal congestion in upper respiratory tract conditions*
SYRUP
Adults. 20 mg dextromethorphan, 4 mg brompheniramine, and 10 mg phenylephrine (10 ml) q 4 hr.

Mechanism of Action
Dextromethorphan suppresses cough by acting directly on the cough center in the medulla of the brain.

Brompheniramine competes with histamine for H_1 receptor sites, antagonizing many histamine effects and reducing allergy signs and symptoms.

Phenylephrine stimulates alpha-adrenergic receptors and inhibits the intracellular enzyme adenyl cyclase, which then inhibits production of cAMP. Inhibition of cAMP causes arterial and venous constriction in nasal passages, which decreases blood flow and mucosal edema caused by allergic response.

Contraindications
Asthma; breastfeeding; chronic bronchitis; emphysema; hypersensitivity to dextromethorphan, brompheniramine or phenylephrine

or their components; hyperthyroidism; narrow-angle glaucoma; productive cough; prostatic hypertrophy; severe hypertension; use of MAO inhibitors within 14 days

Interactions

DRUGS

dextromethorphan, brompheniramine and phenylephrine

MAO inhibitors: Possibly prolonged and intensified anticholinergic effects of brompheniramine and overall effects of dextromethorphan and phenylephrine

dextromethorphan and brompheniramine

CNS depressants: Additive CNS effects

dextromethorphan component

amiodarone, fluoxetine, paroxetine, quinidine: Decreased dextromethorphan metabolism, which may result in increased plasma dextromethorphan level and adverse reactions

brompheniramine component

anticholinergics: Potentiated anticholinergic effects

phenylephrine component

alpha blockers, haloperidol, loxapine, phenothiazines, thioxanthenes: Possibly decreased vasoconstrictor effect of phenylephrine

antihypertenisves, diuretics: Possibly decreased antihypertensive effects

atropine: Possibly enhanced vasopressor effect of phenylephrine

beta blockers: Decreased therapeutic effects of both drugs

bretylium: Possibly potentiated vaopressor effect and arrhythmias

doxapram: Increased vasopressor effect of both drugs

ergot alkaloids: Possibly cerebral blood vessel rupture, increased vasopressor effect, peripheral vascular ischemia, and gangrene (with ergotamine)

guanadrel, guanethidine: Increased vasopressor effect of phenylephrine; increased risk of severe hypertension and arrhythmias

hydrocarbon inhalation anesthetics: Increased risk of serious arrhythmias

maprotiline, tricyclic antidepressants: Increased risk of severe cardiovascular effects (including arrhythmias, hyperpyrexia, severe hypertension)

mecamylamine, methyldopa: Decreased hypotensive effects of these drugs; increased vasopressor effect of phenylephrine

nitrates: Possibly decreased vasopressor effect of phenylephrine and decreased antianginal effect of nitrates

oxytocin: Possibly severe, persistent hypertension

phenoxybenzamine: Decreased vasoconstrictor effect of phenylephrine, possibly hypotension and tachycardia
theophylline: Possibly enhanced toxicity (including cardiac toxicity)
thyroid hormones: Increased cardiovascular effects of each drug
ACTIVITIES
dextromethorphan and brompheniramine
alcohol use: Additive CNS effects
dextromethorphan component
smoking: Possibly increased respiratory secretion retention

Adverse Reactions
CNS: Confusion, dizziness, drowsiness, fever, hallucinations,
headache, hyperactivity, insomnia, nervousness, paresthesia, rest-
lessness, sedation, seizures, tiredness, tremor, weakness
CV: Angina, arrhythmias, bradycardia, edema, hypertension, hy-
potension, palpitations, peripheral vasoconstriction that may lead
to necrosis or gangrene, tachycardia, ventricular arrhythmias
EENT: Dry mouth, sore throat
GI: Abdominal pain, constipation, nausea, vomiting
GU: Urinary hesitancy, urine retention
HEME: Unusual bleeding or bruising
RESP: Dyspnea, respiratory depression
Other: Anaphylaxis, emotional and physical dependence (pro-
longed use with high doses)

Nursing Considerations
• Use cautiously in patients with bladder neck obstruction, cardiovascular disease, hypertension, glaucoma, or urine retention.
• Also use cautiously in patient with diabetes because some products contain sugar, which may disrupt blood glucose control; in
patients with impaired hepatic function because dextromethorphan is metabolized by the liver; and in patients with respiratory depression because dextromethorphan adversely affects
respirations.
• Monitor patients who may be more susceptible to dizziness, sedation, and hypotension, such as the elderly.
• Assess patient regularly for bleeding or bruising abnormalities
because of brompheniramine component.
• Regularly evaluate effectiveness of dextromethorphan, brompheniramine, and phenylephrine in relieving cough and reducing nasal congestion.
• Be aware that patient shouldn't have intradermal allergen tests
within 72 hours of receiving drug because results may be altered.

PATIENT TEACHING
- Instruct patient to use a calibrated measuring device when measuring dextromethorphan, brompheniramine, and phenylephrine to ensure an accurate dose.
- Stress importance of taking drug exactly as prescribed and not increasing dose or frequency without consulting prescriber.
- Urge patient to avoid alcohol and other antidepressants while taking drug.
- Instruct patient to avoid potentially hazardous activities until drug's CNS effects are known.
- Suggest that patient relieve dry mouth with frequent rinsing and use of sugarless gum or hard candy.

dextromethorphan hydrobromide, brompheniramine maleate, and pseudoephedrine hydrochloride

AccuHist DM, Anaplex-DM, Andehist-DM, Bromatane DX, Bromfed DM, Carbodex DM, Carbofed DM, Coldec DM, Dimetapp-DM, Robitussin Allergy & Cough, Rondamine DM, Rondec-DM, Sildec-DM

Class and Category

Chemical: D-isomer codeine analogue of levorphanol (dextromethorphan), propylamine derivative (brompheniramine), sympatho-mimetic amine (pseudoephedrine)
Therapeutic: Antitussive (dextromethorphan), antihistamine (brompheniramine), decongestant (pseudoephedrine)
Pregnancy category: C

Indications and Dosages

▶ *To relieve cough and persistent runny nose, sneezing, and nasal congestion caused by upper respiratory infections, sinus inflammation, or hay fever*
ORAL SOLUTION
Adults. 20 to 30 mg dextromethorphan, 4 mg brompheniramine, and 60 mg pseudoephedrine (5 or 10 ml depending on product) q 4 to 6 hr. Or, 15 mg dextromethorphan, 4 mg brompheniramine and 45 to 60 mg pseudoephedrine (5 ml) q.i.d. *Maximum:* 4 doses daily.
SYRUP
Adults and children age 12 and over. 20 to 30 mg dextromethorphan, 4 mg brompheniramine, and 60 mg pseudo-

ephedrine (5 or 10 ml depending on product) q 4 to 6 hr. Or, 15 mg dextromethorphan, 4 mg brompheniramine, and 45 to 60 mg pseudoephedrine (5 ml) q.i.d. *Maximum:* 4 doses daily.
Children ages 6 to 12. 10 mg dextromethorphan, 2 mg brompheniramine, and 30 mg pseudoephedrine (5 ml) q 4 hr. *Maximum:* 4 doses daily.
Children ages 2 to 6. 5 mg dextromethorphan, 1 mg brompheniramine, and 15 mg pseudoephedrine (2.5 ml) q 4 hr. *Maximum:* 4 doses daily.
DROPS
Children ages 12 months to 24 months. 4 mg dextromethorphan, 1 mg brompheniramine, and 15 mg pseudoephedrine (1 ml) q.i.d.
Children ages 6 months to 12 months. 3 mg dextromethorphan, 0.75 mg brompheniramine, and 11.25 mg pseudoephedrine (0.75 ml) q.i.d.
Infants ages 3 months to 6 months. 2 mg dextromethorphan, 0.5 mg brompheniramine, and 7.5 mg pseudoephedrine (0.5 ml) q.i.d.
Infants ages 1 month to 3 months. 1 mg dextromethorphan, 0.25 mg brompheniramine, and 3.75 mg pseudoephedrine (0.25 ml) q.i.d.

Mechanism of Action
Dextromethorphan suppresses cough by acting directly on the cough center in the medulla of the brain.

Brompheniramine competes with histamine for H_1 receptor sites, antagonizing many histamine effects and reducing allergy signs and symptoms.

Pseudoephedrine acts on $alpha_1$-adrenergic receptors in the mucosa of the respiratory tract to produce vasoconstriction. This process shrinks swollen nasal mucous membranes; reduces tissue hyperemia, edema, and nasal congestion; and increases nasal airway patency. It also may increase drainage of sinus secretions and open obstructed eustachian ostia.

Contraindications
Asthma; breastfeeding; chronic bronchitis; emphysema; hypersensitivity or idiosyncratic reactions to dextromethorphan, brompheniramine, pseudoephedrine, or their components; hyperthyroidism; narrow-angle glaucoma; productive cough; prostatic hypertrophy; severe coronary artery disease or hypertension; urine retention; use within 14 days of MAO inhibitor therapy

Interactions
DRUGS
dextromethorphan and pseudoephedrine
MAO inhibitors: Increased and prolonged cardiac stimulation, increased vasopressor effect, increased risk of severe cardiovascular and cerebrovascular effects, hyperpyrexia, and vomiting
dextromethorphan and brompheniramine
CNS depressants: Additive CNS effects
dextromethorphan component
amiodarone, fluoxetine, paroxetine, quinidine: Decreased metabolism of dextromethorphan, which may result in increased plasma dextromethorphan levels and adverse reactions
brompheniramine component
anticholinergics: Additive anticholinergic effects
MAO inhibitors: Prolonged and intensified anticholinergic (drying) effects of brompheniramine
pseudoephedrine component
antacids: Increased pseudoephedrine absorption
antihypertensives, diuretics: Possibly decreased antihypertensive effects
beta blockers: Decreased therapeutic effects of both drugs
citrates: Possibly inhibited urinary pseudoephedrine excretion and prolonged duration of action
CNS stimulant, other sympathomimetics: Possibly increased additive CNS stimulation to excessive levels
cocaine (mucosal-local): Possibly increased cardiovascular effects of either drug and CNS stimulation
digoxin, levodopa: Increased risk of cardiac arrhythmias
hydrocarbon inhalation anesthetics: Increased risk of serious arrhythmias
kaolin: Decreased pseudoephedrine absorption
nitrates: Reduced antianginal effects of nitrates
rauwolfia alkaloids: Possibly inhibited pseudoephedrine action
thyroid hormones: Increased cardiovascular effects of both drugs
ACTIVITIES
dextromethorphan and brompheniramine
alcohol use: Additive CNS effects
dextromethorphan component
smoking: Possibly increased respiratory secretion retention

Adverse Reactions
CNS: Anxiety, chills, confusion, coordination disturbance, dizziness, drowsiness, fatigue, fear, hallucinations, headache, hyperac-

tivity, hysteria, insomnia, irritability, light-headedness, nervousness, numbness, restlessness, sedation, seizures, tenseness, trembling, vertigo, weakness

CV: Arrhythmias, chest tightness, hypertension, palpitations, tachycardia

EENT: Blurred or double vision; dry mouth, nose, and throat; nasal congestion, tinnitus

ENDO: Early menstruation

GI: Abdominal pain, anorexia, constipation, diarrhea, nausea, stomach upset or pain, vomiting

GU: Dysuria, frequent urination, urinary hesitancy, urine retention

HEME: Anemia, unusual bleeding or bruising

RESP: Dyspnea, increased chest congestion, respiratory depression, wheezing

SKIN: Diaphoresis, pallor, photosensitivity, rash, urticaria

Other: Anaphylaxis, emotional and physical dependence (prolonged use with high doses)

Nursing Considerations

- Use cautiously in patients with asthma, cardiovascular disease, emphysema or other chronic lung disease, hypertension, or peptic ulcer.
- Also use cautiously in patients with diabetes because some products contain sugar, which may interfere with blood glucose control; in those with impaired hepatic function because dextromethorphan is metabolized by the liver; and in those with respiratory depression because dextromethorphan adversely affect respirations.
- Monitor patients who may be more susceptible to dizziness, sedation, and hypotension, such as the elderly.
- Monitor renal function, as ordered, because pseudoephedrine is substantially excreted by the kidneys.
- Regularly evaluate effectiveness of dextromethorphan, brompheniramine, and pseudoephedrine in relieving cough and reducing upper respiratory symptoms.
- Be aware that patient shouldn't have intradermal allergen tests within 72 hours of receiving drug because results may be altered.

PATIENT TEACHING

- Instruct patient to use a calibrated measuring device when using syrup or oral solution form of dextromethorphan, brompheniramine, and pseudoephedrine to ensure accurate dose.

- Caution patient not to exceed prescribed dose or frequency without consulting prescriber.
- Urge patient to avoid alcohol and other antidepressants while taking drug.
- Instruct patient to avoid potentially hazardous activities until drug's CNS effects are known.
- Suggest that patient relieve dry mouth with frequent rinsing and use of sugarless gum or hard candy.
- Tell patient to take last dose of the day a few hours before bedtime if dextromethorphan, brompheniramine and pseudoephedrine makes him nervous or restless.

dextromethorphan hydrobromide, carbinoxamine maleate, and pseudoephedrine hydrochloride

Andehist DM NR, Balamine DM, Carbinoxamine Compound, Carbodex DM, Carbofed DM, Cardec DM, C.P.-DM, Cydec-DM, Pediatex-DM, Pseudo-Car DM, Rondec-DM, Sildec-DM, Tussafed

Class and Category

Chemical: D-isomer codeine analogue of levorphanol (dextromethorphan), ethanolamine derivative (carbinoxamine), sympathomimetic amine (pseudoephedrine)
Therapeutic: Antitussive (dextromethorphan), antihistamine (carbinoxamine), decongestant (pseudoephedrine)
Pregnancy category: C

Indications and Dosages

▶ *To relieve cough, persistent runny nose, sneezing, and nasal congestion caused by upper respiratory tract infections, sinus inflammation, or hay fever*
ORAL SOLUTION
Adults and children age 6 and over. 15 mg dextromethorphan, 2 mg carbinoxamine, and 15 mg pseudoephedrine (5 ml) q.i.d.
Children ages 18 months to 6 years. 7.5 mg dextromethorphan, 1 mg carbinoxamine, and 7.5 mg psuedoephedrine (0.25 ml) q.i.d.
SYRUP
Adults and children age 6 and over. 12.5 or 15 mg dextromethorphan, 4 mg carbinoxamine, and 60 mg pseudoephedrine (5 ml) q 4 to 6 hr *Maximum:* 4 doses daily.

Children ages 18 months to 6 years. 6.25 to 7.5 mg dextromethorphan, 2 mg carbinoxamine, and 30 mg pseudoephedrine (2.5 ml) q 4 to 6 hr. *Maximum:* 4 doses daily.

DROPS (ANDEHIST DM NR, C.P.-DM, CARBOFED DM, RONDEC-DM)
Children ages 12 months to 24 months. 4 mg dextromethorphan, 1 mg carbinoxamine, and 15 mg pseudoephedrine (1 ml) q.i.d.

Children ages 6 months to 12 months. 3 mg dextromethorphan, 0.75 mg carbinoxamine, and 11.25 mg pseudoephedrine (0.75 ml) q.i.d.

Infants ages 3 months to 6 months. 2 mg dextromethorphan, 0.5 mg carbinoxamine, and 7.5 mg pseudoephedrine (0.5 ml) q.i.d.

Infants ages 1 month to 3 months. 1 mg dextromethorphan, 0.25 mg carbinoxamine, and 3.75 mg pseudoephedrine (0.25 ml) q.i.d.

DROPS (BALAMINE DM, CARBINOXAMINE COMPOUND, CARBODEX DM, CYDEC-DM, SILDEC-DM, TUSSAFED)
Children ages 9 months to 18 months. 3.5 or 4 mg dextromethorphan, 2 mg carbinoxamine, and 15 or 25 mg pseudoephedrine (1 ml) q.i.d.

Children ages 6 months to 9 months. 2.6 or 3 mg dextromethorphan, 1.5 mg carbinoxamine, and 18.75 or 11.25 mg pseudoephedrine (0.75 ml) q.i.d.

Infants ages 3 months to 6 months. 1.75 or 2 mg dextromethorphan, 1 mg carbinoxamine, and 12.5 or 7.5 mg pseudoephedrine (0.5 ml) q.i.d.

Infants ages 1 month to 3 months. 0.875 or 1 mg dextromethorphan, 0.5 mg carbinoxamine and 6.25 or 3.75 mg pseudoephedrine (0.25 ml) q.i.d.

Mechanism of Action
Dextromethorphan suppresses cough by directly acting on the cough center in the medulla of the brain.

Carbinoxamine competes with histamine for H_1 receptor sites, thereby antagonizing many histamine effects and reducing allergy signs and symptoms.

Pseudoephedrine acts on alpha$_1$-adrenergic receptors in the mucosa of the respiratory tract to produce vasoconstriction. This process shrinks swollen nasal mucous membranes; reduces tissue hyperemia, edema, and nasal congestion; and increases nasal airway patency.

Contraindications

Acute MI; angina; asthma; breastfeeding; chronic bronchitis; emphysema; hypersensitivity or idiosyncractic reactions to dextromethorphan, carbinoxamine, pseudoephedrine, or their components; hyperthyroidism; narrow-angle glaucoma; productive cough; severe coronary artery disease or hypertension; tachycardia; urine retention; use within 14 days of MAO inhibitor therapy

Interactions

DRUGS

dextromethorphan, carbinoxamine and pseudoephedrine

MAO inhibitors: Increased and prolonged cardiac stimulation, increased vasopressor effect, increased risk of severe cardiovascular and cerebrovascular effects, hyperpyrexia, and vomiting

dextromethorphan and carbinoxamine

CNS depressants: Additive CNS effects

dextromethorphan component

amiodarone, fluoxetine, paroxetine, quinidine: Decreased metabolism of dextromethorphan which may result in increased plasma dextromethorphan levels and incidence of adverse reactions

carbinoxamine component

anticholinergics: Additive anticholinergic effects

pseudoephedrine component

antacids: Increased pseudoephedrine absorption

antihypertensives, diuretics: Possibly decreased antihypertensive effects

beta blockers: Decreased therapeutic effects of both drugs

citrates: Possibly inhibited urinary pseudoephedrine excretion and prolonged duration of action

CNS stimulant, other sympathomimetics: Possibly increased additive CNS stimulation to excessive levels

cocaine (mucosal-local): Possibly increased cardiovascular effects of either drug and CNS stimulation

digoxin, levodopa: Increased risk of cardiac arrhythmias

hydrocarbon inhalation anesthetics: Increased risk of serious arrhythmias

kaolin: Decreased pseudoephedrine absorption

nitrates: Reduced antianginal effects of nitrates

rauwolfia alkaloids: Possibly inhibited pseudoephedrine action

thyroid hormones: Increased cardiovascular effects of both drugs

ACTIVITIES

dextromethorphan and carbinoxamine

alcohol use: Additive CNS effects

dextromethorphan component
smoking: Possibly increased respiratory secretion retention

Adverse Reactions

CNS: Anxiety, chills, confusion, coordination disturbance, dizziness, drowsiness, excitation (children), fatigue, fear, hallucinations, headache, hyperactivity, hysteria, insomnia, irritability, light-headedness, nervousness, numbness, restlessness, sedation, seizures, tenseness, trembling, vertigo, weakness
CV: Arrhythmias, chest tightness, hypertension, palpitations, tachycardia
EENT: Blurred or double vision; dry mouth, nose, and throat; nasal congestion, tinnitus
ENDO: Early menstruation
GI: Abdominal pain, anorexia, constipation, diarrhea, nausea, stomach upset or pain, vomiting
GU: Dysuria, frequent urination, urinary hesitancy, urine retention
HEME: Anemia, unusual bleeding or bruising
RESP: Dyspnea, increased chest congestion, respiratory depression, wheezing
SKIN: Diaphoresis, pallor, photosensitivity, rash, urticaria
Other: Anaphylaxis, emotional and physical dependence (prolonged use with high doses)

Nursing Considerations

- Use cautiously in patients with diabetes because some products contain sugar, which may disrupt blood glucose control; in those with impaired hepatic function because dextromethorphan is metabolized by the liver; and in those with respiratory depression because dextromethorphan adversely affects respirations.
- Monitor patients who may be more susceptible to dizziness, sedation, and hypotension, such as the elderly.
- Monitor renal function, as ordered, because pseudoephedrine is substantially excreted by the kidneys.
- Regularly evaluate effectiveness of dextromethorphan, carbinoxamine, and pseudoephedrine in reducing upper respiratory symptoms.
- Be aware that patient shouldn't have intradermal allergen tests within 72 hours of receiving drug because results may be altered.

PATIENT TEACHING
- Instruct patient to use a calibrated measuring device when measuring syrup to ensure accurate dose.

- Stress importance of taking drug exactly as prescribed and not increasing dose or frequency without consulting prescriber.
- Urge patient to avoid alcohol and other antidepressants while taking dextromethorphan, carbinoxamine, and pseudoephedrine.
- Instruct patient to avoid potentially hazardous activities until drug's CNS effects are known.
- Suggest that patient relieve dry mouth with frequent rinsing and use of sugarless gum or hard candy.
- Tell patient to take last dose of the day a few hours before bedtime if dextromethorphan, carbinoxamine and pseudoephedrine makes her nervous or restless.

dextromethorphan hydrobromide, chlorpheniramine maleate, phenylephrine hydrochloride, and guaifenesin

Donatussin

Class and Category

Chemical: D-isomer codeine analog of levorphanol (dextromethorphan), propylamine derivative (chlorpheniramine), sympathomimetic amine (phenylephrine), glyceryl guaiacolate (guaifenesin)

Therapeutic: Antitussive (dextromethorphan), antihistaminic (chlorpheniramine), decongestant (phenylephrine), and expectorant (guaifenesin)

Pregnancy category: C

Indications and Dosages

▶ *To provide symptomatic relief of cough and nasal congestion associated with upper respiratory tract conditions*

SYRUP

Adults and children age 12 and over. 7.5 mg dextromethorphan, 2 mg chlorpheniramine, 10 mg phenylephrine, and 100 mg guaifenesin (5 ml) q 4 to 6 hr.

Children ages 6 to 12. 3.75 mg dextromethorphan, 1 mg chlorpheniramine, 5 mg phenylephrine, and 50 mg guaifenesin (2.5 ml) q 4 to 6 hr.

Children ages 2 to 6. 1.82 mg dextromethorphan, 0.5 mg chlorpheniramine, 2.5 mg phenylephrine, and 25 mg guaifenesin (1.25 ml) q 4 to 6 hr.

Mechanism of Action

Dextromethorphan suppresses cough by acting directly on the cough center in the medulla of the brain.

Chlorpheniramine competes with histamine for H_1 receptor sites, thereby antagonizing many histamine effects to reduce allergy signs and symptoms.

Phenylephrine stimulates alpha-adrenergic receptors and inhibits the intracellular enzyme adenyl cyclase, which then inhibits production of cAMP. Inhibition of cAMP causes arterial and venous constriction in nasal passages, which decreases blood flow and mucosal edema caused by allergic response.

Guaifenesin increases fluid and mucus removal from the upper respiratory tract by increasing the volume of secretions and reducing their adhesiveness and surface tension.

Contraindications

Asthma; breastfeeding; chronic bronchitis; emphysema; hypersensitivity to dextromethorphan, chlorpheniramine, phenylephrine, guaifenesin, or their components; productive cough; use of MAO inhibitors within 14 days

Interactions

DRUGS

dextromethorphan, chlorpheniramine and phenylephrine

MAO inhibitors: Increased and prolonged cardiac stimulation, increased vasopressor effect, increased risk of severe cardiovascular and cerebrovascular effects, hyperpyrexia, and vomiting

dextromethorphan and chlorpheniramine

CNS depressants: Additive CNS effects

dextromethorphan component

amiodarone, fluoxetine, quinidine: Decreased metabolism of dextromethorphan, which may result in increased plasma dextromethorphan level and adverse reactions

chlorpheniramine component

anticholinergics: Potentiated anticholinergic effects

phenytoin: Possibly increased serum phenytoin levels and toxicity

phenylephrine component

alpha blockers, haloperidol, loxapine, phenothiazines, thioxanthenes: Possibly decreased vasoconstrictor effect of phenylephrine

antihypertenisves, diuretics: Possibly decreased antihypertensive effects

atropine: Possibly enhanced vasopressor effect of phenylephrine

beta blockers: Decreased therapeutic effects of both drugs

bretylium: Possibly potentiated vaopressor effect and arrhythmias
doxapram: Increased vasopressor effect of both drugs
ergot alkaloids: Possibly cerebral blood vessel rupture, increased vasopressor effect, peripheral vascular ischemia, and gangrene (with ergotamine)
guanadrel, guanethidine: Increased vasopressor effect of phenylephrine; increased risk of severe hypertension and arrhythmias
hydrocarbon inhalation anesthetics: Increased risk of serious arrhythmias
maprotiline, tricyclic antidepressants: Increased risk of severe cardiovascular effects (including arrhythmias, hyperpyrexia, severe hypertension)
mecamylamine, methyldopa: Decreased hypotensive effects of these drugs; increased vasopressor effect of phenylephrine
nitrates: Possibly decreased vasopressor effect of phenylephrine and decreased antianginal effect of nitrates
oxytocin: Possibly severe, persistent hypertension
phenoxybenzamine: Decreased vasoconstrictor effect of phenylephrine and possibly hypotension and tachycardia
theophylline: Possibly enhanced toxicity (including cardiac toxicity)
thyroid hormones: Increased cardiovascular effects of each drug
ACTIVITIES
dextromethorphan and chlorpheniramine
alcohol use: Additive CNS effects
dextromethorphan component
smoking: Possibly increased respiratory secretion retention

Adverse Reactions

CNS: Confusion, dizziness, drowsiness, fever, hallucinations, headache, hyperactivity, insomnia, nervousness, paresthesia, restlessness, sedation, seizures, tiredness, tremor, weakness
CV: Angina, arrhythmias, bradycardia, edema, hypertension, hypotension, palpitations, peripheral vasoconstriction that may lead to necrosis or gangrene, tachycardia, ventricular arrhythmias
EENT: Dry mouth, sore throat
GI: Abdominal pain, constipation, nausea, vomiting
GU: Urinary hesitancy, urine retention
RESP: Dyspnea, respiratory depression
SKIN: Rash, urticaria
Other: Anaphylaxis, emotional and physical dependence (prolonged use with high doses)

Nursing Considerations
- Use cautiously in patients with bladder neck obstruction, cardiovascular disease, hypertension, hyperthyroidism, glaucoma, prostatic hypertrophy, or urine retention.
- Also use cautiously in patients with diabetes because products containing sugar may disrupt blood glucose control, in those with hepatic impairment because dextromethorphan is metabolized by the liver, and in those with respiratory depression because dextromethorphan adversely affect respirations.
- Monitor patients who may be more susceptible to experiencing dizziness, sedation, and hypotension, such as the elderly.
- Regularly evaluate effectiveness of dextromethorphan, chlorpheniramine, phenylephrine, and guaifenesin in relieving cough and reducing nasal congestion.
- Be aware that patient shouldn't have intradermal allergen tests within 72 hours of receiving drug because results may be altered.

PATIENT TEACHING
- Instruct patient to use a calibrated measuring device when measuring dextromethorphan, brompheniramine, phenylephrine, and guaifenesin to ensure accurate dose.
- Stress importance of taking drug exactly as prescribed and not increasing dose or frequency without consulting prescriber.
- Urge patient to avoid alcohol and other antidepressants while taking drug.
- Instruct patient to avoid potentially hazardous activities until drug's CNS effects are known.
- Suggest that patient relieve dry mouth with frequent rinsing and use of sugarless gum or hard candy.

dextromethorphan tannate, chlorpheniramine tannate, and pseudoephedrine tannate
Tanafed DM
dextromethorphan tannate, dexchlorpheniramine tannate, and pseudoephedrine tannate
Tanafed DMX

Class and Category
Chemical: D-isomer codeine analogue of levorphanol (dextromethorphan),

alkylamine (chlorpheniramine, dexchlorpheniramine), sympathomimetic amine (pseudoephedrine)
Therapeutic: Antitussive (dextromethorphan), antihistamine
(chlorpheniramine, dexchlorpheniramine), decongestant (pseudoephedrine)
Pregnancy category: C

Indications and Dosages

▶ *To relieve cough, persistent runny nose, sneezing, and nasal congestion
caused by upper respiratory infection, sinus inflammation or hay fever*
SUSPENSION (TANAFED DM)
Adults. 50 to 100 mg dextromethorphan, 9 to 18 mg chlorpheniramine, and 150 to 300 mg pseudoephedrine (10 to 20 ml)
q 12 hr. *Maximum:* 40 ml daily.
SUSPENSION (TANAFED DMX)
Adults. 50 to 100 mg dextromethorphan, 5 to 10 mg chlorpheniramine, and 150 to 300 mg pseudoephedrine (10 to 20 ml)
q 12 hr. *Maximum:* 40 ml daily.

Mechanism of Action

Dextromethorphan suppresses cough by directly acting on the cough center
in the medulla of the brain.

Chlorpheniramine and dexchlorpheniramine compete with histamine for H_1
receptor sites, thereby antagonizing many histamine effects and reducing allergy signs and symptoms.

Pseudoephedrine acts on $alpha_1$-adrenergic receptors in the mucosa of the
respiratory tract to produce vasoconstriction. This process shrinks swollen
nasal mucous membranes; reduces tissue hyperemia, edema, and nasal congestion; and increases nasal airway patency. It also may increase drainage of
sinus secretions and open obstructed eustachian ostia.

Contraindications

Asthma; breastfeeding; chronic bronchitis; emphysema; hypersensitivity or idiosyncratic reactions to dextromethorphan, chlorpheniramine, dexchlorpheniramine, pseudoephedrine, or their
components; hyperthyroidism; narrow-angle glaucoma; productive cough; severe coronary artery disease or hypertension; urine
retention; use within 14 days of MAO inhibitor therapy

Interactions

DRUGS
**dextromethorphan, chlorpheniramine,
dexchlorpheniramine, and pseudoephedrine**

MAO inhibitors: Increased and prolonged cardiac stimulation, increased vasopressor effect, increased risk of severe cardiovascular and cerebrovascular effects, hyperpyrexia, and vomiting

dextromethorphan, chlorpheniramine, and dexchlorpheniramine

CNS depressants: Additive CNS effects

dextromethorphan component

amiodarone, fluoxetine, quinidine: Decreased metabolism of dextromethorphan, which may result in increased plasma dextromethorphan level and adverse effects

chlorpheniramine and dexchlorpheniramine component

anticholinergics: Additive anticholinergic effects

phenytoin: Possibly increased serum phenytoin level and toxicity

pseudoephedrine component

antacids: Increased pseudoephedrine absorption

antihypertensives, diuretics: Possibly decreased antihypertensive effects

beta blockers: Decreased therapeutic effects of both drugs

citrates: Possibly inhibited urinary pseudoephedrine excretion and prolonged duration of action

CNS stimulant, other sympathomimetics: Possibly increased additive CNS stimulation to excessive levels

cocaine (mucosal-local): Possibly increased cardiovascular effects of either drug and CNS stimulation

digoxin, levodopa: Increased risk of cardiac arrhythmias

hydrocarbon inhalation anesthetics: Increased risk of serious arrhythmias

kaolin: Decreased pseudoephedrine absorption

nitrates: Reduced antianginal effects of nitrates

rauwolfia alkaloids: Possibly inhibited pseudoephedrine action

thyroid hormones: Increased cardiovascular effects of both drugs

ACTIVITIES

dextromethorphan, chlorpheniramine, and dexchlorpheniramine

alcohol use: Additive CNS effects

dextromethorphan component

smoking: Possibly increased respiratory secretion retention

Adverse Reactions

CNS: Anxiety, chills, confusion, coordination disturbance, dizziness, drowsiness, fatigue, fear, hallucinations, headache, hyperactivity, hysteria, insomnia, irritability, light-headedness, nervousness, numbness, restlessness, sedation, seizures, tenseness, trembling, vertigo, weakness

CV: Arrhythmias, chest tightness, hypotension, palpitations, tachycardia

EENT: Blurred or double vision; dry mouth, nose, and throat; nasal congestion; tinnitus

ENDO: Early menstruation

GI: Abdominal pain, anorexia, constipation, diarrhea, nausea, stomach upset or pain, vomiting

GU: Dysuria, frequent urination, urinary hesitancy, urine retention

HEME: Anemia, unusual bleeding or bruising

RESP: Dyspnea, increased chest congestion, respiratory depression, wheezing

SKIN: Diaphoresis, pallor, photosensitivity, rash, urticaria

Other: Anaphylaxis, emotional and physical dependence (prolonged use with high doses)

Nursing Considerations

• Use cautiously in patients with cardiovascular disease or peptic ulcer.
• Also use cautiously in patient with diabetes because some products contain sugar, which may disrupt blood glucose control; in those with impaired hepatic function because dextromethorphan is metabolized by the liver; and in those with respiratory depression because dextromethorphan adversely affects respirations.
• Monitor patients who may be more susceptible to dizziness, sedation, and hypotension, such as the elderly.
• Monitor renal function, as ordered, because pseudoephedrine is substantially excreted by the kidneys.
• Regularly evaluate effectiveness of drug in relieving cough and reducing upper respiratory symptoms.
• Be aware that patient shouldn't have intradermal allergen tests within 72 hours of receiving drug because results may be altered.

PATIENT TEACHING

• Instruct patient to use a calibrated measuring device to ensure accurate dose.
• Caution patient not to exceed dose or frequency without consulting prescriber.
• Urge patient to avoid alcohol and other antidepressants while taking drug.

- Instruct patient to avoid potentially hazardous activities until drug's CNS effects are known.
- Suggest that patient relieve dry mouth with frequent rinsing and use of sugarless gum or hard candy.
- Tell patient to take last dose of the day a few hours before bedtime if drug makes her nervous or restless.

dextromethorphan hydrobromide, chlorpheniramine tannate, pseudoephedrine hydrochloride, guaifenesin, and potassium guaiacolsulfonate

Lemotussin-DM

Class and Category

Chemical: D-isomer codeine analog of levorphanol (dextromethorphan), alkylamine (chlorpheniramine), sympathomimetic amine (pseudoephedrine), glyceryl guaiacolate (guaifenesin), unclassified (potassium guaiacolsulfonate)

Therapeutic: Antitussive (dextromethorphan), antihistamine (chlorpheniramine), decongestant (pseudoephedrine), expectorants (guaifenesin, potassium guaiacolsulfonate)

Pregnancy category: C

Indications and Dosages

▶ *To relieve cough, persistent runny nose, sneezing, and nasal congestion caused by upper respiratory infection, sinus inflammation, or hay fever*

ORAL SOLUTION

Adults. 7.5 to 15 mg dextromethorphan, 2 to 4 mg chlorpheniramine, 10 to 20 mg pseudoephedrine, 50 to 100 mg guaifenesin and 50 to 100 mg potassium guaiacolsulfonate (5 to 10 ml) q 6 to 8 hr.

Contraindications

Acute MI; angina; asthma; breastfeeding; chronic bronchitis; emphysema; hyperkalemia, hypersensitivity or idiosyncractic reactions to dextromethorphan, chlorpheniramine, pseudoephedrine, guafenesin, potassium guaiacolsulfonate, or their components; hyperthyroidism; narrow-angle glaucoma; productive cough; severe coronary artery disease or hypertension; urine retention; use within 14 days of MAO inhibitor therapy

---

Mechanism of Action

Dextromethorphan suppresses cough by directly acting on the cough center in the medulla of the brain.

Chlorpheniramine competes with histamine for H_1 receptor sites, thereby antagonizing many histamine effects and reducing allergy effects.

Pseudoephedrine acts on alpha$_1$-adrenergic receptors in the mucosa of the respiratory tract to produce vasoconstriction. This process shrinks swollen nasal mucous membranes; reduces tissue hyperemia, edema, and nasal congestion; and increases nasal airway patency. It also may increase drainage of sinus secretions and open obstructed eustachian ostia.

Guaifenesin increases fluid and mucus removal from the upper respiratory tract by increasing the volume of secretions and reducing their adhesiveness and surface tension.

Interactions

DRUGS

dextromethorphan and pseudoephedrine
MAO inhibitors: Increased and prolonged cardiac stimulation, increased vasopressor effect, increased risk of severe cardiovascular and cerebrovascular effects, hyperpyrexia, and vomiting

dextromethorphan and chlorpheniramine
CNS depressants: Additive CNS effects

dextromethorphan component
amiodarone, fluoxetine, paroxetine, quinidine: Decreased metabolism of dextromethorphan, which may result in increased plasma dextromethorphan levels and adverse reactions

chlorpheniramine component
anticholinergics: Additive anticholinergic effects
MAO inhibitors: Prolonged and intensified anticholinergic (drying) effects of chlorpheniramine
phenytoin: Possibly increased serum phenytoin level and toxicity

pseudoephedrine component
antacids: Increased pseudoephedrine absorption
antihypertensives, diuretics: Possibly decreased antihypertensive effects
beta blockers: Decreased therapeutic effects of both drugs
citrates: Possibly inhibited urinary pseudoephedrine excretion and prolonged duration of action

CNS stimulant, other sympathomimetics: Possibly increased additive CNS stimulation to excessive levels

cocaine (mucosal-local): Possibly increased cardiovascular effects of either drug and CNS stimulation

digoxin, levodopa: Increased risk of cardiac arrhythmias

hydrocarbon inhalation anesthetics: Increased risk of serious arrhythmias

kaolin: Decreased pseudoephedrine absorption

nitrates: Reduced antianginal effects of nitrates

rauwolfia alkaloids: Possibly inhibited pseudoephedrine action

thyroid hormones: Increased cardiovascular effects of both drugs

potassium guaiacolsulfonate component

potassium-sparing diuretics, potassium-containing drugs, potassium supplements: Increased risk of hyperkalemia

ACTIVITIES

dextromethorphan and chlorpheniramine

alcohol use: Additive CNS effects

dextromethorphan component

smoking: Possibly increased respiratory secretion retention

Adverse Reactions

CNS: Anxiety, chills, confusion, coordination disturbance, dizziness, drowsiness, fatigue, fear, hallucinations, headache, hyperactivity, hysteria, insomnia, irritability, light-headedness, nervousness, numbness, restlessness, sedation, seizures, tenseness, trembling, vertigo, weakness

CV: Arrhythmias, chest tightness, hypertension, palpitations, tachycardia

EENT: Blurred or double vision; dry mouth, nose, and throat; nasal congestion; tinnitus

ENDO: Early menstruation

GI: Abdominal pain, anorexia, constipation, diarrhea, nausea, stomach upset or pain, vomiting

GU: Dysuria, frequent urination, urinary hesitancy, urine retention

HEME: Anemia, unusual bleeding or bruising

RESP: Dyspnea, increased chest congestion, respiratory depression, wheezing

SKIN: Diaphoresis, pallor, photosensitivity, rash, urticaria

Other: Anaphylaxis, emotional and physical dependence (prolonged use with high doses), hyperkalemia

Nursing Considerations

- Use cautiously in patients with cardiovascular disease, hypertension, or peptic ulcer.
- Also use cautiously in patients with diabetes because some products contain sugar, which may disrupt blood glucose control; in those with impaired hepatic function because dextromethorphan is metabolized by the liver; and in those with respiratory depression because dextromethorphan adversely affect respirations.
- Monitor patients who may be more susceptible to dizziness, sedation, and hypotension, such as the elderly.
- Monitor renal function, as ordered, because pseudoephedrine is substantially excreted by the kidneys.
- Regularly evaluate effectiveness of drug in relieving cough and reducing upper respiratory symptoms.
- Be aware that patient shouldn't have intradermal allergen tests within 72 hours of receiving drug because results may be altered.

PATIENT TEACHING

- Instruct patient to use a calibrated measuring device to ensure accurate dose.
- Caution patient not to exceed dose or frequency without consulting prescriber.
- Urge patient to avoid alcohol, CNS depressants, and potassium supplements while taking drug.
- Instruct patient to avoid potentially hazardous activities until drug's CNS effects are known.
- Suggest that patient relieve dry mouth with frequent rinsing and use of sugarless gum or hard candy.
- Tell patient to take last dose of the day a few hours before bedtime if drug makes him nervous or restless.
- Advise patient to increase his fluid intake to help loosen mucus and thin secretions if not contraindicated by a fluid-restrictive condition such as heart failure or liver or renal disease.

dextromethorphan hydrobromide and guaifenesin

Allfen-DM, Aquatab DM, Dex GG TR, Duratuss DM,
Gani-Tuss-DM NR, GFN 1000/DM 60, GFN 1200/DM 60,
Guaifenesin DM, Guaifenesin-DM NR, Guaifenex DM,
Guiadrine DM, Humibid DM, Hydro-Tussin DM, Iobid DM,
Maxi-tuss DM, Muco-Fen DM, Respa-DM, Robitussin-DM,

Sudal-DM, SU-TUSS DM, Touro DM, TUSS-bid, Tussi-Organidin-DM NR, Z-Cof LA

Class and Category

Chemical: D-isomer codeine analog of levorphanol (dextromethorphan), glyceryl guaiacolate (guaifenesin)

Therapeutic: Antitussive (dextromethorphan), expectorant (guaifenesin)

Pregnancy category: C

Indications and Dosages

▶ *To relieve cough caused by minor throat and bronchial irritation, especially when secretions are thick*

ELIXIR, ORAL LIQUID

Adults and children age 12 and over. 20 mg dextromethorphan and 200 mg guaifenesin (5 or 10 ml depending on product) q 4 hr.

Children ages 6 to 12. 10 mg dextromethorphan and 100 mg guaifenesin (5 ml) q 4 hr.

Children ages 2 to 6. 5 mg dextromethorphan and 50 mg guaifenesin (2.5 ml) q 4 hr.

Children ages 6 months to 2 years. 1.25 to 2.5 mg dextromethorphan and 12.5 to 25 mg guaifenesin (0.6 to 1.25 ml) q 4 hr.

E.R. TABLETS

Adults and children age 12 and over. 28 to 60 mg dextromethorphan and 600 to 1,300 mg guaifenesin (1 or 2 tablets depending on product) q 12 hr.

Children ages 6 to 12. 30 mg dextromethorphan and 575 or 600 mg guaifenesin (1 tablet) q 12 hr.

Children ages 2 to 6. 15 mg dextromethorphan and 287.5 or 300 mg guaifenesin (½ tablet) q 12 hr.

Mechanism of Action

Dextromethorphan suppresses cough by acting directly on the cough center in the medulla of the brain.

Guaifenesin increases fluid and mucus removal from the upper respiratory tract by increasing the volume of secretions and reducing their adhesiveness and surface tension.

Contraindications

Asthma; chronic bronchitis; emphysema; hypersensitivity to dextromethorphan, guaifenesin, or their components; productive cough

Interactions
DRUGS
dextromethorphan component
amiodarone, fluoxetine, paroxetine, quinidine: Decreased metabolism of dextromethorphan, which may result in increased plasma dextromethorphan level and adverse effects
CNS depressants: Additive CNS effects
MAO inhibitors: Increased and prolonged cardiac stimulation, increased vasopressor effect, increased risk of severe cardiovascular and cerebrovascular effects, hyperpyrexia, and vomiting
ACTIVITIES
dextromethorphan component
smoking: Possibly increased respiratory secretion retention

Adverse Reactions
CNS: Confusion, dizziness, drowsiness, hallucinations, headache, hyperactivity
GI: Abdominal pain, constipation, nausea, vomiting
RESP: Respiratory depression
SKIN: Rash, urticaria
Other: Emotional and physical dependence (prolonged use with high doses), serotonin syndrome

Nursing Considerations
- Use cautiously in patients with diabetes because some products contain sugar, which may disrupt blood glucose control.
- Also use cautiously in patients with impaired hepatic function because dextromethorphan is metabolized by the liver and in those with respiratory depression because dextromethorphan adversely affect respirations.

PATIENT TEACHING
- Stress importance of taking dextromethorphan and guaifenesin exactly as prescribed and not increasing dose or frequency without consulting prescriber.
- Instruct patient to use a calibrated measuring device to ensure accurate dose when using liquid or elixir form of drug.
- Caution patient not to use other CNS depressants while taking dextromethorphan and guaifenesin.
- Advise patient to avoid potentially hazardous activities until drug's CNS effects are known.
- To prevent constipation, encourage patient to consume plenty of fluids and high-fiber foods, if not contraindicated by another condition.

- Advise patient to notify prescriber if she becomes short of breath or has difficulty breathing.
- Advise patient to increase her fluid intake to help loosen mucus and thin secretions if not contraindicated by a fluid-restrictive condition such as heart failure or liver or renal disease

dextromethorphan hydrobromide, phenylephrine hydrochloride, and guaifenesin

Tussafed Ex

Class and Category

Chemical: D-isomer codeine analog of levorphanol (dextromethorphan), sympathomimetic amine (phenylephrine), glyceryl guaiacolate (guaifenesin)

Therapeutic: Antitussive (dextromethorphan), decongestant (phenylephrine), expectorant (guaifenesin)

Pregnancy category: C

Indications and Dosages

▶ *To relieve cough and other upper respiratory symptoms of the common cold and allergies*

SYRUP

Adults. 30 mg dextromethorphan, 10 mg phenylephrine, and 200 mg guaifenesin (5 ml) q.i.d.

Mechanism of Action

Dextromethorphan suppresses cough by acting directly on the cough center in the medulla of the brain.

Phenylephrine stimulates alpha-adrenergic receptors and inhibits the intracellular enzyme adenyl cyclase, which then inhibits production of cAMP. Inhibition of cAMP causes arterial and venous constriction in nasal passages, which decreases blood flow and mucosal edema caused by allergic response.

Guaifenesin increases fluid and mucus removal from the upper respiratory tract by increasing the volume of secretions and reducing their adhesiveness and surface tension.

Contraindications

Angina; asthma; chronic bronchitis; emphysema; hypersensitivity to dextromethorphan, bisulfites, guaifenesin, phenylephrine, or their components; severe coronary artery disease or hypertension;

use within 14 days of MAO inhibitor therapy; urine retention; ventricular tachycardia

Interactions

DRUGS

dextromethorphan and phenylephrine

MAO inhibitors: Increased and prolonged cardiac stimulation, increased vasopressor effect, increased risk of severe cardiovascular and cerebrovascular effects, hyperpyrexia, and vomiting

dextromethorphan component

amiodarone, fluoxetine, paroxetine, quinidine: Decreased dextromethorphan metabolism, which may result in increased plasma dextromethorphan level and adverse effects

CNS depressants: Additive CNS effects

phenylephrine component

alpha blockers, haloperidol, loxapine, phenothiazines, thioxanthenes: Possibly decreased vasoconstrictor effect of phenylephrine

antihypertenisves, diuretics: Possibly decreased antihypertensive effects

atropine: Possibly enhanced vasopressor effect of phenylephrine

beta blockers: Decreased therapeutic effects of both drugs

bretylium: Possibly potentiated vaopressor effect and arrhythmias

doxapram: Increased vasopressor effect of both drugs

ergot alkaloids: Possibly cerebral blood vessel rupture, increased vasopressor effect, peripheral vascular ischemia, and gangrene (with ergotamine)

guanadrel, guanethidine: Increased vasopressor effect of phenylephrine; increased risk of severe hypertension and arrhythmias

hydrocarbon inhalation anesthetics: Increased risk of serious arrhythmias

maprotiline, tricyclic antidepressants: Increased risk of severe cardiovascular effects (including arrhythmias, hyperpyrexia, severe hypertension)

mecamylamine, methyldopa: Decreased hypotensive effects of these drugs; increased vasopressor effect of phenylephrine

nitrates: Possibly decreased vasopressor effect of phenylephrine and decreased antianginal effect of nitrates

oxytocin: Possibly severe, persistent hypertension

phenoxybenzamine: Decreased vasoconstrictor effect of phenylephrine, possibly hypotension and tachycardia

theophylline: Possibly enhanced toxicity (including cardiac toxicity)

thyroid hormones: Increased cardiovascular effects of each drug

ACTIVITIES

dextromethorphan component

smoking: Possibly increased respiratory secretion retention

Adverse Reactions

CNS: Anxiety, confusion, dizziness, drowsiness, hallucinations, headache, hyperactivity, insomnia, nervousness, paresthesia, restlessness, tremor, weakness

CV: Angina, bradycardia, hypertension, palpitations, peripheral vasoconstriction that may lead to necrosis or gangrene, tachycardia, ventricular arrhythmia

GI: Abdominal pain, constipation, nausea, vomiting

RESP: Dyspnea, respiratory depression

SKIN: Pallor, rash, urticaria

Other: Allergic reaction, emotional and physical dependence (prolonged use with high doses), serotonin syndrome

Nursing Considerations

- Assess patient for signs and symptoms of angina, arrhythmias, and hypertension because phenylephrine may increase myocardial oxygen demand and the risk of proarrhythmias and blood pressure changes.
- Use cautiously in patients with diabetes because some products contain sugar, which may disrupt blood glucose control; in those with impaired hepatic function because dextromethorphan is metabolized by the liver; and in those with respiratory depression because dextromethorphan adversely affect respirations.
- **WARNING** Monitor patient with thyroid disease for increased sensitivity to catecholamines and possibly thyrotoxicity or cardiotoxicity.
- Regularly evaluate effectiveness of dextromethorphan, phenylephrine, and guaifenesin in relieving upper respiratory symptoms. Notify prescriber if symptoms persist or worsen.

PATIENT TEACHING

- Stress importance of taking drug exactly as prescribed and not increasing dose or frequency without consulting prescriber.
- Caution patient not to use other CNS depressants while taking dextromethorphan, phenylephrine, and guaifenesin.
- Instruct patient to increase fluid intake (unless contraindicated) to help thin secretions.
- Advise patient to avoid potentially hazardous activities until drug's CNS effects are known.

dextromethomethorphan, pseudoephedrine hydrochloride, and guaifenesin

Aquatab C, GFN 600/PSE 60/DM 30, GFN 1200/CM 60/PSE 120, Maxifed DM, Medent-DM, Profen Forte DM, PanMist-DM, Profen II DM, Protuss DM, Robitussin-CF, Robitussin Cough and Cold, Touro CC, Tussafed-LA, Z-Cof DM

Class and Category

Chemical: D-isomer codeine analog of levorphanol (dextromethorphan), sympathomimetic amine (pseudoephedrine), glyceryl guaiacolate (guaifenesin)

Therapeutic: Antitussive (dextromethomethorphan), decongestant (pseudoephedrine), expectorant (guaifenesin)

Pregnancy category: C

Indications and Dosages

▶ *To treat nasal congestion and cough, especially nonproductive cough caused by the common cold, acute respiratory infections, acute and chronic bronchitis, hay fever, and sinusitis*

SYRUP

Adults. 15 to 30 mg dextromethorphan, 40 to 80 mg pseudoephedrine, and 100 to 400 mg guaifenesin (5 to 10 ml depending on product) q 4 to 6 hr. *Maximum:* 4 doses daily.

E.R. TABLETS

Adults. 30 to 64 mg dextromethorphan, 45 to 120 mg pseudoephedrine, and 550 to 1,200 mg guaifenesin (1 or 2 tablets depending on product) q 12 hr.

Mechanism of Action

Dextromethorphan suppresses cough by acting directly on the cough center in the medulla of the brain.

Pseudoephedrine acts on alpha$_1$-adrenergic receptors in respiratory mucosa, producing vasoconstriction that shrinks swollen nasal mucous membranes; reduces tissue hyperemia, edema, and nasal congestion; and increases nasal airway patency. It also may increase sinus drainage and open obstructed eustachian ostia.

Guaifenesin increases fluid and mucus removal from the upper respiratory tract by increasing the volume of secretions and reducing their adhesiveness and surface tension.

Contraindications

Acute MI; angina; asthma; cardiac arrhythmias; chronic bronchitis; emphysema; hypersensitivity or idiosyncractic reactions to dextromethorphan, pseudoephedrine, guaifenesin, or their components; hyperthyroidism; narrow-angle glaucoma; prostatic hypertrophy; severe coronary artery disease or hypertension; urine retention; use within 14 days of MAO inhibitor therapy

Interactions

DRUGS

dextromethorphan and pseudoephedrine

MAO inhibitors: Increased and prolonged cardiac stimulation, increased vasopressor effect, increased risk of severe cardiovascular and cerebrovascular effects, hyperpyrexia, and vomiting

dextromethorphan component

amiodarone, fluoxetine,paroxetine, quinidine: Decreased dextromethorphan metabolism, which may result in increased plasma dextromethorphan level and adverse effects

CNS depressants: Additive CNS effects

pseudoephedrine component

antacids: Increased pseudoephedrine absorption

antihypertensives, diuretics: Possibly decreased antihypertensive effects

beta blockers: Decreased therapeutic effects of both drugs

citrates: Possibly inhibited urinary pseudoephedrine excretion and prolonged duration of action

CNS stimulant, other sympathomimetics: Possibly increased additive CNS stimulation to excessive levels

cocaine (mucosal-local): Possibly increased cardiovascular effects of either drug and CNS stimulation

digoxin, levodopa: Increased risk of cardiac arrhythmias

hydrocarbon inhalation anesthetics: Increased risk of serious arrhythmias

kaolin: Decreased pseudoephedrine absorption

nitrates: Reduced antianginal effects of nitrates

rauwolfia alkaloids: Possibly inhibited pseudoephedrine action

thyroid hormones: Increased cardiovascular effects of both drugs

ACTIVITIES

dextromethorphan component

smoking: Possibly increased respiratory secretion retention

Adverse Reactions

CNS: Anxiety, confusion, dizziness, drowsiness, excitability, hallucinations, headache, hyperactivity, insomnia, irritability, light-headedness, nervousness, restlessness, trembling, weakness

CV: Angina, hypertension, palpitations, tachycardia
GI: Abdominal pain, constipation, nausea, vomiting
GU: Dysuria
RESP: Respiratory depression
SKIN: Diaphoresis, pallor, rash, urticaria
Other: Emotional and physical dependence (prolonged use with high doses), serotonin syndrome

Nursing Considerations

- Use cautiously in patients with diabetes, hypertension, increased intraocular pressure, ischemic heart disease, stenosing peptic ulcer, or pyloroduodenal obstruction because of the vaso-constictive action of pseudoepherine.
- Evaluate therapeutic response. Notify prescriber if cough and other symptoms persist or worsen despite use of dextromethorphan, pseudoephedrine, and guaifenesin.
- Monitor renal function, as ordered, because pseudoephedrine is substantially excreted by the kidneys.

PATIENT TEACHING

- Instruct patient to take dextromethorphan, pseudoephedrine, and guaifenesin exactly as prescribed and not to increase dose or frequency without consulting prescriber.
- Instruct patient to use a calibrated measuring device to ensure accurate dose of syrup.
- To minimize nausea, suggest that patient take drug with food and a full glass of water.
- Advise patient not to break, crush, or chew E.R. tablets but to swallow them whole.
- Advise patient to avoid alcohol or other CNS depressants while taking drug.
- Advise patient to avoid potentially hazardous activities until drug's CNS effects are known.
- Instruct patient to increase fluid intake (unless contraindicated) to help thin secretions.

ephedrine hydrochloride and guaifenesin

Bronkaid, Broncholate, Primatene

Class and Category
Chemical: Sympathomimetic amine (ephedrine), glyceryl guaiacolate (guaifenesin)
Therapeutic: Bronchodilator (ephedrine), expectorant (guaifenesin)
Pregnancy category: C

Indications and Dosages
▶ *To relieve upper respiratory symptoms of the common cold and seasonal allergies*
SYRUP
Adults and children age 12 and over. 12.5 to 25 mg ephedrine and 200 to 400 mg guaifenesin (10 to 20 ml) q 4 hr.
Children ages 6 to 12. 6.25 to 12.5 mg ephedrine and 100 to 200 mg guaifenesin (5 to 10 ml) q 4 hr.
Children ages 2 to 6. 3.125 to 6.25 mg ephedrine and 50 to 100 mg guaifenesin (2.5 to 5 ml) q 4 hr.

Mechanism of Action
Ephedrine stimulates beta-adrenergic receptors in the lungs to relax bronchial smooth muscle, which relieves bronchospasm. It also stimulates alpha-adrenergic receptors in nasal passages to produce vasoconstriction and a drying effect on nasal mucous membranes.

Guaifenesin increases fluid and mucus removal from the upper respiratory tract by increasing the volume of secretions and reducing their adhesiveness and surface tension.

Contraindications
Breastfeeding; cardiac disease, including arrhythmias; hypersensitivity to ephedrine, guaifenesin, or their components; hypertension; hyperthyroidism; pregnancy; prostatic hypertrophy; uncontrolled seizure disorder; use within 14 days of MAO inhibitor therapy

Interactions
DRUGS
ephedrine component
alpha blockers, haloperidol, loxapine, phenothiazines, thioxanthenes: Possibly decreased vasoconstrictor effect of ephedrine
beta blockers: Decreased therapeutic effects of each drug
ergot alkaloids: Possibly cerebral blood vessel rupture, increased vasopressor effect, peripheral vascular ischemia, and gangrene (with ergotamine)

guanadrel, guanethidine: Possibly decreased hypotensive effects of these agents

guanethidine, methyldopa, reserpine: Reduced pressor response of ephedrine

hydrocarbon inhalation anesthetics: Increased risk of serious arrhythmias

MAO inhibitors: Increased pressor effect of ephedrine; possibly increased risk of severe hypertensive crisis

theophylline: Possibly enhanced toxicity, especially increased nausea, nervousness and insomnia

thyroid hormones: Increased cardiovascular effects of each drug

tricyclic antidepressants: Possibly increased pressor response

urinary acidifers: May decrease half-life of ephedrine, which may lead to decreased effects

urinary alkalizers: May increase half-life of ephedrine, which may lead to increased effects

Adverse Reactions

CNS: Anxiety, confusion, dizziness, headache, insomnia, nervousness, seizures, tremor, vertigo

CV: Arrhythmias, hypertension, palpitations, tachycardia

ENDO: Hyperglycemia

GI: Abdominal pain, anorexia, diarrhea, nausea, vomiting

MS: Muscle cramps

SKIN: Diaphoresis, rash, urticaria

Nursing Considerations

• Evaluate effectiveness of ephedrine in relieving respiratory symptoms, and notify prescriber if symptoms worsen.

• Monitor patient's blood glucose level closely because ephedrine can cause hyperglycemia.

PATIENT TEACHING

• Caution patient to take drug exactly as prescribed and not to increase dose or frequency without consulting prescriber.

• Instruct patient to avoid potentially hazardous activities until drug's CNS effects are known.

• Tell patient to take last dose of the day a few hours before bedtime if drug makes her nervous.

• Instruct patient with diabetes to monitor blood glucose level closely during drug therapy.

• Advise patient to increase fluid intake (if not contraindicated) to help loosen mucus and thin secretions.

fexofenadine hydrochloride and pseudoephedrine hydrochloride

Allegra-D 12 Hour, Allegra-D 24 Hour

Class and Category

Chemical: Terfenadine metabolite (fexofenadine), (sympatho-mimetic amine (pseudoephedrine)

Therapeutic: Antihistaminic (fexofenadine), decongestant (pseudo-ephedrine)

Pregnancy category: C

Indications and Dosages

▶ *To relieve symptoms of seasonal allergic rhinitis*

TABLETS (ALLEGRA-D 12 HOUR)

Adults and children age 12 and over. 60 mg fexofenadine and 120 mg pseudoephedrine (1 tablet) b.i.d.

DOSAGE ADJUSTMENT For patients with renal impairment, dosage frequency decreased to once daily.

TABLETS (ALLEGRA-D 24 HOUR)

Adults and children age 12 and over. 180 mg fexofenadine and 240 mg pseudoephedrine (1 tablet) daily.

Mechanism of Action

Fexofenadine competes with histamine for histamine H_1 receptor sites on effector cells and antagonizes the vasodilator effect of endogenously released histamine. This prevents vascular engorgement, mucosal edema, sneezing, and profuse watery secretion and irritation that normally result from histamine action on peripheral afferent nerve terminals.

Pseudoephedrine acts on $alpha_1$-adrenergic receptors in the mucosa of the respiratory tract to produce vasoconstriction. This process shrinks swollen nasal mucous membranes; reduces tissue hyperemia, edema, and nasal congestion; and increases nasal airway patency. It also may increase drainage of sinus secretions and open obstructed eustachian ostia.

Contraindications

Hypersensitivity or idiosyncratic reactions to fexofenadine, pseudoephedrine, or their components; hyperthyroidism; narrow-angle glaucoma; severe coronary artery disease or hypertension; urine retention; use within 14 days of MAO inhibitor therapy

Interactions

DRUGS

fexofenadine component

aluminum and magnesium containing antacids: Decreased fexofenadine absorption

erythromycin, ketoconazole: Enchanced fexofenadine absorption which increased plasma fexofenadine levels

psuedoephedrine component

antacids: Increased pseudoephedrine absorption

antihypertensives, diuretics: Possibly decreased antihypertensive effects

beta blockers: Decreased therapeutic effects of both drugs

citrates: Possibly inhibited urinary pseudoephedrine excretion and prolonged duration of action

CNS stimulant, other sympathomimetics: Possibly increased additive CNS stimulation to excessive levels

cocaine (mucosal-local): Possibly increased cardiovascular effects of either drug and CNS stimulation

digoxin, levodopa: Increased risk of cardiac arrhythmias

hydrocarbon inhalation anesthetics: Increased risk of serious arrhythmias

kaolin: Decreased pseudoephedrine absorption

MAO inhibitors: Increased and prolonged cardiac stimulation, increased vasopressor effect, increased risk of severe cardiovascular and cerebrovascular effects, hyperpyrexia, vomiting

nitrates: Reduced antianginal effects of nitrates

rauwolfia alkaloids: Possibly inhibited pseudoephedrine action

thyroid hormones: Increased cardiovascular effects of both drugs

FOODS

fexofenadine component

all foods: Decreased fexofenadine absorption

fruit juices: Possibly decreased fexofenadine absorption

Adverse Reactions

CNS: Anxiety, excitability, dizziness, drowsiness, fear, hallucinations, headache, insomnia, light-headedness, nervousness, paranoia, restlessness, seizures, sleep disturbances, trembling, weakness

CV: Arrhythmias, hypertension, palpitations, tachycardia

EENT: Dry mouth, throat irritation

GI: Abdominal pain, nausea, vomiting

GU: Dysuria

MS: Back pain

RESP: Dyspnea, upper respiratory tract infection

SKIN: Pallor, pruritis, rash, urticaria

Other: Anaphylaxis, angioedema

Nursing Considerations
- Be aware that Allegra-D 24 Hour isn't recommended for patients with renal insufficiency.
- Use cautiously in patients with diabetes, hypertension, increased intraocular pressure, ischemic heart disease, prostatic hypertrophy, stenosing peptic ulcer, or pyloroduodenal obstruction because of the vasoconstrictive action of pseudoepherine.
- Monitor elderly patients closely for CNS effects because they're more likely to develop these adverse effects.
- Monitor renal function, as ordered, because pseudoephedrine is substantially excreted by the kidneys.
- Evaluate effectiveness of fexofenadine and pseudoepherine in relieving symptoms of seasonal allergic rhinitis, such as sneezing, rhinorrhea, pruritus, lacrimation, and nasal congestion.
- Be aware that patient shouldn't have intradermal allergen tests within 4 days of receiving drug because results may be altered.

PATIENT TEACHING
- Instruct patient to take fexofenadine and pseudoephedrine only with water on an empty stomach and to swallow the tablet whole without crushing or chewing it.
- Caution patient not to exceed dosage prescribed.
- Advise patient that if she experiences nervousness, dizziness, or sleeplessness, she should stop taking fexofenadine and pseudoephedrine and consult the prescriber.
- Urge patient to avoid alcohol, other antidepressants, and OTC drugs containing other antihistamines or sympathomimetics while taking fexofenadine and pseudoephedrine.
- Instruct patient to avoid potentially hazardous activities until drug's CNS effects are known.

fluticasone propionate and salmeterol
Advair Diskus 100/50, Advair Diskus 250/50,
Advair Diskus 500/50

Class and Category
Chemical: Corticorsteroid (fluticasone), beta$_2$-adrengeric receptor agonist (salmeterol)
Therapeutic: Anti-inflammatory agent (fluticasone), bronchodilator (salmeterol)
Pregnancy category: C

Indications and Dosages

▶ *To provide long-term maintenance treatment of asthma*
INHALATION

Adults and children age 12 and over not using an inhaled corticosteroid. 100 mcg fluticasone and 50 mcg salmeterol b.i.d.
Adults and children age 12 and over taking beclomethasone dipropionate or triamcinolone acetonide by inhalation. 100 or 250 mcg fluticasone and 50 mcg salmeterol b.i.d.
Adults and children age 12 and over taking budesonide or fluticasone propionate by inhalation. 100, 250, or 500 mcg fluticasone and 50 mcg salmeterol b.i.d.
Adults and children age 12 and over taking flunisolide. 100 or 250 mcg fluticasone and 50 mcg salmeterol b.i.d.
Children ages 4 to 12 who are symptomatic despite using an inhaled corticosteroid. 100 mcg fluticasone and 50 mcg salmeterol b.i.d.

▶ *To provide maintenance treatment of COPD with chronic bronchitis*
INHALATION

Adults. 250 mcg fluticasone and 50 mcg salmeterol b.i.d.

Mechanism of Action

Fluticasone inhibits cells involved in the inflammatory response of asthma, such as mast cells, eosinophils, basophils, lymphocytes, macrophages, and neutrophils. It also inhibits production or secretion of chemical mediators, such as histamine, eicosanoids, leukotrienes, and cytokines.

Salmeterol attaches to beta$_2$ receptors on bronchial cell membranes, stimulating the intracellular enzyme adenylate cyclase to convert adenosine triphosphate to cAMP. The resulting increase in intracellular cAMP level relaxes bronchial smooth-muscle cells, stabilizes mast cells, and inhibits histamine release.

Contraindications

Hypersensitivity to fluticasone, salmeterol, or their components; primary treatment of status asthmaticus or other acute asthma or COPD episodes that require intensive measures; untreated nasal mucosal infection (nasal suspension)

Interactions

DRUGS
fluticasone component
ketoconazole, ritonavir, and other strong CYP 3A4 inhibitors (long-term use): Possibly increased blood fluticasone level

salmeterol component

beta blockers: Mutual inhibition of therapeutic effects

loop or thiazide diuretics: Increased risk of hypokalemia and potentially life-threatening arrhythmias

MAO inhibitors, tricyclic antidepressants: Potentiated adverse vascular effects, such as hypertensive crisis

Adverse Reactions

CNS: Aggressiveness, agitation, depression, difficulty speaking, dizziness, fatigue, fever, headache, insomnia, malaise, nervousness, paresthesia, restlessness, tremor

CV: Tachycardia

EENT: Allergic rhinitis; cataracts; conjunctivitis; dry mouth, nose, and throat; eye irritation; glaucoma; laryngitis; laryngeal spasm, irritation, or swelling; loss of voice; nasal congestion or discharge; oropharyngeal candidiasis; otitis media; pharyngitis; sinus problems; tonsillitis

ENDO: Adrenal insufficiency, cushingoid symptoms, hyperglycemia

GI: Abdominal pain, diarrhea, indigestion, nausea, vomiting

GU: Dysmenorrhea

HEME: Easy bruising

MS: Arthralgia, myalgia

RESP: Asthma exacerbation, bronchitis, chest congestion and tightness, cough, dyspnea, paradoxical bronchospasm, upper respiratory tract infection, wheezing

SKIN: Dermatitis, ecchymosis, eczema, rash, urticaria

Other: Angioedema, flulike symptoms, generalized aches and pains, weight gain

Nursing Considerations

• Use fluticasone and salmeterol cautiously in patients with ocular herpes simplex, pulmonary tuberculosis, or untreated systemic bacterial, fungal, parasitic, or viral infection because fluticasone can mask signs and symptoms and severity of condition.

• Be aware that fluticasone and salmeterol shouldn't be used to relieve bronchospasm quickly because of its prolonged onset of action. As prescribed, give a fast-acting inhaled bronchodilator if bronchospsm occurs.

• Monitor effectiveness of fluticasone and salmeterol. Notify prescriber if patient needs more short-acting inhalations than usual or the patient develops a significant decrease in lung function. Have patient reassessed, and expect his medication regimen to change, which may include increasing the strength of fluticasone and salmeterol combination (never the number of inhalations) or adding an inhaled or systemic corticosteroid.

• **WARNING** Be aware that a recent study suggests asthma-related deaths may be increased in African-American patients taking salmeterol. Monitor this patient population closely throughout therapy, and notify prescriber immediately of any changes in patient's respiratory status.

• Watch for arrhythmias and changes in blood pressure after use in patients with cardiovascular disorders, including ischemic cardiac disease, hypertension, and arrhythmias, because of drug's beta-adrengeric effects.

• Monitor patient for immediate hypersensitivity reaction after giving fluticasone and salmeterol. Reaction may include urticaria, rash, angioedema, bronchospasm, or laryngeal spasm, irritation, or swelling. Notify prescriber immediately, and expect to provide supportive care and to discontinue drug.

• Assess patient for risk factors for decreased bone mineral content, such as smoking, advanced age, sedentary lifestyle, poor nutrition, family history of osteoporosis, or chronic use of drugs that can reduce bone mass, such as anticonvulsants and corticosteroids. If present, have the patient undergo a bone mineral density study, as prescribed, because chronic use of any drug containing fluticasone may adversely affect bone density.

• Be aware that systemic absorption may occur with inhalation of fluticasone and salmeterol with the potential to suppress the hypothalamic-pituitary-adrenal axis with long-term use. Don't stop drug abruptly but withdraw gradually, as prescribed, to prevent acute adrenal insufficiency.

PATIENT TEACHING

• Advise patient to take doses 12 hours apart for optimum effect. Caution against using fluticasone and salmeterol more than every 12 hours or stopping it abruptly.

• Teach patient how to use the diskus by instructing him to slide the lever only once when preparing dose to avoid wasting doses. Advise him to exhale immediately before using the diskus and then to place the mouthpiece to his lips, holding it in a level, horizontal position, and inhale through his mouth, not his nose. Then he should remove the mouthpiece from his mouth, hold his breath for at least 10 seconds, and exhale slowly. Then tell patient to close the diskus, which will also reset the dose lever for the next scheduled dose.

- Warn patient not to use fluticasone and salmeterol combination to treat acute bronchospasm but instead to use a short-acting bronchodilator as prescribed.
- Advise patient to rinse his mouth with water after each dose to minimize dry mouth.
- Advise patient to discard diskus 1 month after removing it from the foil overwrap or when dose indicator reads zero, whichever comes first.
- Urge patient to carry medical identification indicating the need for supplemental systemic corticosteroids during stress or severe asthma attack.
- Caution patient to report exposure to chickenpox, measles, or other infectious diseases because prophylactic treatment may be required.

guaifenesin and codeine phosphate

Brontex, Cheracol, Endal, Gani-Tuss NR, Guiatuss AC Syrup, Halotussin AC Liquid, Mytussin AC Cough Syrup, Robafen AC, Robitussin A-C Syrup, Romilar AC Liquid, Tussi-Organidin NR Liquid, Tussi-Organidin-S NR Liquid

Class, Category, and Schedule

Chemical: Glyceryl guaiacolate (guaifenesin), phenanthrene derivative (codeine)
Therapeutic: Expectorant (guaifenesin), antitussive (codeine)
Pregnancy category: C
Controlled substance: Schedule V (oral solution), III (tablets)

Indications and Dosages

▶ *To relieve cough and chest congestion*

ORAL SOLUTION, SYRUP (ALL BRANDS EXCEPT BRONTEX)

Adults and children age 12 and over. 100 to 200 mg guaifenesin and 10 to 20 mg codeine (5 or 10 ml depending on product) q 4 to 6 hr. *Maximum:* 6 doses daily.

Children ages 6 to 12. 50 to 100 mg guaifenesin and 5 to 10 mg codeine (5 ml) q 6 to 8 hr. *Maximum:* 6 doses daily.

Children ages 2 to 6. 50 mg guaifenesin and 5 mg codeine (2.5 ml) q 6 to 8 hr.

ORAL SOLUTION (BRONTEX)

Adults and children age 12 and over. 300 mg guaifenesin and 10 mg codeine (20 ml) q 4 hr. *Maximum:* 6 doses daily.

Children ages 6 to 12. 150 mg guaifenesin and 5 mg codeine (10 ml) q 4 hr.

TABLETS (BRONTEX)
Adults and children age 12 and over. 300 mg guaifenesin and
10 mg codeine (1 tablet) q 4 hr.

Mechanism of Action

Guaifenesin increases fluid and mucus removal from the upper respiratory
tract by increasing the volume of secretions and reducing their adhesiveness
and surface tension.

    Codeine suppresses cough by directly acting on opiate receptors in the
medulla's cough center.

Contraindications

Hypersensitivity to guaifenesin, codeine, other opioids, or their
components; irritable bowel syndrome; paralytic ileus; significant
respiratory depression

Interactions

DRUGS

codeine component

anticholinergics, paregoric: Possibly intensified anticholinergic adverse effects

antidiarrheals: Increased risk of severe constipation

antihypertensives, diuretics: Potentiated hypotensive effects

buprenorphine: Decreased codeine effectiveness

CNS depressants: Additive CNS depression

hydroxyzine: Increased codeine analgesic effect; increased CNS depressant and hypotensive effects

MAO inhibitors: Increased risk of unpredictable, severe, and sometimes fatal reactions with codeine

metoclopramide: Antagonized effect of metoclopramide on GI
motility

naloxone: Antagonized codeine analgesic effect

naltrexone: Precipitated withdrawal symptoms in codeine-dependent patients

neuromuscular blockers: Additive respiratory depressant effects

opioids: Additive CNS and respiratory depressants effects and hypotensive effects

ACTIVITIES

codeine component

alcohol use: Additive CNS depression

Adverse Reactions

CNS: Coma, delirium, depression, disorientation, dizziness,

drowsiness, euphoria, hallucinations, headache, lack of coordination, lethargy, light-headedness, mental and physical impairment, mood changes, restlessness, sedation, seizures, tremor
CV: Bradycardia, heart block, hypertension, orthostatic hypotension, palpitations, tachycardia
EENT: Altered taste, blurred vision, diplopia, dry mouth, laryngeal edema, laryngospasm, miosis
GI: Abdominal cramps and pain, anorexia, constipation, flatulence, gastroesophageal reflux, ileus, indigestion, nausea, vomiting
GU: Decreased libido, difficult ejaculation, dysuria, impotence, oliguria, ureteral spasm, urinary incontinence, urine retention
MS: Muscle rigidity
RESP: Apnea, bronchoconstriction, bronchospasm, depressed cough reflex, respiratory depression
SKIN: Diaphoresis, flushing, pallor, pruritus, rash, urticaria
Other: Anaphylaxis, facial edema, physical and psychological dependence

Nursing Considerations

- Evaluate patient for therapeutic response, including decreased cough. Notify prescriber if symptoms persist or worsen despite use of guaifenesin and codeine.
- Take safety precautions, if needed, because codeine can cause excessive drowsiness.
- Monitor respiratory depth, effort, and rate. Notify prescriber immediately if respiratory rate drops below 10 breaths/minute.
- Assess urine output; decreasing output may signal urine retention.
- **WARNING** Assess patient for evidence of physical and psychological dependence.

PATIENT TEACHING

- Instruct patient to take guaifenesin and codeine exactly as prescribed and not to increase dose or frequency without consulting prescriber.
- Tell patient to take drug with a full glass of water.
- Advise patient to avoid alcohol or other CNS depressants while taking drug.
- To minimize nausea, suggest that patient take drug with food.
- Advise patient to avoid potentially hazardous activities until drug's CNS effects are known.
- Caution patient to get up slowly from a sitting or lying position.

- To prevent constipation, encourage patient to consume plenty of fluids and high-fiber foods, if not contraindicated.
- Advise patient to notify prescriber if she becomes short of breath or has difficulty breathing.

guaifenesin, codeine phosphate, and pseudoephedrine hydrochloride

Cycofed, Dihistine Expectorant, Guiatuss DAC, Halotussin DAC, KG-Fed Expectorant, Mytussin DAC, Novagest Expectorant with Codeine, Nucofed Expectorant, Nucofed Pediatric Expectorant, Nucotuss Expectorant, Nucotuss Pediatric Expectorant, Robitussin DAC, Ryna-CX

Class, Category, and Schedule

Chemical: Glyceryl guaiacolate (guaifenesin), phenanthrene derivative (codeine), sympathomimetic amine (pseudoephedrine)
Therapeutic: Expectorant (guaifenesin), antitussive (codeine), decongestant (pseudoephedrine)
Pregnancy category: C
Controlled substance: Schedule V (all except Nucofed and Nucotuss Expectorant Syrup), III (Nucofed and Nucotuss Expectorant Syrup)

Indications and Dosages

▶ *To relieve cough and chest congestion*
ORAL SOLUTION, SYRUP
Adults and children age 12 and over. 200 mg guaifenesin, 20 mg codeine, and 60 mg pseudoephedrine (available as either 5 ml or 10 ml depending on brand) q 4 to 6 hr. *Maximum:* 4 doses daily
Children ages 6 to 12. 100 mg guaifenesin, 10 mg codeine, and 30 mg pseudoephedrine (5 ml) q 6 hr. *Maximum:* 4 doses daily.
Children ages 2 to 6. 50 mg guaifenesin, 5 mg codeine, and 15 mg pseudoephedrine (2.5 ml) q 6 hr. *Maximum:* 4 doses daily.

Contraindications

Hypersensitivity or idiosyncractic reactions to guaifenesin, codeine, pseudoephedrine, other opioids, or their components; hyperthyroidism; narrow-angle glaucoma; prostatic hypertrophy; severe coronary artery disease or hypertension; significant respiratory depression; urine retention; use within 14 days of MAO inhibitor therapy

Mechanism of Action

Guaifenesin increases fluid and mucus removal from the upper respiratory tract by increasing the volume of secretions and reducing their adhesiveness and surface tension.

Codeine suppresses cough by directly acting on opiate receptors in the medulla's cough center.

Pseudoephedrine acts on alpha$_1$-adrenergic receptors in the mucosa of the respiratory tract to produce vasoconstriction. This process shrinks swollen nasal mucous membranes; reduces tissue hyperemia, edema, and nasal congestion; and increases nasal airway patency. It also may increase drainage of sinus secretions and open obstructed eustachian ostia.

Interactions

DRUGS

codeine and pseudoephedrine components

MAO inhibitors: Increased and prolonged cardiac stimulation, increased vasopressor effect, increased risk of severe cardiovascular and cerebrovascular effects, hyperpyrexia, vomiting

codeine component

anticholinergics, paregoric: Possibly intensified anticholinergic adverse effects

antidiarrheals: Increased risk of severe constipation

antihypertensives, diuretics: Potentiated hypotensive effects

buprenorphine: Decreased codeine effectiveness

CNS depressants: Additive CNS depression

hydroxyzine: Increased codeine analgesic effect; increased CNS depressant and hypotensive effects

metoclopramide: Antagonized effect of metoclopramide on GI motility

naloxone: Anatagonized codeine analgesic effect

naltrexone: Precipitated withdrawal symptoms in codeine-dependent patients

neuromuscular blockers: Additive respiratory depressant effects

opioids: Additive CNS and respiratory depressants effects and hypotensive effects

pseudoephedrine component

antacids: Increased pseudoephedrine absorption

antihypertensives, diuretics: Possibly decreased antihypertensive effects

beta blockers: Decreased therapeutic effects of both drugs

citrates: Possibly inhibited urinary pseudoephedrine excretion and prolonged duration of action

CNS stimulant, other sympathomimetics: Possibly increased additive CNS stimulation to excessive levels

cocaine (mucosal-local): Possibly increased cardiovascular effects of either drug and CNS stimulation

digoxin, levodopa: Increased risk of cardiac arrhythmias

hydrocarbon inhalation anesthetics: Increased risk of serious arrhythmias

kaolin: Decreased pseudoephedrine absorption

nitrates: Reduced antianginal effects of nitrates

rauwolfia alkaloids: Possibly inhibited pseudoephedrine action

thyroid hormones: Increased cardiovascular effects of both drugs

ACTIVITIES

codeine component

alcohol use: Additive CNS depression

Adverse Reactions

CNS: Coma, delirium, depression, disorientation, dizziness, drowsiness, euphoria, hallucinations, headache, insomnia, lack of coordination, lethargy, light-headedness, mental and physical impairment, mood changes, nervousness, restlessness, sedation, seizures, tremor, weakness

CV: Bradycardia, heart block, hypertension, orthostatic hypotension, palpitations, tachycardia

EENT: Altered taste, blurred vision, diplopia, dry mouth, laryngeal edema, laryngospasm, miosis

GI: Abdominal cramps and pain, anorexia, constipation, flatulence, gastroesophageal reflux, ileus, indigestion, nausea, vomiting

GU: Decreased libido, difficult ejaculation, dysuria, impotence, oliguria, ureteral spasm, urinary incontinence, urine retention

MS: Muscle rigidity

RESP: Apnea, bronchoconstriction, bronchospasm, depressed cough reflex, respiratory depression

SKIN: Diaphoresis, flushing, pallor, pruritus, rash, urticaria

Other: Anaphylaxis, facial edema, physical and psychological dependence

Nursing Considerations

- Use cautiously in patients with diabetes, hypertension, hyperthyroidism, increased intraocular pressure, ischemic heart disease, prostatic hypertrophy, stenosing peptic ulcer or pyloroduodenal obstruction because of the vasoconstictive action of pseudoepherine.

- Watch for therapeutic response, including decreased cough. Notify prescriber if symptoms persist or worsen despite use of guaifenesin, codeine, and pseudoephedrine.
- Monitor renal function, as ordered, because pseudoephedrine is substantially excreted by the kidneys.
- Take safety precautions, if needed because codeine component of drug can cause excessive drowsiness.
- Monitor respiratory depth, effort, and rate. Notify prescriber immediately if respiratory rate drops below 10 breaths/minute.
- Assess urine output; decreasing output may signal urine retention.
- **WARNING** Assess patient for evidence of physical and psychological dependence.

PATIENT TEACHING
- Instruct patient to take guaifenesin, codeine, and pseudoephedrine exactly as prescribed and not to increase dosage or frequency without consulting prescriber.
- Tell patient to take each dose with a full glass of water.
- Advise patient to avoid alcohol or other CNS depressants while taking drug.
- To minimize nausea, suggest that patient take drug with food.
- Advise patient to avoid potentially hazardous activities until drug's CNS effects are known.
- Caution patient to get up slowly from a sitting or lying position.
- To prevent constipation, encourage patient to consume plenty of fluids and high-fiber foods, if not contraindicated.
- Advise patient to notify prescriber if he becomes short of breath or has difficulty breathing.

guaifenesin and hydrocodone bitartrate
Codiclear DH, Co-Tuss V, Hycosin Expectorant,
Hycotuss Expectorant, Hydrocodone GF, Kwelcof, Pneumotussin,
Vicodin Tuss, Vitussin

Class, Category, and Schedule
Chemical: Glyceryl guaiacolate (guaifenesin), opioid and phenanthrene derivative (hydrocodone)
Therapeutic: Expectorant (guaifenesin), antitussive (hydrocodone)
Pregnancy category: C
Controlled substance: Schedule III

Indications and Dosages

▶ *To relieve cough and other symptoms of allergies and the common cold*

ORAL SOLUTION, SYRUP

Adults and children age 12 and over. 100 to 400 mg guaifenesin and 5 mg hydrocodone (5 or 10 ml) q 4 to 6 hr.

Children ages 2 to 12. 50 to 100 mg guaifenesin and 2.5 to 5 mg hydrocodone (2.5 or 5 ml) q 4 to 6 hr.

TABLETS

Adults. 300 to 600 mg guaifenesin and 2.5 to 5 mg hydrocodone (1 or 2 tablets) q 4 to 6 hr. *Maximum:* 4 doses daily.

Mechanism of Action

Guaifenesin increases fluid and mucus removal from the upper respiratory tract by increasing the volume of secretions and reducing their adhesiveness and surface tension.

Hydrocodone suppresses cough by directly acting on opiate receptors in the medulla's cough center.

Contraindications

Hypersensitivity or idiosyncractic reactions to guaifenesin, hydrocodone, other opioids, or their components; respiratory depression

Interactions

DRUGS

hydrocodone component

anticholinergics, paregoric: Possibly intensified anticholinergic adverse effects

antidiarrheals: Increased risk of severe constipation or paralytic ileus

antihypertensives, diuretics: Potentiated hypotensive effects

buprenorphine: Decreased hydrocodone effectiveness

CNS depressants: Additive CNS depression

hydroxyzine: Increased hydrocodone analgesic effect; increased CNS depressant and hypotensive effects

MAO inhibitors: Increased and prolonged cardiac stimulation, increased vasopressor effect, increased risk of severe cardiovascular and cerebrovascular effects, hyperpyrexia, vomiting

metoclopramide: Antagonized effect of metoclopramide on GI motility

naloxone: Antagonized hydrocodone analgesic effect

naltrexone: Precipitated withdrawal symptoms in hydrocodone-dependent patients

neuromuscular blockers: Additive respiratory depressant effects

opioids: Additive CNS and respiratory depressants effects and hypotensive effects

ACTIVITIES

hydrocodone component

alcohol use: Additive CNS effects

Adverse Reactions

CNS: Coma, delirium, depression, disorientation, dizziness, drowsiness, euphoria, hallucinations, headache, lack of coordination, lethargy, light-headedness, mental and physical impairment, mood changes, restlessness, sedation, seizures, tremor

CV: Bradycardia, heart block, hypertension, orthostatic hypotension, palpitations, tachycardia

EENT: Altered taste, blurred vision, diplopia, dry mouth, laryngeal edema, laryngospasm, miosis

GI: Abdominal cramps and pain, anorexia, constipation, flatulence, gastroesophageal reflux, ileus, indigestion, nausea, vomiting

GU: Decreased libido, difficult ejaculation, dysuria, impotence, oliguria, ureteral spasm, urinary incontinence, urine retention

MS: Muscle rigidity

RESP: Apnea, bronchoconstriction, bronchospasm, depressed cough reflex, respiratory depression

SKIN: Diaphoresis, flushing, pallor, pruritus, rash, urticaria

Other: Anaphylaxis, facial edema, physical and psychological dependence

Nursing Considerations

• Watch for therapeutic response, including decreased cough. Notify prescriber if symptoms persist or worsen despite use of guaifenesin and hydrocodone.

• Monitor respiratory depth, effort, and rate. Notify prescriber immediately if respiratory rate drops below 10 breaths/minute.

• Assess urine output; decreasing output may signal urine retention.

• **WARNING** Assess patient for evidence of physical and psychological dependence.

PATIENT TEACHING

• Instruct patient to take guaifenesin and hydrocodone exactly as prescribed and not to increase dose or frequency without consulting prescriber.

- Instruct patient to use a calibrated measuring device to ensure accurate dose when using liquid form of drug.
- Tell patient to take each dose with a full glass of water.
- Advise patient to avoid alcohol or other CNS depressants while taking drug.
- To minimize nausea, suggest that patient take drug with food.
- Advise patient to avoid potentially hazardous activities until drug's CNS effects are known.
- Caution patient to get up slowly from a sitting or lying position.
- Advise patient to notify prescriber if she becomes short of breath or has difficulty breathing.

guaifenesin and hydromorphone hydrochloride
Dilaudid Cough Syrup

Class, Category, and Schedule
Chemical: Glyceryl guaiacolate (guaifenesin), opioid and phenanthrene derivative (hydromorphone)
Therapeutic: Expectorant (guaifenesin), antitussive (hydromorphone)
Pregnancy category: C
Controlled substance: Schedule II

Indications and Dosages
▶ *To relieve cough and other symptoms of allergies and the common cold*
SYRUP
Adults. 1 mg hydromorphone and 100 guaifenesin (5 ml) q 3 to 4 hr.

Mechanism of Action
Guaifenesin increases fluid and mucus removal from the upper respiratory tract by increasing the volume of secretions and reducing their adhesiveness and surface tension.

Hydromorphone suppresses cough by acting directly on opiate receptors in the medulla's cough center.

Contraindications
Hypersensitivity or idiosyncractic reactions to guaifenesin, hydro-

morphone, other opioids, or their components; respiratory depression

Interactions

DRUGS

hydromorphone component

anticholinergics, paregoric: Possibly intensified anticholinergic adverse effects

antihypertensives, diuretics: Potentiated hypotensive effects

buprenorphine: Decreased hydromorphone effectiveness

CNS depressants: Additive CNS depression

hydroxyzine: Increased hydromorphone analgesic effect; increased CNS depressant and hypotensive effects

MAO inhibitors: Increased and prolonged cardiac stimulation, increased vasopressor effect, increased risk of severe cardiovascular and cerebrovascular effects, hyperpyrexia, vomiting

metoclopramide: Antagonized effect of metoclopramide on GI motility

naloxone: Antagonized hydromorphone analgesic effect

naltrexone: Precipitated withdrawal symptoms in hydromorphone-dependent patients

neuromuscular blockers: Additive respiratory depressant effects

opioids: Additive CNS and respiratory depressants effects and hypotensive effects

ACTIVITIES

hydromorphone component

alcohol use: Additive CNS effects

Adverse Reactions

CNS: Coma, delirium, depression, disorientation, dizziness, drowsiness, euphoria, hallucinations, headache, lack of coordination, lethargy, light-headedness, mental and physical impairment, mood changes, restlessness, sedation, seizures, tremor

CV: Bradycardia, heart block, hypertension, orthostatic hypotension, palpitations, tachycardia

EENT: Altered taste, blurred vision, diplopia, dry mouth, laryngeal edema, laryngospasm, miosis

GI: Abdominal cramps and pain, anorexia, constipation, flatulence, gastroesophageal reflux, ileus, indigestion, nausea, vomiting

GU: Decreased libido, difficult ejaculation, dysuria, impotence, oliguria, ureteral spasm, urinary incontinence, urine retention

MS: Muscle rigidity

RESP: Apnea, bronchoconstriction, bronchospasm, depressed cough reflex, respiratory depression
SKIN: Diaphoresis, flushing, pallor, pruritus, rash, urticaria
Other: Anaphylaxis, facial edema, physical and psychological dependence

Nursing Considerations

- Evaluate therapeutic response, including decreased cough. If symptoms persist or worsen despite use of guaifenesin and hydromorphone, notify prescriber.
- Monitor respiratory depth, effort, and rate. If respiratory rate drops below 10 breaths/minute, notify prescriber immediately.
- Assess urine output; decreasing output may signal urine retention.
- **WARNING** Assess patient for evidence of physical and psychological dependence.

PATIENT TEACHING

- Instruct patient to take guaifenesin and hydromorphone exactly as prescribed and not to increase dose or frequency without consulting prescriber.
- Instruct patient to use a calibrated measuring device to ensure accurate dose.
- Advise patient to avoid alcohol or other CNS depressants while taking drug.
- To minimize nausea, suggest that patient take drug with food.
- Advise patient to avoid potentially hazardous activities until drug's CNS effects are known.
- Caution patient to get up slowly from a sitting or lying position.
- Advise patient to notify prescriber if he becomes short of breath or has difficulty breathing.

guaifenesin and pseudoephedrine hydrochloride

Anatussin LA, AquatabD, Coldmist JR, Coldmist LA, Congess SR, Deconsal II, Defen-LA, Durasal II, Duratuss, Duratuss GP, Dynex, Entex PSE, GP-500, GFN/PSE, GP-500, GP 1200/60, Guaifed, Guaifenex GP, Guaifenex PSE, Guaifenex PSE 60, Guaifenex PSE 120, Guaifenex-Rx, H 9600 SR, GuaiMAX-D, Guaipax PSE, Guiatuss PE, Guai-Vent/PSE, Iosal II, Maxifed, Maxifed-G, Miraphen PSE, Nasatab LA, PanMist JR, PanMist LA, PanMist-S, Profen Forte, Profen II, Pseudovent, Pseudovent-PED, Respa-1st, Respaire-60 SR, Respaire-120 SR, Robafen PE, Robitussin PE, Robitussin Severe

Congestion, Ru-Tuss, Ru-Tuss DE, Severe Congestion Tussin, Sinufed Timecelles, Sinutab Non-Drying, Stamoist E, Sudal 60/500, Sudafed Non-Drowsy Non-Drying Sinus, Thera-Hist Expectorant Chest Congestion, Triacting, Triaminic Chest Congestion, Touro LA, Tuss-LA, V-Dec M, Versacaps, Sudal 60/500, Sudal 120/600, Zephrex, Zephrex-LA

Class and Category

Chemical: Sympathomimetic amine (pseudoephedrine), glyceryl guaiacolate (guaifenesin)
Therapeutic: Decongestant (pseudoephedrine), expectorant (guaifenesin)
Pregnancy category: C

Indications and Dosages

▶ *To relieve symptoms of seasonal allergic rhinitis*
SYRUP
Adults and children age 12 and over. 100 to 400 mg guaifenesin and 30 to 80 mg pseudoephrine (5 to 10 ml depending on product) q.i.d.
Children ages 6 to 12. 100 to 200 mg guaifenesin and 30 mg pseudoephedrine (2.5 to 5 ml depending on product) q 4 to 6 hr. *Maximum:* 4 doses daily.
Children ages 2 to 6. 50 to 100 mg and 15 mg pseudoephedrine (1.25 to 2.5 ml depending on product) q 4 to 6 hr. *Maximum:* 4 doses daily.
ORAL SOLUTION
Adults and children age 12 and over. 200 mg guaifenesin and 60 mg pseudoephedrine (10 ml) q 4 hr. *Maximum:* 4 doses daily.
Children ages 6 to 12. 30 mg pseudoephedrine and 100 mg guaifenesin (10 ml) q 4 to 6 hr. *Maximum:* 4 doses daily.
Children ages 2 to 6. 50 mg guaifenesin and 15 mg pseudoephedrine (5 ml) q 4 to 6 hr. *Maximum:* 4 doses daily.
E.R. CAPSULES
Adults and children age 12 and over. 200 to 600 mg guaifenesin and 60 to 120 mg pseudoephrine (1 or 2 capsules depending on product) q 12 hr.
Children ages 6 to 12. 300 mg quaifenesin and 60 mg pseudoephedrine (1 capsule) q 12 hr.
LIQUID CAPSULES
Adults. 240 to 400 mg guaifenesin and 60 mg pseudoephedrine (2 capsules) q 4 hr. *Maximum:* 8 capsules daily.

E.R. TABLETS
Adults and children age 12 and over. 400 to 1,200 mg guaifenesin and 45 to 120 mg pseudoephedrine (1 or 2 tablets depending on product) q 12 hr.
Children ages 6 to 12. 200 to 600 mg guaifenesin and 30 to 60 mg pseudoephedrine (½ to 2 tablets depending on product) q 12 hr.
Children ages 2 to 6. 150 to 300 mg guaifenesin and 15 to 30 mg pseudoephedrine (1/2 to 1 tablet depending on product) q 12 hr.
TABLETS
Adults. 400 mg guaifenesin and 60 mg pseudoephedrine (1 tablet) q 6 hr.

Mechanism of Action
Pseudoephedrine acts on alpha$_1$-adrenergic receptors in the mucosa of the respiratory tract to produce vasoconstriction. This process shrinks swollen nasal mucous membranes; reduces tissue hyperemia, edema, and nasal congestion; and increases nasal airway patency. It also may increase drainage of sinus secretions and open obstructed eustachian ostia.

Guaifenesin increases fluid and mucus removal from the upper respiratory tract by increasing the volume of secretions and reducing their adhesiveness and surface tension.

Contraindications
Hypersensitivity or idiosyncratic reactions to pseudoephedrine, guaifenesin, or their components; hyperthyroidism; narrow-angle glaucoma; prostatic hypertrophy; severe coronary artery disease or hypertension; urine retention; use within 14 days of MAO inhibitor therapy

Interactions
DRUGS
pseudoephedrine component
antacids: Increased pseudoephedrine absorption
antihypertensives, diuretics: Possibly decreased antihypertensive effects
beta blockers: Decreased therapeutic effects of both drugs
citrates: Possibly inhibited urinary pseudoephedrine excretion and prolonged duration of action
CNS stimulant, other sympathomimetics: Possibly increased additive CNS stimulation to excessive levels

cocaine (mucosal-local): Possibly increased cardiovascular effects of either drug and CNS stimulation

digoxin, levodopa: Increased risk of cardiac arrhythmias

hydrocarbon inhalation anesthetics: Increased risk of serious arrhythmias

kaolin: Decreased pseudoephedrine absorption

MAO inhibitors: Increased and prolonged cardiac stimulation, increased vasopressor effect, increased risk of severe cardiovascular and cerebrovascular effects, hyperpyrexia, vomiting

nitrates: Reduced antianginal effects of nitrates

rauwolfia alkaloids: Possibly inhibited pseudoephedrine action

thyroid hormones: Increased cardiovascular effects of both drugs

Adverse Reactions

CNS: Dizziness, headache, insomnia, light-headedness, nervousness, restlessness, trembling, weakness

CV: Angina, hypertension, palpitations, tachycardia

GI: Nausea, vomiting

GU: Dysuria

SKIN: Diaphoresis, pallor, rash, urticaria

Nursing Considerations

- Use cautiously in patients with diabetes, hypertension, increased intraocular pressure, ischemic heart disease, stenosing peptic ulcer, or pyloroduodenal obstruction because of the vasoconstrictive action of pseudoepherine.
- Evaluate therapeutic response. Notify prescriber if symptoms persist or worsen despite use of guaifenesin and pseudoephedrine.
- Monitor renal function, as ordered, because pseudoephedrine is substantially excreted by the kidneys.

PATIENT TEACHING

- Instruct patient to take guaifenesin and pseudoephedrine exactly as prescribed and not to increase dose or frequency without consulting prescriber.
- To minimize nausea, suggest that patient take drug with food and to take each dose with a full glass of water.
- Advise patient not to break, crush, or chew E.R. tablets or capsules but to swallow them whole.
- Advise patient to avoid alcohol or other CNS depressants while taking drug.
- Advise patient to avoid potentially hazardous activities until drug's CNS effects are known.

• Instruct patient to increase fluid intake (unless contraindicated) to help thin secretions.

hydrocodone bitartrate, brompheniramine maleate, and pseudoephedrine hydrochloride
Anaplex HD

Class, Category, and Schedule
Chemical: Opioid and phenanthrene derivative (hydrocodone), alkylamine (brompheniramine), sympathomimetic amine (pseudoephedrine)
Therapeutic: Antitussive (hydrocodone), antihistamine (brompheniramine), decongestant (pseudoephedrine)
Pregnancy category: C
Controlled substance: Schedule III

Indications and Dosages
▶ *To relieve cough and upper respiratory symptoms caused by hay fever, other upper respiratory allergies, or allergic rhinitis*
ORAL SOLUTION
Adults. 3.4 mg hydrocodone, 4 mg brompheniramine, and 60 mg pseudoephedrine (10 ml) t.i.d. or q.i.d. *Maximum:* 40 ml daily.

Mechanism of Action
Hydrocodone suppresses cough by directly acting on opiate receptors in the medulla's cough center.

Brompheniramine competes with histamine for H_1 receptor sites, thereby antagonizing many histamine effects and reducing allergy effects.

Pseudoephedrine acts on alpha$_1$-adrenergic receptors in the mucosa of the respiratory tract to produce vasoconstriction. This process shrinks swollen nasal mucous membranes; reduces tissue hyperemia, edema, and nasal congestion; and increases nasal airway patency. It also may increase drainage of sinus secretions and open obstructed eustachian ostia.

Contraindications
Hypersensitivity or idiosyncractic reactions to hydrocodone, other opioids, brompheniramine, pseudoephedrine, or their components; hyperthyroidism; narrow-angle glaucoma; prostatic hypertrophy; respiratory depression; severe asthma or coronary artery

disease; severe or uncontrolled hypertension; upper airway obstruction, urine retention; use of MAO inhibitors within 14 days

Interactions

DRUGS

hydrocodone, brompheniramine, and pseudoephedrine
MAO inhibitors: Increased and prolonged cardiac stimulation, increased vasopressor effect, increased risk of severe cardiovascular and cerebrovascular effects, hyperpyrexia, and vomiting

hydrocodone and brompheniramine
anticholinergics, paregoric: Possibly intensified anticholinergic adverse effects
CNS depressants: Additive CNS effects

hydrocodone component
antihypertensives, diuretics: Potentiated hypotensive effects
buprenorphine: Decreased hydrocodone effectiveness
hydroxyzine: Increased hydrocodone analgesic effect; increased CNS depressant and hypotensive effects
metoclopramide: Antagonized effect of metoclopramide on GI motility
naloxone: Antagonized hydrocodone analgesic effect
naltrexone: Precipitated withdrawal symptoms in hydrocodone-dependent patients
neuromuscular blockers: Additive respiratory depressant effects
opioids: Additive CNS and respiratory depressants effects and hypotensive effects
tricyclic antidepressants: Possibly increased effect of either the antidepressant or hydrocodone

pseudoephedrine component
antacids: Increased pseudoephedrine absorption
antihypertensives, diuretics: Possibly decreased antihypertensive effects
beta blockers: Decreased therapeutic effects of both drugs
citrates: Possibly inhibited urinary pseudoephedrine excretion and prolonged duration of action
CNS stimulant, other sympathomimetics: Possibly increased additive CNS stimulation to excessive levels
cocaine (mucosal-local): Possibly increased cardiovascular effects of either drug and CNS stimulation
digoxin, levodopa: Increased risk of cardiac arrhythmias
hydrocarbon inhalation anesthetics: Increased risk of serious arrhythmias
kaolin: Decreased pseudoephedrine absorption

nitrates: Reduced antianginal effects of nitrates
rauwolfia alkaloids: Possibly inhibited pseudoephedrine action
thyroid hormones: Increased cardiovascular effects of both drugs
ACTIVITIES
hydrocodone and brompheniramine
alcohol use: Additive CNS effects

Adverse Reactions

CNS: Asthenia, anxiety, confusion, dizziness, depression, drowsiness, dyskinesia, euphoria, excitability, faintness, headache, insomnia, irritability, light-headedness, nervousness, restlessness, sedation, syncope, tiredness, tremor, vertigo, weakness
CV: Bradycardia, hypertension, hypotension, orthostatic hypotension, palpitation, tachycardia
ENDO: Decreased lactation, early menses, gynecomastia, hyperglycemia, hypoglycemia
EENT: Blurred vision; diplopia; dry mouth, pharynx, and respiratory passages; hypermetropia; increased lacrimation; labyrinthitis; laryngismus; mydriasis; nasal stuffiness; photophobia; tinnitus
GI: Abdominal distention or pain, acute pancreatitis, anorexia, constipation, diarrhea, dyspepsia, epigastric distress, esophageal reflux, increased appetite, nausea, vomiting
GU: Dysuria, increased libido, urinary frequency or hesitancy, urine retention, ureteral spasm
RESP: Dyspnea, respiratory depression, wheezing
SKIN: Dermatitis, diaphoresis, erythema, flushing, pallor, pruritus, rash, urticaria
Other: Drug fever, emotional or physical dependence

Nursing Considerations

• Use cautiously in patients with recent head injury and those with Addison's disease, mildly to moderately severe asthma or other chronic respiratory disease, increased intraocular pressure, or liver or renal impairment.
• **WARNING** Monitor respiratory function because hydrocodone, brompheniramine, and pseudoephedrine may suppress cough reflex and cause thickening of bronchial secretions, aggravating such conditions as asthma and COPD. Rarely, it may depress respirations and induce apnea. Notify prescriber immediately if respiratory rate drops below 10 breaths/minute.
• Monitor patients who may be more susceptible to dizziness, sedation, and hypotension, such as the elderly.
• Monitor renal function, as ordered, because pseudoephedrine is substantially excreted by the kidneys.

- Regularly evaluate effectiveness of hydrocodone, brompheniramine, and pseudoephedrine in reducing symptoms.
- Be aware that patient shouldn't have intradermal allergen tests within 72 hours of receiving drug because results may be altered.

PATIENT TEACHING
- Tell patient that hydrocodone, brompheniramine, and pseudoephedrine must not be diluted with fluids or mixed with other drugs.
- Urge patient to avoid alcohol and other antidepressants while taking hydrocodone, brompheniramine, and pseudoephedrine.
- Instruct patient to avoid potentially hazardous activities until drug's CNS effects are known.
- Suggest that patient relieve dry mouth with frequent rinsing and use of sugarless gum or hard candy.
- Tell patient to take last dose of the day a few hours before bedtime if hydrocodone, brompheniramine, and pseudoephedrine makes him nervous or restless.

hydrocodone bitartrate, carbinoxamine maleate, and pseudoephedrine hydrochloride

Histex HC

Class, Category, and Schedule

Chemical: Opioid and phenanthrene derivative (hydrocodone), ethanolamine derivative (carbinoxamine), sympathomimetic amine (pseudoephedrine)
Therapeutic: Antitussive (hydrocodone), antihistamine (carbinoxamine), decongestant (pseudoephedrine)
Pregnancy category: C
Controlled substance: Schedule III

Indications and Dosages

▶ *To relieve cough and upper respiratory symptoms caused by hay fever, other upper respiratory allergies, or allergic rhinitis*
ORAL SOLUTION
Adults. 5 to 10 mg hydrocodone, 2 to 4 mg carbinoxamine, and 30 to 60 mg pseudoephedrine (5 to 10 ml) q 4 to 6 hr.

Contraindications

Hypersensitivity or idiosyncractic reactions to hydrocodone, other opioids, carbinoxamine, pseudoephedrine, or their components;

hyperthyroidism; narrow-angle glaucoma; prostatic hypertrophy; respiratory depression; severe asthma or coronary artery disease; severe or uncontrolled hypertension; upper airway obstruction, urine retention; use of MAO inhibitors within 14 days

---

Mechanism of Action

Hydrocodone suppresses cough by acting directly on opiate receptors in the medulla's cough center.

Carbinoxaminecompetes with histamine for H_1 receptor sites, thereby antagonizing many histamine effects and reducing allergy signs and symptoms.

Pseudoephedrine acts on $alpha_1$-adrenergic receptors in the mucosa of the respiratory tract to produce vasoconstriction. This process shrinks swollen nasal mucous membranes; reduces tissue hyperemia, edema, and nasal congestion; and increases nasal airway patency. It also may increase drainage of sinus secretions and open obstructed eustachian ostia.

Interactions

DRUGS

hydrocodone, carbinoxamine and pseudoephedrine

MAO inhibitors: Increased and prolonged cardiac stimulation, increased vasopressor effect, increased risk of severe cardiovascular and cerebrovascular effects, hyperpyrexia, and vomiting

hydrocodone and carbinoxamine

anticholinergics, paregoric: Possibly intensified anticholinergic adverse effects

CNS depressants: Additive CNS effects

hydrocodone component

antihypertensives, diuretics: Potentiated hypotensive effects

buprenorphine: Decreased hydrocodone effectiveness

hydroxyzine: Increased hydrocodone analgesic effect; increased CNS depressant and hypotensive effects

metoclopramide: Antagonized effect of metoclopramide on GI motility

naloxone: Antagonized hydrocodone analgesic effect

naltrexone: Precipitated withdrawal symptoms in hydrocodone-dependent patients

neuromuscular blockers: Additive respiratory depressant effects

opioids: Additive CNS and respiratory depressants effects and hypotensive effects

tricyclic antidepressants: Possibly increased effect of either the antidepressant or hydrocodone

pseudoephedrine component

antacids: Increased pseudoephedrine absorption

antihypertensives, diuretics: Possibly decreased antihypertensive effects

beta blockers: Decreased therapeutic effects of both drugs

citrates: Possibly inhibited urinary pseudoephedrine excretion and prolonged duration of action

CNS stimulant, other sympathomimetics: Possibly increased additive CNS stimulation to excessive levels

cocaine (mucosal-local): Possibly increased cardiovascular effects of either drug and CNS stimulation

digoxin, levodopa: Increased risk of cardiac arrhythmias

hydrocarbon inhalation anesthetics: Increased risk of serious arrhythmias

kaolin: Decreased pseudoephedrine absorption

nitrates: Reduced antianginal effects of nitrates

rauwolfia alkaloids: Possibly inhibited pseudoephedrine action

thyroid hormones: Increased cardiovascular effects of both drugs

ACTIVITIES

hydrocodone and carbinoxamine

alcohol use: Additive CNS effects

Adverse Reactions

CNS: Asthenia, anxiety, confusion, dizziness, depression, drowsiness, dyskinesia, euphoria, excitability, faintness, headache, insomnia, irritability, light-headedness, nervousness, restlessness, sedation, syncope, tiredness, tremor, vertigo, weakness

CV: Bradycardia, hypertension, hypotension, orthostatic hypotension, palpitation, tachycardia

ENDO: Decreased lactation, early menses, gynecomastia, hyperglycemia, hypoglycemia

EENT: Blurred vision; diplopia; dry mouth, pharynx, and respiratory passages; hypermetropia; increased lacrimation; labyrinthitis; laryngismus; mydriasis; nasal stuffiness; photophobia; tinnitus

GI: Abdominal distention or pain, acute pancreatitis, anorexia, constipation, diarrhea, dyspepsia, epigastric distress, esophageal reflux, increased appetite, nausea, vomiting

GU: Dysuria, increased libido, urinary frequency or hesitancy, urine retention, ureteral spasm

RESP: Dyspnea, respiratory depression, wheezing

SKIN: Dermatitis, diaphoresis, erythema, flushing, pallor, pruritus, rash, urticaria

Other: Drug fever, emotional or physical dependence

Nursing Considerations

- Use cautiously in patients with recent head injury and those with Addison's disease, mildly to moderately severe asthma or other chronic respiratory disease, increased intraocular pressure, or liver or renal impairment.
- **WARNING** Monitor respiratory function because hydrocodone, carbinoxamine, and pseudoephedrine may suppress cough reflex and cause thickening of bronchial secretions, aggravating such conditions as asthma and COPD. Rarely, it may depress respirations and induce apnea. Notify prescriber immediately if respiratory rate drops below 10 breaths/minute.
- Monitor patients who may be more susceptible to dizziness, sedation, and hypotension, such as the elderly.
- Monitor renal function, as ordered, because pseudoephedrine is substantially excreted by the kidneys.
- Regularly evaluate effectiveness of hydrocodone, carbinoxamine, and pseudoephedrine in reducing symptoms.
- Be aware that patient shouldn't have intradermal allergen tests within 72 hours of receiving drug because results may be altered.

PATIENT TEACHING

- Instruct patient to use calibrated measuring spoon to ensure accurate dosage.
- Tell patient that hydrocodone, carbinoxamine, and pseudoephedrine must not be diluted with fluids or mixed with other drugs.
- Urge patient to avoid alcohol and other antidepressants while taking hydrocodone, carbinoxamine, and pseudoephedrine.
- Instruct patient to avoid potentially hazardous activities until drug's CNS effects are known.
- Suggest that patient relieve dry mouth with frequent rinsing and use of sugarless gum or hard candy.
- Tell patient to take last dose of the day a few hours before bedtime if hydrocodone, carbinoxamine, and pseudoephedrine makes her nervous or restless.

hydrocodone bitartrate, chlorpheniramine maleate, phenylephrine hydrochloride, acetaminophen, and caffeine

Hycomine Compound

Class, Category, and Schedule
Chemical: Opioid and phenanthrene derivative (hydrocodone),
alkylamine (chlorpheniramine), sympathomimetic amine
(phenylephrine), acetamide (acetaminophen), and methylxantine
derivative (caffeine)
Therapeutic: Antitussive (hydrocodone), antihistamine (chlorpheniramine), decongestant (phenylephrine), analgesic and antipyretic (acetaminophen), and centrally acting stimulant (caffeine)
Pregnancy category: C
Controlled substance: Schedule III

Indications and Dosages
▶ *To relieve cough, nasal congestion, and discomfort from upper
respiratory tract infections*
TABLETS
Adults and children age 12 and over. 5 mg hydrocodone,
2 mg chlorpheniramine, 10 mg phenylephrine, 250 mg acetaminophen, and 30 mg caffeine (1 tablet) q.i.d.
Children ages 6 to 12. 2.5 mg hydrocodone, 1 mg chlorpheniramine, 5 mg phenylephrine, 125 mg acetaminophen, and 15 mg
caffeine (½ tablet) q.i.d.

Mechanism of Action
Chlorpheniramine competes with histamine for H_1 receptor sites, thereby antagonizing many histamine effects and reducing allergy signs and symptoms.

Hydrocodone suppresses cough by acting directly on opiate receptors in
the medulla's cough center.

Phenylephrine stimulates alpha-adrenergic receptors and inhibits the intracellular enzyme adenyl cyclase, which then inhibits production of cAMP. Inhibition of cAMP causes arterial and venous constriction in nasal passages,
which decreases blood flow and mucosal edema caused by allergic response.

Acetaminophen inhibits the enzyme cyclooxygenase, thereby blocking prostaglandin production and interfering with pain impulse generation in the peripheral nervous system.

Caffeine is a competitive, nonselective antagonist of adenosine receptor
sites that stimulates the CNS and counteracts the sedative properties of hydrocodone and chlorpheniramine.

Contraindications
Breastfeeding; diabetes mellitus; heart disease; hypersensitivity to
hydrocodone, other opioids, chlorpheniramine, other antihistamines, phenylephrine, other sympathomimetic amines, acetamin-

ophen, caffeine, or their components; hypertension; hyperthy-roidism; presence of intracranial lesion and increased intracranial pressure; respiratory depression; severe asthma or hepatic impairment; upper airway obstruction, use of MAO inhibitor within 14 days

Interactions
DRUGS
hydrocodone, chlorpheniramine, and acetaminophen
anticholinergics: Possibly intensified anticholinergic adverse effects (hydrocondone, chlorpheniramine, phenylephrine); decreased onset of acetaminophen action
CNS depressants: Additive CNS effects
hydrocodone, chlorpheniramine, and phenylephrine
MAO inhibitors: Increased and prolonged cardiac stimulation, increased vasopressor effect, increased risk of severe cardiovascular and cerebrovascular effects, hyperpyrexia, and vomiting
hydrocodone component
antihypertensives, diuretics: Potentiated hypotensive effects
buprenorphine: Decreased hydrocodone effectiveness
hydroxyzine: Increased hydrocodone analgesic effect; increased CNS depressant and hypotensive effects
metoclopramide: Antagonized effect of metoclopramide on GI motility
naloxone: Antagonized hydrocodone analgesic effect
naltrexone: Precipitated withdrawal symptoms in hydrocodone-dependent patients
neuromuscular blockers: Additive respiratory depressant effects
opioids: Additive CNS and respiratory depressants effects and hypotensive effects
chlorpheniramine component
phenytoin: Possibly increased serum phenytoin levels and toxicity
phenylephrine component
alpha blockers, haloperidol, loxapine, phenothiazines, thioxanthenes: Possibly decreased vasoconstrictor effect of phenylephrine
antihypertenisves, diuretics: Possibly decreased antihypertensive effects
atropine: Possibly enhanced vasopressor effect of phenylephrine
beta blockers: Decreased therapeutic effects of both drugs
bretylium: Possibly potentiated vaopressor effect and arrhythmias
doxapram: Increased vasopressor effect of both drugs
ergot alkaloids: Possibly cerebral blood vessel rupture, increased va-

sopressor effect, peripheral vascular ischemia, and gangrene (with ergotamine)

guanadrel, guanethidine: Increased vasopressor effect of phenylephrine, increased risk of severe hypertension and arrhythmias

hydrocarbon inhalation anesthetics: Increased risk of serious arrhythmias

maprotiline, tricyclic antidepressants: Increased risk of severe cardiovascular effects (including arrhythmias, hyperpyrexia, severe hypertension)

mecamylamine, methyldopa: Decreased hypotensive effects of these drugs, increased vasopressor effect of phenylephrine

nitrates: Possibly decreased vasopressor effect of phenylephrine and decreased antianginal effect of nitrates

oxytocin: Possibly severe, persistent hypertension

phenoxybenzamine: Decreased vasoconstrictor effect of phenylephrine, possibly hypotension and tachycardia

theophylline: Possibly enhanced toxicity (including cardiac toxicity)

thyroid hormones: Increased cardiovascular effects of each drug

acetaminophen component

barbiturates, carbamazepine, hydantoins, isoniazid, rifampin, sulfinpyrazone: Decreased therapeutic effects and increased hepatotoxic effects of acetaminophen

lamotrigine, loop diuretics: Possibly decreased therapeutic effects of these drugs

oral contraceptives: Decreased effectiveness of acetaminophen

probenecid: Possibly increased therapeutic effects of acetaminophen

propranolol: Possibly increased action of acetaminophen

zidovudine: Possibly decreased effects of zidovudine

caffeine component

beta-adrenergic agonists: Possibly enhanced cardiac inotropic effects of beta-adrenergic agonists

disulfiram: Decreased blood clearance of caffeine

ACTIVITIES

hydrocodone, chlorpheniramine, and acetaminophen

alcohol use: Additive CNS effects; increased risk of hepatotoxicity (acetaminophen)

Adverse Reactions

CNS: Anxiety, coma, confusion, decreased mental and physical performance, delirium, depression, disorientation, dizziness, drowsiness, excitation (children), euphoria, faintness, fear, hallucinations, headache, insomnia, lack of coordination, lethargy, light-headedness, mental and physical impairment, mood changes, nervousness, paresthesia, restlessness, sedation, seizures, tiredness, tremor, weakness

CV: Angina, bradycardia, chest tightness, heart block, hypertension, hypotension, palpitations, peripheral vasoconstriction, tachycardia, ventricular arrhythmias

EENT: Altered taste, blurred vision, diplopia, dry mouth, laryngeal edema, laryngospasm, miosis

ENDO: Hypoglycemic coma

GI: Abdominal cramps and pain, anorexia, constipation, flatulence, gastroesophageal reflux, jaundice, hepatotoxicity, indigestion, nausea, paralytic ileus, toxic megacolon, vomiting

GU: Decreased libido, difficult ejaculation, dysuria, frequent urination, impotence, oliguria, ureteral spasm, urinary hesitancy, urinary incontinence, urine retention

HEME: Hemolytic anemia (with long-term use), leukopenia, neutropenia, pancytopenia, thrombocytopenia

MS: Muscle rigidity

RESP: Apnea, bronchoconstriction, bronchospasm, depressed cough reflex, dyspnea, respiratory depression, shortness of breath, slow or irregular breathing, wheezing

Skin: Diaphoresis, facial flushing, pallor, pruritis, rash, uriticaria

Other: Angioedema, anaphylaxis, physical or psychological dependence

Nursing Considerations

- Use cautiously in patients with recent head injury and in those with Addison's disease, mildly to moderately severe asthma or other chronic respiratory disease, increased intraocular pressure, or liver or renal impairment.
- Monitor children for excitation and elderly patients for dizziness, sedation, and hypotension; such patients may have an increased risk for these effects.
- Regularly evaluate effectiveness of hydrocodone, chlorpheniramine, phenylephrine, acetaminophen, and caffeine in reducing cough and upper respiratory symptoms.
- Know that the daily dose of acetaminophen shouldn't exceed 4 grams.
- **WARNING** Assess patient for evidence of physical and psychological dependence.
- Monitor urine output; decreasing output may signal urine retention.
- Be aware that patient shouldn't have intradermal allergen tests within 72 hours of receiving drug because results may be altered.

PATIENT TEACHING

• Instruct patient to take drug with food or after meals to minimize stomach upset.

• Instruct patient to take drug exactly as prescribed and not to adjust dose or frequency without consulting prescriber because drug can become habit-forming.

• Urge patient to avoid alcohol and other antidepressants while taking drug and also to contact prescriber before taking other prescription or OTC drugs that may contain similar ingredients, possibly causing toxicity.

• Advise patient to notify prescriber if he becomes short of breath or has difficulty breathing.

• Instruct patient to avoid potentially hazardous activities until drug's CNS effects are known.

• Suggest that patient relieve dry mouth with frequent rinsing and use of sugarless gum or hard candy.

• Tell patient to take last dose of the day a few hours before bedtime if drug makes him nervous or restless.

hydrocodone bitartrate, guaifenesin, and pseudoephedrine hydrochloride

Duratuss HD, Hydro-Tussin HD, Nalex Expectorant, Pancof-XP, Su-Tuss HD

Class, Category, and Schedule

Chemical: Opioid and phenanthrene derivative (hydrocodone), glyceryl guaiacolate (guaifenesin), sympathomimetic amine (pseudoephedrine)

Therapeutic: Antitussive (hydrocodone), expectorant (guaifenesin), decongestant (pseudoephedrine)

Pregnancy category: C

Controlled substance: Schedule III

Indications and Dosages

▶ *To relieve cough and other symptoms caused by allergies and the common cold*

ORAL SOLUTION

Adults. 3 to 5 mg hydrocodone, 100 to 200 mg guaifenesin, and 15 to 60 mg pseudoephedrine (5 to 10 ml depending on product) q 4 to 6 hr. Or, doses may be given q.i.d.

ELIXIR
Adults. 5 mg hydrocodone, 200 mg guaifenesin, and 60 mg pseudoephedrine (10 ml) q 4 to 6 hr. *Maximum:* 4 doses daily.

Mechanism of Action

Hydrocodone suppresses cough by acting directly on opiate receptors in the medulla's cough center.

Guaifenesin increases fluid and mucus removal from the upper respiratory tract by increasing the volume of secretions and reducing their adhesiveness and surface tension.

Pseudoephedrine acts on $alpha_1$-adrenergic receptors in the mucosa of the respiratory tract to produce vasoconstriction. This process shrinks swollen nasal mucous membranes; reduces tissue hyperemia, edema, and nasal congestion; and increases nasal airway patency. It also may increase drainage of sinus secretions and open obstructed eustachian ostia.

Contraindications

Hypersensitivity or idiosyncractic reactions to hydrocodone, other opioids, guaifenesin, pseudoephedrine, or their components; hyperthyroidism; narrow-angle glaucoma; respiratory depression; severe asthma, coronary artery disease or hypertension; upper airway obstruction; urine retention; use of MAO inhibitors within 14 days

Interactions

DRUGS

hydrocodone and pseudoephedrine
MAO inhibitors: Increased and prolonged cardiac stimulation, increased vasopressor effect, increased risk of severe cardiovascular and cerebrovascular effects, hyperpyrexia, vomiting
hydrocodone component
anticholinergics, paregoric: Possibly intensified anticholinergic adverse effects
antihypertensives, diuretics: Potentiated hypotensive effects
buprenorphine: Decreased hydrocodone effectiveness
CNS depressants: Additive CNS depression
hydroxyzine: Increased hydrocodone analgesic effect; increased CNS depressant and hypotensive effects
metoclopramide: Antagonized effect of metoclopramide on GI motility
naloxone: Antagonized hydrocodone analgesic effect

naltrexone: Precipitated withdrawal symptoms in hydrocodone-dependent patients

neuromuscular blockers: Additive respiratory depressant effects

opioids: Additive CNS and respiratory depressants effects and hypotensive effects

pseudoephedrine component

antacids: Increased pseudoephedrine absorption

antihypertensives, diuretics: Possibly decreased antihypertensive effects

beta blockers: Decreased therapeutic effects of both drugs

citrates: Possibly inhibited urinary pseudoephedrine excretion and prolonged duration of action

CNS stimulant, other sympathomimetics: Possibly increased additive CNS stimulation to excessive levels

cocaine (mucosal-local): Possibly increased cardiovascular effects of either drug and CNS stimulation

digoxin, levodopa: Increased risk of cardiac arrhythmias

hydrocarbon inhalation anesthetics: Increased risk of serious arrhythmias

kaolin: Decreased pseudoephedrine absorption

nitrates: Reduced antianginal effects of nitrates

rauwolfia alkaloids: Possibly inhibited pseudoephedrine action

thyroid hormones: Increased cardiovascular effects of both drugs

ACTIVITIES

hydrocodone component

alcohol use: Additive CNS effects

Adverse Reactions

CNS: Confusion, dizziness, drowsiness, euphoria, faintness, headache, insomnia, light-headedness, nervousness, restlessness, seizures, tiredness, trembling, weakness

CV: Bradycardia, hypotension, palpitations, tachycardia

EENT: Blurred or double vision, dry mouth, laryngeal edema, laryngospasm

GI: Anorexia, constipation, nausea, paralytic ileus, toxic megacolon, vomiting

GU: Dysuria, frequent urination

RESP: Dyspnea, shortness of breath, slow or irregular breathing, wheezing

Skin: Diaphoresis, facial flushing, pallor, pruritis, rash, uriticaria

Other: Angioedema, atelectasis

Nursing Considerations

- Use cautiously in patients with hypertension, diabetes mellitus, ischemic heart disease, increased intraocular pressure, or renal impairment because of the pseudoepherine component.
- Monitor renal function, as ordered, because pseudoephedrine is substantially excreted by the kidneys.
- Regularly evaluate effectiveness of hyrdocodone, guaifenesin, and pseudoephedrine in reducing cough and allergy symptoms.
- Be aware that patient shouldn't have intradermal allergen tests within 72 hours of receiving drug because results may be altered.

PATIENT TEACHING

- Instruct patient to use a calibrated measuring device to ensure an accurate dose.
- Urge patient to avoid alcohol and other antidepressants while taking hydrocodone, guaifenesin, and pseudoephedrine.
- Instruct patient to avoid potentially hazardous activities until drug's CNS effects are known.
- Suggest that patient relieve dry mouth with frequent rinsing and use of sugarless gum or hard candy.
- Tell patient to take last dose of the day a few hours before bedtime if hydrocodone, guaifenesin, and pseudoephedrine makes her nervous or restless.

hydrocodone bitartrate and homatropine methylbromide

Hycodan, Hydromet, Hydromide, Hydropane, Tussigon

Class, Category, and Schedule

Chemical: Opioid and phenanthrene derivative (hydrocodone), quaternary ammonium compound (homatropine)
Therapeutic: Antitussive (hydrocodone), anticholinergic (homatropine)
Pregnancy category: C
Controlled substance: Schedule III

Indications and Dosages

▶ *To relieve cough, persistent runny nose, and nasal congestion caused by upper respiratory infections, sinus inflammation, or hay fever*
SYRUP, TABLETS
Adults and children age 12 and over. 5 mg hydrocodone and 1.5 mg homatropine (5 ml or 1 tablet) q 4 to 6 hr.

Children age 6 to 12. 2.5 mg hydrocodone and 0.75 mg homatropine (2.5 ml or ½ tablet) q 4 to 6 hr.

Mechanism of Action

Hydrocodone suppresses cough by acting directly on opiate receptors in the medulla's cough center.

Homatropine competitively inhibits acetylcholine at autonomic postganglionic cholinergic receptors. Because the most sensitive receptors are in the salivary, bronchial, and sweat glands, this action reduces secretions from these glands. It also reduces nasal, oropharyngeal, and bronchial secretions and decreases airway resistance by relaxing smooth muscles in the bronchi and bronchioles.

Contraindications

Cardiac disease, such as arrhythmias, severe hypertension, and mitral stenosis; esophageal reflux; hemorrhage with hemodynamic instability; hypersensitivity to hydrocodone, other opioids, homatropine, or their components; ileus; intestinal atony; myasthenia gravis; narrow-angle glaucoma; obstructive GI or uropathic disease; significant respiratory depression; ulcerative colitis; urine retention

Interactions
DRUGS
hydrocodone and homatropine
anticholinergics, paregoric: Possibly intensified anticholinergic adverse effects
metoclopramide: Possibly antagonized metoclopramide effects on GI motility
hydrocodone component
antihypertensives, diuretics: Potentiated hypotensive effects
buprenorphine: Decreased hydrocodone effectiveness
CNS depressants: Additive CNS effects
hydroxyzine: Increased hydrocodone analgesic effect; increased CNS depressant and hypotensive effects
MAO inhibitors: Increased and prolonged cardiac stimulation, increased vasopressor effect, increased risk of severe cardiovascular and cerebrovascular effects, hyperpyrexia, and vomiting
naloxone: Antagonized hydrocodone analgesic effect
naltrexone: Precipitated withdrawal symptoms in hydrocodone-dependent patients
neuromuscular blockers: Additive respiratory depressant effects

opioids: Additive CNS and respiratory depressants effects and hypotensive effects

homatropine component

antacids, adsorbent antidiarrheals: Possibly reduced absorption of anticholinergics

antimyasthenics: Possibly reduced intestinal motility

haloperidol: Possibly decreased antipsychotic effectiveness of haloperidol

ketoconazole: Possibly significant decreased ketoconazole absorption

opioid (narcotic) analgesics: Increased risk of severe constipation, paralytic ileus, and urine retention

potassium chloride: Possibly increased severity of potassium chloride induced GI lesions

urinary alkalizers such as calcium and or magnesium-containing antacids, carbonic anhydrase inhibitors, citrates, and sodium bicarbonate: Delayed urinary excretion of homatropine with increased therapeutic effects and incidence of adverse reactions

ACTIVITIES

hydrocodone component

alcohol use: Additive CNS effects

Adverse Reactions

CNS: Confusion, dizziness, drowsiness, euphoria, faintness, hallucinations, headache, insomnia, light-headedness, mania, mood changes, nervousness, restlessness, seizures, tiredness, weakness

CV: Bradycardia, hypotension, palpitations, tachycardia

EENT: Blurred or double vision; dry eyes, mouth, nose, and throat; laryngeal edema; laryngospasm

GI: Anorexia, constipation, nausea, paralytic ileus, toxic megacolon, vomiting

GU: Dysuria, frequent urination, urinary hesitancy, urine retention

RESP: Dyspnea, shortness of breath, slow or irregular breathing, wheezing

Skin: Decreased sweating, diaphoresis, dry skin, facial flushing, pruritis, rash, uriticaria

Other: Angioedema, anaphylaxis

Nursing Considerations

- Regularly evaluate effectiveness of hydrocodone and homatropine in relieving cough and upper respiratory symptoms.
- Take safety precautions as needed.
- Monitor respiratory depth, effort, and rate. Notify prescriber immediately if respiratory rate drops below 10 breaths/minute.

- Assess urine output; decreasing output may signal urine retention.
- **WARNING** Assess patient for evidence of physical and psychological dependence.

PATIENT TEACHING
- Instruct patient to use a calibrated measuring device to ensure accurate dose of syrup form.
- Caution patient to take drug exactly as prescribed and not to adjust dose or frequency without consulting prescriber.
- Urge patient to avoid alcohol and other antidepressants while taking hydrocodone and homatropine.
- Instruct patient to avoid potentially hazardous activities until drug's CNS effects are known.
- Suggest that patient relieve dry mouth with frequent rinsing and use of sugarless gum or hard candy and to use lubricating eye drops for dry eyes.
- To prevent constipation, encourage patient to consume plenty of fluids and high-fiber foods, if not contraindicated by another condition.
- Advise patient to notify prescriber if he becomes short of breath or has difficulty breathing or if he develops persistent or severe diarrhea, constipation, or has difficulty urinating.

hydrocodone bitartrate and phenylephrine hydrochloride
Lortus-HD, Nalex DH, Tusdec HC

Class, Category, and Schedule
Chemical: Opioid and phenanthrene derivative (hydrocodone), sympathomimetic amine (phenylephrine)
Therapeutic: Antitussive (hydrocodone), decongestant (phenylephrine)
Pregnancy category: C
Controlled substance: Schedule III

Indications and Dosages
▶ *To relieve cough and other upper respiratory symptoms caused by the common cold and allergies*
ELIXIR
Adults and children age 12 and over. 3.75 to 5 mg hydrocodone and 7.5 to 10 mg phenylephrine (10 ml) q 4 to 6 hr. *Maximum:* 4 doses daily.

Children ages 6 to 12. 1.67 mg hydrocodone and 5 mg phenylephrine (5 ml) q 4 to 6 hr. *Maximum:* 4 doses daily.
Children ages 2 to 6. 0.84 to 1.67 mg hydrocodone and 2.5 to 5 mg phenylephrine (2.5 to 5 ml) q 4 to 6 hr. *Maximum:* 4 doses daily.

Mechanism of Action

Hydrocodone suppresses cough by acting directly on opiate receptors in the medulla's cough center.

Phenylephrine stimulates alpha-adrenergic receptors and inhibits the intracellular enzyme adenyl cyclase, which then inhibits production of cAMP. Inhibition of cAMP causes arterial and venous constriction in nasal passages, which decreases blood flow and mucosal edema caused by allergic response.

Contraindications

Hypersensitivity to hydrocodone, other opioids, bisulfites, phenylephrine, or their components; severe coronary artery disease or hypertension; significant respiratory depression; use of an MAO inhibitor within 14 days; ventricular tachycardia

Interactions

DRUGS

hydrocodone and phenylephrine

MAO inhibitors: Increased and prolonged cardiac stimulation, increased vasopressor effect, increased risk of severe cardiovascular and cerebrovascular effects, hyperpyrexia, and vomiting

hydrocodone component

anticholinergics, paregoric: Possibly intensified anticholinergic adverse effects

antihypertensives, diuretics: Potentiated hypotensive effects

buprenorphine: Decreased hydrocodone effectivess

CNS depressants: Additive CNS effects

hydroxyzine: Increased hydrocodone analgesic effect; increased CNS depressant and hypotensive effects

metoclopramide: Possibly antagonized metoclopramide effects on GI motility

naloxone: Antagonized hydrocodone analgesic effect

naltrexone: Precipitated withdrawal symptoms in hydrocodone-dependent patients

neuromuscular blockers: Additive respiratory depressant effects

opioids: Additive CNS and respiratory depressants effects and hypotensive effects

phenylephrine component

alpha blockers, haloperidol, loxapine, phenothiazines, thioxanthenes: Possibly decreased vasoconstrictor effect of phenylephrine

antihyperten isves, diuretics: Possibly decreased antihypertensive effects

atropine: Possibly enhanced vasopressor effect of phenylephrine

beta blockers: Decreased therapeutic effects of both drugs

bretylium: Possibly potentiated vaopressor effect and arrhythmias

doxapram: Increased vasopressor effect of both drugs

ergot alkaloids: Possibly cerebral blood vessel rupture, increased vasopressor effect, peripheral vascular ischemia, and gangrene (with ergotamine)

guanadrel, guanethidine: Increased vasopressor effect of phenylephrine; increased risk of severe hypertension and arrhythmias

hydrocarbon inhalation anesthetics: Increased risk of serious arrhythmias

maprotiline, tricyclic antidepressants: Increased risk of severe cardiovascular effects (including arrhythmias, hyperpyrexia, severe hypertension)

mecamylamine, methyldopa: Decreased hypotensive effects of these drugs; increased vasopressor effect of phenylephrine

nitrates: Possibly decreased vasopressor effect of phenylephrine and decreased antianginal effect of nitrates

oxytocin: Possibly severe, persistent hypertension

phenoxybenzamine: Decreased vasoconstrictor effect of phenylephrine, possibly hypotension and tachycardia

theophylline: Possibly enhanced toxicity (including cardiac toxicity)

thyroid hormones: Increased cardiovascular effects of each drug

ACTIVITIES

hydrocodone component

alcohol use: Additive CNS effects

Adverse Reactions

CNS: Confusion, dizziness, drowsiness, euphoria, faintness, headache, insomnia, light-headedness, nervousness, paresthesia, restlessness, seizures, tiredness, tremor, weakness

CV: Angina, bradycardia, hypertension, hypotension, palpitations, peripheral vasoconstriction that may lead to necrosis or gangrene, tachycardia, ventricular arrhythmia

EENT: Blurred or double vision, dry mouth, laryngeal edema, laryngospasm

GI: Anorexia, constipation, nausea, paralytic ileus, toxic megacolon, vomiting

GU: Dysuria, frequent urination
RESP: Dyspnea, shortness of breath, slow or irregular breathing, wheezing
SKIN: Diaphoresis, facial flushing, pallor, pruritis
Other: Angioedema, anaphylaxis

Nursing Considerations

* Assess patient for signs and symptoms of angina, arrhythmias, and hypertension because phenylephrine may increase myocardial oxygen demand and the risk of proarrhythmias and blood pressure changes.
* **WARNING** Monitor patient with thyroid disease for increased sensitivity to catecholamines and possible thyrotoxicity or cardiotoxicity.
* Regularly evaluate effectiveness of hydrocodone and phenylephrine in relieving upper respiratory symptoms. Notify prescriber if symptoms persist or worsen.
* Take safety precautions as needed.
* Monitor patient's respiratory depth, effort, and rate. Notify prescriber immediately if respiratory rate drops below 10 breaths/ minute.
* **WARNING** Assess patient for evidence of physical and psychological dependence.

PATIENT TEACHING
* Instruct patient to use a calibrated measuring device to ensure accurate dose.
* Caution patient to take drug exactly as prescribed and not to adjust dose or frequency without consulting prescriber.
* Urge patient to avoid alcohol and other antidepressants while taking hydrocodone and phenylephrine.
* Instruct patient to avoid potentially hazardous activities until drug's CNS effects are known.
* Suggest that patient relieve dry mouth with frequent rinsing and use of sugarless gum or hard candy.
* To prevent constipation, encourage patient to consume plenty of fluids and high-fiber foods, if not contraindicated.
* Advise patient to notify prescriber if she becomes short of breath or has difficulty breathing or if she develops persistent or severe diarrhea, constipation or has difficulty urinating.
* Instruct patient to increase fluid intake (unless contraindicated) to help thin secretions.

hydrocodone bitartrate, phenylephrine hydrochloride, and guaifenesin

Atuss-G, Donatussin DC, Entex HC, Levall 5.0, Tussafed HC, Tussafed HCG

Class, Category, and Schedule

Chemical: Opioid and phenanthrene derivative (hydrocodone), sympathomimetic amine (phenylephrine), glyceryl guaiacolate (guaifenesin)

Therapeutic: Antitussive (hydrocodone), decongestant (phenylephrine), expectorant (guaifenesin)

Pregnancy category: C

Controlled substance: Schedule III

Indications and Dosages

▶   *To relieve cough and other upper respiratory symptoms related to the common cold and allergies*

SYRUP

Adults. 4 to 5 mg hydrocodone, 12 to 20 mg phenylephrine, and 100 to 200 mg guaifenesin (10 ml) q 4 to 6 hr.

ORAL SOLUTION

Adults. 5 to 10 mg hydrocodone, 7.5 to 20 mg phenylephrine, and 100 to 450 mg guaifenesin (5 or 10 ml depending on product) q 4 to 6 hr.

Mechanism of Action

Hydrocodone suppresses cough by acting directly on opiate receptors in the medulla's cough center.

Phenylephrine stimulates alpha-adrenergic receptors and inhibits the intracellular enzyme adenyl cyclase, which then inhibits production of cAMP. Inhibition of cAMP causes arterial and venous constriction in nasal passages, which decreases blood flow and mucosal edema caused by allergic response.

Guaifenesin increases fluid and mucus removal from the upper respiratory tract by increasing the volume of secretions and reducing their adhesiveness and surface tension.

Contraindications

Hypersensitivity to hydrocodone, other opioids, bisulfites, phenylephrine, guaifenesin, or their components; severe coronary artery disease or hypertension; significant respiratory depression; use within 14 days of MAO inhibitor therapy; ventricular tachycardia

Interactions
DRUGS
hydrocodone and phenylephrine
MAO inhibitors: Increased and prolonged cardiac stimulation, increased vasopressor effect, increased risk of severe cardiovascular and cerebrovascular effects, hyperpyrexia, and vomiting
hydrocodone component
anticholinergics, paregoric: Possibly intensified anticholinergic adverse effects
antihypertensives, diuretics: Potentiated hypotensive effects
buprenorphine: Decreased effectiveness of hydrocodone
CNS depressants: Additive CNS effects
hydroxyzine: Increased hydrocodone analgesic effect; increased CNS depressant and hypotensive effects
metoclopramide: Possibly antagonized metoclopramide effects on GI
motility naloxone: Anatagonized hydrocodone analgesic effect
naltrexone: Precipitated withdrawal symptoms in hydrocodone-dependent patients
neuromuscular blockers: Additive respiratory depressant effects
opioids: Additive CNS and respiratory depressants effects and hypotensive effects
phenylephrine component
alpha blockers, haloperidol, loxapine, phenothiazines, thioxanthenes: Possibly decreased vasoconstrictor effect of phenylephrine
antihypertenisves, diuretics: Possibly decreased antihypertensive effects
atropine: Possibly enhanced vasopressor effect of phenylephrine
beta blockers: Decreased therapeutic effects of both drugs
bretylium: Possibly potentiated vaopressor effect and arrhythmias
doxapram: Increased vasopressor effect of both drugs
ergot alkaloids: Possibly cerebral blood vessel rupture, increased vasopressor effect, peripheral vascular ischemia, and gangrene (with ergotamine)
guanadrel, guanethidine: Increased vasopressor effect of phenylephrine, increased risk of severe hypertension and arrhythmias
hydrocarbon inhalation anesthetics: Increased risk of serious arrhythmias
maprotiline, tricyclic antidepressants: Increased risk of severe cardiovascular effects (including arrhythmias, hyperpyrexia, severe hypertension)
mecamylamine, methyldopa: Decreased hypotensive effects of these drugs, increased vasopressor effect of phenylephrine

nitrates: Possibly decreased vasopressor effect of phenylephrine and decreased antianginal effect of nitrates

oxytocin: Possibly severe, persistent hypertension

phenoxybenzamine: Decreased vasoconstrictor effect of phenylephrine, possibly hypotension and tachycardia

theophylline: Possibly enhanced toxicity (including cardiac toxicity)

thyroid hormones: Increased cardiovascular effects of each drug

ACTIVITIES

hydrocodone component

alcohol use: Additive CNS effects

Adverse Reactions

CNS: Confusion, dizziness, drowsiness, euphoria, faintness, headache, insomnia, light-headedness, nervousness, paresthesia, restlessness, seizures, tiredness, tremor, weakness

CV: Angina, bradycardia, hypertension, hypotension, palpitations, peripheral vasoconstriction that may lead to necrosis or gangrene, tachycardia, ventricular arrhythmia

EENT: Blurred or double vision, dry mouth, laryngeal edema, laryngospasm

GI: Anorexia, constipation, nausea, paralytic ileus, toxic megacolon, vomiting

GU: Dysuria, frequent urination

RESP: Dyspnea, shortness of breath, slow or irregular breathing, wheezing

SKIN: Diaphoresis, facial flushing, pallor, pruritis, rash, urticaria

Other: Angioedema, anaphylaxis

Nursing Considerations

• Assess patient for signs and symptoms of angina, arrhythmias, and hypertension because phenylephrine may increase myocardial oxygen demand and the risk of proarrhythmias and blood pressure changes.

• **WARNING** Monitor patient with thyroid disease for increased sensitivity to catecholamines and possible thyrotoxicity or cardiotoxicity.

• Regularly evaluate effectiveness of hydrocodone, phenylephrine, and guaifenesin in relieving upper respiratory symptoms. Notify prescriber if symptoms persist or worsen.

• Take safety precautions as needed.

• Monitor respiratory depth, effort, and rate. Notify prescriber immediately if respiratory rate drops below 10 breaths/minute.

• Assess urine output; decreasing output may signal urine retention.

- **WARNING** Assess patient for evidence of physical and psychological dependence.

PATIENT TEACHING
- Instruct patient to use a calibrated measuring device to ensure accurate dose.
- Caution patient to take drug exactly as prescribed and not to adjust dose or frequency without consulting prescriber.
- Urge patient to avoid alcohol and other antidepressants while taking hydrocodone, phenylephrine, and guaifenesin.
- Instruct patient to avoid potentially hazardous activities until drug's CNS effects are known.
- Suggest that patient relieve dry mouth with frequent rinsing and use of sugarless gum or hard candy.
- To prevent constipation, encourage patient to consume plenty of fluids and high-fiber foods, if not contraindicated by another condition.
- Advise patient to notify prescriber if he becomes short of breath or has difficulty breathing or if he develops persistent or severe diarrhea, constipation, or trouble urinating.
- Instruct patient to increase fluid intake (unless contraindicated) to help thin secretions.

hydrocodone bitartrate, phenylephrine hydrochloride, and pyrilamine maleate

Codal-DH, Codimal DH, Dicomal-DH, Mintuss MR

Class, Category, and Schedule

Chemical: Opioid and phenanthrene derivative (hydrocodone), sympathomimetic amine (phenylephrine), ethylenediamine derivative (pyrilamine)
Therapeutic: Antitussive (hydrocodone), decongestant (phenylephrine), antihistaminic (pyrilamine)
Pregnancy category: C
Schedule Category: III

Indications and Dosages

▶ *To relieve cough and upper respiratory symptoms caused by hay fever, other upper respiratory allergies, or allergic rhinitis*

SYRUP
Adults. 1.66 to 10 mg hydrocodone, 5 to 10 mg phenylephrine and 5 to 16.66 mg pyrilamine (5 to 10 ml depending on product) q 4 hr.

Mechanism of Action

Hydrocodone suppresses cough by acting directly on opiate receptors in the medulla's cough center.

Phenylephrine stimulates alpha-adrenergic receptors and inhibits the intracellular enzyme adenyl cyclase, which then inhibits production of cAMP. Inhibition of cAMP causes arterial and venous constriction in nasal passages, which decreases blood flow and mucosal edema caused by allergic response.

Pyrilamine competes with histamine for H_1 receptor sites, thereby antagonizing many histamine effects to reduce allergy signs and symptoms.

Contraindications

Breastfeeding; hypersensitivity to hydrocodone, other opioids, phenylephrine, pyrilamine, or their components; respiratory depression; severe asthma; upper airway obstruction; use of an MAO inhibitor within 14 days

Interactions

DRUGS

hydrocodone, phenylephrine, and pyrilamine

MAO inhibitors: Increased and prolonged cardiac stimulation, increased vasopressor effect, increased risk of severe cardiovascular and cerebrovascular effects, hyperpyrexia, and vomiting

hydrocodone and pyrilamine

anticholinergics, paregoric: Possibly intensified anticholinergic adverse effects

CNS depressants: Additive CNS effects

hydrocodonecomponent

antihypertensives, diuretics: Potentiated hypotensive effects

buprenorphine: Decreased hydrocodone effectiveness

hydroxyzine: Increased hydrocodone analgesic effect; increased CNS depressant and hypotensive effects

metoclopramide: Antagonized effect of metoclopramide on GI motility

naloxone: Antagonized hydrocodone analgesic effect

naltrexone: Precipitated withdrawal symptoms in hydrocodone-dependent patients

neuromuscular blockers: Additive respiratory depressant effects

opioids: Additive CNS and respiratory depressants effects and hypotensive effects

tricyclic antidepressants: Possibly increased effect of either the antidepressant or hydrocodone

phenylephrine component

alpha blockers, haloperidol, loxapine, phenothiazines, thioxanthenes: Possibly decreased vasoconstrictor effect of phenylephrine

antihypertenisves, diuretics: Possibly decreased antihypertensive effects

atropine: Possibly enhanced vasopressor effect of phenylephrine

beta blockers: Decreased therapeutic effects of both drugs

bretylium: Possibly potentiated vaopressor effect and arrhythmias

doxapram: Increased vasopressor effect of both drugs

ergot alkaloids: Possibly cerebral blood vessel rupture, increased vasopressor effect, peripheral vascular ischemia, and gangrene (with ergotamine)

guanadrel, guanethidine: Increased vasopressor effect of phenylephrine; increased risk of severe hypertension and arrhythmias

hydrocarbon inhalation anesthetics: Increased risk of serious arrhythmias

maprotiline, tricyclic antidepressants: Increased risk of severe cardiovascular effects (including arrhythmias, hyperpyrexia, severe hypertension)

mecamylamine, methyldopa: Decreased hypotensive effects of these drugs; increased vasopressor effect of phenylephrine

nitrates: Possibly decreased vasopressor effect of phenylephrine and decreased antianginal effect of nitrates

oxytocin: Possibly severe, persistent hypertension

phenoxybenzamine: Decreased vasoconstrictor effect of phenylephrine, possibly hypotension and tachycardia

theophylline: Possibly enhanced toxicity (including cardiac toxicity)

thyroid hormones: Increased cardiovascular effects of each drug
ACTIVITIES

hydrocodone and pyrilamine
alcohol use: Additive CNS effects

Adverse Reactions
CNS: Asthenia, anxiety, confusion, dizziness, depression, drowsiness, dyskinesia, euphoria, faintness, headache, insomnia, irritability, light-headedness, nervousness, paresthesia, restlessness, sedation, syncope, tiredness, tremor, vertigo, weakness
CV: Angina, bradycardia, hypertension, hypotension, orthostatic hypotension, palpitations, peripheral vasoconstriction that may lead to necrosis or gangrene, tachycardia, ventricular arrhythmias
ENDO: Decreased lactation, early menses, gynecomastia, hyperglycemia, hypoglycemia
EENT: Blurred vision; diplopia; dry mouth, pharynx, and respira-

tory passages; hypermetropia; increased lacrimation; labyrinthitis; laryngismus; mydriasis; nasal stuffiness; photophobia; tinnitus

GI: Abdominal distention or pain, acute pancreatitis, anorexia, constipation, diarrhea, dyspepsia, epigastric distress, esophageal reflux, increased appetite, nausea, vomiting

GU: Dysuria, increased libido, urinary frequency or hesitancy, urine retention, ureteral spasm

RESP: Dyspnea, respiratory depression, wheezing

SKIN: Dermatitis, diaphoresis, erythema, flushing, pruritus, rash, urticaria

Other: Drug fever, emotional or physical dependence

Nursing Considerations

- Use cautiously in patients with recent head injury and those with Addison's disease, mildly to moderately severe asthma or other chronic respiratory disease, cardiovascular disease, diabetes, hypertension, liver or renal impairment, narrow-angle glaucoma, prostatic hypertrophy, or thyroid imbalance.
- **WARNING** Monitor respiratory function because hydrocodone, phenylephrine, and pyrilamine may suppress cough reflex and cause thickening of bronchial secretions, aggravating such conditions as asthma and COPD. Rarely, it may depress respirations and induce apnea. Notify prescriber immediately if respiratory rate drops below 10 breaths/minute.
- Monitor patients who may be more susceptible to dizziness, sedation, and hypotension, such as the elderly.
- Regularly evaluate effectiveness of hydrocodone, phenylephrine, and pyrilamine in reducing cough and upper respiratory symptoms.
- Be aware that patient shouldn't have intradermal allergen tests within 72 hours of receiving drug because results may be altered.

PATIENT TEACHING

- Instruct patient to use a calibrated measuring device to ensure accurate dose.
- Urge patient to avoid alcohol and other antidepressants while taking hydrocodone, phenylephrine, and pyrilamine.
- Instruct patient to avoid potentially hazardous activities until drug's CNS effects are known.
- Suggest that patient relieve dry mouth with frequent rinsing and use of sugarless gum or hard candy.
- Tell patient to take last dose of the day a few hours before bedtime if hydrocodone, phenylephrine, and pyrilamine makes her nervous or restless.

hydrocodone bitartrate and potassium guaiacolsulfonate

Cotuss EX, Entuss, Hydron EX, Hydron KGS, Marcof Expectorant, Prolex DH

Class, Category, and Schedule

Chemical: Opioid and phenanthrene derivative (hydrocodone), unclassified (potassium guaiacolsulfonate)

Therapeutic: Antitussive (hydrocodone), expectorant (potassium guaiacolsulfonate

Pregnancy category: C

Controlled substance: Schedule III

Indications and Dosages

▶ *To relieve cough caused by minor throat and bronchial irritation, especially when secretions are thick*

ORAL SOLUTION, SYRUP

Adults. 4.5 mg hydrocodone and 120 to 450 mg potassium guaiacolsulfonate (5 to 15 ml depending on product) q 4 to 6 hr or q.i.d. (depending on product).

Mechanism of Action

Hydrocodone suppresses cough by acting directly on opiate receptors in the medulla's cough center.

Potassium guaiacolsulfonate is thought to act by increasing the fluid volume in respiratory tract secretions. This decreases the viscosity of bronchial secretions, making it easier to remove them from the respiratory tract.

Contraindications

Hyperkalemia; hypersensitivity or idiosyncractic reactions to hydrocodone, potassium guaiacolsulfonate, other opioids, or their components; respiratory depression

Interactions

DRUGS

hydrocodone component

anticholinergics, paregoric: Possibly intensified anticholinergic adverse effects

antihypertensives, diuretics: Potentiated hypotensive effects

buprenorphine: Decreased hydrocodone effectiveness

CNS depressants: Additive CNS depression

hydroxyzine: Increased hydrocodone analgesic effect; increased CNS depressant and hypotensive effects

MAO inhibitors: Increased and prolonged cardiac stimulation, increased vasopressor effect, increased risk of severe cardiovascular and cerebrovascular effects, hyperpyrexia, vomiting
metoclopramide: Antagonized effect of metoclopramide on GI motility
naloxone: Antagonized hydrocodone analgesic effect
naltrexone: Precipitated withdrawal symptoms in hydrocodone-dependent patients
neuromuscular blockers: Additive respiratory depressant effects
opioids: Additive CNS and respiratory depressants effects and hypotensive effects
potassium guaiacolsulfonate component
drugs that increase potassium levels such as ACE inhibitors, potassium-sparing diuretics, potassium-containing drugs, potassium supplements: Increased risk of hyperkalemia
ACTIVITIES
hydrocodone component
alcohol use: Additive CNS effects

Adverse Reactions

CNS: Coma, delirium, depression, disorientation, dizziness, drowsiness, euphoria, hallucinations, headache, lack of coordination, lethargy, light-headedness, mental and physical impairment, mood changes, restlessness, sedation, seizures, tremor
CV: Bradycardia, heart block, hypertension, orthostatic hypotension, palpitations, tachycardia
EENT: Altered taste, blurred vision, diplopia, dry mouth, laryngeal edema, laryngospasm, miosis
GI: Abdominal cramps and pain, anorexia, constipation, flatulence, gastroesophageal reflux, ileus, indigestion, nausea, vomiting
GU: Decreased libido, difficult ejaculation, dysuria, impotence, oliguria, ureteral spasm, urinary incontinence, urine retention
MS: Muscle rigidity
RESP: Apnea, bronchoconstriction, bronchospasm, depressed cough reflex, respiratory depression
SKIN: Diaphoresis, flushing, pallor, pruritus, rash, urticaria
Other: Anaphylaxis, facial edema, hyperkalemia, physical and psychological dependence

Nursing Considerations

• Evaluate for therapeutic response, such as decreased cough. Notify prescriber if symptoms persist or worsen despite use of hydrocodone and potassium guaiacolsulfonate.

- Monitor respiratory depth, effort, and rate. Notify prescriber immediately if respiratory rate drops below 10 breaths/minute.
- Assess urine output; decreasing output may signal urine retention.
- **WARNING** Assess patient for evidence of physical and psychological dependence.

PATIENT TEACHING
- Instruct patient to take hydrocodone and potassium guaiacolsulfonate exactly as prescribed and not to increase dose or frequency without consulting prescriber.
- Advise patient to avoid alcohol or other CNS depressants while taking drug.
- To minimize nausea, suggest that patient take drug with food.
- Advise patient to avoid potentially hazardous activities until drug's CNS effects are known.
- Caution patient to get up slowly from a sitting or lying position.
- Advise patient to notify prescriber if she becomes short of breath or has difficulty breathing.

hydrocodone bitartrate and pseudoephedrine hydrochloride

Detussin, Histussin D, Pancof HC, P-V Tussin Tablets, Tyrodone

Class, Category, and Schedule

Chemical: Opioid and phenanthrene derivative (hydrocodone), sympathomimetic amine (pseudoephedrine)
Therapeutic: Antitussive (hydrocodone), decongestant (pseudoephedrine)
Pregnancy category: C
Controlled substance: Schedule III

Indications and Dosages

▶ *To relieve cough and other symptoms caused by allergies and the common cold*

SYRUP
Adults. 3 to 6 mg hydrocodone and 15 to 60 mg pseudoephedrine (5 to 10 ml depending on product) q.i.d.
TABLETS
Adults. 5 mg hydrocodone and 60 mg pseudoephedrine (1 tablet) q 4 to 6 hr. *Maximum:* 4 doses daily.

Contraindications

Hypersensitivity or idiosyncractic reactions to hydrocodone, other opioids, pseudoephedrine, or their components; hyperthyroidism; narrow-angle glaucoma; prostatic hypertrophy; respiratory depression; severe asthma, coronary artery disease or hypertension; upper airway obstruction; urine retention; use of an MAO inhibitor within 14 days

---

Mechanism of Action

Hydrocodone suppresses cough by acting directly on opiate receptors in the medulla's cough center.

Pseudoephedrine acts on alpha$_1$-adrenergic receptors in the mucosa of the respiratory tract to produce vasoconstriction. This process shrinks swollen nasal mucous membranes; reduces tissue hyperemia, edema, and nasal congestion; and increases nasal airway patency. It also may increase drainage of sinus secretions and open obstructed eustachian ostia.

Interactions

DRUGS

hydrocodone and pseudoephedrine

MAO inhibitors: Increased and prolonged cardiac stimulation, increased vasopressor effect, increased risk of severe cardiovascular and cerebrovascular effects, hyperpyrexia, and vomiting

hydrocodone component

anticholinergics, paregoric: Possibly intensified anticholinergic adverse effects

antidiarrheals: Increased risk of severe constipation

antihypertensives, diuretics: Potentiated hypotensive effects

buprenorphine: Decreased hydrocodone effectiveness

CNS depressants: Additive CNS depression

hydroxyzine: Increased hydrocodone analgesic effect; increased CNS depressant and hypotensive effects

metoclopramide: Antagonized effect of metoclopramide on GI motility

naloxone: Antagonized hydrocodone analgesic effect

naltrexone: Precipitated withdrawal symptoms in hydrocodone-dependent patients

neuromuscular blockers: Additive respiratory depressant effects

opioids: Additive CNS and respiratory depressants effects and hypotensive effects

pseudoephedrine component

antacids: Increased pseudoephedrine absorption

antihypertensives, diuretics: Possibly decreased antihypertensive effects

beta blockers: Decreased therapeutic effects of both drugs
citrates: Possibly inhibited urinary pseudoephedrine excretion and prolonged duration of action
CNS stimulant, other sympathomimetics: Possibly increased additive CNS stimulation to excessive levels
cocaine (mucosal-local): Possibly increased cardiovascular effects of either drug and CNS stimulation
digoxin, levodopa: Increased risk of cardiac arrhythmias
hydrocarbon inhalation anesthetics: Increased risk of serious arrhythmias
kaolin: Decreased absorption of pseudoephedrine
nitrates: Reduced antianginal effects of nitrates
rauwolfia alkaloids: Possibly inhibited action of pseudoephedrine
thyroid hormones: Increased cardiovascular effects of both drugs
ACTIVITIES
hydrocodone component
alcohol use: Additive CNS effects

Adverse Reactions

CNS: Confusion, dizziness, drowsiness, euphoria, faintness, headache, insomnia, light-headedness, nervousness, restlessness, seizures, tiredness, trembling, weakness
CV: Bradycardia, hypotension, palpitations, tachycardia
EENT: Blurred or double vision, dry mouth, laryngeal edema, laryngospasm
GI: Anorexia, constipation, nausea, paralytic ileus, toxic megacolon, vomiting
GU: Dysuria, frequent urination
RESP: Dyspnea, shortness of breath, slow or irregular breathing, wheezing
Skin: Diaphoresis, facial flushing, pallor, pruritis, rash, uriticaria
Other: Angioedema, atelectasis

Nursing Considerations

- Use cautiously in patients with hypertension, diabetes mellitus, ischemic heart disease, increased intraocular pressure, or renal impairment because of the pseudoepherine component.
- Monitor renal function, as ordered, because pseudoephedrine is substantially excreted by the kidneys.
- Regularly evaluate effectiveness of hyrdocodone and pseudoephedrine in reducing cough and allergy symptoms.

PATIENT TEACHING
- Instruct patient to use a calibrated measuring device to ensure accurate dose of hydrocodone and pseudoephedrine.

- Urge patient to avoid alcohol and other antidepressants while taking hydrocodone and pseudoephedrine.
- Instruct patient to avoid potentially hazardous activities until drug's CNS effects are known.
- Suggest that patient relieve dry mouth with frequent rinsing and use of sugarless gum or hard candy.
- Tell patient to take last dose of the day a few hours before bedtime if hydrocodone and pseudoephedrine makes him nervous or restless.

hydrocodone bitartrate, pseudoephedrine hydrochloride, and potassium guaiacolsulfonate

Protuss-D

Class, Category, and Schedule

Chemical: Opioid and phenanthrene derivative (hydrocodone), sympathomimetic amine (pseudoephedrine), unclassified (potassium guaiacolsulfonate)
Therapeutic: Antitussive (hydrocodone), decongestant (pseudoephedrine), expectorant (potassium guaiacolsulfonate)
Pregnancy category: C
Controlled substance: Schedule III

Indications and Dosages

▶ *To relieve cough and other symptoms caused by allergies and the common cold*
ORAL SOLUTION
Adults and children age 12 and over. 5 to 7.5 mg hydrocodone, 30 to 45 mg pseudoephedrine, and 300 to 450 mg potassium guaiacolsulfonate (5 to 7.5 ml) q 6 hr.
Children ages 6 to 12. 2.5 to 5 mg hydrocodone, 15 to 30 mg pseudoephedrine, and 150 to 300 mg potassium guaiacolsulfonate (2.5 to 5 ml) q 6 hr.
Children ages 2 to 6. 1.25 to 2.5 mg hydrocodone, 7.5 to 15 mg pseudoephedrine, and 75 to 150 mg potassium guaiacolsulfonate (1.25 to 2.5 ml) q 6 hr.

Contraindications

Hypersensitivity or idiosyncractic reactions to hydrocodone, other opioids, pseudoephedrine, potassium guaiacolsulfonate, or their components; hyperkalemia; hyperthyroidism; narrow-angle glaucoma; prostatic hypertrophy; respiratory depression; severe asthma, coronary artery disease or hypertension; upper airway obstruction, urine retention; use of an MAO inhibitor within 14 days

---

Mechanism of Action

Hydrocodone suppresses cough by directly acting on opiate receptors in the medulla's cough center.

Pseudoephedrine acts on alpha$_1$-adrenergic receptors in the mucosa of the respiratory tract to produce vasoconstriction. This process shrinks swollen nasal mucous membranes; reduces tissue hyperemia, edema, and nasal congestion; and increases nasal airway patency. It also may increase drainage of sinus secretions and open obstructed eustachian ostia.

Potassium guaiacolsulfonate is thought to act by increasing the fluid volume contained in respiratory tract secretions. This decreases the viscosity of bronchial secretions making it easier to remove them from the respiratory tract.

Interactions
DRUGS
hydrocodone and pseudoephedrine
MAO inhibitors: Increased and prolonged cardiac stimulation, increased vasopressor effect, increased risk of severe cardiovascular and cerebrovascular effects, hyperpyrexia, vomiting
hydrocodone component
anticholinergics, paregoric: Possibly intensified anticholinergic adverse effects
antihypertensives, diuretics: Potentiated hypotensive effects
buprenorphine: Decreased hydrocodone effectiveness
CNS depressants: Additive CNS depression
hydroxyzine: Increased hydrocodone analgesic effect; increased CNS depressant and hypotensive effects
metoclopramide: Antagonized effect of metoclopramide on GI motility
naloxone: Antagonized hydrocodone analgesic effect
naltrexone: Precipitated withdrawal symptoms in hydrocodone-dependent patients
neuromuscular blockers: Additive respiratory depressant effects
opioids: Additive CNS and respiratory depressants effects and hypotensive effects
pseudoephedrine component
antacids: Increased pseudoephedrine absorption

antihypertensives, diuretics: Possibly decreased antihypertensive effects

beta blockers: Decreased therapeutic effects of both drugs

citrates: Possibly inhibited urinary pseudoephedrine excretion and prolonged duration of action

CNS stimulant, other sympathomimetics: Possibly increased additive CNS stimulation to excessive levels

cocaine (mucosal-local): Possibly increased cardiovascular effects of either drug and CNS stimulation

digoxin, levodopa: Increased risk of cardiac arrhythmias

hydrocarbon inhalation anesthetics: Increased risk of serious arrhythmias

kaolin: Decreased absorption of pseudoephedrine

nitrates: Reduced antianginal effects of nitrates

rauwolfia alkaloids: Possibly inhibited action of pseudoephedrine

thyroid hormones: Increased cardiovascular effects of both drugs

potassium guaiacolsulfonate component

drugs that increase potassium levels, such as ACE inhibitors, potassium-sparing diuretics, potassium-containing drugs, potassium supplements: Increased risk of hyperkalemia

ACTIVITIES

hydrocodone component

alcohol use: Additive CNS effects

Adverse Reactions

CNS: Confusion, dizziness, drowsiness, euphoria, faintness, headache, insomnia, light-headedness, nervousness, restlessness, seizures, tiredness, trembling, weakness

CV: Bradycardia, hypotension, palpitations, tachycardia

EENT: Blurred or double vision, dry mouth, laryngeal edema, laryngospasm

GI: Anorexia, constipation, nausea, paralytic ileus, toxic megacolon, vomiting

GU: Dysuria, frequent urination

RESP: Dyspnea, shortness of breath, slow or irregular breathing, wheezing

Skin: Diaphoresis, facial flushing, pallor, pruritis, rash, uriticaria

Other: Angioedema, atelectasis, hyperkalemia

Nursing Considerations

• Use cautiously in patients with hypertension, diabetes mellitus, ischemic heart disease, increased intraocular pressure, or renal impairment because of the pseudoepherine component.

* Monitor renal function, as ordered, because pseudoephedrine is substantially excreted by the kidneys.
* Regularly evaluate effectiveness of hyrdocodone, pseudo-ephedrine, and potassium guaiacolsulfonate in reducing cough and allergy symptoms.

PATIENT TEACHING

* Instruct patient to use a calibrated measuring device to ensure accurate dose of hydrocodone, pseudoephedrine, and potassium guaiacolsulfonate.
* Urge patient to avoid alcohol and other antidepressants while taking hydrocodone, pseudoephedrine, and potassium guaiacol-sulfonate.
* Instruct patient to avoid potentially hazardous activities until drug's CNS effects are known.
* Suggest that patient relieve dry mouth with frequent rinsing and use of sugarless gum or hard candy.
* Tell patient to take last dose of the day a few hours before bed-time if hydrocodone, pseudoephedrine, and potassium guaiacol-sulfonate makes her nervous or restless.

ipratropium bromide and albuterol sulfate

Combivent, DuoNeb

Class and Category

Chemical: Quarternary N-methyl isopropyl derivative of noratropine (ipratropium); selective beta$_2$-adrenergic agonist, sympathomimetic (albuterol)
Therapeutic: Bronchodilator
Pregnancy category: C

Indications and Dosages

▶ *To treat bronchospasm in patients with COPD who need more than one bronchodilator*

INHALATION AEROSOL (COMBIVENT)

Adults. 2 inhalations (36 mcg ipratropium, 180 mcg albuterol base) q.i.d. and as needed. *Maximum:* 12 inhalations (216 mcg ipratropium, 1.08 g albuterol base) in 24 hr.

INHALATION SOLUTION FOR NEBULIZER (DUONEB)

Adults. 3 ml (0.5 mg ipratropium, 2.5 mg albuterol base) q.i.d. *Maximum:* 2 additional 3-ml doses in 24 hr, p.r.n.

Mechanism of Action

Ipratropium prevents acetylcholine (after its release from cholinergic fibers) from attaching to muscarinic receptors on membranes of smooth-muscle cells. By blocking acetylcholine's effects in the bronchi and bronchioles, ipratropium relaxes smooth muscles and causes bronchodilation.

Albuterol attaches to $beta_2$ receptors on bronchial cell membranes, which stimulates the intracellular enzyme adenylate cyclase to convert adenosine triphosphate to cyclic adenosine monophosphate (cAMP). This reaction decreases intracellular calcium level and increases intracellular cAMP. Together, these effects relax bronchial smooth-muscle cells and inhibit histamine release.

Contraindications

Hypersensitivity to albuterol, ipratropium, or their components; hypersensitivity to atropine or its derivatives; hypersensitivity to peanuts, soya lecithin, soybeans, or related products (with aerosol inhaler)

Interactions

DRUGS

anticholinergics, such as atropine: Possibly additive effects of ipratropium

beta blockers: Possibly mutual inhibition of therapeutic effects

MAO inhibitors, tricyclic antidepressants: Possibly potentiation of albuterol's adverse cardiovascular effects

non–potassium-sparing diuretics, such as loop and thiazide diuretics: Increased risk of hypokalemia

sympathomimetic bronchodilators, such as theophylline: Increased risk of adverse cardiovascular effects

Adverse Reactions

CNS: Drowsiness, headache, nervousness, tremor

CV: Chest pain, increased heart rate, palpitations

EENT: Acute eye pain, altered taste, blurred vision, dry mouth, pharyngitis, sinusitis, sore throat, voice alterations, worsened angle-closure glaucoma

GI: Constipation, diarrhea, indigestion, nausea

GU: UTI

MS: Back pain, leg cramps, muscle aches

RESP: Bronchitis, cough, exacerbation of COPD, paradoxical bronchospasm, pneumonia, upper respiratory tract infection, wheezing

SKIN: Flushing
Other: Hypokalemia

Nursing Considerations

- Prime the aerosol inhaler with three priming sprays if using it for the first time or if it hasn't been used for more than 24 hours.
- As prescribed, administer nebulized dose using a mouthpiece or properly fitted face mask attached to a jet nebulizer connected to an air compressor with adequate airflow.
- **WARNING** Avoid spraying drug directly into patient's eyes because it may cause vision disturbances. In a patient with angle-closure glaucoma, be aware that spraying drug directly into his eyes may precipitate an acute attack or worsen the condition.
- Monitor urine output if patient has a history of prostatic hyperplasia or bladder-neck obstruction because drug may aggravate these conditions and cause urine retention.
- Monitor heart rate and rhythm and blood pressure often in patients with a history of arrhythmias, coronary artery insufficiency, or hypertension because the drug may cause adverse cardiovascular effects in these patients. If adverse cardiovascular effects occur, expect to discontinue drug.
- Monitor serum potassium level because drug may cause transient hypokalemia.
- Although immediate hypersensitivity reactions are rare, monitor patient for angioedema, bronchospasm, oropharyngeal edema, pruritus, rash, urticaria, and anaphylaxis.

PATIENT TEACHING

- Teach patient how to use inhaler or nebulizer properly. Instruct him to shake aerosol inhaler well before use and to wait 1 minute between inhalations.
- Instruct patient to rinse mouth after each nebulizer or inhaler treatment to help minimize throat dryness and irritation.
- Advise patient to keep drug out of his eyes because it may cause irritation or blurred vision. If drug contacts his eyes, instruct patient to flush them with cool tap water and to contact prescriber immediately.
- Caution patient not to exceed prescribed dose because of possible serious adverse reactions or death. Advise patient to contact prescriber immediately if doses become less effective.
- Advise patient to contact prescriber before using other inhaled drugs.

loratadine and pseudoephedrine sulfate
Claritin-D 12 Hour, Claritin-D 24 Hour

Class and Category
Chemical: Azatadine devirative (loratadine), sympathomimetic amine (pseudoephedrine)
Therapeutic: Antihistamine (loratadine), decongestant (pseudoephedrine)
Pregnancy category: B

Indications and Dosages
▶ *To relieve symptoms of seasonal allergic rhinitis*
E.R. TABLETS (CLARITIN-D 12)

Adults and children age 12 and over. 5 mg loratadine and 120 mg pseudoephedrine (1 tablet) q 12 hr.

DOSAGE ADJUSTMENT For patients with renal impairment (creatinine clearance less than 30 ml/min/1.73 m^2) dosage reduced to 5 mg loratadine and 120 mg psuedoephedrine (1 tablet) q 24 hr.

E.R. TABLETS (CLARITIN-D 24)

Adults and children age 12 and over. 10 mg loratadine and 240 mg pseudoephedrine (1 tablet) q 24 hr.

DOSAGE ADJUSTMENT For patients with renal impairment (creatinine clearance less than 30 ml/min/1.73 m^2) dosage reduced to 10 mg loratadine and 240 mg psuedoephedrine (1 tablet) q 48 hr.

Mechanism of Action
Loratadine competes with histamine for histamine H_1 receptor sites on effector cells and antagonizes the vasodilator effect of endogenously released histamine. This prevents vascular engorgement, mucosal edema, profuse watery secretion, local irritation, and sneezing that normally result from histamine action on afferent nerve terminals in nasal passages.

Pseudoephedrine acts on alpha$_1$-adrenergic receptors in the mucosa of the respiratory tract to produce vasoconstriction. This process shrinks swollen nasal mucous membranes; reduces tissue hyperemia, edema, and nasal congestion; and increases nasal airway patency. It also may increase drainage of sinus secretions and open obstructed eustachian ostia.

Contraindications
Hepatic insufficiency; history of dysphagia or abnormal esophageal peristalsis; hypersensitivity or idiosyncractic reactions

to loratadine, pseudoephedrine, or their components; narrow-angle glaucoma; severe coronary artery disease or hypertension; urine retention; use of an MAO inhibitor within 14 days

Interactions
DRUGS
loratadine component
barbiturates, CNS depressants, tricyclic antidepressants: Additive effects
pseudoephedrine component
antacids: Increased pseudoephedrine absorption
beta blockers, diuretics, methyldopa, mecamylamine, reserpine, veratum alkaloids: Decreased antihypertensive effects of these agents
citrates: Possibly inhibited urinary excretion and prolonged duration of action of pseudoephedrine
CNS stimulant, other sympathomimetics: Possibly increased additive CNS stimulation to excessive levels
cocaine (mucosal-local): Possibly increased cardiovascular effects of either drug and CNS stimulation
digoxin, levodopa: Increased risk of cardiac arrhythmias
hydrocarbon inhalation anesthetics: Increased risk of serious arrhythmias
kaolin: Decreased pseudoephedrine absorptino
MAO inhibitors: Increased and prolonged cardiac stimulation, increased vasopressor effect, increased risk of severe cardiovascular and cerebrovascular effects, hyperpyrexia, vomiting
nitrates: Reduced antianginal effects of nitrates
rauwolfia alkaloids: Possibly inhibited pseudoephedrine action
thyroid hormones: Increased cardiovascular effects of both drugs
ACTIVITIES
loratadine component
alcohol use: Additive effects

Adverse Reactions
CNS: Dizziness, fatigue, headache, insomnia, light-headedness, nervousness, restlessness, seizures, somnolence, trembling, weakness
CV: Palpitations, tachycardia
EENT: Dry mouth, pharyngitis
ENDO: Dysmenorrhea
GI: Anorexia, nausea, vomiting
GU: Dysuria, urine retention
RESP: Bronchospasm, coughing, dyspnea
SKIN: Diaphoresis, pallor

Nursing Considerations

• Be aware that because a previously marketed formulation of loratadine and pseudoepherine caused esophageal obstruction and perforation, the current formulation of the drug isn't recommended for patients who have a history of trouble swallowing tablets or who have been diagnosed with upper-GI narrowing or abnormal esophageal peristalsis.
• Use cautiously in patients with diabetes, hypertension, hyperthyroidism, increased intraocular pressure, ischemic heart disease, prostatic hypertrophy, or renal disease because of the pseudoepherine component.
• Monitor elderly patients closely because they are more prone to developing adverse effects.
• Monitor renal function, as ordered, because pseudoephedrine is substantially excreted by the kidneys.
• Regularly evaluate effectiveness of loratadine and pseudoepherine in relieving seasonal allergic rhinitis.
• Be aware that patient shouldn't have intradermal allergen tests within 4 days of receiving drug because results may be altered.

PATIENT TEACHING

• Instruct patients to take loratadine and pseudoepherine with a full glass of water.
• Urge patient to avoid alcohol, other antidepressants, and OTC drugs containing other antihistamines or sympathomimetics while taking loratadine and pseudoepherine.
• Instruct patient to avoid potentially hazardous activities until drug's CNS effects are known.
• Suggest that patient relieve dry mouth with frequent rinsing and use of sugarless gum or hard candy.

phenylephrine hydrochloride and chlorpheniramine maleate

Dallergy-JR, Ed A-Hist

phenylephrine tannate and chlorpheniramine tannate

Ed A-Hist, Rescon JR, Rynatan, Rynatan Pediatric

Class and Category

Chemical: Sympathomimetic amine (phenylephrine), propylamine derivative (chlorpheniramine)

Therapeutic: Decongestant (phenylephrine), antihistaminic (chlorpheniramine)
Pregnancy category: C

Indications and Dosages

▶ *To provide symptomatic relief of nasal congestion caused by the common cold, sinusitis, allergic rhinitis, and other upper respiratory tract conditions*

ER CAPSULES (DALLERGY JR)

Adults and children age 12 and over. 40 mg phenylephrine and 8 mg chlorpheniramine (1 capsule) q 12 hr.

Children ages 6 to 12. 20 mg phenylephrine and 4 mg chlorpheniramine (1 capsule) q 12 hr.

E.R. TABLETS (ED A HIST, RESCON JR)

Adults and children age 12 and over. 20 to 40 mg phenylephrine and 4 to 8 mg chlorpheniramine (1 to 2 tablets) q 12 hr.

Children ages 6 to 12. 20 mg phenylephrine and 4 mg chlorpheniramine (1 tablet) q 12 hr.

SUSPENSION (RYNATAN, RYNATAN PEDIATRIC)

Adults and children age 6 and over. 5 to 10 mg phenylephrine and 4.5 to 9 mg chlorpheniramine (5 to 10 ml) q 12 hr.

Children ages 2 to 6. 2.5 to 5 mg phenylephrine and 2.25 to 4.5 mg chlorpheniramine (2.5 to 5 ml) q 12 hr.

Mechanism of Action

Phenylephrine stimulates alpha-adrenergic receptors and inhibits activity of the intracellular enzyme adenyl cyclase, which then inhibits production of cAMP. The inhibition of cAMP causes arterial and venous constriction in nasal passages, which decreases blood flow and mucosal edema caused by an allergic response.

Chlorpheniramine competes with histamine for H_1 receptor sites, thereby antagonizing many histamine effects to reduce allergy signs and symptoms.

Contraindications

Breastfeeding, hypersensitivity to phenylephrine, chlorpheniramine or their components; use of an MAO inhibitor within 14 days

Interactions

DRUGS

phenylephrine and chlorpheniramine

MAO inhibitors: Possibly prolonged and intensified anticholinergic effects of chlorpheniramine and overall effects of phenylephrine

phenylephrine component

alpha blockers, haloperidol, loxapine, phenothiazines, thioxanthenes: Possibly decreased vasoconstrictor effect of phenylephrine

antihypertenisves, diuretics: Possibly decreased antihypertensive effects

atropine: Possibly enhanced vasopressor effect of phenylephrine

beta blockers: Decreased therapeutic effects of both drugs

bretylium: Possibly potentiated vaopressor effect and arrhythmias

doxapram: Increased vasopressor effect of both drugs

ergot alkaloids: Possibly cerebral blood vessel rupture, increased vasopressor effect, peripheral vascular ischemia, and gangrene (with ergotamine)

guanadrel, guanethidine: Increased vasopressor effect of phenylephrine, increased risk of severe hypertension and arrhythmias

hydrocarbon inhalation anesthetics: Increased risk of serious arrhythmias

maprotiline, tricyclic antidepressants: Increased risk of severe cardiovascular effects (including arrhythmias, hyperpyrexia, severe hypertension)

mecamylamine, methyldopa: Decreased hypotensive effects of these drugs; increased vasopressor effect of phenylephrine

nitrates: Possibly decreased vasopressor effect of phenylephrine and decreased antianginal effect of nitrates

oxytocin: Possibly severe, persistent hypertension

phenoxybenzamine: Decreased vasoconstrictor effect of phenylephrine, possibly hypotension, and tachycardia

theophylline: Possibly enhanced toxicity (including cardiac toxicity)

thyroid hormones: Increased cardiovascular effects of each drug

chlorpheniramine component

CNS depressants: Additive CNS effects

phenytoin: Possibly increased serum phenytoin levels and toxicity

ACTIVITIES

chlorpheniramine component

alcohol use: Additive CNS effects

Adverse Reactions

CNS: Dizziness, drowsiness, excitation (children), headache, insomnia, nervousness, paresthesia, restlessness, sedation, somnolence, tremor, weakness

CV: Angina, bradycardia, hypertension, hypotension, palpitations, peripheral vasoconstriction that may lead to necrosis or gangrene, tachycardia, ventricular arrhythmias

EENT: Dry mouth

GI: Anorexia, constipation, nausea, vomiting
GU: Urinary hesitancy, urine retention
RESP: Asthma exacerbation, dyspnea

Nursing Considerations

- Use cautiously in patients with cardiovascular disease, diabetes, hypertension, hyperthyroidism, narrow-angle glaucoma, and prostatic hypertrophy.
- Monitor children for excitation and elderly patients for dizziness, sedation, and hypotension; such patients may have an increased risk for these effects.
- Regularly evaluate effectiveness of phenylephrine and chlorpheniramine in reducing nasal congestion.
- Be aware that patient shouldn't have intradermal allergen tests within 72 hours of receiving drug because results may be altered.

PATIENT TEACHING

- Instruct patient to use a calibrated measuring device when using suspension form of phenylephrine and chlorpheniramine to ensure accurate dose.
- Urge patient to avoid alcohol and other antidepressants while taking phenylephrine and chlorpheniramine.
- Instruct patient to avoid potentially hazardous activities until drug's CNS effects are known.
- Suggest that patient relieve dry mouth with frequent rinsing and use of sugarless gum or hard candy.

phenylephrine hydrochloride, chlorpheniramine tannate, and guaifenesin

Decolate, Donatussin

Class and Category

Chemical: Sympathomimetic amine (phenylephrine), propylamine derivative (chlorpheniramine), glyceryl guaiacolate (guaifenesin)
Therapeutic: Decongestant (phenylephrine), antihistaminic (chlorpheniramine), expectorant (guaifenesin)
Pregnancy category: C

Indications and Dosages

▶ *To provide symptomatic relief of upper respiratory symptoms caused by the common cold, sinusitis, allergic rhinitis, and other upper respiratory tract conditions*

TABLETS
Adults. 5 mg phenylephrine, 4 mg chlorpheniramine, and
100 mg guaifenesin (1 tablet) t.i.d. or q.i.d.
ORAL SOLUTION (DROPS)
Children ages 1 to 2. 2 to 4 mg phenylephrine, 1 to 2 mg
chlorpheniramine, and 20 to 40 mg guaifenesin (1 to 2 ml) q 4 to
6 hr.
Children ages 6 months to 1 year. 1 to 2 mg phenylephrine,
0.6 to 1 mg chlorpheniramine, and 10 to 20 mg guaifenesin
(0.6 to 1 ml) q 4 to 6 hr.
Infants ages 3 to 6 months. 0.3 to 0.6 ml (1 ml, containing
2 mg phenylephrine, 1 mg chlorpheniramine, and 20 mg guaifenesin) q 4 to 6 hr.
Infants under age 3 months. 2 to 3 drops/month of age (1 ml
containing 2 mg phenylephrine, 1 mg chlorpheniramine, and
20 mg guaifenesin) q 4 to 6 hr.

Mechanism of Action

Phenylephrine stimulates alpha-adrenergic receptors and inhibits the intracellular enzyme adenyl cyclase, which then inhibits production of cAMP. Inhibition of cAMP causes arterial and venous constriction in nasal passages,
which decreases blood flow and mucosal edema caused by allergic response.

Chlorpheniramine competes with histamine for H_1 receptor sites, thereby
antagonizing many histamine effects to reduce allergy signs and symptoms.

Guaifenesin increases fluid and mucus removal from the upper respiratory
tract by increasing the volume of secretions and reducing their adhesiveness
and surface tension.

Contraindications

Breastfeeding, hypersensitivity to phenylephrine, chlorpheniramine, guaifenesin, or their components; use of MAO inhibitors
within 14 days

Interactions

DRUGS
phenylephrine and chlorpheniramine
MAO inhibitors: Possibly prolonged and intensified anticholinergic
effects of chlorpheniramine and overall effects of phenylephrine
phenylephrine component
alpha blockers, haloperidol, loxapine, phenothiazines, thioxanthenes:
Possibly decreased vasoconstrictor effect of phenylephrine

antihypertenisves, diuretics: Possibly decreased antihypertensive effects

atropine: Possibly enhanced vasopressor effect of phenylephrine

beta blockers: Decreased therapeutic effects of both drugs

bretylium: Possibly potentiated vaopressor effect and arrhythmias

doxapram: Increased vasopressor effect of both drugs

ergot alkaloids: Possibly cerebral blood vessel rupture, increased vasopressor effect, peripheral vascular ischemia, and gangrene (with ergotamine)

guanadrel, guanethidine: Increased vasopressor effect of phenylephrine, increased risk of severe hypertension and arrhythmias

hydrocarbon inhalation anesthetics: Increased risk of serious arrhythmias

maprotiline, tricyclic antidepressants: Increased risk of severe cardiovascular effects (including arrhythmias, hyperpyrexia, severe hypertension)

mecamylamine, methyldopa: Decreased hypotensive effects of these drugs, increased vasopressor effect of phenylephrine

nitrates: Possibly decreased vasopressor effect of phenylephrine and decreased antianginal effect of nitrates

oxytocin: Possibly severe, persistent hypertension

phenoxybenzamine: Decreased vasoconstrictor effect of phenylephrine, possibly hypotension and tachycardia

theophylline: Possibly enhanced toxicity (including cardiac toxicity)

thyroid hormones: Increased cardiovascular effects of each drug

chlorpheniramine component

CNS depressants: Additive CNS effects

phenytoin: Possibly increased serum phenytoin levels and toxicity

ACTIVITIES

chlorpheniramine component

alcohol use: Additive CNS effects

Adverse Reactions

CNS: Dizziness, drowsiness, excitation (children), headache, insomnia, nervousness, paresthesia, restlessness, sedation, tremor, weakness

CV: Angina, bradycardia, hypertension, hypotension, palpitations, peripheral vasoconstriction that may lead to necrosis or gangrene, tachycardia, ventricular arrhythmias

EENT: Dry mouth

GI: Constipation, nausea, vomiting

GU: Urinary hesitancy, urine retention

RESP: Dyspnea

SKIN: Rash, urticaria

Nursing Considerations

- Use cautiously in patients with cardiovascular disease, diabetes, hypertension, hyperthyroidism, narrow-angle glaucoma, or prostatic hypertrophy.
- Monitor patients who may be more susceptible to dizziness, sedation, and hypotension, such as the elderly.
- Regularly evaluate effectiveness of phenylephrine, chlorpheniramine, and guaifenesin in reducing upper respiratory symptoms.
- Be aware that patient shouldn't have intradermal allergen tests within 72 hours of receiving drug because results may be altered.

PATIENT TEACHING

- Instruct patient to take each dose with a full glass of water.
- Urge patient to avoid alcohol and other antidepressants while taking phenylephrine, chlorpheniramine, and guaifenesin.
- Instruct patient to avoid potentially hazardous activities until drug's CNS effects are known.
- Suggest that patient relieve dry mouth with frequent rinsing and use of sugarless gum or hard candy.
- Instruct patient to increase fluid intake (unless contraindicated) to help thin secretions.

phenylephrine hydrochloride, chlorpheniramine maleate, and methscopolamine nitrate

AH-Chew, D.A. Chewable, Dallergy, Dehistine Syrup, DriHist SR, Duradryl, Duradryl JR, Dura-Vent/DA, Extendryl, Extendryl JR, Extendryl SR, Ex-Histine, Hista-Vent DA, OMNhist L.A., Pre-Hist-D

Class and Category

Chemical: Sympathomimetic amine (phenylephrine), alkylamine derivative (chlorpheniramine), hyoscine methobromide (methscopolamine)
Therapeutic: Decongestant (phenylephrine), antihistaminic (chlorpheniramine), anticholinergic (methscopolamine)
Pregnancy category: C

Indications and Dosages

▶ *To relieve nasal congestion caused by the common cold, sinusitis, allergic rhinitis, and other upper respiratory tract conditions*

SYRUP

Adults and children age 12 and over. 10 to 20 mg phenylephrine, 2 to 4 mg chlorpheniramine, and 1.25 or 2.5 mg methscopolamine (5 or 10 ml depending on product) q 4 to 6 hr. *Maximum:* 4 doses daily.

Children ages 6 to 12. 10 mg phenylephrine, 2 mg chlorpheniramine, and 0.625 mg methscopolamine (5 ml) q 4 to 6 hr.

CHEWABLE TABLETS

Adults and children age 12 and over. 10 to 20 mg phenylephrine, 4 to 8 mg chlorpheniramine and 1.25 to 2.5 mg methscopolamine (1 or 2 tablets depending on product) q 4 hr.

Children age 6 to 12. 10 mg phenylephrine, 4 mg chlorpheniramine, and 1.25 mg methscopolamine (1 tablet) q 4 hr.

TABLETS

Adults and children age 12 and over. 10 mg phenylephrine, 4 mg chlorpheniramine, and 1.25 mg methscopolamine (1 tablet) q 4 to 6 hr. *Maximum:* 4 tablets daily.

Children ages 6 to 12. 5 mg phenylephrine, 2 mg chlorpheniramine, and 0.625 mg methscopolamine (½ tablet) q 4 to 6 hr.

E.R. TABLETS

Adults. 20 mg phenylephrine, 8 to 12 mg chlorpheniramine, and 2.5 mg methscopolamine (1 tablet) q 12 hr.

Children ages 6 to 12. 10 mg phenylephrine, 4 to 6 mg chlorpheniramine, and 1.25 mg methscopolamine (½ tablet) q 12 hr.

E.R. CAPSULES

Adults and children age 12 and over. 20 mg phenylephrine, 8 to 12 mg chlorpheniramine, and 2.5 mg methscopolamine (1 capsule) q 12 hr.

Mechanism of Action

Phenylephrine stimulates alpha-adrenergic receptors and inhibits the intracellular enzyme adenyl cyclase, which then inhibits production of cAMP. Inhibition of cAMP causes arterial and venous constriction in nasal passages, which decreases blood flow and mucosal edema caused by allergic response.

Chlorpheniramine competes with histamine for H_1 receptor sites, thereby antagonizing many histamine effects to reduce allergy signs and symptoms.

Methscopolamine competitively inhibits acetylcholine at autonomic postganglionic cholinergic receptors. Because the most sensitive receptors are in the salivary, bronchial, and sweat glands, this action reduces secretions from these glands. It also reduces nasal, oropharyngeal, and bronchial secretions and decreases airway resistance by relaxing smooth muscles in the bronchi and bronchioles.

Contraindications

Angle-closure glaucoma; breastfeeding; cardiac disease, such as arrhythmias, congestive heart failure, coronary artery disease, and mitral stenosis; hemorrhage with hemodynamic instability; hepatic dysfunction; hypersensitivity to phenylephrine, chlorpheniramine, methscopolamine, or their components; ileus; intestinal atony; myasthenia gravis; myocardial ishcemia; obstructive GI or uropathic disease; prostatic hypertrophy; reflux esophagitis; renal impairment; tachycardia; toxic megacolon; ulcerative colitis; use of an MAO inhibitor within 14 days

Interactions

DRUGS

phenylephrine and chlorpheniramine

MAO inhibitors: Possibly prolonged and intensified anticholinergic effects of chlorpheniramine and overall effects of phenylephrine

chlorpheniramine and methscopolamine

anticholinergics (other): Possibly intensified anticholinergic effects

CNS depressants: Additive CNS effects

phenylephrine component

alpha blockers, haloperidol, loxapine, phenothiazines, thioxanthenes: Possibly decreased vasoconstrictor effect of phenylephrine

antihypertenisves, diuretics: Possibly decreased antihypertensive effects

atropine: Possibly enhanced vasopressor effect of phenylephrine

beta blockers: Decreased therapeutic effects of both drugs

bretylium: Possibly potentiated vaopressor effect and arrhythmias

doxapram: Increased vasopressor effect of both drugs

ergot alkaloids: Possibly cerebral blood vessel rupture, increased vasopressor effect, peripheral vascular ischemia, and gangrene (with ergotamine)

guanadrel, guanethidine: Increased vasopressor effect of phenylephrine; increased risk of severe hypertension and arrhythmias

hydrocarbon inhalation anesthetics: Increased risk of serious arrhythmias

maprotiline, tricyclic antidepressants: Increased risk of severe cardiovascular effects (including arrhythmias, hyperpyrexia, severe hypertension)

mecamylamine, methyldopa: Decreased hypotensive effects of these drugs, increased vasopressor effect of phenylephrine

nitrates: Possibly decreased vasopressor effect of phenylephrine and decreased antianginal effect of nitrates

oxytocin: Possibly severe, persistent hypertension

phenoxybenzamine: Decreased vasoconstrictor effect of phenylephrine; possibly hypotension and tachycardia
theophylline: Possibly enhanced toxicity (including cardiac toxicity)
thyroid hormones: Increased cardiovascular effects of each drug
chlorpheniramine component
phenytoin: Possibly increased serum phenytoin level and toxicity
methscopolamine component
adsorbent antidiarrheals, antacids: Decreased absorption and therapeutic effects of methscopolamine
antimyasthenics: Possibly reduced intestinal motility
haloperidol: Decreased antipsychotic effect of haloperidol
ketoconazole: Decreased ketoconazole absorption
lorazepam (parenteral): Possibly hallucinations, irrational behavior, and sedation
metoclopramide: Possibly antagonized effect of metoclopramide on GI motility
opioid analgesics: Increased risk of severe constipation and ileus
potassium chloride: Possibly increased severity of potassium chloride–induced GI lesions
sildenafil, tadalafil, vardenafil: Possibly increased risk of hypotension
urinary alkalizers (antacids, carbonic anhydrase inhibitors, citrates, sodium bicarbonate): Delayed excretion of methscopolamine, possibly leading to increased therapeutic and adverse effects
ACTIVITIES
chlorpheniramine and methscopolamine
alcohol use: Additive CNS effects

Adverse Reactions

CNS: Anxiety, dizziness, drowsiness, euphoria, fear, headache, insomnia, irritability, memory loss, nervousness, paradoxical stimulation, paresthesia, restlessness, sedation, tremor, weakness
CV: Angina, bradycardia, hypertension, hypotension, palpitations, peripheral vasoconstriction that may lead to necrosis or gangrene, tachycardia, ventricular arrhythmias
EENT: Blurred vision; dry eyes, mouth, nose, and throat; mydriasis
GI: Constipation, dysphagia, nausea, vomiting
GU: Urinary hesitancy, urine retention
RESP: Dyspnea
SKIN: Decreased sweating, dry skin, flushing

Nursing Considerations

• Use cautiously in patients with diabetes, hypertension, and hyperthyroidism.

- Monitor patients who may be more susceptible to dizziness, sedation, and hypotension, such as the elderly.
- Assess patient for bladder distention and monitor urine output because methscopolamine's antimuscarinic effects can cause urine retention.
- Regularly evaluate effectiveness of phenylephrine, chlorpheniramine, and methoscopolamine in reducing upper respiratory symptoms.
- Be aware that patient shouldn't have intradermal allergen tests within 72 hours of receiving drug because results may be altered.

PATIENT TEACHING
- Instruct patient to use a calibrated measuring device when using liquid form of phenylephrine, chlorpheniramine, and methscopolamine to ensure accurate dose.
- Urge patient to avoid alcohol, other antidepressants, and OTC cough and cold preparations without consulting prescriber first while taking phenylephrine, chlorpheniramine, and methscopolamine.
- Instruct patient to avoid potentially hazardous activities until drug's CNS effects are known.
- Suggest that patient relieve dry mouth with frequent rinsing and use of sugarless gum or hard candy and to use lubricating eye drops for dry eyes.

phenylephrine hydrochloride, chlorpheniramine maleate, and phenyltoloxamine citrate
Comhist, Nalex-A

Class and Category
Chemical: Sympathomimetic amine (phenylephrine), propylamine derivative (chlorpheniramine), ethanolamine derivative (phenyltoloxamine)
Therapeutic: Decongestant (phenylephrine), antihistamines (chlorpheniramine, phenyltoloxamine)
Pregnancy category: C

Indications and Dosages
▶ *To relieve nasal congestion caused by the common cold, sinusitis, allergic rhinitis, and other upper respiratory tract conditions*
TABLETS
Adults. 10 to 20 mg phenylephrine, 2 to 4 mg chlorphenira-

mine, and 25 to 50 mg phenyltoloxamine (1 to 2 tablets) q 8 hr.

E.R. TABLETS

Adults and children age 12 and over. 10 to 20 mg phenylephrine, 2 to 4 mg chlorpheniramine, and 20 to 40 mg phenyltoloxamine (½ to 1 tablet) q 8 to 12 hr.

Children ages 6 to 12. 10 mg phenylephrine, 2 mg chlorpheniramine, and 20 mg phenyltoloxamine (½ tablet) q 8 to 12 hr.

SOLUTION (NALEX A)

Adults and children age 12 and over. 10 mg phenylephrine, 5 mg chlorpheniramine, and 15 mg phenyltoloxamine (10 ml) q 4 hr.

Children ages 6 to 12. 5 mg phenylephrine, 2.5 mg chlorpheniramine, and 7.5 mg phenyltoloxamine (5 ml) q 4 hr.

Children up to age 6. 1.25 to 2.5 mg phenylephrine, 0.625 to 1.25 mg chlorpheniramine, and 1.87 to 3.75 mg phenyltoloxamine (1.25 to 2.5 ml) q 4 hr.

Mechanism of Action

Phenylephrine stimulates alpha-adrenergic receptors and inhibits the intracellular enzyme adenyl cyclase, which then inhibits production of cAMP. Inhibition of cAMP causes arterial and venous constriction in nasal passages, which decreases blood flow and mucosal edema caused by allergic response.

Chlorpheniramine and phenyltoloxamine compete with histamine for H_1 receptor sites, thereby antagonizing many histamine effects to reduce allergy signs and symptoms.

Contraindications

Breastfeeding, hypersensitivity to phenylephrine, chlorpheniramine, phenyltoloxamine, or their components; use of an MAO inhibitor within 14 days

Interactions

DRUGS

phenylephrine, chlorpheniramine, and phenyltoloxamine
MAO inhibitors: Increased and prolonged cardiac stimulation, increased vasopressor effect, increased risk of severe cardiovascular and cerebrovascular effects, hyperpyrexia, and vomiting

chlorpheniramine and phenyltoloxamine
CNS depressants: Additive CNS effects
phenytoin: Possibly increased serum phenytoin levels and toxicity

phenylephrine component

alpha blockers, haloperidol, loxapine, phenothiazines, thioxanthenes: Possibly decreased vasoconstrictor effect of phenylephrine

antihypertenisves, diuretics: Possibly decreased antihypertensive effects

atropine: Possibly enhanced vasopressor effect of phenylephrine

beta blockers: Decreased therapeutic effects of both drugs

bretylium: Possibly potentiated vaopressor effect and arrhythmias

doxapram: Increased vasopressor effect of both drugs

ergot alkaloids: Possibly cerebral blood vessel rupture, increased vasopressor effect, peripheral vascular ischemia, and gangrene (with ergotamine)

guanadrel, guanethidine: Increased vasopressor effect of phenylephrine, increased risk of severe hypertension and arrhythmias

hydrocarbon inhalation anesthetics: Increased risk of serious arrhythmias

maprotiline, tricyclic antidepressants: Increased risk of severe cardiovascular effects (including arrhythmias, hyperpyrexia, severe hypertension)

mecamylamine, methyldopa: Decreased hypotensive effects of these drugs, increased vasopressor effect of phenylephrine

nitrates: Possibly decreased vasopressor effect of phenylephrine and decreased antianginal effect of nitrates

oxytocin: Possibly severe, persistent hypertension

phenoxybenzamine: Decreased vasoconstrictor effect of phenylephrine, possibly hypotension and tachycardia

theophylline: Possibly enhanced toxicity (including cardiac toxicity)

thyroid hormones: Increased cardiovascular effects of each drug

ACTIVITIES

chlorpheniramine and phenyltoloxamine

alcohol use: Additive CNS effects

Adverse Reactions

CNS: Dizziness, drowsiness, excitation (children), headache, insomnia, nervousness, paresthesia, restlessness, sedation, tremor, weakness

CV: Angina, bradycardia, hypertension, hypotension, palpitations, peripheral vasoconstriction that may lead to necrosis or gangrene, tachycardia, ventricular arrhythmias

EENT: Dry mouth

GI: Constipation, nausea, vomiting

GU: Urinary hesitancy, urine retention

RESP: Dyspnea

Nursing Considerations
- Use cautiously in patients with cardiovascular disease, diabetes, hypertension, hyperthyroidism, narrow-angle glaucoma, or prostatic hypertrophy.
- Monitor patients who may be more susceptible to dizziness, sedation, and hypotension, such as the elderly.
- Regularly evaluate effectiveness of phenylephrine, chlorpheniramine, and phenyltoloxamine in reducing nasal congestion.
- Be aware that patient shouldn't have intradermal allergen tests within 72 hours of receiving drug because results may be altered.

PATIENT TEACHING
- Instruct patient to take drug exactly as prescribed and not to increase dosage or frequency without consulting prescriber.
- Urge patient to avoid alcohol and other antidepressants while taking phenylephrine, chlorpheniramine, and phenyltoloxamine.
- Instruct patient to avoid potentially hazardous activities until drug's CNS effects are known.
- Suggest that patient relieve dry mouth with frequent rinsing and use of sugarless gum or hard candy.

phenylephrine tannate, chlorpheniramine tannate, and pyrilamine tannate

AlleRx, Atrohist Pediatric, R-Tannamine, R-Tannamine Pediatric, R-Tannate, Rhinatate Pediatric, Tri-Tannate, Triotann, Triotann Pediatric, Triotann-S Pediatric

Class and Category
Chemical: Sympathomimetic amine (phenylephrine), propylamine derivative (chlorpheniramine), ethylenediamine derivative (pyrilamine)
Therapeutic: Decongestant (phenylephrine), antihistaminic (chlorpheniramine, pyrilamine)
Pregnancy category: C

Indications and Dosages
▶ *To relieve nasal congestion caused by the common cold, sinusitis, allergic rhinitis, and other upper respiratory tract conditions*
SUSPENSION
Adults. 30 mg phenylephrine, 10 to 12 mg chlorpheniramine, and 62.5 to 75 mg pyrilamine (30 ml) q 12 hr.
Children age 6 and over. 5 to 10 mg phenylephrine, 2 to 4 mg

chlorpheniramine, and 12.5 to 25 mg pyrilamine (5 to 10 ml)
q 12 hr.
Children ages 2 to 6. 2.5 to 5 mg phenylephrine, 1 to 2 mg
chlorpheniramine, and 6.25 to 12.5 mg pyrilamine (2.5 to 5 ml)
q 12 hr.
TABLETS
Adults. 25 to 50 mg phenylephrine, 8 to 16 mg chlorpheniramine, and 25 to 50 mg pyrilamine (1 to 2 tablets) q 12 hr.

Mechanism of Action

Phenylephrine stimulates alpha-adrenergic receptors and inhibits the intracellular enzyme adenyl cyclase, which then inhibits production of cAMP. Inhibition of cAMP causes arterial and venous constriction in nasal passages,
which decreases blood flow and mucosal edema caused by allergic response.
   Chlorpheniramine and pyrilamine compete with histamine for H_1 receptor
sites, antagonizing many histamine effects and reducing allergy effects.

Contraindications

Breastfeeding, hypersensitivity to phenylephrine, chlorpheniramine, pyrilamine or their components; use of MAO inhibitors
within 14 days

Interactions

DRUGS
phenylephrine, chlorpheniramine and pyrilamine
MAO inhibitors: Possibly prolonged and intensified anticholinergic
effects of chlorpheniramine and overall effects of phenylephrine
phenylephrine component
alpha blockers, haloperidol, loxapine, phenothiazines, thioxanthenes:
Possibly decreased vasoconstrictor effect of phenylephrine
antihypertenisves, diuretics: Possibly decreased antihypertensive effects
atropine: Possibly enhanced vasopressor effect of phenylephrine
beta blockers: Decreased therapeutic effects of both drugs
bretylium: Possibly potentiated vaopressor effect and arrhythmias
doxapram: Increased vasopressor effect of both drugs
ergot alkaloids: Possibly cerebral blood vessel rupture, increased vasopressor effect, peripheral vascular ischemia, and gangrene (with
ergotamine)
guanadrel, guanethidine: Increased vasopressor effect of phenylephrine, increased risk of severe hypertension and arrhythmias
hydrocarbon inhalation anesthetics: Increased risk of serious arrhythmias

maprotiline, tricyclic antidepressants: Increased risk of severe cardiovascular effects (including arrhythmias, hyperpyrexia, severe hypertension)

mecamylamine, methyldopa: Decreased hypotensive effects of these drugs; increased vasopressor effect of phenylephrine

nitrates: Possibly decreased vasopressor effect of phenylephrine and decreased antianginal effect of nitrates

oxytocin: Possibly severe, persistent hypertension

phenoxybenzamine: Decreased vasoconstrictor effect of phenylephrine; possibly hypotension and tachycardia

theophylline: Possibly enhanced toxicity (including cardiac toxicity)

thyroid hormones: Increased cardiovascular effects of each drug

chlorpheniramine component

CNS depressants: Additive CNS effects

phenytoin: Possibly increased serum phenytoin levels and toxicity

ACTIVITIES

chlorpheniramine component

alcohol use: Additive CNS effects

Adverse Reactions

CNS: Dizziness, drowsiness, headache, insomnia, nervousness, paresthesia, restlessness, sedation, tremor, weakness

CV: Angina, bradycardia, hypertension, hypotension, palpitations, peripheral vasoconstriction that may lead to necrosis or gangrene, tachycardia, ventricular arrhythmias

EENT: Dry mouth

GI: Constipation, nausea, vomiting

GU: Urinary hesitancy, urine retention

RESP: Dyspnea

Nursing Considerations

- Use cautiously in patients with cardiovascular disease, diabetes, hypertension, hyperthyroidism, narrow-angle glaucoma, or prostatic hypertrophy.
- Monitor patients who may be more susceptible to dizziness, sedation, and hypotension, such as the elderly.
- Regularly evaluate effectiveness of phenylephrine, chlorpheniramine, and pyrilamine in reducing nasal congestion.
- Be aware that patient shouldn't have intradermal allergen tests within 72 hours of receiving drug because results may be altered.

PATIENT TEACHING

- Instruct patient to use a calibrated device when measuring dose of phenylephrine, chlorpheniramine, and pyrilamine to ensure accurate dose.

- Urge patient to avoid alcohol and other antidepressants while taking phenylephrine, chlorpheniramine, and pyrilamine.
- Instruct patient to avoid potentially hazardous activities until drug's CNS effects are known.
- Suggest that patient relieve dry mouth with frequent rinsing and use of sugarless gum or hard candy.

phenylephrine hydrochloride and guaifenesin

Crantex ER, Deconsall II, Endal, Entex, Entex ER, Entex LA, GFN 600/Phenylephrine 20, Guaifed, Guaifed-PD, Liquibid-D, Liquibid PD, PhenaVent LA, SINUvent PE

Class and Category

Chemical: Sympathomimetic amine (phenylephrine), glyceryl guaiacolate (guaifenesin)
Therapeutic: Decongestant (phenylephrine), expectorant (guaifenesin)
Pregnancy category: C

Indications and Dosages

▶ *To relieve upper respiratory symptoms caused by the common cold or allergies*

ORAL SOLUTION

Adults. 7.5 to 15 mg phenylephrine and 100 to 200 mg guaifenesin (5 to 10 ml) q 4 to 6 hr. *Maximum:* 40 ml daily.

E.R. CAPSULES

Adults. 7.5 to 20 mg phenylephrine and 200 to 800 mg guaifenesin (1 or 2 capsules depending on product) q 12 hr.

Children age 12 and over. 10 mg phenylephrine and 300 mg guaifenesin (1 capsule) q 12 hr.

Children ages 6 to 12. 7.5 mg phenylephrine and 200 mg guaifenesin (1 capsule) q 12 hr.

E.R. TABLETS

Adults and children age 12 and over. 20 to 50 mg phenylephrine and 275 to 1200 mg guaifenesin (1 or 2 tablets depending on product) q 12 hr.

Children ages 6 to 12. 12.5 to 25 mg phenylephrine and 275 to 600 mg guaifenesin (½ tablet) q 12 hr.

Contraindications

Hypersensitivity to bisulfites, guaifenesin, phenylephrine, or their components; severe coronary artery disease or hypertension; use within 14 days of MAO inhibitor therapy; ventricular tachycardia

---

Mechanism of Action

Phenylephrine stimulates alpha-adrenergic receptors and inhibits the intracellular enzyme adenyl cyclase, which then inhibits production of cAMP. Inhibition of cAMP causes arterial and venous constriction in nasal passages, which decreases blood flow and mucosal edema caused by allergic response.

Guaifenesin increases fluid and mucus removal from the upper respiratory tract by increasing the volume of secretions and reducing their adhesiveness and surface tension.

Interactions
DRUGS
phenylephrine component
alpha blockers, haloperidol, loxapine, phenothiazines, thioxanthenes: Possibly decreased vasoconstrictor effect of phenylephrine
antihypertenisves, diuretics: Possibly decreased antihypertensive effects
atropine: Possibly enhanced vasopressor effect of phenylephrine
beta blockers: Decreased therapeutic effects of both drugs
bretylium: Possibly potentiated vaopressor effect and arrhythmias
doxapram: Increased vasopressor effect of both drugs
ergot alkaloids: Possibly cerebral blood vessel rupture, increased vasopressor effect, peripheral vascular ischemia, and gangrene (with ergotamine)
guanadrel, guanethidine: Increased vasopressor effect of phenylephrine; increased risk of severe hypertension and arrhythmias
hydrocarbon inhalation anesthetics: Increased risk of serious arrhythmias
MAO inhibitors: Increased and prolonged cardiac stimulation, increased vasopressor effect, increased risk of severe cardiovascular and cerebrovascular effects, hyperpyrexia, vomiting
maprotiline, tricyclic antidepressants: Increased risk of severe cardiovascular effects (including arrhythmias, hyperpyrexia, severe hypertension)
mecamylamine, methyldopa: Decreased hypotensive effects of these drugs; increased vasopressor effect of phenylephrine
nitrates: Possibly decreased vasopressor effect of phenylephrine and decreased antianginal effect of nitrates
oxytocin: Possibly severe, persistent hypertension

phenoxybenzamine: Decreased vasoconstrictor effect of phenyle-phrine; possibly hypotension and tachycardia
theophylline: Possibly enhanced toxicity (including cardiac toxicity)
thyroid hormones: Increased cardiovascular effects of each drug

Adverse Reactions

CNS: Dizziness, hallucinations, headache, insomnia, nervousness, paresthesia, restlessness, seizures, tremor, weakness
CV: Angina, bradycardia, hypertension, hypotension, palpitations, peripheral vasoconstriction that may lead to necrosis or gangrene, tachycardia, ventricular arrhythmia
GI: Nausea, vomiting
RESP: Dyspnea
SKIN: Pallor, rash, urticaria
Other: Allergic reaction

Nursing Considerations

• Assess patient for signs and symptoms of angina, arrhythmias, and hypertension because phenylephrine may increase myocardial oxygen demand and the risk of proarrhythmias and blood pressure changes.
• **WARNING** Monitor patient with thyroid disease for increased sensitivity to catecholamines and possible thyrotoxicity or cardiotoxicity.
• Regularly evaluate effectiveness of phenylephrine and guaifenesin in relieving upper respiratory symptoms. Notify prescriber if symptoms persist or worsen.
• Watch for signs of more serious condition, such as cough that lasts longer than 1 week, fever, persistent headache, and rash.
PATIENT TEACHING
• Instruct patient to take each dose with a full glass of water.
• Advise patient not to break, crush, or chew E.R. tablets or capsules but to swallow them whole.
• Instruct patient to increase fluid intake (unless contraindicated) to help thin secretions.
• Advise patient to avoid potentially hazardous activities until drug's CNS effects are known.

phenylephrine tannate and pyrilamine tannate

Duonate-12, P-Tanna 12, R-Tannic-S A/D, Ryna-12, Viravan-S

Class and Category

Chemical: Sympathomimetic amine (phenylephrine), ethylene-diamine derivative (pyrilamine)

Therapeutic: Decongestant (phenylephrine), antihistaminic (pyrilamine)

Pregnancy category: C

Indications and Dosages

▶ *To relieve nasal congestion caused by the common cold, sinusitis, allergic rhinitis, and other upper respiratory tract conditions*

SUSPENSION

Adults. 12.5 mg phenylephrine and 30 mg pyrilamine or 25 mg phenylephrine and 60 mg pyrilamine (5 or 10 ml) q 12 hr.

Children age 6 and over. 5 to 10 mg phenylephrine and 30 to 60 mg pyrilamine (5 or 10 ml) q 12 hr.

Children ages 2 to 6. 2.5 to 5 mg phenylephrine and 15 to 30 mg pyrilamine (2.5 ml or 5 ml) q 12 hr.

CHEWABLE TABLETS

Adults. 25 mg phenylephrine and 30 mg pyrilamine (1 tablet) q 12 hr.

Children ages 6 to 12. 12.5 mg phenylephrine and 15 mg pyrilamine (½ tablet) q 12 hr.

TABLETS

Adults. 25 to 50 mg phenylephrine and 60 to 120 mg pyrilamine (1 or 2 tablets) q 12 hr.

Children ages 6 to 12. 12.5 to 25 mg phenylephrine and 30 to 60 mg pyrilamine (½ to 1 tablet) q 12 hr.

Mechanism of Action

Phenylephrine stimulates alpha-adrenergic receptors and inhibits the intracellular enzyme adenyl cyclase, which then inhibits production of cAMP. Inhibition of cAMP causes arterial and venous constriction in nasal passages, which decreases blood flow and mucosal edema caused by allergic response.

Pyrilamine competes with histamine for H_1 receptor sites, thereby antagonizing many histamine effects to reduce allergy signs and symptoms.

Contraindications

Breast-feeding; hypersensitivity to phenylephrine, pyrilamine, or their components; use of an MAO inhibitor within 14 days

Interactions

DRUGS

phenylephrine and pyrilamine

MAO inhibitors: Possibly prolonged and intensified anticholinergic effects of pyrilamine and overall effects of phenylephrine

phenylephrine component

alpha blockers, haloperidol, loxapine, phenothiazines, thioxanthenes: Possibly decreased vasoconstrictor effect of phenylephrine

antihypertenisves, diuretics: Possibly decreased antihypertensive effects

atropine: Possibly enhanced vasopressor effect of phenylephrine

beta blockers: Decreased therapeutic effects of both drugs

bretylium: Possibly potentiated vaopressor effect and arrhythmias

doxapram: Increased vasopressor effect of both drugs

ergot alkaloids: Possibly cerebral blood vessel rupture, increased vasopressor effect, peripheral vascular ischemia, and gangrene (with ergotamine)

guanadrel, guanethidine: Increased vasopressor effect of phenylephrine; increased risk of severe hypertension and arrhythmias

hydrocarbon inhalation anesthetics: Increased risk of serious arrhythmias

maprotiline, tricyclic antidepressants: Increased risk of severe cardiovascular effects (including arrhythmias, hyperpyrexia, severe hypertension)

mecamylamine, methyldopa: Decreased hypotensive effects of these drugs; increased vasopressor effect of phenylephrine

nitrates: Possibly decreased vasopressor effect of phenylephrine and decreased antianginal effect of nitrates

oxytocin: Possibly severe, persistent hypertension

phenoxybenzamine: Decreased vasoconstrictor effect of phenylephrine; possibly hypotension and tachycardia

theophylline: Possibly enhanced toxicity (including cardiac toxicity)

thyroid hormones: Increased cardiovascular effects of each drug

pyrilamine component

CNS depressants: Additive CNS effects

ACTIVITIES

pyrilamine component

alcohol use: Additive CNS effects

Adverse Reactions

CNS: Dizziness, drowsiness, excitation (children), headache, insomnia, nervousness, paresthesia, restlessness, sedation, tremor, weakness

CV: Angina, bradycardia, hypertension, hypotension, palpitations, peripheral vasoconstriction that may lead to necrosis or gangrene, tachycardia, ventricular arrhythmias

EENT: Dry mouth
GI: Constipation, nausea, vomiting
GU: Urinary hesitancy, urine retention
RESP: Dyspnea

Nursing Considerations

- Use cautiously in patients with cardiovascular disease, diabetes, hypertension, hyperthyroidism, narrow-angle glaucoma, or prostatic hypertrophy.
- Monitor children for excitation and elderly patients for dizziness, sedation, and hypotension; such patients may have an increased risk for these effects.
- Regularly evaluate effectiveness of phenylephrine and pyrilamine in reducing nasal congestion.
- Be aware that patient shouldn't have intradermal allergen tests within 72 hours of receiving drug because results may be altered.

PATIENT TEACHING

- Instruct patient to use a calibrated measuring device to ensure accurate dose of phenylephrine and pyrilamine suspension.
- Tell patient to swallow nonchewable tablets whole.
- Urge patient to avoid alcohol and other antidepressants while taking phenylephrine and pyrilamine.
- Instruct patient to avoid potentially hazardous activities until drug's CNS effects are known.
- Suggest that patient relieve dry mouth with frequent rinsing and use of sugarless gum or hard candy.

promethazine hydrochloride and codeine phosphate

Phenergan with Codeine, Prometh with Codeine

Class, Category, and Schedule

Chemical: Phenothiazine derivative (promethazine), phenanthrene derivative (codeine)
Therapeutic: Antihistamine (promethazine), analgesic and antitussive (codeine)
Pregnancy category: C
Controlled substance: Schedule V

Indications and Dosages

▶ *To relieve cough and other symptoms caused by allergies and the common cold*

SYRUP

Adults and children age 12 and over. 6.25 mg promethazine and 10 mg codeine (5 ml) q 4 to 6 hr. *Maximum:* 30 ml daily.

Children ages 6 to 12. 3.125 to 6.25 mg promethazine and 5 to 10 mg codeine (2.5 to 5 ml) q 4 to 6 hr. *Maximum:* 30 ml daily.

Children ages 2 to 6. 1.56 to 3.125 promethazine and 2.5 to 5 mg codeine (1.25 to 2.5 ml) q 4 to 6 hr. *Maximum:* 0.5 ml/kg/day for children weighing 12 to 18 kg; 6 ml/day for children weighing less than 12 kg.

DOSAGE ADJUSTMENT For patient with renal insufficiency (creatinine clearance of 10 to 50 ml/min/1.73 m^2), dosage reduced by 75%.

Mechanism of Action

Promethazine competes with histamine for H$_1$ receptor sites, thereby antagonizing many histamine effects and reducing allergy signs and symptoms.

Codeine suppresses cough by directly acting on opiate receptors in the medulla's cough center.

Contraindications

Angle-closure glaucoma; benign prostatic hyperplasia; bladder neck obstruction; bone marrow depression; breastfeeding; children under age 2; coma; hypersensitivity to promethazine, codeine, other opioids, or their components; hypertensive crisis; pyloroduodenal obstruction; stenosing peptic ulcer; significant respiratory depression; use of large quantities of CNS depressants

Interactions

DRUGS

promethazine and codeine

anticholinergics: Possibly intensified anticholinergic adverse effects

CNS depressants: Additive CNS depression

MAO inhibitors: Possibly prolonged and intensified anticholinergic and CNS depressant effects of promethazine; increased risk of unpredictable, severe, and sometimes fatal reactions with codeine

promethazine component

amphetamines: Decreased stimulant effect of amphetamines

anticonvulsants: Lowered seizure threshold

appetite suppressants: Possibly antagonized anorectic effect of appetite suppressants

beta blockers: Increased risk of additive hypotensive effects, irreversible retinopathy, arrhythmias, and tardive dyskinesia

bromocriptine: Decreased bromocriptine effectiveness
dopamine: Possibly antagonized peripheral vasoconstriction (with high doses of dopamine
ephedrine, metaraminol, methoxamine: Decreased vasopressor response to these drugs
epinephrine: Blocked alpha-adrenergic effects of epinephrine, increased risk of hypotension
guanadrel, guanethidine: Decreased antihypertensive effects of these drugs
hepatotoxic drugs: Increased risk of hepatotoxicity
hypotension-producing drugs: Possibly severe hypotension with syncope
levodopa: Inhibited antidyskinetic effects of levodopa
metrizamide: Increased risk of seizures
ototoxic drugs: Possibly masking of some symptoms of ototoxicity, such as dizziness, tinnitus, and vertigo
quinidine: Additive cardiac effects
riboflavin: Increased riboflavin requirements
codeine component
antihypertensives, diuretics: Potentiated hypotensive effects
buprenorphine: Decreased codeine effectiveness
hydroxyzine: Increased codeine analgesic effect; increased CNS depressant and hypotensive effects
metoclopramide: Antagonized effect of metoclopramide on GI motility
naloxone: Antagonized codeine analgesic effect
naltrexone: Precipitated withdrawal symptoms in codeine-dependent patients
neuromuscular blockers: Additive respiratory depressant effects
opioids: Additive CNS and respiratory depressant effects and hypotensive effects
paregoric: Increased risk of severe constipation
ACTIVITIES
promethazine and codeine
alcohol use: Additive CNS depression

Adverse Reactions
CNS: Akathisia, CNS stimulation, coma, confusion, delirium, depression, disorientation, dizziness, drowsiness, dystonia, euphoria, excitation, fatigue, hallucinations, headache, hysteria, insomnia, irritability, lack of coordination, lethargy, light-headedness, mental and physical impairment, mood changes, nervousness, neuroleptic malignant syndrome, paradoxical stimulation, pseudo-

parkinsonism, restlessness, sedation, seizures, syncope, tardive dyskinesia, tremor

CV: Bradycardia, heart block, hypertension, orthostatic hypotension, palpitations, tachycardia

EENT: Altered taste; blurred vision; diplopia; dry mouth, nose, and throat; laryngeal edema; laryngospasm; miosis; nasal congestion; tinnitus; vision changes

ENDO: Hyperglycemia

GI: Abdominal cramps and pain, anorexia, constipation, flatulence, gastroesophageal reflux, ileus, indigestion, nausea, vomiting

GU: Decreased libido, difficult ejaculation, dysuria, impotence, oliguria, ureteral spasm, urinary incontinence, urine retention

HEME: Agranulocytosis, leukopenia, thrombocytopenia, thrombocytopenic purpura

MS: Muscle rigidity

RESP: Apnea, bronchoconstriction, bronchospasm, depressed cough reflex, respiratory depression, tenacious bronchial secretions

SKIN: Dermatitis, diaphoresis, flushing, jaundice, pallor, photosensitivity, pruritus, rash, urticaria

Other: Anaphylaxis, angeioedema, paradoxical reactions, physical and psychological dependence

Nursing Considerations

- Use cautiously in patients with a head injury or who have peptic ulcer or other abdominal obstruction (except for pyloroduodenal obstruction, which is a contraindication), cardiovascular disease, liver or kidney impairment, fever, seizures, hypothyroidism, intestinal inflammation, or Addison's disease.
- Use cautiously in children age 2 and over because of risk for respiratory depression.
- Be aware that cautious use is also required in patients who have recently undergone stomach, intestinal, or urinary tract surgery.
- Monitor effectiveness of promethazine and codeine in relieving allergy symptoms and cough. Notify prescriber if symptoms persist or worsen.
- **WARNING** Monitor respiratory function because promethazine and codeine may suppress cough reflex and cause thickening of bronchial secretions, aggravating such conditions as asthma and COPD. Rarely, it may depress respirations and induce apnea. Notify prescriber immediately if respiratory rate

drops below 10 breaths/minute.
- Monitor patient's hematologic status as ordered because promethazine may cause bone marrow depression. Assess patient for signs and symptoms of infection or bleeding.
- **WARNING** Monitor patient for signs and symptoms of neuroleptic malignant syndrome, such as fever, hypertension or hypotension, involuntary motor activity, mental changes, muscle rigidity, tachycardia, and tachypenia. Be prepared to provide supportive treatment and additional drug therapy, as prescribed.
- Take safety precautions, if needed, because promethazine and codeine can cause considerable drowsiness and many other adverse CNS effects.
- Be aware that patient shouldn't have intradermal allergen tests within 72 hours of receiving promethazine and codeine because drug may significantly alter flare response.

PATIENT TEACHING
- Tell patient to take only the dosage prescribed and not to increase dose or frequency without consulting prescriber.
- Instruct patient to use a calibrated measuring device to ensure accurate dose of liquid formulation.
- Advise patient to contact prescriber if symptoms, including cough, aren't better after 5 days of therapy.
- Instruct patient to avoid potentially hazardous activities until drug's CNS effects are known.
- Warn patient to avoid alcoholic beverages and OTC antihistamine and CNS depressant drugs while taking promethazine and codeine.
- Caution patient to drink plenty of fluids and increase fiber in diet because codeine can cause or worsen constipation.
- Tell patient to rise slowly from a lying or sitting position to minimize dizziness or light-headedness.
- Alert female patients that promethazine and codeine may affect pregnancy test results.
- Instruct diabetic patient to monitor her blood glucose level closely while taking promethazine and codeine.
- Tell patient to report any involuntary muscle movements or unusual sensitivity to sunlight to the prescriber because drug may need to be discontinued.
- Advise patient to avoid excessive sun exposure and to use sunscreen when outdoors.

promethazine hydrochloride and dextromethorphan hydrobromide

Phenergan with Dextromethorphan, Promethazine DM

Class and Category

Chemical: Phenothiazine derivative (promethazine), D-isomer codeine analogue of levorphanol (dextromethorphan)

Therapeutic: Antihistamine (promethazine), antitussive (dextromethorphan)

Pregnancy category: C

Indications and Dosages

▶ *To relieve cough and allergic signs and symptoms caused by upper respiratory conditions such as the common cold and seasonal allergies*

SYRUP

Adults and children age 12 and over. 6.25 mg promethazine and 15 mg dextromethorphan (5 ml) q 4 to 6 hr. *Maximum:* 30 ml q 24 hr.

Children ages 6 to 12. 3.125 to 6.25 mg promethazine and 7.5 to 15 mg dextromethorphan (2.5 to 5 ml) q 4 to 6 hr. *Maximum:* 20 ml q 24 hr.

Children ages 2 to 6. 1.5 to 3.125 mg promethazine and 3.75 to 7.5 mg dextromethorphan (1.25 to 2.5 ml) q 4 to 6 hr. *Maximum:* 10 ml q 24 hr.

ORAL SOLUTION

Adults. 6.25 mg promethazine and 15 mg dextromethorphan (5 ml) q 4 to 6 hr. *Maximum:* 30 ml q 24 hr.

Mechanism of Action

Promethazine competes with histamine for H$_1$ receptor sites, thereby antagonizing many histamine effects and reducing allergy signs and symptoms.

Dextromethorphan suppresses cough by directly acting on the cough center in the medulla of the brain.

Contraindications

Angle-closure glaucoma; asthma; benign prostatic hyperplasia; bladder neck obstruction; bone marrow depression; breastfeeding; chronic bronchitis; coma; emphysema; hypersensitivity to promethazine, dextromethorphan, or their components; hypertensive crisis; productive cough; pyloroduodenal obstruction; stenosing peptic ulcer; use of large quantities of CNS depressants; use of an MAO inhibitor within 14 days

Interactions
DRUGS
promethazine and dextromethorphan
CNS depressants: Additive CNS depression
MAO inhibitors: Possibly prolonged and intensified anticholinergic and CNS depressant effects of promethazine; increased risk of unpredictable, severe, and sometimes fatal reactions with dextromethorphan
promethazine component
amphetamines: Decreased stimulant effect of amphetamines
anticonvulsants: Lowered seizure threshold
anticholinergics: Possibly intensified anticholinergic adverse effects
appetite suppressants: Possibly antagonized anorectic effect of appetite suppressants
beta blockers: Increased risk of additive hypotensive effects, irreversible retinopathy, arrhythmias, and tardive dyskinesia
bromocriptine: Decreased effectiveness of bromocriptine
dopamine: Possibly antagonized peripheral vasoconstriction (with high doses of dopamine
ephedrine, metaraminol, methoxamine: Decreased vasopressor response to these drugs
epinephrine: Blocked alpha-adrenergic effects of epinephrine; increased risk of hypotension
guanadrel, guanethidine: Decreased antihypertensive effects of these drugs
hepatotoxic drugs: Increased risk of hepatotoxicity
hypotension-producing drugs: Possibly severe hypotension with syncope
levodopa: Inhibited antidyskinetic effects of levodopa
metrizamide: Increased risk of seizures
ototoxic drugs: Possibly masking of some symptoms of ototoxicity, such as dizziness, tinnitus, and vertigo
quinidine: Additive cardiac effects
riboflavin: Increased riboflavin requirements
dextromethorphan component
amiodarone, fluoxetine, quinidine: Decreased metabolism of dextromethorphan, which may increase plasma dextromethorphan levels and adverse reactions
CNS depressants: Additive CNS effects
ACTIVITIES
promethazine and dextromethorphan
alcohol use: Additive CNS depression

dextromethorphan component
smoking: Possibly increased respiratory secretion retention

Adverse Reactions

CNS: Akathisia, CNS stimulation, confusion, dizziness, drowsiness, dystonia, euphoria, excitation, fatigue, hallucinations, hyperactivity, hysteria, insomnia, irritability, nervousness, neuroleptic malignant syndrome, paradoxical stimulation, pseudoparkinsonism, restlessness, sedation, seizures, syncope, tardive dyskinesia, tremor
CV: Bradycardia, hypertension, hypotension, tachycardia
EENT: Blurred vision; diplopia; dry mouth, nose, and throat; nasal congestion; tinnitus; vision changes
GI: Abdominal pain, anorexia, constipation, ileus, nausea, vomiting
GU: Dysuria
HEME: Agranulocytosis, leukopenia, thrombocytopenia, thrombocytopenic purpura
RESP: Apnea, respiratory depression, tenacious bronchial secretions
SKIN: Dermatitis, diaphoresis, jaundice, photosensitivity, rash, urticaria
Other: Angioedema, emotional and physical dependence (prolonged use with high doses), paradoxical reactions

Nursing Considerations

- Use promethazine and dextromethorphan cautiously in patients with cardiovascular disease or hepatic dysfunction because of potential adverse effects.
- Use cautiously in children age 2 and over because of risk for respiratory depression.
- Also use cautiously in patients with diabetes because some products contain sugar, which may disrupt blood glucose control; in those with impaired hepatic function because dextromethorphan is metabolized by the liver; in those with respiratory depression because dextromethorphan adversely affects respirations; and in those with seizure disorders or those who use medication that may affect seizure threshold because promethazine may lower patient's seizure threshold.
- **WARNING** Monitor respiratory function because drug may suppress cough reflex and cause thickening of bronchial secretions. It also may depress respirations and induce apnea.
- Monitor patient's hematologic status as ordered because promethazine may cause bone marrow depression, especially

when used with other marrow-toxic agents. Assess patient for signs and symptoms of infection or bleeding.

- **WARNING** Monitor patient for evidence of neuroleptic malignant syndrome, such as fever; hypertension or hypotension, involuntary motor activity, mental changes, muscle rigidity, tachycardia, and tachypenia. Be prepared to provide supportive treatment and additional drug therapy, as prescribed.
- Take safety precautions, if needed, because promethazine and dextromethorphan can cause drowsiness and many other adverse CNS effects.
- Be aware that patient shouldn't have intradermal allergen tests within 72 hours of receiving promethazine and dextromethorphan because drug may significantly alter flare response.

PATIENT TEACHING
- Instruct patient to use a calibrated measuring device to ensure accurate dose.
- Stress importance of taking promethazine and dextromethorphan exactly as prescribed and not increasing dose or frequency without consulting prescriber.
- Warn patient to avoid alcoholic beverages and OTC antihistamines and CNS depressants while taking promethazine and dextromethorphan.
- Tell patient to rise slowly from a lying or sitting position to minimize dizziness or light-headedness.
- Instruct diabetic patient to monitor his blood glucose level closely while taking promethazine and dextromethorphan.
- Tell patient to report involuntary muscle movements or unusual sensitivity to sunlight because drug may need to be stopped.
- Advise patient to avoid excessive sun exposure and to use sunscreen when outdoors.

promethazine hydrochloride and phenylephrine hydrochloride
Phenameth VC, Phenergan VC, Prometh VC Plain, Promethazine VC

Class and Category
Chemical: Phenothiazine derivative (promethazine), sympathomimetic amine (phenylephrine)
Therapeutic: Antihistamine (promethazine), decongestant (phenylephrine)

Pregnancy category: C

Indications and Dosages

▶ *To relieve cough and other symptoms caused by allergies and the common cold*

SYRUP

Adults and children age 12 and over. 6.25 mg promethazine and 5 mg phenylephrine (5 ml) q 4 to 6 hr. *Maximum:* 30 ml q 24 hr.

Children ages 6 to 12. 3.125 to 6.25 mg promethazine and 2.5 to 5 mg phenylephrine (2.5 to 5 ml) q 4 to 6 hr. *Maximum:* 15 ml q 24 hr

Children ages 2 to 6. 1.56 to 3.125 promethazine and 1.25 to 2.5 mg phenylephrine (1.25 to 2.5 ml) q 4 to 6 hr. *Maximum:* 7.5 ml q 24 hr.

Mechanism of Action

Promethazine competes with histamine for H_1 receptor sites, thereby antagonizing many histamine effects and reducing allergy signs and symptoms.

Phenylephrine stimulates alpha-adrenergic receptors, constricting local vessels and decreasing blood flow and mucosal edema to relieve nasal congestion.

Contraindications

Angle-closure glaucoma; benign prostatic hyperplasia; bladder neck obstruction; bone marrow depression; breastfeeding; children under age 2; coma; hypersensitivity to bisulfites, promethazine, phenylephrine, or their components; lower respiratory disorders (including asthma); pyloroduodenal obstruction; severe coronary artery disease or hypertension; stenosing peptic ulcer; use of large quantities of CNS depressants; use of MAO inhibitor within 14 days; ventricular tachycardia

Interactions

DRUGS

promethazine and phenylephrine components

guanadrel, guanethidine: Decreased antihypertensive effects of these drugs; increased risk of severe hypertension and arrhythmias; increased vasopressor effect of phenylephrine

MAO inhibitors: Possibly prolonged and intensified anticholinergic and CNS depressant effects of promethazine; increased and prolonged cardiac stimulation, increased vasopressor effect, increased

risk of severe cardiovascular and cerebrovascular effects, hyperpyrexia, and vomiting with phenylephrine

promethazine component

amphetamines: Decreased stimulant effect of amphetamines

anticholinergics: Possibly intensified anticholinergic adverse effects

anticonvulsants: Lowered seizure threshold

appetite suppressants: Possibly antagonized anorectic effect of appetite suppressants

beta blockers: Increased risk of additive hypotensive effects, irreversible retinopathy, arrhythmias, and tardive dyskinesia

bromocriptine: Decreased effectiveness of bromocriptine

CNS depressants: Additive CNS depression

dopamine: Possibly antagonized peripheral vasoconstriction (with
high doses of dopamine

ephedrine, metaraminol, methoxamine: Decreased vasopressor response to these drugs

epinephrine: Blocked alpha-adrenergic effects of epinephrine; increased risk of hypotension

hepatotoxic drugs: Increased risk of hepatotoxicity

hypotension-producing drugs: Possibly severe hypotension with syncope

levodopa: Inhibited antidyskinetic effects of levodopa

metrizamide: Increased risk of seizures

ototoxic drugs: Possibly masking of some symptoms of ototoxicity,
such as dizziness, tinnitus, and vertigo

quinidine: Additive cardiac effects

riboflavin: Increased riboflavin requirements

phenylephrine component

alpha blockers, haloperidol, loxapine, phenothiazines, thioxanthenes:
Possibly decreased vasoconstrictor effect of phenylephrine

antihypertenisves, diuretics: Possibly decreased antihypertensive effects

atropine: Possibly enhanced vasopressor effect of phenylephrine

beta blockers: Decreased therapeutic effects of both drugs

bretylium: Possibly potentiated vaopressor effect and arrhythmias

doxapram: Increased vasopressor effect of both drugs

ergot alkaloids: Possibly cerebral blood vessel rupture, increased vasopressor effect, peripheral vascular ischemia, and gangrene (with
ergotamine)

hydrocarbon inhalation anesthetics: Increased risk of serious arrhythmias

maprotiline, tricyclic antidepressants: Increased risk of severe cardiovascular effects (including arrhythmias, hyperpyrexia, severe hypertension)

mecamylamine, methyldopa: Decreased hypotensive effects of these drugs, increased vasopressor effect of phenylephrine
nitrates: Possibly decreased vasopressor effect of phenylephrine and decreased antianginal effect of nitrates
oxytocin: Possibly severe, persistent hypertension
phenoxybenzamine: Decreased vasoconstrictor effect of phenylephrine, possibly hypotension and tachycardia
theophylline: Possibly enhanced toxicity (including cardiac toxicity)
thyroid hormones: Increased cardiovascular effects of each drug
ACTIVITIES
promethazine component
alcohol use: Additive CNS depression

Adverse Reactions

CNS: Akathisia, CNS stimulation, confusion, dizziness, drowsiness, dystonia, euphoria, excitation, fatigue, hallucinations, headache, hysteria, insomnia, irritability, lack of coordination, nervousness, neuroleptic malignant syndrome, paradoxical stimulation, pseudoparkinsonism, restlessness, sedation, seizures, syncope, tardive dyskinesia, tremor, weakness
CV: Angina, bradycardia, hypertension, orthostatic hypotension, palpitations, peripheral vasoconstriction, tachycardia, ventricular arrhythmias
EENT: Blurred vision; diplopia; dry mouth, nose, and throat; nasal congestion; tinnitus; vision changes
ENDO: Hyperglycemia
GI: Anorexia, ileus, nausea, vomiting
GU: Dysuria
HEME: Agranulocytosis, leukopenia, thrombocytopenia, thrombocytopenic purpura
RESP: Apnea, dyspnea, respiratory depression, tenacious bronchial secretions
SKIN: Dermatitis, diaphoresis, jaundice, pallor, photosensitivity, rash, urticaria
Other: Angioedema, paradoxical reactions

Nursing Considerations

• Use cautiously in patients with cardiovascular disease, hepatic dysfunction, or sleep apnea because of potential adverse effects.
• Use cautiously in children age 2 and over because of risk of respiratory depression.
• Use cautiously in patients who have seizure disorders or receive drugs that lower the seizure threshold, such as opioids and anesthetics.

- Monitor effectiveness of promethazine and phenylephrine in relieving allergy symptoms. Notify prescriber if symptoms persist or worsen.
- **WARNING** Monitor respiratory function because promethazine and phenylephrine may suppress cough reflex and cause thickening of bronchial secretions, aggravating such conditions as asthma and COPD. Rarely, it may depress respirations and induce apnea. Notify prescriber immediately if respiratory rate drops below 10 breaths/minute.
- Monitor patient's hematologic status as ordered because promethazine may cause bone marrow depression. Assess patient for signs and symptoms of infection or bleeding.
- **WARNING** Monitor patient for evidence of neuroleptic malignant syndrome, such as fever, hypertension or hypotension, involuntary motor activity, mental changes, muscle rigidity, tachycardia, and tachypenia. Be prepared to provide supportive treatment and additional drug therapy, as prescribed.
- Take safety precautions, if needed, because promethazine and phenylephrine can cause considerable drowsiness and multiple other adverse CNS effects.
- Be aware that patient shouldn't have intradermal allergen tests within 72 hours of receiving promethazine and phenylephrine because drug may significantly alter flare response.

PATIENT TEACHING
- Tell patient to take only the dosage prescribed and not to increase dose or frequency without consulting prescriber.
- Instruct patient to use a calibrated measuring device to ensure accurate dose.
- Advise patient to contact prescriber if signs and symptoms persist after 5 days of therapy.
- Instruct patient to avoid potentially hazardous activities until drug's CNS effects are known.
- Warn patient to avoid alcoholic beverages and OTC decongestants and CNS depressants while taking promethazine and phenylephrine.
- Tell patient to rise slowly from a lying or sitting position to minimize dizziness or light-headedness.
- Instruct diabetic patient to monitor her blood glucose level closely while taking promethazine and phenylephrine.
- Tell patient to report involuntary muscle movements or unusual sensitivity to sunlight because drug may need to be stopped.
- Advise patient to avoid excessive sun exposure and to use sunscreen when outdoors.

promethazine hydrochloride, phenylephrine hydrochloride, and codeine phosphate

Phenergan VC with Codeine, Prometh VC with Codeine, Promethazine VC with Codeine

Class, Category, and Schedule

Chemical: Phenothiazine derivative (promethazine), sympathomimetic amine (phenylephrine), and phenanthrene alkaloid of opium (codeine)
Therapeutic: Antihistamine (promethazine), decongestant (phenylephrine) and analgesic and antiussive (codeine)
Pregnancy category: C
Controlled substance: Schedule V

Indications and Dosages

▶ *To relieve cough and other symptoms caused by allergies and the common cold*

SYRUP

Adults and children age 12 and over. 6.25 mg promethazine, 5 mg phenylephrine, and 10 mg codeine (5 ml) q 4 to 6 hr. *Maximum:* 30 ml q 24 hr.

Children ages 6 to 12. 3.125 to 6.25 mg promethazine, 2.5 to 5 mg phenylephrine, and 5 to 10 mg codeine (2.5 to 5 ml) q 4 to 6 hr. *Maximum:* 15 ml q 24 hr.

Children ages 2 to 6. 1.56 to 3.125 promethazine, 1.25 to 2.5 mg phenylephrine, and 2.5 to 5 mg codeine (1.25 to 2.5 ml) q 4 to 6 hr. *Maximum:* 9 ml q 24 hr for children weighing 18 kg (40 lb) or more, 8 ml q 24 hr for children weighing 16 to 18 kg (35 to 40 lb), 7 ml q 24 hr for children weighing 14 to 16 kg (30 to 35 lb), and 6 ml q 24 hr for children weighing 12 to 14 kg (25 to 30 lb).

Contraindications

Angle-closure glaucoma; benign prostatic hyperplasia; bladder neck obstruction; bone marrow depression; breastfeeding; children under age 2; coma; hypersensitivity to bisulfites, promethazine, phenylephrine, codeine, other opioids, or their components; lower respiratory disorders (including asthma); pyloroduodenal obstruction; severe coronary artery disease or hypertension; stenosing peptic ulcer; significant respiratory depression; use of large quantities of CNS depressants; use of an MAO inhibitor within 14 days; ventricular tachycardia

Mechanism of Action

Promethazine competes with histamine for H_1 receptor sites, thereby antagonizing many histamine effects and reducing allergy signs and symptoms.

Phenylephrine stimulates alpha-adrenergic receptors, constricting local vessels and decreasing blood flow and mucosal edema to relieve nasal congestion.

Codeine suppresses cough by acting on opiate receptors in the medulla.

Interactions

DRUGS

promethazine, phenylephrine, and codeine

MAO inhibitors: With promethazine, possibly prolonged and intensified anticholinergic and CNS depressant effects; with phenylephrine and codeine, increased and prolonged cardiac stimulation, increased vasopressor effect, increased risk of severe cardiovascular and cerebrovascular effects (including hypertensive crisis), hyperpyrexia, and vomiting

promethazine and phenylephrine components

guanadrel, guanethidine: Decreased antihypertensive effects of these drugs; increased risk of severe hypertension and arrhythmias; increased vasopressor effect of phenylephrine

promethazine and codeine components

anticholinergics: Possibly intensified anticholinergic adverse effects
CNS depressants: Additive CNS depression

promethazine component

amphetamines: Decreased stimulant effect of amphetamines
anticonvulsants: Lowered seizure threshold
appetite suppressants: Possibly antagonized anorectic effect of appetite suppressants
beta blockers: Increased risk of additive hypotensive effects, irreversible retinopathy, arrhythmias, and tardive dyskinesia
bromocriptine: Decreased effectiveness of bromocriptine
dopamine: Possibly antagonized peripheral vasoconstriction with high doses of dopamine
ephedrine, metaraminol, methoxamine: Decreased vasopressor response to these drugs
epinephrine: Blocked alpha-adrenergic effects of epinephrine; increased risk of hypotension
hepatotoxic drugs: Increased risk of hepatotoxicity
hypotension-producing drugs: Possibly severe hypotension and syncope
levodopa: Inhibited antidyskinetic effects of levodopa

metrizamide: Increased risk of seizures

ototoxic drugs: Possibly masking of some symptoms of ototoxicity, such as dizziness, tinnitus, and vertigo

quinidine: Additive cardiac effects

riboflavin: Increased riboflavin requirements

phenylephrine component

alpha blockers, haloperidol, loxapine, phenothiazines, thioxanthenes: Possibly decreased vasoconstrictor effect of phenylephrine

antihypertenisves, diuretics: Possibly decreased antihypertensive effect

atropine: Possibly enhanced vasopressor effect of phenylephrine

beta blockers: Decreased therapeutic effects of both drugs

bretylium: Possibly potentiated vaopressor effect and arrhythmias

doxapram: Increased vasopressor effect of both drugs

ergot alkaloids: Possibly cerebral blood vessel rupture, increased vasopressor effect, peripheral vascular ischemia, and gangrene (with ergotamine)

hydrocarbon inhalation anesthetics: Increased risk of serious arrhythmias

maprotiline, tricyclic antidepressants: Increased risk of severe cardiovascular effects (including arrhythmias, hyperpyrexia, severe hypertension)

mecamylamine, methyldopa: Decreased hypotensive effects of these drugs; increased vasopressor effect of phenylephrine

nitrates: Possibly decreased vasopressor effect of phenylephrine and decreased antianginal effect of nitrates

oxytocin: Possibly severe, persistent hypertension

phenoxybenzamine: Decreased vasoconstrictor effect of phenylephrine, possibly hypotension and tachycardia

theophylline: Possibly enhanced toxicity (including cardiac toxicity)

thyroid hormones: Increased cardiovascular effects of each drug

codeine component

antihypertensives, diuretics: Potentiated hypotensive effects

buprenorphine: Decreased effectiveness of codeine

hydroxyzine: Increased codeine analgesic effect; increased CNS depressant and hypotensive effects

metoclopramide: Antagonized effect of metoclopramide on GI motility

naloxone: Antagonized codeine analgesic effect

naltrexone: Precipitated withdrawal symptoms in codeine-dependent patients

neuromuscular blockers: Additive respiratory depressant effects

opioids: Additive CNS and respiratory depressants effects and hypotensive effects

paregoric: Increased risk of severe constipation

ACTIVITIES

promethazine and codeine components
alcohol use: Additive CNS depression

Adverse Reactions

CNS: Akathisia, CNS stimulation, coma, confusion, delirium, depression, disorientation, dizziness, drowsiness, dystonia, euphoria, excitation, fatigue, hallucinations, headache, hysteria, insomnia, irritability, lack of coordination, lethargy, light-headedness, mental and physical impairment, mood changes, nervousness, neuroleptic malignant syndrome, paradoxical stimulation, paresthesia, pseudoparkinsonism, restlessness, sedation, seizures, syncope, tardive dyskinesia, tremor, weakness

CV: Angina, bradycardia, heart block, hypertension, orthostatic hypotension, palpitations, peripheral vasoconstriction, tachycardia, ventricular arrhythmias

EENT: Altered taste; blurred vision; diplopia; dry mouth, nose, and throat; laryngeal edema; laryngospasm; miosis; nasal congestion; rhinitis, tinnitus; vision changes

ENDO: Hyperglycemia

GI: Abdominal cramps and pain, anorexia, constipation, flatulence, gastroesophageal reflux, ileus, indigestion, nausea, vomiting

GU: Decreased libido, difficult ejaculation, dysuria, impotence, oliguria, ureteral spasm, urinary incontinence, urine retention

HEME: Agranulocytosis, leukopenia, thrombocytopenia, thrombocytopenic purpura

MS: Muscle rigidity

RESP: Apnea, bronchoconstriction, bronchospasm, depressed cough reflex, dyspnea, respiratory depression, tenacious bronchial secretions

SKIN: Dermatitis, diaphoresis, flushing, jaundice, pallor, photosensitivity, pruritus, rash, urticaria

Other: Anaphylaxis, angioedema, paradoxical reactions, physical and psychological dependence

Nursing Considerations

- Use cautiously in children age 2 and over because of risk for respiratory depression.
- Use cautiously in patients with a head injury or who have cardiovascular disease, liver or kidney impairment, fever, seizures, hypothyroidism, intestinal inflammation, or Addison's disease.
- Be aware that cautious use is also required in patients who have recently had stomach, intestinal, or urinary tract surgery.

- Monitor effectiveness of promethazine, phenylephrine, and codeine in relieving allergy symptoms and cough. Notify prescriber if symptoms persist or worsen.
- **WARNING** Monitor respiratory function because promethazine, phenylephrine, and codeine may suppress cough reflex and cause thickening of bronchial secretions, aggravating such conditions as asthma and COPD. In rare cases, it may depress respirations and induce apnea. Notify prescriber immediately if respiratory rate drops below 10 breaths/minute.
- Monitor patient's hematologic status as ordered because promethazine may cause bone marrow depression. Assess patient for signs and symptoms of infection or bleeding.
- **WARNING** Monitor patient for evidence of neuroleptic malignant syndrome, such as fever, hypertension or hypotension, involuntary motor activity, mental changes, muscle rigidity, tachycardia, and tachypenia. Be prepared to provide supportive treatment and additional drug therapy, as prescribed.
- Take safety precautions, if needed, because promethazine, phenylephrine, and codeine can cause considerable drowsiness and many other adverse CNS effects.
- Be aware that patient shouldn't have intradermal allergen tests within 72 hours of receiving promethazine, phenylephrine, and codeine because drug may significantly alter flare response.

PATIENT TEACHING

- Tell patient to take only the dosage prescribed and not to increase dose or frequency without consulting prescriber.
- Instruct patient to use a calibrated measuring device to ensure accurate dose.
- Advise patient to contact prescriber if symptoms, including cough, are not better after 5 days of therapy.
- Instruct patient to avoid potentially hazardous activities until drug's CNS effects are known.
- Warn patient to avoid alcoholic beverages and OTC antihistamine and CNS depressant drugs while taking promethazine, phenylephrine, and codeine.
- Caution patient to drink plenty of fluids and increase fiber in diet because codeine can cause or worsen constipation.
- Tell patient to rise slowly from a lying or sitting position to minimize dizziness or light-headedness.
- Alert female patients that promethazine, phenylephrine, and codeine may affect pregnancy test results.
- Instruct diabetic patient to monitor his blood glucose level closely while taking promethazine, phenylephrine, and codeine.

- Tell patient to report involuntary muscle movements or unusual sensitivity to sunlight because drug may need to be stopped.
- Advise patient to avoid excessive sun exposure and to use sunscreen when outdoors.

pseudoephedrine hydrochloride and methscopolamine nitrate
AlleRx-D, PSE 120/MSC 2.5

Class and Category
Chemical: Sympathomimetic amine (pseudoephedrine), hyoscine methobromide (methscopolamine)
Therapeutic: Decongestant (pseudoephedrine), anticholinergic (methscopolamine)
Pregnancy category: C

Indications and Dosages
▶ *To relieve nasal congestion caused by the common cold, sinusitis, allergic rhinitis, and other upper respiratory tract conditions*
E. R. TABLETS
Adults. 120 mg pseudoephedrine and 2.5 mg methscopolamine (1 tablet) q 12 hr.

Mechanism of Action
Pseudoephedrine acts on alpha$_1$-adrenergic receptors in the mucosa of the respiratory tract to produce vasoconstriction. This process shrinks swollen nasal mucous membranes; reduces tissue hyperemia, edema, and nasal congestion; and increases nasal airway patency. It also may increase drainage of sinus secretions and open obstructed eustachian ostia.

Methscopolamine competitively inhibits acetylcholine at autonomic postganglionic cholinergic receptors. Because the most sensitive receptors are in the salivary, bronchial, and sweat glands, this action reduces secretions from these glands. It also reduces nasal, oropharyngeal, and bronchial secretions and decreases airway resistance by relaxing smooth muscles in the bronchi and bronchioles.

Contraindications
Breastfeeding; cardiac disease, such as arrhythmias, heart failure, coronary artery disease, and mitral stenosis; hemorrhage with hemodynamic instability; hepatic dysfunction; hypersensitivity or idiosyncratic reactions to pseudoephedrine, methscopolamine, or their components; hyperthyroidism; ileus; intestinal atony; myasthenia

gravis; myocardial ischemia; narrow-angle glaucoma; obstructive GI or uropathic disease; renal impairment; tachycardia; toxic megacolon; ulcerative colitis; severe coronary artery disease or hypertension; urine retention; use of an MAO inhibitor within 14 days

Interactions
DRUGS

pseudoephedrine component

antacids: Increased pseudoephedrine absorption

antihypertensives, diuretics: Possibly decreased antihypertensive effect

beta blockers: Decreased therapeutic effects of both drugs

citrates: Possibly inhibited urinary pseudoephedrine excretion and prolonged duration of action

CNS stimulant, other sympathomimetics: Possibly increased additive CNS stimulation to excessive levels

cocaine (mucosal-local): Possibly increased cardiovascular effects of either drug and CNS stimulation

digoxin, levodopa: Increased risk of cardiac arrhythmias

hydrocarbon inhalation anesthetics: Increased risk of serious arrhythmias

kaolin: Decreased pseudoephedrine absorption

MAO inhibitors: Increased and prolonged cardiac stimulation; increased vasopressor effect; increased risk of severe cardiovascular and cerebrovascular effects, such as hypertensive crisis, hyperpyrexia, and vomiting

nitrates: Reduced antianginal effects of nitrates

rauwolfia alkaloids: Possibly inhibited pseudoephedrine action

thyroid hormones: Increased cardiovascular effects of both drugs

methscopolamine component

adsorbent antidiarrheals, antacids: Decreased absorption and therapeutic effects of methoscopolamine

anticholinergics (other): Possibly intensified anticholinergic effects

antimyasthenics: Possibly reduced intestinal motility

CNS depressants: Possibly potentiated effects of either drug, resulting in additive sedation

haloperidol: Decreased antipsychotic effect of haloperidol

ketoconazole: Decreased ketoconazole absorption

lorazepam (parenteral): Possibly hallucinations, irrational behavior, and sedation

metoclopramide: Possibly antagonized effect of metoclopramide on GI motility

opioid analgesics: Increased risk of severe constipation and ileus

potassium chloride: Possibly increased severity of potassium chloride-induced GI lesions, *urinary alkalizers (antacids, carbonic anhydrase inhibitors, citrates, sodium bicarbonate):* Delayed excretion of methscopolamine, possibly leading to increased therapeutic and adverse effects

ACTIVITIES

methscopolamine component
alcohol use: Additive CNS effects

Adverse Reactions

CNS: Dizziness, drowsiness, euphoria, headache, insomnia, lightheadedness, memory loss, nervousness, paradoxical stimulation, restlessness, trembling, weakness

CV: Palpitations, tachycardia

EENT: Blurred vision; dry eyes, mouth, nose, and throat; mydriasis

GI: Constipation, dysphagia, nausea, vomiting

GU: Dysuria, urinary hesitancy, urine retention

SKIN: Decreased sweating, diaphoresis, dry skin, flushing, pallor

Nursing Considerations

- Monitor renal function, as ordered, because pseudoephedrine is substantially excreted by the kidneys.
- Monitor patients who may be more susceptible to dizziness, drowsiness, and weakness, such as the elderly.
- Monitor renal function, as ordered, because pseudoephedrine is substantially excreted by the kidneys.
- Regularly evaluate effectiveness of pseudoephedrine and methscopolamine in reducing upper respiratory symptoms.

PATIENT TEACHING

- Tell patient to take last dose of the day a few hours before bedtime if drug makes her nervous or restless.
- Instruct patient to swallow tablets whole and not to break, crush, or chew them.
- Urge patient to avoid alcohol, other antidepressants, or OTC preparations without consulting prescriber while taking pseudoephedrine and methscopolamine.
- Instruct patient to avoid potentially hazardous activities until drug's CNS effects are known.
- Suggest frequent rinsing and use of sugarless gum or hard candy for dry mouth; suggest lubricating drops for dry eyes.

theophylline and guaifenesin
Bronchial, Glyceryl-T, Mudrane GG-2, Quibron, Quibron-300, Slo-Phyllin GG

dyphylline and guaifenesin

Dilor-G, Dyflex-G, Dyline GG, Lyfyllin-GG, Panfil G

Class and Category

Chemical: Xanthine derivative (theophylline, dyphylline), glyceryl guaiacolate (guaifenesin)

Therapeutic: Bronchodilator (theophylline, dyphylline), expectorant (guaifenesin)

Pregnancy category: C

Indications and Dosages

▶ *To treat or prevent bronchial spasm; to treat chronic bronchitis and emphysema*

CAPSULES (BRONCHIAL, QUIBRON-300, QUIBRON)

Adults. Highly individualized based on theophylline need. 150 or 300 mg theophylline and 90 or 180 mg guaifenesin per capsule, depending on product used. Number of capsules based on individual dosage calculated to provide 16 mg/kg/day or 400 mg theophylline/day (whichever is less) in divided doses q 6 to 8 hr.

CAPSULES (GLYCERYL-T)

Adults. 150 to 300 mg theophylline and 90 to 180 mg guaifenesin (1 or 2 capsules) b.i.d. or t.i.d.

CAPSULES (SLO-PHYLLIN GG)

Adults. Highly individualized based on theophylline need. 150 mg theophylline and 90 mg guaifenesin per capsule. Number of capsules based on individual dosage calculated to provide 3 mg/kg of theophylline in divided doses q 6 to 8 hr.

TABLETS (MUDRANE GG-2)

Adults. 111 mg theophylline and 100 mg guaifenesin t.i.d. or q.i.d.

TABLETS (DYFLEX-G, DYLINE G.G., LUFYLLIN-GG, PANFIL G)

Adults. 200 to 400 mg dyphylline and 100 to 400 mg guaifenesin (1 to 2 tablets depending on product used) t.i.d. or q.i.d.

ORAL SOLUTION (THEOLATE, GLYCERYL-T)

Adults. 150 mg theophylline and 90 mg guaifenesin (15 ml) q 6 to 8 hr.

ORAL SOLUTION (SLO-PHYLLIN, SYNOPHYLATE-GG)

Adults. Highly individualized based on theophylline need. 150 mg theophylline and 90 or 100 mg guaifenesin per 15 ml. Number of ml based on individual dosage calculated to provide 3 mg/kg of theophylline in divided doses q 8 hr.

ORAL SOLUTION (ELIXOPHYLLIN GG)

Adults. Highly individualized based on theophylline need. 100 mg theophylline and 100 mg guaifenesin per 15 ml. Number of ml prescribed based on individual dosage calculated to provide 3 mg/kg of theophylline in divided doses q 8 hr.

ORAL SOLUTION (DILOR-G, DYLINE-GG)
Adults. 100 mg dyphylline and 100 mg guaifenesin per 5 ml or 200 mg dyphylline and 200 mg guaifenesin per 10 ml t.i.d. or q.i.d.
ORAL SOLUTION (PANFIL G)
Adults. 200 mg dyphylline and 100 mg guaifenesin/10 ml t.i.d. or q.i.d.
ORAL SOLUTION (DYPHYLLINE-GG)
Adults. 200 mg dyphylline and 200 mg guaifenesin (30 ml) q.i.d.

Mechanism of Action
Theophylline and dyphylline inhibit phosphodiesterase enzymes, causing bronchodilation. Normally, these enzymes inactivate cAMP and cGMP, which are responsible for bronchial smooth muscle relaxation. These agents also may cause calcium translocation, antagonize prostaglandins and adenosine receptors, stimulate catecholamines, and inhibit cGMP metabolism.

Guaifenesin increases fluid and mucus removal from the upper respiratory tract by increasing the volume of secretions and reducing their adhesiveness and surface tension.

Contraindications
Hypersensitivity to theophylline, dyphylline, guaifenesin or their components; peptic ulcer disease; uncontrolled seizure disorder

Interactions
DRUGS
theophylline and dyphylline components
adenosine: Decreased adenosine effectiveness
allopurinol, cimetidine, ciprofloxacin, clarithromycin, disulfiram, enoxacin, erythromycin, fluvoxamine, interferon alpha (human recombinant), methotrexate, mexiletine, pentoxifylline, propafenone, propranolol, tacrine, thiabendazole, ticlopidine, troleandomycin, verapamil: Increased blood theophylline or dyphylline level and risk of toxicity
aminoglutethimide, carbamazepine, isoproterenol (I.V.), moricizine, oral contraceptives (containing estrogen), phenobarbital, phenytoin, rifampin: Decreased blood theophylline or dyphylline level and possibly drug effectiveness
benzodiazepines: Possibly reversal of benzodiazepine sedation
beta blockers: Possibly decreased bronchodilator effect of theophylline or dyphylline
ephedrine: Increased adverse effects, including insomnia, nausea, and nervousness
halothane anesthetics: Increased risk of ventricular arrhythmias

ketamine: Lowered seizure threshold
lithium: Decreased lithium effectiveness
neuromuscular blockers: Possibly antagonized neuromuscular blockage
sucralfate: Decreased absorption of theophylline or dyphylline
FOODS
theophylline and dyphylline components
caffeine (large amounts): Possibly increased risk of adverse reactions
high-carbohydrate, low-protein diet: Possibly decreased theophylline or dyphylline elimination
low-carbohydrate, high-protein diet; daily intake of charbroiled beef: Possibly increased theophyllin or dyphylline elimination
ACTIVITIES
theophylline and dyphylline components
alcohol use: Increased blood theophylline or dyphylline level and risk of toxicity
smoking: Increased drug clearance, decreased drug effectiveness

Adverse Reactions
CNS: Agitation, behavioral changes, confusion, disorientation, dizziness, headache, insomnia, nervousness, seizures, tremor
CV: Hypotension, tachycardia, ventricular arrhythmias
ENDO: Hyperglycemia
GI: Abdominal pain, diarrhea, heartburn, nausea, vomiting
GU: Increased urine output
SKIN: Rash, urticaria

Nursing Considerations
- Be aware that ideal body weight is used to calculate theophylline and dyphylline dosages; drug doesn't bind well in body fat.
- Be aware that E.R. capsules and tablets shouldn't be used for oral loading doses.
- Monitor blood theophylline (dyphylline) levels as ordered to gauge therapeutic level and detect toxicity.
- Suspect toxicity if patient develops nausea, vomiting, irritability, and restlessness, and be prepared to obtain blood theophylline (dyphylline) level.
- Assess heart rate and rhythm often because theophylline and dyphylline can worsen existing arrhythmias.
- Be especially alert for signs of toxicity in patient with acute pulmonary edema, hypothyroidism, influenza vaccination, prolonged fever, sepsis with multiple organ failure, shock, or viral pulmonary infection because of decreased drug clearance. Also monitor patients with uncorrected acidemia because they have an increased risk of toxicity.

- Evaluate effectiveness of theophylline or dyphylline and guaifenesin in relieving respiratory symptoms, and notify prescriber if symptoms worsen.

PATIENT TEACHING

- Instruct patient prescribed oral solution or syrup to use a calibrated measuring device to ensure accurate dose.
- Teach patient to swallow theophylline or dyphylline and guaifenesin tablets whole and not to chew or crush them, unless scored for breaking.
- Explain that patient may open capsules and mix contents with soft food but that he shouldn't chew or crush granules.
- Instruct patient to take drug with a full glass of water on an empty stomach (30 to 60 minutes before meals or 2 hours after meals). If he develops GI distress, suggest taking drug with food or antacids.
- Encourage patient to take drug at the same times every day.
- Stress importance of not interchanging brands because concentration of drug varies among manufacturers.
- Urge patient to avoid alcohol while taking drug.
- Instruct patient to avoid potentially hazardous activities until drug's CNS effects are known.
- Tell patient to take last dose of the day a few hours before bedtime if drug makes him nervous.
- Advise patient to notify prescriber if he develops a fever, makes a significant dietary change, or starts or stops smoking or taking other drugs because these factors may alter blood theophylline and dyphylline level.
- Instruct patient to notify prescriber if his underlying respiratory condition worsens.

theophylline and potassium iodide

Elixophyllin-KI, Theophylline KI

Class and Category

Chemical: Xanthine derivative (theophylline), iodine (potassium iodide)

Therapeutic: Bronchodilator (theophylline), expectorant (potassium iodide

Pregnancy category: D

Indications and Dosages

▶ *To relieve bronchospasm caused by asthma, bronchitis, or emphysema; to treat chronic bronchitis and emphysema*

ELIXIR
Adults. Highly individualized based on theophylline need. 80 mg theophylline and 130 mg potassium iodide per 15 ml. Number of ml prescribed based on individual dosage calculated to provide 3 mg/kg of theophylline in divided doses q 8 hr.

Mechanism of Action
Theophylline inhibits phosphodiesterase enzymes, causing bronchodilation. Normally, these enzymes inactivate cAMP and cGMP, which are responsible for bronchial smooth muscle relaxation. These agents also may cause calcium translocation, antagonize prostaglandins and adenosine receptors, stimulate catecholamines, and inhibit cGMP metabolism.

Potassium iodide increases fluid and mucus removal from the upper respiratory tract by increasing the volume of secretions and reducing their adhesiveness and surface tension.

Contraindications
Acute bronchitis; Addison's disease; dehydration; heat cramps; hyperkalemia; hyperthyroidism; hypersensitivity to theophylline, iodide, or their components; peptic ulcer disease; iodism; renal impairment; tuberculosis; uncontrolled seizure disorder

Interactions
DRUGS
theophylline component
adenosine: Decreased adenosine effectiveness
allopurinol, cimetidine, ciprofloxacin, clarithromycin, disulfiram, enoxacin, erythromycin, fluvoxamine, interferon alfa (human recombinant), methotrexate, mexiletine, pentoxifylline, propafenone, propranolol, tacrine, thiabendazole, ticlopidine, troleandomycin, verapamil: Increased blood theophylline level and risk of toxicity
aminoglutethimide, carbamazepine, hormonal contraceptives (containing estrogen), isoproterenol (I.V.), moricizine, phenobarbital, phenytoin, rifampin: Decreased blood theophylline level and possibly drug effectiveness
benzodiazepines: Possibly reversal of benzodiazepine sedation
beta blockers: Possibly decreased bronchodilator effect of theophylline
ephedrine: Increased adverse effects, including insomnia, nausea, and nervousness
halothane anesthetics: Increased risk of ventricular arrhythmias
ketamine: Lowered seizure threshold

lithium: Decreased lithium effectiveness
neuromuscular blockers: Possibly antagonized neuromuscular blockage
sucralfate: Decreased absorption of theophylline
potassium iodide component
antithyroid drugs, lithium: Increased risk of hypothyroidism and goiter
captopril, enalapril, lisinopril, potassium-sparing diuretics: Increased risk of hyperkalemia
FOODS
theophylline component
caffeine (high amounts): Increased risk of adverse reactions
high-carbohydrate, low-protein diet: Possibly decreased theophylline elimination
low-carbohydrate, high-protein diet; daily intake of charbroiled beef: Possibly increased theophyllin elimination
ACTIVITIES
theophylline component
alcohol use: Increased blood theophylline level and risk of toxicity
smoking: Increased drug clearance, decreased drug effectiveness

Adverse Reactions
CNS: Agitation, behavioral changes, confusion, disorientation, dizziness, fatigue, headache, heaviness or weakness in legs, insomnia, nervousness, paresthesia, seizures, tremor
CV: Hypotension, irregular heartbeat, tachycardia, ventricular arrhythmias
ENDO: Hyperglycemia
EENT: Burning in mouth or throat, increased salivation, metallic taste, sore teeth or gums
GI: Abdominal pain, diarrhea, epigastric pain, heartburn, indigestion, nausea, vomiting
GU: Increased urine output
HEME: Eosinophilia
MS: Arthralgia
SKIN: Acneiform lesions, urticaria
Other: Angioedema, lymphadenopathy

Nursing Considerations
- Use with caution in pregnant or breastfeeding mothers because potassium iodide can cause hypothyroidism and goiter in the fetus and newborn or rash and thyroid suppression in the nursing infant because it is excreted in breast milk.
- Be aware that ideal body weight is used to calculate theophylline dosages because drug doesn't bind well in body fat.

- Monitor blood theophylline levels, as ordered, to gauge therapeutic level and detect toxicity.
- Suspect theophylline toxicity if patient develops nausea, vomiting, irritability, or restlessness; be prepared to obtain blood theophylline level.
- Monitor serum potassium level regularly in patients with renal impairment because of the risk of hyperkalemia.
- Assess heart rate and rhythm often because theophylline and potassium iodide may worsen existing arrhythmias.
- Be especially alert for signs of toxicity in patient with acute pulmonary edema, hypothyroidism, influenza vaccination, prolonged fever, sepsis with multiple organ failure, shock, or viral pulmonary infection because of decreased drug clearance. Also monitor patients with uncorrected acidemia because they have an increased risk of toxicity.
- Evaluate effectiveness of theophylline and potassium iodide in relieving respiratory symptoms; notify prescriber if symptoms worsen.

PATIENT TEACHING

- Instruct patient to use a calibrated measuring device to ensure accurate dose.
- Instruct patient to take drug with a full glass of water on an empty stomach (30 to 60 minutes before meals or 2 hours after meals). If she develops GI distress, suggest taking drug with food or antacids.
- Encourage patient to take drug at the same times every day.
- Urge patient to avoid alcohol while taking drug.
- Instruct patient to avoid potentially hazardous activities until drug's CNS effects are known.
- Tell patient to take last dose of the day a few hours before bedtime if drug makes her nervous.
- Advise patient to notify prescriber if she develops a fever, makes a significant dietary change, or starts or stops smoking or taking other drugs because these factors may alter blood theophylline level.
- Instruct patient to notify prescriber if her underlying respiratory condition worsens.

ANTINEOPLASTIC COMBINATION THERAPY FOR SELECTED COMMON CANCERS

This table lists common cancers for which combination chemotherapy is standard therapy. Specific regimens, dosages, and protocols depend on the stage of the cancer, presence of metastasis, and the patient's physical condition at the time of therapy.

Cancer Type	Combination Therapy Used
Breast (Female)	**Node-Negative Patients** • CMF: cyclophosphamide, methotrexate, and fluorouracil • FAC/CAF: fluorouracil, doxorubicin, and cyclophosphamide • AC: doxorubicin and cyclophosphamide **Node-Positive Patients** • FAC (CAF): fluorouracil, doxorubicin, and cyclophosphamide • CEF: cyclophosphamide, epirubicin, and fluorouracil • AC: doxorubicin and cyclophosphamide • EC: epirubicin and cyclophosphamide • TAC: docetaxel, doxorubicin, cyclophosphamide, with or without filgrastim support • CMF: cyclophosphamide, methotrexate, and fluorouracil • A-CMF: doxorubicin followed by cyclophosphamide, methotrexate, and fluorouracil • AC-T: doxorubicin and cyclophosphamide followed by paclitaxel or docetaxel • A-T-C: doxorubicn followed by paclitaxel followed by cyclophosphamide
Lung	**General Combinations** • paclitaxel and carboplatin • cisplatin and vinorelbine • cisplatin and etoposide • carboplatin and etoposide **Non–Small-Cell Lung Cancer** • gemcitabine, cisplatin, and vinorelbine • etoposide, cisplatin **Small-Cell Lung Cancer (limited stage)** • etoposide, cisplatin • etoposide, cisplatin, and vincristine

(continued)

ANTINEOPLASTIC COMBINATION THERAPY FOR SELECTED COMMON CANCERS *(continued)*

Cancer Type	Combination Therapy Used
Lung *(continued)*	**Small-Cell Lung Cancer (extensive stage)** • cyclophosphamide, doxorubicin, and vincristine • cyclophosphamide, doxorubicin, and etoposide • etoposide and cisplatin or carboplatin • ifosfamide, carboplatin, and etoposide • cyclophosphamide, methotrexate, and lomustine • cyclophosphamide, methotrexate, lomustine, and vincristine • cyclophosphamide, etoposide, and vincristine • cyclophosphamide, doxorubicn, etoposide, and vincristine • cyclophosphamide, doxorubicin, etoposide, and vincristine
Colon	• irinotecan, fluorouracil, leucovorin • folic acid, fluorouracil, irinotecan • oxaliplatin, leucovorin, fluorouracil • fluorouracil, levamisole • fluorouracil, leucovorin
Melanoma	• dacarbazine, carmustine, cisplatin, and tamoxifen • dacarbazine, carmustine and cisplatin • cisplatin, vinblastine, and dacarbazine
Bladder *(invasive)*	• MVAC: methotrexate, vinblastine, doxorubicin [adriamycin], and cisplatin • CMV: cisplatin, methotrexate, and vincristine • CISCA: cisplatin, cyclophosphamide, and doxorubicin • GC: gemcitabine and cisplatin

ANTINEOPLASTIC COMBINATION THERAPY FOR SELECTED COMMON CANCERS *(continued)*

Cancer Type	Combination Therapy Used
Non-Hodgkin's Lymphoma	• CHOP: cyclophosphamide, doxorubin or hydroxydoxorubicin, vincristine, and prednisone • CHOP-R: cyclophosphamide, doxorubin or hydroxydoxorubicin, vincristine, and prednisone plus rituxan • CVP: cyclophosphamide, vincristine, and prednisolone • BACOD: bleomycin, doxorubicin, cyclophosphamide, vincristine, and dexamethasone • MACOP-B: methotrexate, doxorubicin, cyclophosphamide, vincristine, prednisone, and bleomycin • Pro-MACE-CytaBOM: prednisone, methotrexate (with leucovorin rescuer), doxorubicin, cyclophosphamide, etoposide, cytarabine, bleomycin, vincristine • EPOCH: etoposide, prednisone, vincristine, cyclophosphamide, fluoxymesterone
Pancreatic	• gemcitabine and erlotinib

COMBINATION ORAL CONTRACEPTIVES

Combination oral contraceptives (COCs) prevent pregnancy mainly by preventing ovulation. They also thicken the cervical mucus, which helps prevent sperm from passing through the cervix. COCs contain estrogen and progesterone in varying amounts and delivery sequence, depending on the manufacturer.

Minor adverse reactions to COCs include spotting or bleeding between menstrual periods, headache, nausea, vomiting, breast tenderness, dizziness, weight or mood changes, and facial acne or melasma. Most of these reactions resolve after the first few months of use. Serious adverse reactions to estrogen-containing contraceptive pills include blood clots, MI, and stroke. Women who smoke have a higher risk of these complications. Therefore, women who smoke should not consider using COCs.

There are several contraindications to COCs, including being age 35 or over, a smoker, or pregnant; being diabetic for 20 years or more; having complications of diabetes; or having a history of active thromboembolic or CV disease, known or suspected breast cancer, active liver disease or tumors, or migraine headaches with visual abnormalities, such as blurring or loss of vision.

Familiarize yourself with the many COCs by reviewing the table that appears on the following pages. Also, give patients the following detailed instructions on how to take prescribed COCs correctly and safely.

GENERAL INSTRUCTIONS

- Take the first pill on any of the first 7 days of your menstrual period (day 1 is the first day of bleeding). Many women find it easiest to take the first pill on the first day of bleeding.
- During the first cycle of pills, use a backup contraceptive method, such as a condom, until you have taken the pills for 2 consecutive days.
- Swallow 1 pill each day at the same time of day, whether or not you have sexual intercourse.
- If you're using a 28-day or 84-day extended cycle packet, don't skip a single day between packets, even if you are still menstruating. Always start a new packet the day after finishing the last packet. If you're using a 21-day packet, wait 7 days after finishing a packet before starting a new packet of pills.
- If this is your first time taking COCs and you have no problems, return to your healthcare provider when you need a new supply of pills. Bring the empty pill packets with you when you return.
- If you've just delivered a baby and you aren't breastfeeding, you may start taking the pill after the third postpartum week, or

COMBINATION ORAL CONTRACEPTIVES *(continued)*

any time you and your healthcare provider confirm that you aren't pregnant.

• If you've just had an abortion, you may start taking the pill on the same day as the abortion or any time you and your healthcare provider confirm that you aren't pregnant.

• If you're ill and have severe vomiting or diarrhea, your pills may not work effectively. Use another contraceptive method or avoid sexual intercourse until you're better and have taken the pills for 7 consecutive days without severe vomiting or diarrhea.

• Some medications interfere with the pill's effectiveness. Check with your healthcare provider if you start taking medication for seizures or convulsions, or you begin taking rifampin (rifampicin)—a drug used to treat tuberculosis. Bring the pill packets with you when you visit your healthcare provider, and explain that you're taking a COC.

If you miss taking a pill

• If you miss day 1, take a pill as soon as you remember. Take the next pill at the regular time, even if this means taking 2 pills on the same day.

• If you miss taking a pill 2 or more days in a row, take a pill as soon as you remember, and continue taking a pill each day. Wait to have sexual intercourse, or use an additional contraceptive method (such as condoms), until you have taken 1 COC pill daily for 7 consecutive days. This will give the pills time to protect you fully against pregnancy.

• If you have trouble remembering to take a pill every day, talk with your healthcare provider about using another method of family planning.

OTHER INSTRUCTIONS

• Usually, your period will start while you're taking the fourth week of pills. If you don't have a period, keep taking the pils as prescribed.

• If you think you could be pregnant, contact your healthcare provider.

• Go to the hospital immediately if you have any of the following signs and symptoms: severe pain in your belly; severe pain in your chest; severe headache, dizziness, weakness, or numbness; blurred or reduced vision; speech problems; yellowing of the skin or eyes (jaundice); severe pain in your leg (calf or thigh).

(continued)

COMBINATION ORAL CONTRACEPTIVES *(continued)*

Trade Names	Estrogen Content	Synthetic Progesterone Content
Monophasic Contraceptives		
Alesse, Levline, Lutera	*21 tablets:* 20 mcg ethinyl estradiol *7 tablets:* placebo	*21 tablets:* 100 mcg levonoregestrel *7 tablets:* placebo
Loestrin 1/20 Fe, Loestrin 24 Fe, Microgestin 1/20	*21 tablets:* 20 mcg ethinyl estradiol *7 tablets:* placebo	*21 tablets:* 1,000 mcg norethindrone *7 tablets:* placebo
Levlen, Levora, Nordette	*21 tablets:* 30 mcg ethinyl estradiol *7 tablets:* placebo	*21 tablets:* 150 mcg levonoregestrel *7 tablets:* placebo
Seasonale (extended cycle of 84 days)	*84 tablets:* 30 mcg ethinyl estradiol	*84 tablets:* 150 mcg levonorgestrel
Seasonique (extended cycle of 84 days)	*84 tablets:* 30 mcg ethinyl estradiol *7 tablets:* 10 mcg ethinyl estradiol	*84 tablets:* 150 mcg levonorgestrel *7 tablets:* no levonorgestrel
Lo-Ovral	*21 tablets:* 30 mcg ethinyl estradiol *7 tablets:* placebo	*21 tablets:* 300 mcg norgestrel *7 tablets:* placebo
Desogen, Ortho-Cept	*21 tablets:* 30 mcg ethinyl estradiol *7 tablets:* placebo	*21 tablets:* 150 mcg desogestrel *7 tablets:* placebo
Loestrin 1.5/30, Microgestin 1.5/30	*21 tablets:* 30 mcg ethinyl estradiol *7 tablets:* placebo	*21 tablets:* 1,500 mcg norethindrone *7 tablets:* placebo
Yasmin	*21 tablets:* 30 mcg ethinyl estradiol *7 tablets:* placebo	*21 tablets:* 3,000 mcg drospirenone *7 tablets:* placebo

COMBINATION ORAL CONTRACEPTIVES *(continued)*

Trade Names	Estrogen Content	Synthetic Progesterone Content
Monophasic Contraceptives *(continued)*		
Ortho-Cyclen	*21 tablets:* 35 mcg ethinyl estradiol *7 tablets:* placebo	*21 tablets:* 250 mcg norgestimate *7 tablets:* placebo
Ovcon-35	*21 tablets:* 35 mcg ethinyl estradiol *7 tablets:* placebo	*21 tablets:* 400 mcg norethindrone *7 tablets:* placebo
Modicon, Brevicon	*21 tablets:* 35 mcg ethinyl estradiol *7 tablets:* placebo	*21 tablets:* 500 mcg norethindrone *7 tablets:* placebo
Ortho-Novum 1/35, Necon, Norethin, Norinyl 1/35	*21 tablets:* 35 mcg ethinyl estradiol *7 tablets:* placebo	*21 tablets:* 1,000 mcg norethindrone *7 tablets:* placebo
Demulen 1/35, Zovia 1/35	*21 tablets:* 35 mcg ethinyl estradiol *7 tablets:* placebo	*21 tablets:* 1,000 mcg ethynodiol diacetate *7 tablets:* placebo
Ovcon 50	*21 tablets:* 50 mcg ethinyl estradiol *7 tablets:* placebo	*21 tablets:* 1,000 mcg norethindrone *7 tablets:* placebo
Ogestrel, Ovral	*21 tablets:* 50 mcg ethinyl estradiol *7 tablets:* placebo	*21 tablets:* 500 mcg norgestrel *7 tablets:* placebo
Demulen 1/50, Zovia 1/50	*21 tablets:* 50 mcg ethinyl estradiol *7 tablets:* placebo	*21 tablets:* 1,000 mcg ethynodiol diacetate *7 tablets:* placebo
Necon 1/50, Norinyl 1/50, Ortho-Novum 1/50	*21 tablets:* 50 mcg mestraol *7 tablets:* placebo	*21 tablets:* 1,000 mcg norethindrone *7 tablets:* placebo

(continued)

COMBINATION ORAL CONTRACEPTIVES (continued)

Trade Names	Estrogen Content	Synthetic Progesterone Content
Multiphasic Contraceptives		
Kariva, Mircette	*21 tablets:* 20 mcg ethinyl estradiol *5 tablets:* 10 mcg ethinyl estradiol *2 tablets:* placebo	*21 tablets:* 150 mcg desogestrel *5 tablets:* 0 mcg desogestrel *2 tablets:* placebo
Cyclessa, Velivet (placebo tablets contain ferric oxide)	*7 tablets:* 25 mcg ethinyl estradiol *7 tablets:* 25 mcg ethinyl estradiol *7 tablets:* 25 mcg ethinyl estradiol *7 tablets:* placebo	*7 tablets:* 100 mcg desogestrel *7 tablets:* 125 mcg desogestrel *7 tablets:* 150 mcg desogestrel *7 tablets:* placebo
TriLevelen, Triphasil, Trivora	*6 tablets:* 30 mcg ethinyl estradiol *5 tablets:* 40 mcg ethinyl estradiol *10 tablets:* 30 mcg ethinyl estradiol *7 tablets:* placebo	*6 tablets:* 50 mcg levonorgestrel *5 tablets:* 75 mcg levonorgestrel *10 tablets:* 125 mcg levonorgestrel *7 tablets:* placebo
Ortho-Novum 10/11	*10 tablets:* 35 mcg ethinyl estradiol *11 tablets:* 35 mcg ethinyl estradiol *7 tablets:* placebo	*10 tablets:* 500 mcg norethindrone *11 tablets:* 1,000 mcg norethindrone *7 tablets:* placebo
Ortho-Novum 7/7/7	*7 tablets:* 35 mcg ethinyl estradiol *7 tablets:* 35 mcg ethinyl estradiol *7 tablets:* 35 mcg ethinyl estradiol *7 tablets:* placebo	*7 tablets:* 500 mcg norethindrone *7 tablets:* 750 mcg norethindrone *7 tablets:* 1,000 mcg norethindrone *7 tablets:* placebo

COMBINATION ORAL CONTRACEPTIVES *(continued)*

Trade Names	Estrogen Content	Synthetic Progesterone Content
Multiphasic Contraceptives *(continued)*		
Ortho Tri Cyclen	*7 tablets:* 35 mcg ethinyl estradiol *7 tablets:* 35 mcg ethinyl estradiol *7 tablets:* 35 mcg ethinyl estadiol *7 tablets:* placebo	*7 tablets:* 180 mcg norgestimate *7 tablets:* 215 mcg norgestimate *7 tablets:* 250 mcg norgestimate *7 tablets:* placebo
Ortho Tri Cyclen Lo	*7 tablets:* 25 mcg ethinyl estradiol *7 tablets:* 25 mcg ethinyl estradiol *7 tablets:* 25 mcg ethinyl estradiol *7 tablets:* placebo	*7 tablets:* 180 mcg norgestimate *7 tablets:* 215 mcg norgestimate *7 tablets:* 250 mcg norgestimate *7 tablets:* placebo

COMPATIBLE DRUGS IN A SYRINGE

The chart below lets you know at a glance whether listed drugs are compatible for at least 15 minutes when mixed together in a syringe for immediate administration. However, keep in mind that drugs listed as compatible when mixed in a syringe may not be compatible when prepared for other routes of administration. Drug combinations pre-

	atropine	chlorpromazine	dexamethasone	diazepam	diphenhydramine	droperidol	furosemide	glycopyrrolate	haloperidol	heparin	hydromorphone
atropine		C	n/a	n/a	C	C	n/a	C	I	n/a	C
chlorpromazine	C		n/a	n/a	C	C	n/a	C	n/a	I	C
dexamethasone	n/a	n/a		n/a	I	n/a	n/a	n/a	n/a	n/a	C
diazepam	n/a	n/a	n/a		n/a	n/a	n/a	I	n/a	I	n/a
diphenhydramine	C	C	I	n/a		C	n/a	C	I	n/a	C
droperidol	C	C	n/a	n/a	C		I	C	n/a	I	n/a
furosemide	n/a	n/a	n/a	n/a	n/a	I		n/a	n/a	C	n/a
glycopyrrolate	C	C	I	C	C	C	n/a		C	n/a	C
haloperidol	n/a	n/a	n/a	n/a	C	n/a	n/a	n/a		I	C
heparin	C	I	n/a	I	n/a	I	C	n/a	I		n/a
hydromorphone	C	C	n/a	n/a	C	n/a	n/a	C	C	n/a	
hydroxyzine	C	C	n/a	n/a	C	C	n/a	C	I	n/a	C
ketorolac	n/a	n/a	n/a	I	n/a	n/a	n/a	n/a	I	n/a	I
lidocaine	n/a	n/a	n/a	n/a	n/a	n/a	n/a	C	n/a	C	n/a
lorazepam	n/a	n/a	n/a	n/a	n/a	n/a	n/a	n/a	n/a	n/a	C
meperidine	C	C	n/a	C	C	C	n/a	C	n/a	I	n/a
metoclopramide	C	C	n/a	n/a	C	C	I	n/a	n/a	C	C
midazolam	C	C	n/a	n/a	C	n/a	n/a	C	C	n/a	C
morphine	C	C	n/a	n/a	C	C	n/a	C	I	C*	n/a
pentobarbital	C	I	n/a	n/a	I	I	n/a	I	n/a	n/a	C
prochlorperazine	C	n/a	n/a	n/a	C	C	n/a	C	n/a	n/a	I
ranitidine	C	I	C	n/a	C	n/a	n/a	C	n/a	n/a	C
scopolamine	C	C	n/a	n/a	C	C	n/a	C	n/a	n/a	C

* Compatible only with morphine doses of 1 mg, 2 mg, and 5 mg.

pared for immediate administration usually require a more concentrated solution than those prepared for infusion.

Key: C = compatible; I = Incompatible; n/a = Compatibility information not available; n = No recommendations can be given

hydroxyzine	ketorolac	lidocaine	lorazepam	meperidine	metoclopramide	midazolam	morphine	pentobarbital	prochlorperazine	ranitidine	scopolamine
C	n/a	n/a	n/a	C	C	C	C	C	C	C	C
C	n/a	n/a	n/a	C	C	C	I	I	C	C	C
n/a	n/a	n/a	n/a	n/a	C	n/a	n/a	n/a	n/a	C	n/a
n/a	I	n/a	n/a	n/a	n/a	n/a	n/a	n/a	n/a	I	n/a
C	n/a	n/a	n/a	C	C	C	C	I	C	C	C
C	n/a	n/a	n/a	C	C	C	C	I	C	n/a	C
n/a	n/a	n/a	n/a	n/a	I	n/a	n/a	n/a	n/a	n	n/a
C	n/a	C	n/a	C	n/a	C	C	I	C	C	C
I	I	n/a	n/a	n/a	n/a	n/a	I	n/a	n/a	n/a	n/a
n/a	n/a	C	n/a	I	C	n/a	C	n/a	n/a	n	n/a
C	I	n/a	C	n/a	n/a	C	n/a	C	I	C	C
	I	C	n/a	C	C	C	C	I	C	C	C
I		n/a	n/a	n/a	n/a	n/a	n/a	I	n/a	n/a	n/a
C	n/a		n/a	n/a	C	n/a	n/a	n/a	n/a	n/a	n/a
n/a	n/a	n/a		n/a	n/a	n/a	n/a	n/a	n/a	I	n/a
C	n/a	n/a	n/a		C	C	I	I	C	C	C
n/a	n/a	C	n/a	C		C	C	n/a	C	C	C
C	n/a	n/a	n/a	C	C		C	I	I	I	C
C	n/a	n/a	n/a	n/a	C	C		I	C	C	C
I	n/a	n/a	n/a	I	I	I	I		I	I	C
C	I	n/a	n/a	C	C	I	C	I		C	C
I	n/a	n/a	I	C	C	I	C	I	C		C
C	n/a	n/a	n/a	C	C	C	C	C	C	C	

DRUG FORMULAS AND CALCULATIONS

When administering drugs, you must be familiar with drug formulas and calculation methods to ensure that your patient receives the prescribed drug in the correct dosage, strength, or flow rate. This appendix will provide you with a quick review of how to calculate solution strengths, drug dosages, and I.V. flow rates.

CALCULATING THE STRENGTH OF A SOLUTION

Most solutions come prepared in the required strength by the pharmacy or medical supply source. But sometimes only the concentrated form is available, and you'll need to dilute the solution or solid to administer the prescribed strength.

When a solid form of a drug is used to prepare a solution, the drug must be completely dissolved. Solid forms, such as tablets, crystals, and powders, are considered 100% strength. (An exception is boric acid, which is only 5% at full strength.) The final diluted solution is stated in terms of liquid measurement. To prepare a solution, you'll need to add the prescribed solid or liquid form of the drug (the solute) to the prescribed amount of diluent (the solvent). Two of the most common diluents used in the clinical setting are normal saline solution and sterile water.

You can use either of two formulas to calculate the strength of a solution, as shown in the examples below.

Method 1: Calculating percentage and volume
Use the following formula:

$$\frac{\text{Weaker solution}}{\text{Stronger solution}} = \frac{\text{Solute}}{\text{Solvent}}$$

Example: You need to dilute a stock solution of 100% strength to a 5% solution. How much solute will you need to add to obtain 500 ml of the 5% solution?

Calculate as follows:

$$\frac{5 \ (\%) \ (\text{Weaker solution})}{100 \ (\%) \ (\text{Stronger solution})} = \frac{X \ (g) \ (\text{Solute})}{500 \ ml \ (\text{Solvent})}$$

$$100 \ X = (500)(5) \text{ or } 2,500$$

$$X = 25 \ g$$

Answer: You'll need to add 25 g of solute to each 500 ml of solvent to prepare a 5% solution.

CALCULATING THE STRENGTH OF A SOLUTION *(continued)*

Method 2: Calculating percentage and volume

Use the following formula:

$$\frac{\text{(Desired strength)}}{\text{(Available strength)}} \times \begin{array}{c}\text{Total amount}\\\text{of desired}\\\text{solution}\end{array} = X \begin{array}{c}\text{(Amount of undiluted}\\\text{drug needed to}\\\text{make solution)}\end{array}$$

Example: You need to make 100 ml of a 20% solution, using an 80% solution. How much of the 80% solution must you add to the sterile water to yield a final volume of 100 ml of a 20% solution?

Calculate as follows:

$$\frac{20\ (\%)\ \text{(Desired strength)}}{80\ (\%)\ \text{(Available strength)}} \times 100\ \text{ml} \begin{array}{c}\text{(Total amount of}\\\text{desired solution)}\end{array} = X$$

$$\frac{0.20}{0.80} = 0.25$$

$$0.25 \times 100\ \text{(ml)} = X$$

$$X = 25\ \text{ml of 80\% solution}$$

Answer: You'll need to add 25 ml of the 80% solution to the water to yield a final volume of 100 ml of a 20% solution.

CALCULATING DRUG DOSAGES
You may be required to calculate drug dosages when you need to administer a drug that's available only in one measure, but prescribed in another. You should also be prepared to convert various units of measure, such as milligrams (mg) to grains (gr), and dry measurements to liquid. You can use three common methods of ratio and proportion to calculate drug dosages, as shown in the examples on the next five pages.

(continued)

DRUG FORMULAS AND CALCULATIONS
(continued)

CALCULATING ORAL DRUG DOSAGES
Example: You need to give a patient 0.25 mg of digoxin, which comes only in 0.125-mg tablets. How many tablets will you need to give him to attain the proper dosage?

Method 1: Using labeled amount of drug
In this method, true proportions between the drug label and the prescribed dose are used to determine ratio and proportion. The drug label, which states the amount of drug in one unit of measurement—in this case, 0.125-mg in each tablet of digoxin—is the first ratio, expressed as follows:

milligrams : tablets = milligrams : tablets

0.125 mg (amount of drug) : 1 tablet (unit of measure)

The prescribed dose—in this case, 0.25-mg—is the second ratio; it must be stated in the same order and units of measure as the first, as follows:

0.125 mg : 1 tablet = 0.25 mg : X (tablets)

Calculate as follows:

$$0.125 \, X = 0.25$$

$$X = \frac{0.25}{0.125}$$

$$X = 2$$

Answer: You'll need to give the patient 2 tablets of digoxin 0.125 mg.

Be sure to use critical thinking to assess whether your answer is correct. Because the amount of drug prescribed is greater than the amount of drug in one tablet, it's reasonable to expect the required number of tablets to be greater than one.

CALCULATING ORAL DRUG DOSAGES *(continued)*

Method 2: Using an established formula

To determine the correct number of digoxin tablets to give using this method, use the following formula:

$$\frac{\text{Prescribed dose}}{\text{Dose available}} \times \text{Quantity (unit of measure)} = X \text{ (unknown quantity to be given)}$$

Calculate as follows:

$$\frac{0.25 \text{ mg}}{0.125 \text{ mg}} \times 1 \text{ tablet} = X \text{ (number of 0.125-mg tablets)}$$

$$\frac{0.25}{0.125} = 2X$$

$$2 = X$$

Answer: You'll need to give the patient 2 tablets of digoxin 0.125 mg.

Method 3: Calculating according to proportion size

This method uses the same components as method #1, but the ratio is based on proportions according to size. To determine the correct number of digoxin tablets to give using this method, use the following formula:

$$\frac{\text{smaller}}{\text{larger}} = \frac{\text{smaller}}{\text{larger}}$$

Substitute 0.125 into the smaller part and 0.25 into the greater part of the first ratio. Critical thinking leads us to believe that you'll need more than 1 tablet of the weaker 0.125-mg strength to equal the stronger 0.25 mg. Set up the proportion as follows:

$$\frac{0.125 \text{ mg}}{0.25 \text{ mg}} = \frac{1 \text{ (tablet)}}{X \text{ (tablets)}}$$

Calculate as follows:

$$0.125 X = 0.25$$

$$X = \frac{0.25}{0.125}$$

$$X = 2 \text{ tablets}$$

Answer: You'll need to give the patient 2 tablets of digoxin 0.125 mg.

(continued)

DRUG FORMULAS AND CALCULATIONS
(continued)

CALCULATING PARENTERAL DRUG DOSAGES
The same methods used for calculating oral drugs and solutions can be used for preparing parenteral injections.

Example: You need to administer a prescribed dose of 1 mg morphine sulfate from a unit-dose cartridge containing 4 mg per 2 ml. How many milliliters will you need to give to equal the prescribed dose of 1 mg?

Method 1: Using labeled amount of drug
Using the same ratio as for oral drugs, the drug label—in this case, 4 mg—is the first ratio, and the prescribed dose—in this case, 1 mg—is the second ratio, expressed as follows:

4 mg (the amount of drug) : 2 ml (the unit of measure)

Calculate as follows:

$$4 \text{ mg} : 2 \text{ ml} = 1 \text{ mg} : X \text{ ml}$$
$$4X = 2$$
$$X = \frac{2}{4}$$
$$X = 0.5 \text{ ml}$$

Answer: You'll need to give 0.5 ml of morphine sulfate to equal the prescribed dose of 1 mg.

Method 2: Using an established formula
Use this formula:

$$\frac{\text{Prescribed dose}}{\text{Dose available}} \times \text{Quantity (unit of measure)} = X \text{ (unknown quantity to be given)}$$

Calculate as follows:

$$\frac{1 \text{ mg}}{4 \text{ mg}} \times 2 \text{ ml} = X \text{ (number of ml)}$$

$$\frac{4}{2} = 0.5$$

Answer: You'll need to give 0.5 ml of morphine sulfate to equal the prescribed dose of 1 mg.

CALCULATING PARENTERAL DRUG DOSAGES *(continued)*

Method 3: Calculating according to proportion size
To determine the correct amount of morphine sulfate to give using this method, use the following formula:

smaller : greater = smaller : greater
milligrams : milligrams = milliliters : milliliters

Critical thinking leads us to believe that 1 mg is less than 4 mg and that you'll need less than 2 ml to give 1 mg of the drug; therefore, 1 mg goes into the smaller part of the first ratio, and X goes into the smaller part of the second ratio. Set up the proportion as follows:

$$1 \text{ mg} : 4 \text{ mg} = X \text{ (ml)} : 2 \text{ ml}$$
$$4X = 2$$
$$X = \frac{2}{4}$$
$$X = 0.5$$

Answer: You'll need to give 0.5 ml of morphine sulfate to equal the prescribed dose of 1 mg.

CALCULATING I.V. FLOW RATES
When an I.V. solution is delivered by gravity, you must calculate the number of drops needed per minute for proper infusion. To calculate I.V. flow rates, you need to know three things:
• the drip factor—or the number of drops contained in 1 ml for the type of I.V. set you'll be using. This information is provided on the individual package label.
• the amount and type of fluid that you'll infuse as prescribed on the physician's order sheet
• the infusion duration time in minutes.
    Once you've gathered this information, you can calculate the I.V. flow rate using the following equation:

$$\frac{\text{Total number of ml}}{\text{Total number of minutes}} \times \text{drip factor (gtt/ml)} = \text{flow rate (gtt/min)}$$

(continued)

DRUG FORMULAS AND CALCULATIONS
(continued)

CALCULATING I.V. FLOW RATES *(continued)*
Example 1: If the physician prescribes 1,000 ml of D_5W to infuse over 10 hours, and the drip rate for your administration set delivers 15 drops (gtt) per ml, calculate as follows:

$$\frac{1,000 \text{ ml}}{10 \text{ hours x 60 minutes}} \times 15 \text{ gtt/ml} = X \text{ gtt/minute}$$

$$\frac{1,000 \text{ ml}}{600 \text{ minutes}} \times 15 \text{ gtt/ml} = X \text{ gtt/minute}$$

$$1.67 \text{ ml/minute} \times 15 \text{ gtt/ml} = X \text{ gtt/minute}$$

$$25.05 \text{ gtt/minute} = X$$

Answer: To infuse, round off 25.05 to 25 gtt/minute or according to your institution's policy.

Example 2: If the physician prescribes 500 ml of 0.45% NS to infuse over 2 hours, and the drip rate for your administration set delivers 10 gtt/ml, calculate as follows:

$$\frac{500 \text{ ml}}{2 \text{ hours} \times 60 \text{ minutes}} \times 10 \text{ gtt/ml} = X \text{ gtt/minute}$$

$$\frac{500 \text{ ml}}{120 \text{ minutes}} \times 10 \text{ gtt/ml} = X \text{ gtt/minute}$$

$$4.17 \text{ ml/minute} \times 10 \text{ gtt/ml} = X \text{ gtt/minute}$$

$$41.7 \text{ gtt/minute} = X$$

Answer: To infuse, round off 41.7 to 42 gtt/minute or according to your institution's policy.

Note: When preparing for I.V. administration using a controlled infusion device, the electronic flow-regulator will either count drops using an electronic eye or use a controlled pumping action to deliver the fluid in milliliters. Your final calculation will be based on the unit of measure used by the device: drops per minute or ml per hour.

WEIGHTS AND EQUIVALENTS

Table 1: Liquid Equivalents Among Household Apothecaries', and Metric Systems

Household	Apothecaries'	Metric
1 teaspoon (tsp)	1 fluid dram	5 milliliters (ml)
1 tablespoon (tbs)	0.5 fluid ounce	15 ml
2 tbs (1 ounce [1 oz])	1 fluid ounce	30 ml
1 cupful	8 fluid ounces	240 ml
1 pint (pt)	16 fluid ounces	473 ml
1 quart (qt)	32 fluid ounces	946 ml (1 liter)

Table 2: Solid Equivalents Among Apothecaries' and Metric Systems

Apothecaries'	Metric
15 grains (gr)	1 gram (g) (1,000 milligrams [mg])
10 gr	0.5 g (500 mg)
7.5 gr	0.5 g (500 mg)
5 gr	0.3 g (300 mg)
3 gr	0.2 g (200 mg)
1.5 gr	0.1 g (100 mg)
1 gr	0.06 g (60 mg) or 0.065 g (65 mg)
0.75 gr	0.05 g (50 mg)
0.5 gr	0.03 g (30 mg)
0.25 gr	0.015 g (15 mg)
1/60 gr	0.001 g (1 mg)
1/100 gr	0.5 mg
1/120 gr	0.5 mg
1/150 gr	0.4 mg

(continued)

WEIGHTS AND EQUIVALENTS *(continued)*

Table 3: Solid Equivalents Among Avoirdupois Apothecaries', and Metric Systems

Avoirdupois	Apothecaries'	Metric
1 gr	1 gr	0.065 g
15.4 gr	15 gr	1 g
1 ounce (1 oz)	480 gr	28.35 g
437.5 gr	1 oz	31 g
1 pound (lb)	1.33 lb	454 g
0.75 lb	1 lb	373 g
2.2 lb	2.7 lb	1 kilogram (kg)

ABBREVIATIONS

The following abbreviations, which are common to nursing practice, are used throughout the book.

ABG	arterial blood gas
a.c.	before meals
ACE	angiotensin-converting enzyme
ADH	antidiuretic hormone
AIDS	acquired immunodeficiency syndrome
ALT	alanine aminotransferase
ANA	antinuclear antibodies
APTT	activated partial thromboplastin time
AST	aspartate aminotransferase
ATP	adenosine triphosphate
AV	atrioventricular
b.i.d.	twice a day
BUN	blood urea nitrogen
°C	degrees Celsius
cAMP	cyclic adenosine monophosphate
(CAN)	Canadian drug trade name
cap	capsule
CBC	complete blood count
cGMP	cyclic guanosine monophosphate
CK	creatine kinase
Cl	chloride
cm	centimeter
CMV	cytomegalovirus
CNS	central nervous system
COPD	chronic obstructive pulmonary disease
C.R.	controlled-release
CSF	cerebrospinal fluid
CV	cardiovascular
CVA	cerebrovascular accident
CYP	cytochrome P-450
D_5LR	dextrose 5% in lactated Ringer's solution
D_5NS	dextrose 5% in normal saline solution
$D_5/0.2NS$	dextrose 5% in quarter-normal saline solution
$D_5/0.45NS$	dextrose 5% in half-normal saline solution
D_5W	dextrose 5% in water
$D_{10}W$	dextrose 10% in water
$D_{50}W$	dextrose 50% in water
dl	deciliter
DNA	deoxyribonucleic acid

(continued)

ABBREVIATIONS *(continued)*

DS	double-strength
EC	enteric-coated
ECG	electrocardiogram
EEG	electroencephalogram
EENT	eyes, ears, nose, and throat
ENDO	endocrine
E.R.	extended-release
°F	degrees Fahrenheit
FDA	Food and Drug Administration
g	gram
GFR	glomerular filtration rate
GI	gastrointestinal
GU	genitourinary
H_1	histamine$_1$
H_2	histamine$_2$
HDL	high-density lipoprotein
HEME	hematologic
HIV	human immunodeficiency virus
HPV	human papilloma virus
hr	hour
h.s.	at bedtime
HSV	herpes simplex virus
HZV	herpes zoster virus
ICP	intracranial pressure
I.D.	intradermal
IgA	immunoglobulin A
IgE	immunoglobulin E
I.M.	intramuscular
INR	international normalized ratio
I.V.	intravenous
IVPB	intravenous piggyback
kg	kilogram
KIU	kallikrein inactivator unit
L	liter
LA	long-acting
LD	lactate dehydrogenase
LDL	low-density lipoprotein
LOC	level of consciousness
LR	lactated Ringer's solution
M	molar
m^2	square meter
MAO	monoamine oxidase

ABBREVIATIONS *(continued)*

mcg	microgram
mEq	milliequivalent
mg	milligram
MI	myocardial infarction
min	minute
ml	milliliter
mm	millimeter
mm³	cubic millimeter
mmol	millimole
mo	month
MS	musculoskeletal
Na	sodium
NaCl	sodium chloride
NG	nasogastric
NPH	human isophane insulin
NPO	nothing by mouth
NS	normal saline solution
0.225NS	quarter-normal saline (0.225%) solution
0.45NS	half-normal saline (0.45%) solution
NSAID	nonsteroidal anti-inflammatory drug
OTC	over the counter
p.c.	after meals
PCA	patient-controlled analgesia
P.O.	by mouth
P.R.	by rectum
p.r.n.	as needed
PSVT	paroxysmal supraventricular tachycardia
PT	prothrombin time
PTCA	percutaneous transluminal coronary angioplasty
PVC	premature ventricular contraction
q	every
q.i.d.	four times a day
RBC	red blood cell
REM	rapid eye movement
RESP	respiratory
RNA	ribonucleic acid
RSV	respiratory syncytial virus
SA	sinoatrial
sec	second
SGOT	serum glutamic oxaloacetic transaminase
S.L.	sublingual

(continued)

ABBREVIATIONS *(continued)*

S.R.	sustained-release
stat	immediately
supp	suppository
tab	tablet
T_3	triiodothyronine
T_4	thyroxine
t.i.d.	three times a day
USP	United States Pharmacopeia
UTI	urinary tract infection
VLDL	very low-density lipoprotein
WBC	white blood cell
wk	week

INDEX

• **Generic and alternate names:** lowercase initial letter
• **Trade names:** uppercase initial letter

A

abacavir sulfate, 1–3, 3–6
abacavir sulfate and lamivudine, 1–3
abacavir sulfate, lamivudine, and zidovudine, 3–6
AccuHist DM, 567
AccuHist Pediatric Drops, 498
Accuretic, 166
Accuzyme, 324
Aceta with Codeine, 192
acetaminophen, 189–192, 192–195, 196–198, 213–217, 263–266, 274–277, 284–287, 291–294, 623–628
acetaminophen and codeine phosphate, 192–195
acetaminophen and hydrocodone bitartrate, 196–198
acetaminophen, caffeine, and butalbital, 189–192
acrivastine, 493–495
acrivastine and pseudoephedrine sulfate, 493–495
Activella, 347
Actonel with Calcium, 396
Actoplus Met, 392
Adderall, Adderall XR, 198
adriamycin, 708
Advair Diskus 500/50, 598
Advair Diskus 100/50, 598
Advair Diskus 250/50, 598
Advicor, 150
Aggrenox, 92
AH-Chew, 664
AK-Poly Bac Ophthalmic, 407
AK-Spore, 426
AK-Spore HC, 428
AK-Trol, 431

Alacol DM, 564
albuterol sulfate, 653–655
Aldactazide, 171
Aldoril 15, 133
Aldoril 25, 133
Aldoril D30, 133
Aldoril D50, 133
alendronate sodium, 331–334
alendronate sodium and cholecalciferol, 331–334
Alesse, 714
Allay, 196
Allegra-D 12 Hour, 596
Allegra-D 24 Hour, 596
AlleRx, 671
AlleRx-D, 697
Allfen-DM, 585
Americet, 189
Amerifed, 531
amiloride hydrochloride, 55–58
amiloride hydrochloride and hydrochlorothiazide, 55–58
amitriptyline hydrochloride, 229–232, 279–284
amlodipine besylate, 58–62, 62–65
amlodipine besylate and atorvastatin calcium, 58–62
amlodipine besylate and benazepril hydrochloride, 62–65
amoxicillin, 466–469
amoxicillin trihydrate, 6–9
amoxicillin trihydrate and clavulanate potassium, 6–9
amphetamine, 198–202
amphetamine and dextroamphetamine, 198–202
ampicillin sodium, 9–12
ampicillin sodium and sulbactam sodium, 9–12
Analpram-HC, 307, 308

D

H

N

S

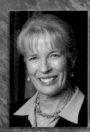

"*Nurse's Handbook of Combination Drugs* is a one-of-a-kind reference you'll want to have at your fingertips. It's a resource you'll use often and confidently because of its accurate, clearly written, and essential information—a vital nursing tool."

Kathleen A. Dracup, RN, FNP, DNSc, FAAN
Dean of Nursing
University of California, San Francisco

The Nurse's Combination Drug Resource

Using one formulation to administer two or more medications simultaneously can simplify a patient's drug regimen and even improve compliance. For the nurse, however, the convenience of combination drugs is linked with the added responsibility to provide safe, effective drug therapy and complete patient teaching about the medications.

Blanchard & Loeb Publishers' **Nurse's Handbook of Combination Drugs** meets your nursing need for accurate, up-to-date, and easy-to-use drug information, preparing you to administer these drugs, teach your patients about them, and provide safe and effective care.

What's Inside

- An organization that groups drugs into body system chapters and alphabetizes the entries for quick finding. In each chapter, you'll find all the combination drugs to treat that system's disorders.
- Concise drug entries that use a consistent format. Use one entry and you'll know how all the others are formatted.
- Comprehensive index listing each generic in the combination and all trade names.
- Vital information on preparation, administration, follow-up, and patient teaching, including:
  - ★ Chemical and therapeutic classes, FDA pregnancy risk category, and controlled substance schedule
  - ★ Indications and dosages, including dosage adjustments when appropriate
  - ★ Mechanism of action presented clearly and concisely
  - ★ Incompatibilities; contraindications; interactions with drugs, food, and activities; and adverse reactions
  - ★ Nursing considerations, including precautions, administration techniques and information, and key patient-teaching points

Special Features

- Dosage adjustment needed for elderly patients, those with renal impairment, and others with special needs
- Warnings you need to know before, during, and after drug administration
- Appendices on antineoplastic combination drugs for selected cancers and on combination oral contraceptives

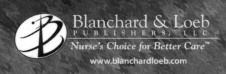

Blanchard & Loeb
PUBLISHERS, LLC
Nurse's Choice for Better Care™
www.blanchardloeb.com

ISBN 13: 978-1-930138-61-2
ISBN 10: 1-930138-61-X

90000

9 781930 138612

Nursing category: Pharmacology and Drug Administration